Child Maltreatment in Residential Care

Adrian V. Rus • Sheri R. Parris
Ecaterina Stativa
Editors

Child Maltreatment in Residential Care

History, Research, and Current Practice

Springer

Editors
Adrian V. Rus
Department of Social and Behavioral Science
Southwestern Christian University
Bethany, OK, USA

Sheri R. Parris
Texas Christian University
Fort Worth, TX, USA

Ecaterina Stativa
Social Pediatrics and Obstetrics Research
Department
National Institute for Mother and Child
Health "Alessandrescu-Rusescu"
Bucuresti, Romania

ISBN 978-3-319-57989-4 ISBN 978-3-319-57990-0 (eBook)
DOI 10.1007/978-3-319-57990-0

Library of Congress Control Number: 2017946616

Printed on acid-free paper

This Springer imprint is published by Springer Nature
The registered company is Springer International Publishing AG
The registered company address is: Gewerbestrasse 11, 6330 Cham, Switzerland

Foreword

This textbook may raise more questions than it answers. It presents multiple views of the role of institutions/residential centers/orphanages/group care or any other name you want to give to the care of children outside of family care that live in group settings with other children. Globally, as you will read throughout these chapters, poverty, civil unrest/social upheaval, and economic insecurity drive child welfare systems, making the most vulnerable children even more at risk – for negative life outcomes, placement outside of their birth family or kinship network, and a host of other negative short-term and long-term impacts. Every country and community develops a way to care for and manage their children who cannot remain in their families. Residential care is an efficient intervention, but many concerns have been raised about its effectiveness in maximizing optimal development of children. In fact, in some countries and locations, there is compelling evidence that residential care for children is deleterious to child development, particularly for infants and toddlers. At the same time, others have demonstrated that institutions can also have protective factors. These contradictory findings present a quandary for policymakers and humanitarians.

It is clear that deprivation early in life creates increased risk for psychopathology and negative adult outcomes. It doesn't matter where that deprivation occurs – North America, Central/South America, Europe, Africa, Asia, or Oceania. It also doesn't matter if children experience deprivation in the family or in residential care, although the nature of deprivation in residential care is more insidious. Residential care clearly poses significant risks for infants and toddlers but may pose different risks and different protections for older children. On the one hand, residential care facilities are not always or mostly safe places for adolescents. Several studies have documented physical abuse, sexual abuse, and emotional abuse or trauma from witnessing abuse or maltreatment, usually perpetrated by another resident but sometimes also by the staff who are supposed to care and protect them. On the other hand, living in the birth family or an extended family may not protect children from experiencing maltreatment if the family also experiences social disorganization with poverty, transient living, substance abuse, mental illness, or health epidemics; then institutions become a safer place to live, have access to medical and social services, and achieve academically.

Given that this is a reality of life for many children worldwide, what can or should be done if this is the only or major intervention for at-risk children? The few scientifically evaluated intervention approaches all aim at improving the caregiver–child relationship and enriching the caregiving environment to mitigate harm. Some interventions may not be cost-effective or sustainable given the low level of resources (training, oversight, foster family availability, or inclination to foster) or the high cost of the alternative models of family care that are created such as some models of foster care. This raises a question of whether resources should emphasize comprehensive family support practices and family alternatives to institutionalization. Interventions that have focused on improving the economic situation of the family through cash transfer and conditional cash transfer programs have experienced a great deal of success in keeping children in families, getting children documented (e.g., birth certificate, healthcare card), improving compliance with inoculations, and enrolling children in education programs. But cash transfer programs are not a panacea and in low resource countries are not sustainable in the long term.

Group facilities are perpetuated around the world and most are tied to faith communities. The argument used to justify the proliferation is post hoc, ergo propter hoc; since as soon as you build an institution it becomes full, then there was a need for the institution. Families make rational choice; they can keep their children and feed them once a day or send them to a residential center where they can get three meals a deal. They can keep their child without sending them to school because of the hidden costs of a "free education" or place them where they will be taught. They can care for them without access to medical care or put them in a center where someone will provide basic medical care.

There is no one "best solution" for at-risk children. Government and organizations, secular and faith-based, need evidence-based interventions that support children in the least restrictive setting. Drawing from the Convention on the Rights of a Child, a child has a right to be raised in a safe family setting. There is a great need for social and economic development to work together so families and communities can care for themselves and for each other. This book continues a dialog about the role of residential care in the life of children, how group care impacts children, and models of intervention to mitigate any negative impact, as well as evidence-based interventions for families parenting children with a history of institutionalization.

Victor Groza
Mandel School of Applied Social Sciences
Case Western Reserve University
Cleveland, OH, USA

Acknowledgments

I would like to express my deepest gratitude and dedicate this book
to my beloved wife, Iulia, and my children, Adyanna and Dennis.
I thank you so much for your support and endless love!
I am grateful to God for this opportunity to give a
voice to those children victimized within
long-term residential centers throughout time
around the globe, including my father.
To my parents.

Adrian Rus

I dedicate this book to my children, Alexander and India; my husband,
Joe Ed; my parents, Ron and Jackie; and God. Thank you for your
support and encouragement. I also want to thank all of the
excellent authors who have shared their important
work in this book. We are honored
to have taken this journey
with each of you.

Sheri Parris

I dedicate this book to my parents, from whom I learned to think freely; my sisters; my husband, Virgil; our children, Ovidiu, Alexandru, Doina; and our nephew, Pavel. I wish to thank Ella Dubreu for the technical support and to my colleagues, who have trusted and supported me to professionally develop, even in the most restricted times. I would like to thank all of the authors of this book for our common belief in nonviolence and respect for the human being. Special thanks also to Adrian Rus and Sheri Parris for the idea of this project and our excellent collaboration.

Ecaterina Stativa

Contents

Introduction

Research studies and investigations of separated or orphaned children who have resided in group or congregate care settings (other terms used to define such settings are orphanages, care institutions, institutional care facilities, residential care facilities, and long-term residential centers) over the past several decades have provided valuable information and continue to provide a growing knowledge base for many fields within the social sciences, such as psychology and social work, or medical sciences, in particular neuroscience. Through ongoing research, we have gained a deeper understanding about the experience of living in institutions, including outcomes that effect children's development in many domains, which often last a lifetime.

In addition, many countries in recent years have moved toward a goal of reducing or eliminating institutionalization and replacing it with other forms of caregiving, mainly foster care, all of which have their own limits. However, even as numbers of institutions are reduced in some countries, many types of group or congregate care settings are still in operation. There are also many children, youth, and adults who have experienced life in institutions and are now either integrated into society as adults in their home countries or as adoptees across the globe. The sad truth is that many of those who have experienced institutionalization, especially early in their lives, cannot integrate well into society to lead productive and independent lives. Many of these adult alumni live in institutions for adults or become homeless. Thus, the topic of institutionalization of children remains a relevant topic, as varying types of institutional care settings continue to be the main source of caregiving for many children around the world.

The topic of maltreatment (i.e., neglect; emotional, physical, and sexual abuse) of institutionalized children has been studied very little compared with maltreatment of children with no histories of institutionalization. However, in recent years, the knowledge base about institutionalized child abuse has steadily grown to the point where we feel that it would be useful to create a resource that brings this information together, from sources around the globe, into one place. *Child Maltreatment in Residential Care: History, Research, and Current Practice* is a compilation of this knowledge, and this textbook was designed to benefit researchers, practitioners, policy-makers, adoptive parents of previously institutionalized children, and others with interest in this topic. Thus, to improve the well-being of children who experience institutionalization, including application of appropriate interventions, there is a need for researchers, practitioners, and policy-makers to look carefully at a comprehensive body of work being produced by researchers across the globe that focus not only on the outcomes of institutionalization (that most often by default imply various forms of neglect) but also *abuse*, *bullying*, *exploitation*, and *polyvictimization* of children placed in long-term residential centers.

For this book, we assembled a team of chapter authors from around the world who are leading researchers of institutionalized children, many of whom took part in important seminal research studies that are cited in peer-reviewed publications and textbooks in psychology, social work, and medical sciences around the globe, and whose research has been used to improve social policy for children and families in various countries.

Child Maltreatment in Residential Care: History, Research, and Current Practice is meant to provide a global perspective on institutionalization with a focus on maltreatment of institutionalized children and to appeal to a worldwide audience. Multiple research teams and authors wrote chapters about societal and institutional changes which have affected institutionalized children's lives or literature reviews and research reports meant to reveal and explain the magnitude of maltreatment or its consequences on various areas of human development. Among the countries in which child protection systems and institutionalized children, adolescents, and alumni were reviewed, studied, and presented in our book are Latin American and Caribbean, African, Asian, Middle-Eastern, and Western and Eastern European countries, as well as the United States of America. Specifically, authors that focused on a specific country or countries summarized previous and current problems of institutionalized children and their lives in that specific country or countries. Additionally, this textbook highlights various child welfare systems; theoretical frameworks regarding the child/childhood and socioeconomic, political, and cultural factors' impact on child welfare systems; how child protection systems have been changed over time; factors that trigger such changes; and preventative interventions aimed at increasing care quality and preventing maltreatment in institutional care.

Child Maltreatment in Residential Care: History, Research, and Current Practice provides a substantive examination of important aspects of institutionalization focusing especially on maltreatment in group or congregate care settings across the globe. We hope that it will be of interest to (1) researchers and professors, including their graduate and undergraduate students (for courses in social work, psychology, and child development, historians of childhood, and sociologists); (2) social workers and psychologists, counselors, and psychotherapists who work with children having a history of institutionalization and their caregivers, adoptive, or foster families; (3) adoption agencies and those providing a variety of services within the adoption field; (4) family service agencies, family court judges, lawyers, medical personnel, child advocates, and policy-makers; and (5) those in the general population with an interest in this topic.

Interested readers can find more supplemental information about the topic of maltreatment of institutionalized children and adolescents, as well as about authors of the chapters, by following the weblink provided here: https://sites.google.com/view/child-maltreatment-texbook/home. Additionally, we would like to receive your comments and recommendations by writing to us at the following email address: institutional.maltreatment@gmail.com.

Chapter 1
An Introduction to Maltreatment of Institutionalized Children

Adrian V. Rus, Sheri R. Parris, Ecaterina Stativa, Anca Bejenaru, Rebecca D. Webster, Jeremy Wente, and Stefan Cojocaru

Childhood should be carefree, playing in the sun; not living a nightmare in the darkness of the soul.

(Pelzer, 1995, p. 98)

1 Defining Child Maltreatment: Early Developments

This section of the chapter presents a short history of the emergence of common definitions of maltreatment. In early research, child maltreatment was simply described based on information gained from case studies of maltreated children.

A.V. Rus (✉) • R. D. Webster • J. Wente
Department of Social and Behavioral Science, Southwestern Christian University, 7210 NW 39th Expressway, Bethany, OK 73008-0340, USA
e-mail: adrian.rus@swcu.edu; aadrianrus@gmail.com; rebecca.webster@swcu.edu; jeremy.wente@swcu.edu

S.R. Parris
Texas Christian University, Fort Worth, TX, USA
e-mail: sheri.parris@gmail.com

E. Stativa
Social Pediatrics and Obstetrics Research Department, The National Institute for Mother and Child Health "Alessandrescu-Rusescu", Bucharest, Romania
e-mail: ecaterina.stativa@gmail.com

A. Bejenaru
Department of Sociology and Social Work, "Lucian Blaga" University of Sibiu, Sibiu, Romania
e-mail: geleriuanca@gmail.com

S. Cojocaru
Department of Sociology and Social Work, Alexandru Ioan Cuza University, Iasi, Romania
e-mail: stefan.cojocaru@expertprojects.ro

A.V. Rus et al. (eds.), *Child Maltreatment in Residential Care*,
DOI 10.1007/978-3-319-57990-0_1

Over time, comparisons were made between maltreated and non-maltreated children. In 1979, a book emerged that was titled *Defining Child Abuse* and that dealt solely with discussions of maltreatment and development of definitions (Giovanni & Becerra, 1979). Then, in 1981 the *National Study of the Incidence and Severity of Child Abuse and Neglect* was published. This was the first national study (in the United States) that provided an operational definition of maltreatment for the purpose of collecting data on its prevalence (National Center on Child Abuse and Neglect, 1981). Later, Zuravin (1991) and Barnett, Manly, and Cicchetti (1993) provided further discussion of defining maltreatment, and in 1991 (volume 3, Issue 1), the journal of *Development and Psychopathology* published an issue devoted to defining maltreatment (see Cicchetti, 1991). The cumulative conclusion from contributors and editors of that issue was that, for definitional purposes, evidence of harmful treatment rather than harm to the child should be sought (see also Hamarman & Bernet, 2000).

In 1993, the National Research Council (NRC, 1993) published their recommendations to improve clarity and precision in maltreatment research. Researchers still struggle with some ambiguity, but progress has been made. Improvements in defining and operationalizing the term *maltreatment* are vital in order to bring comparability across studies and improve researchers' ability to combine and build upon each other's knowledge. The NRC reported that there were no clear, reliable, valid, and useful definitions of child abuse and neglect. In finding a definition, the NRC cited difficulties such as lack of consensus regarding (a) acceptable parenting practices; (b) whether to base definitions on adult characteristics, adult behavior, child outcomes, environmental context, or some combination; (c) whether standards of endangerment or harm should be included; and (d) whether definitions should vary based on use for scientific, legal, or clinical purposes (for a complete review of the historical evolution of *maltreatment* definitions, see Herrenkohl, 2005). Even to the present time, the effort to provide an operational definition of maltreatment is ongoing.

However, four general categories of child maltreatment have emerged that have been widely accepted by researchers. These include (a) neglect (failure to provide minimum standards of care or adequate supervision); (b) emotional maltreatment (persistent and extreme thwarting of a child's basic emotional needs); (c) sexual abuse (sexual contact or attempted sexual contact between a caregiver or other responsible adult and a child, for the purposes of the caregiver's sexual gratification or financial benefit); and (d) physical abuse (injuries by non-accidental means) (Cicchetti & Valentino, 2006).

One effort to produce a widely applicable description of maltreatment resulted in the development of the Maltreatment Classification Scheme (MCS; Barnett et al., 1993). The MCS provides a systematic method to capture data from Child Protective Services records, but the "*ultimate goal was to integrate multiple informants and multiple sources of information within a developmental psychopathology framework to capture aspects of children's experiences that would be likely to impact their development*" (Manly, 2005, p. 427). Since its creation, the MCS has been applied to CPS records, clinical treatment records, medical records, foster care placement histories, and records from other organizations.

In developing their initial working definition for maltreatment within the Maltreatment Classification System, Barnett et al. (1993) determined that three primary components must be addressed: conceptualization of the phenomenon, subtypes, and severity range. They stated that creating specific definitions for the different types of maltreatment, including neglect, is important in order to have objective means to determine when it is necessary to intervene in family's lives, which can have life-changing effects for children and families. Definitions also provide criteria for meeting societal goals of ensuring the physical and emotional well-being of future generations. Where a society draws the line between maltreatment and non-maltreatment, including neglect and non-neglect, has a significant effect on services provided by health-care professionals, social scientists, law enforcement, and legal professionals. However, defining maltreatment has been difficult in part because cultural norms change over time, and changing political and economic conditions can also influence societal views regarding what should be considered maltreatment.

In addition, Barnett, Manly, and Cicchetti (1991) developed an assessment system based on six subtypes of maltreatment (i.e., physical abuse, sexual abuse, physical neglect, lack of supervision, moral/legal/educational maltreatment, and emotional maltreatment). For each subtype, they developed measures for six dimensions that can impact developmental functioning: (1) severity, (2) frequency, (3) chronicity, (4) developmental stage, (5) perpetrator, and (6) separations or placements outside the home. However, they recommend the use of this scale as a guide and not to create definitive, immovable standards that would apply universally. Instead, they conclude that researchers should consider these guidelines while also considering other factors that may impact the population they are studying, such as cultural norms. These guidelines can also be used in the ongoing development of theoretical and empirical knowledge, including issues of classification and measurement regarding psychological maltreatment.

English and LONGSCAN investigators (1997) proposed the Modified Maltreatment Classification System (MMCS) (a modification of the Maltreatment Classification System; Barnett et al., 1993) used in the Longitudinal Studies of Child Abuse and Neglect (LONGSCAN; English, Bangdiwala, & Runyan, 2005), where neglect is presented in detail. The MMCS describes four categories of maltreatment, which are physical abuse, sexual abuse, emotional abuse, and neglect. Neglect is divided into two categories: failure to provide (i.e., food, hygiene, clothing, shelter, and medical) and lack of supervision (i.e., environment, substitute care). Other child maltreatment measurement tools include Adverse Childhood Experiences (ACEs), Adverse Childhood Experiences International Questionnaire (ACE-IQ), Child Abuse and Neglect Inventory Schedule (CANIS-R), Checklist for Child Abuse Evaluation (CCAE), Checklist of Sexual Abuse and Related Stressors (C-SARS), Child Maltreatment History Self-Report (CMHSR), and many others (for a complete list of measurement tools and references, see Meinck et al., 2016).

2 Defining Child Maltreatment: Recent Developments

2.1 United Nations and World Health Organization

In 1989, the General Assembly of the United Nations adopted the Convention on the Rights of the Child (UNCRC), which was an effort to achieve global consensus and participation in addressing the issue of violence toward children. The UNCRC obliges governments, "*to protect the child from all forms of physical or mental violence, injury or abuse, neglect or negligent treatment, maltreatment or exploitation, including sexual abuse...*" (General Assembly of the United Nations, 1989, Part 1, Article 19.1). Furthermore, the World Health Organization (WHO, 1999) developed a definition of child maltreatment to improve assessment and intervention efforts. They defined it as "all forms of physical and/or emotional ill-treatment, sexual abuse, neglect or negligent treatment or commercial or other exploitation, resulting in actual or potential harm to the child's health, survival, development or dignity in the context of a relationship of responsibility, trust or power" (p. 16). This definition not only provided the categories of maltreatment (i.e., physical and emotional abuse, as well as neglect and negligent treatment) but also highlighted the context of it.

2.2 Diagnostic and Statistical Manual and International Classification of Disease

For the first time, the latest edition of the Diagnostic and Statistical Manual (DSM-5; American Psychiatric Association, 2013) separates maltreatment into four separate categories: physical abuse, sexual abuse, neglect, and psychological abuse. Previously, only three categories were identified, with psychological abuse being the newest addition. Also for the first time, the DSM-5 includes definitions for each category, including delineations between threshold and suboptimal but non-abusive parenting (Slep, Heyman, & Foran, 2015). Importantly, the WHO is developing definitions for neglect and other forms of maltreatment for inclusion in the next version of the *International Classification of Disease* (ICD-11) (see http://www.who.int/classifications/icd/en/).

2.3 Trauma

In recent years, there has been a growing body of research that identifies the various forms of maltreatment as either single or ongoing instances of trauma. Complex trauma has been described as "*recurrent interpersonal trauma perpetrated by caregivers early in life*" (Greeson et al., 2011, p. 92) and includes physical, sexual, and emotional abuse, neglect, and domestic violence (Greeson et al., 2011). Youth with histories of complex trauma have significantly higher rates of internalizing problems, posttraumatic stress, and clinical diagnoses than those who have experienced other types of trauma. Trauma screening measures may be helpful for assessing children who have been, or may have been, exposed to maltreatment. Commonly used trauma screening measures include the Childhood Trauma Questionnaire (CTQ) and Childhood Trauma Questionnaire Short Form (CTQ-SF). These measures screen for emotional and physical neglect, emotional abuse, physical abuse, and sexual abuse (Bernstein et al., 1994, 2003). The Childhood Trauma Interview includes questions for respondents about whether they have experiences that fall into the categories of emotional neglect, emotional abuse, physical abuse, and/or sexual abuse (Vrshek-Schallhorn et al. 2014). In one study, Fusco and Cahalane (2013) found that neglect was the maltreatment type most strongly associated with trauma symptoms. Another study found that posttraumatic stress symptoms are found at comparable rates in both neglected children and those who have experienced other forms of abuse (Kolko et al., 2010). Thus, the link between trauma and maltreatment should be considered as part of the ongoing research and practice regarding maltreatment.

3 Child Maltreatment and Sociocultural Issues

It is recognized that an abuse is experienced as a trauma by the person suffering it, no matter their nationality, ethnicity, or religion (Hoff, 2009). Sociocultural factors, however, play an important role in determining the causes that lead to and support violent behavior and the response to the abuse. Maltreatment is seen, in this perspective, as a predominantly "social phenomenon" (Hoff, 2009; Olson, Stroud, & NRC, 2012) or "a public health problem" (IOM & NRC, 2013) with strong effects at individual and social levels (Hoff, 2009).

The focus on sociocultural factors directs attention to issues related to valuing children within each society; parenting styles that are accepted and further transmitted within different ethnic, racial, and religious groups (IOM & NRC, 2013); the maltreatment practices and rituals perpetuated within some cultures; the availability of resources; the status of minority/majority; etc. For instance, there are societies such as Guatemala, who value children less than adults, and among children in Peru or India, little girls have a lower status than boys (Carson, Foster, & Tripathi, 2013; WHO, 2009). In many African and some Middle Eastern countries, genital mutilation of young girls is accepted as a cultural custom (Shetty, 2014). Using punishments in children's education is widely accepted in some countries (see, e.g., Turkey, Ethiopia, India) (Deb, 2006; WHO, 2009), while in other countries these behaviors are accepted among a preponderance of some racial or ethnic groups (Lee, Guterman, & Lee, 2008). Research regarding maltreatment practices and of social and cultural factors that may influence the prevalence, personal consequences, and social response to it has increased over the last 30 years. Furthermore, analyses have gone from single, isolated factors to complex, multifactorial, and multilevel analyses. Sociocultural and developmental factors have been included in ecological models (Belsky, 1980) and later the focus of attention was directed on the interaction between these factors, defining the transactional models (Cicchetti & Rizley, 1981). Currently, ecological-transactional models are frequently used to capture simultaneously the interaction of multiple risk factors and their influence on child development. *Specifically, an ecological-transactional model explains how transacting cultural, community, and family factors* (i.e., *macro-, exo-, and microsystems*), *in conjunction with characteristics of the individual, exert reciprocal influences on each other and shape the course of child development* (Cicchetti, Toth, & Maughan, 2000, p. 695).

Currently, the empirical studies that test these models and show the role of each factor in different constellations are still limited (MacKenzie, Kotch, & Lee, 2011). However, the utility and the complexity of the ecological-transactional model are internationally recognized. Many countries have developed and currently use risk assessment tools built on this model. For example, England has developed the *Framework for the Assessment of Children in Need and their Families* containing three dimensions of assessment: (1) the developmental needs of children, (2) the capacities of parents or caregivers to respond appropriately to those needs and the impact of wider family, and (3) the environmental factors on parenting capacity and children (Department of Health, Department for Education and Employment and Home Office, 2000). These dimensions are analyzed and evaluated in interaction with each other, in the process of decision-making. The adoption of a sociocultural perspective brings changes to the development of interventions. Therapeutic models are considered to be effective if they are integrated into broader intervention strategies that include social intervention, are culturally adapted, and are implemented at different levels (NRC, 1993).

4 Consequences of Child Maltreatment

It is well documented that maltreatment has a relatively early impact on a wide range of domains that effect children's well-being (i.e., behavioral, neurological, and molecular) and can have lasting effects on biological, psychological, academic, and social functioning into adolescence and adulthood. For instance, studies have shown an association between early-life maltreatment and adolescents' school absenteeism and anticipation of attending college, as well as high levels of aggression, anxiety/depression, dissociation, posttraumatic stress disorder symptoms, social problems, thought problems, and social withdrawal (Friedrich, Urquiza, Bilke, 1986; Lansford et al., 2002; Livingston, 1987). In addition, a large study spanning across eight eastern European countries found that adverse childhood experiences were associated with health-harming behaviors into young adulthood (e.g., smoking, physical inactivity, multiple sexual partners, engagement in early sexual activities, drug abuse, problematic alcohol use, and attempted suicide) (Bellis et al., 2014).

Regarding specific types of childhood abuse and their effects into adulthood, physical abuse, physical neglect, teasing, and father's level of care have shown to be significant predictors of antisocial personality disorder symptomologies, with physical abuse and physical neglect predicting the greatest variance in APD symptoms (Krastins, Francis, Field, & Carr, 2014), and physical and sexual abuse are associated with increased risk of suicide attempts (Hardt et al., 2008). Sexual abuse has been associated with hypertension and insomnia and has shown to induce or exacerbate any psychiatric disorder (Goodwin & Stein, 2004; Lind, Aggen, Kendler, York, & Amstadter, 2016; Suglia, Clark, Boynton-Jarrett, Kressin, & Koenen, 2014; Yuce et al., 2015). Research conducted by Raghavan and Kingston (2006) indicates an association between child sexual abuse in the general population and early substance use. Childhood sexual abuse is also associated with the increased risk of adult revictimization and other forms of trauma in adulthood. While those who experience sexual abuse at one point during their lifetime have an increased incidence of adverse mental health outcomes, those who experience sexual abuse at multiple points during their lifetime have an even higher incidence of such adverse outcomes, including depression, disassociation, avoidance, intrusions, anxious arousal, and impaired self-reference (Banyard, Williams, & Siegel, 2001). Traumatic sexualization, a term used by Finkelhor and Browne (1985), is a negative outcome specific to childhood sexual abuse. This term refers to developmentally inappropriate expression of sexual feelings, attitudes, and behaviors.

Neglect is also associated with many pervasive, long-term consequences, including physical injury; toxic ingestions; illness; psychosocial problems; cognitive/developmental delays; problems with physical and social-emotional development, including internalizing and externalizing behavior problems and greater difficulties in relationships than other children; and even death (APSAC, 2008; Egeland, Sroufe, & Erickson, 1983; Smith & Fong, 2004). Relative to children who have experienced physical abuse, neglected children have been found to have more severe cognitive and academic deficits, social withdrawal and limited peer interactions, and internalizing behaviors (Hildyard & Wolfe, 2002). In severe cases, young children who have experienced global neglect exhibit nonorganic failure to thrive syndrome (NFTT) or psychosocial dwarfism (PSD) (also called psychosocial short stature [PSS] or Kaspar Hauser syndrome). NFTT is characterized by children (1) who have fallen below the fifth percentile in weight, and often height; (2) who were once within the expected norm for height and weight; and (3) who demonstrate delay in psychomotor development (Crosson-Tower, 2002). Children with PSD may exhibit disturbances in growth, development, speech, and social relationships (Faller et al., 1981 as cited on page 73 of Crosson-Tower 2002). The type and severity of outcomes due to neglect are linked to many variables, such as the duration and severity of neglect, age of child, resilience of child, or availability of other caring adults in the child's life (Shaughnessy, 2014). In one study, even after controlling for other types of abuse, adults who experienced emotional abuse or emotional neglect in childhood had high rates of psychopathology, depression, anxiety, and posttraumatic stress symptoms and higher rates of health-care utilization and continued to experience high rates of lifetime trauma exposure (e.g., Bernet & Stein,

1999; Spertus, Yehuda, Wong, Halligan, & Seremetis, 2003). In addition, because children who experience physical and sexual abuse often experience concurrent emotional abuse and neglect, the latter should not be overlooked even when the other more outwardly severe forms of abuse are present (Spertus et al., 2003).

Childhood maltreatment has also been associated with neurological, musculoskeletal, cardiovascular, and respiratory diseases in adulthood as shown by a meta-analytic review (for more information, see Wegman & Stetler, 2009). It can also affect brain structure and function, including deficits in brain volume, gray and white matter, neural network abnormalities, and deficits in memory and attention (for more information see Hart & Rubia, 2012) and lead to dysregulation of the stress system (e.g., Twardosz & Lutzker, 2010). For a more thorough review of neurobiological effects, see Grassi-Oliveira, Ashy, and Stein (2008). In addition, maltreatment has an effect at the molecular level. For instance, early severe social deprivation of institutionalized children has been linked to shorter telomere length in middle childhood and adolescence (e.g., Drury et al., 2012; Humphreys et al., 2016), and physical maltreatment has shown to change gene expression leading to the onset of mental and physical disorders (e.g., Romens, McDonald, Svaren, & Pollak, 2015). However, in some instances the risk for chronic health conditions in adults who experienced childhood trauma may be mediated by having good mental health and adequate socioeconomic status (Mock & Arai, 2011). In sum, the consequences of abuse are far reaching, and this section provides just a sampling of the growing body of literature in this area.

5 Maltreatment of Children Placed in Long-Term Residential Centers

In this section of the chapter, we present the forms of maltreatment as defined by the World Health Organization (WHO, 1999) (i.e., neglect and negligent behavior; emotional, physical, and sexual abuse; witnessing violence) and how they were manifested within various long-term institutional settings around the globe. We should note that institutional settings where separated or orphaned children receive care are described by various terms: orphanages, care institutions, institutional care facilities, residential care facilities, and long-term residential centers. These terms are often used interchangeably in the literature.

5.1 Neglect and Negligent Behavior in Institutional Settings

The World Health Organization (1999) adopted a broad definition of neglect and negligent behavior, describing it as "*the failure to provide for the development of the child in all spheres: health, education, emotional development, nutrition, shelter, and safe living conditions, in the context of resources reasonably available to the family or caretakers and causes or has a high probability of causing harm to the child's health or physical, mental, spiritual, moral, or social development. This includes the failure to properly supervise and protect children from harm as much as is feasible*" (p. 15). The terms *neglect, privation,* and/or *deprivation* are often used interchangeably, though in certain contexts meanings may have slight variations. Neglect is considered chronic if (a) one or more needs basic to a child's healthy development are not met, (b) it is perpetrated by a parent or caregiver, and (c) it happens on a recurring or enduring basis (Child Welfare Information Gateway, 2013).

As a form of maltreatment, institutional structural neglect (or the neglect experienced by children placed in long-term residential centers) can be considered one of the most prevalent forms of chronic neglect and has been described as a very harsh living condition that "*includes minimum physical resources, unfavorable and unstable staffing patterns, and socially and emotionally inadequate caregiver-child interactions*" (van IJzendoorn et al., 2011, p. 8). Gunnar (2001) described four categories of needs and stated that levels of neglect children experience correspond with how these needs are met (or not) in institutional settings. The four categories of needs are (1) health and nutrition (the most basic needs); (2) physical and mental stimulation which support sensorimotor, cognitive, and language development; (3) adult-child and child-child social stimulation; and (4) stable and consistent relationships. In addition, studies have defined three levels of privation that could be found within institutions. First, *global privation* occurs when the entire range of needs are not met (Rutter, 1998). In this category, we could include some Romanian orphanages in the 1990s (McCall, 2011). Second, some institutions provide acceptable health and nutrition, but fail to provide stimulation and relationships. These can be called *psychologically depriving institutions.* Rosas and McCall showed that among institutions described in the literature, nearly all lack adequate socioemotional environments, with children having many caregivers that continually change and who provide impersonal, perfunctory caregiving with little talking, sensitivity, or responsivity to children (Rosas & McCall, 2009 as cited in McCall et al., 2010). Finally, some institutions meet all needs except the need for long-term relationships with consistent caregivers (Gunnar, 2001). With this third level of care, or *quality institutions*, children only lack a regular family life embedded in a regular social environment (van IJzendoorn et al., 2011). An example of such institutions would be some SOS Children's Villages (as presented by van IJzendoorn et al., 2011).

Romanian institutionalized children were often presented in scientific literature as experiencing one of the most severe forms of institutional structural neglect (including global privation) soon after the collapse of the communist regime (December 1989) when volunteers, researchers, and adoptive parents could visit, adopt, or work with them. It should be highlighted that for a long time, especially during the communist regime (1947–1989), these residential care facilities were closed to the general public. However, the levels of privation in these Romanian institutions, as described above, were almost always indirectly documented. That is, many of the observed conditions were not quantified, but they were published accounts that were qualitative in nature, such as eyewitness and incidental reports, stories, and descriptions of the living conditions (witnesses were sometimes researchers, but most often adoptive parents, western adoptive parents, and volunteers working temporarily with children in these institutions) (e.g., Castle et al., 1999; Children's Health Care Collaborative Study Group, 1992; Johnson et al., 1992; Misca, 2003; NACPA & UNICEF, 2004; Rutter et al., 2007; Stephenson et al., 1993) (for a quantitative description of the neglect in Romanian institutions in 1999, see Chap. 2). Although conditions varied across time periods and institutional settings, certain features were often found within long-term residential centers (these centers were organized based on children's age and the presence of a chronic diseases; thus, institutionalized children could be housed in nurseries, residential centers for preschool-aged and school-aged children, and centers for children with severe disabilities). Below we present a list of some characteristics of Romanian institutional settings in the 1990s, as reported by various studies or eyewitnesses. These characteristics do not describe the current Romanian child protection system which has been massively restructured and now includes smaller public and residential care settings operating according to new standards of care and safety (Bejenaru & Tucker, 2014).

Many institutions housed large numbers of children (400–500 children) in relatively large buildings until the late 1990s, (NACPA & UNICEF, 2004). These included former castles, casernes, and old prisons or old orphanages often in advanced states of deterioration, or in relatively new, three- or four-story buildings with 14–20 bedrooms (about 8–10 beds per room). Typically, even these buildings had no personal spaces for children, as well as having communal bathrooms and toilets on each floor offering no privacy. Additionally, these buildings were surrounded by fences with an inside courtyard (Misca, 2003; Stativa, Anghelescu, Palicari, Stanescu, & Nanu, 2002). Overall, these buildings were inadequate for the purpose they served. Thus, many children experienced overcrowding (Stativa et al., 2002); sparse access to toys and educational activities (Rutter et al., 2007); only subsistence levels of clothing, shelter (Johnson et al., 1992), and food (McMullan & Fisher, 1992); as well as high ratios of children to caregivers (Ames & Carter, 1992; McMullan & Fisher, 1992; NACPA & UNICEF, 2004; Rosenberg, Pajer, & Rancurello, 1992). Based on our observation, children's clothes were purchased without asking for their preferences regarding colors, styles, or sizes. Thus, most often children's clothes had dark colors (i.e., blue and gray). During late 1990s, children's alimentation was controlled in terms of its calories and proteins, and children had three meals and two snacks during a day, but it lacked variation. Children had to take their meals using aluminum or enameled plates and bowls and use tables with no tablecloths, all of this suggesting disrespect for children (Stativa et al., 2002).

Additionally, heating, plumbing, bathing, and washing facilities were often inadequate (Groze & Ileana, 1996; Morrison, 2004). There were also deficiencies in the provision and preservation of administrative records, such as birth dates, medical information, and personal information about the biological parents (Groze & Ileana, 1996).

Inconsistency in caregivers was due to work schedules with rotating shifts. Also, caregivers had little interaction with children during meals and playtime (Smyke, Zeanah, Fox, & Nelson, 2009; Zeanah et al., 2003). Thus, caregivers also had a lack of psychological investment in the children due to their minimal communication with them (McMullan & Fisher, 1992; Rutter et al., 2007).

There was little interaction between children and their peers, with toilet training and meal time severely restricted (Johnson et al., 1992), and sparse individualized developmental programming (Children's Health Care Collaborative Study Group, 1992; Groze & Ileana, 1996).

Until 1997, the management of institutions was led by medical personnel (Castle et al., 1999), particularly in nurseries (cradles) housing children 0–3 years of age, yet there was a lack of nonmedical specialists (psychologists, physical therapists, or social workers) (Rosenberg, Pajer, & Rancurello, 1992; Stephenson et al., 1993; Williams, 1990) and teachers for children placed in institutions for school-aged children. This organizational culture was facilitated by the abolishment of social work (1969), sociology, psychology, and pedagogy (1977) as academic disciplines across all Romanian universities by the communist regime due to political and ideological reasons until 1989 (Universitatea Babes-Bolyai, Facultatea de Psychologie si Stiinte ale Educatiei, n.d.; Universitatea Bucuresti, Facultatea de Sociologie si Asistenta Sociala, n.d.).

Additionally, many institutionalized children experienced not only deprivation but also high levels of physical abuse (Gavrilovici & Groza 2007; Stativa et al., 2002), including severe punishment and beatings by orphanage staff (Rus et al., 2013; Stativa et al., 2002), children being witness or forced to do various chores or odd jobs, steal, beg, and give away personal belongings (e.g., money, food, clothing, school supplies) for the benefit of older institutionalized peers (Rus et al.,2017; Stativa et al., 2002), or children being aware or victims of sexual abuse in institutions (Stativa et al., 2002).

Even though attempts were made to describe and classify institutional neglect as a heterogeneous phenomenon, it is still difficult to conceptually define or measure, and researchers follow different theoretical approaches and employ different instruments to measure institutional neglect (e.g., Embleton et al., 2014; Groark, McCall, & Fish, 2011; McCall, Groark, & Fish, 2010; St. Petersburg-USA Orphanage Research Team, 2008; Tirella et al., 2008). Thus, we can find variation in children's quality of life across the globe and time periods. In addition to the Romanian institutions of the 1990s, institutions have also shown to provide inadequate care in recent times. For instance, institutions in Central America have been found to provide very little warm, sensitive, responsive, and contingent caregiver–child interaction and a limited amount of furniture, toys, and organized activities beyond routine care (Groark et al., 2011). Moreover, relatively recent studies have presented long-term residential settings as having lower quality conditions for children than family settings in countries like Romania, Greece, and Ukraine (e.g., Dobrova-Krol, van

IJzendoorn, Bakermans-Kranenburg, & Juffer, 2010; Smyke et al., 2007; Stativa et al., 2002; Vorria et al., 2003), even though Embleton et al. (2014) in Kenya and Davidson-Arad and colleagues in Israel (Davidson-Arad, Dekel, & Wozner, 2004) showed the opposite trend. These two studies show that children had better life conditions in these institutions than children reared in biological families. Other children (21.2% of those studied) were presented as experiencing some levels of neglect regarding their clothing, medical care, nutrition, and supervision in Kazakhstan (Haarr, 2011) or having good physical environments, toys, and equipment as well as acceptable medical care, sanitation, and nutrition in orphanages in the Russian Federation (St. Petersburg–USA Orphanage Research Team, 2005, 2008).

Both chronic neglect and institutionalization can occur over a period of years, thus dramatically effecting children's development. In the majority of cases of non-institutionalized children, neglect is characterized by "subthreshold" events and chronic conditions that do not produce "critical events" that would trigger a response from child protective services or law enforcement. Therefore, it is the chronicity of this type of maltreatment that causes long-term damage to children (APSAC, 2008). Regarding institutionalized children, there is strong evidence that having this type of personal history (i.e., some type of deprivation) is associated with social, thought, and attention problems (Gunnar & van Dulmen, 2007), externalizing (Juffer & van IJzendoorn, 2005), and psychiatric disorders (Zeanah et al., 2009) among many other health-related issues (for more information about psychopathology following severe deprivation, see also Chap. 6). Additionally, for more information about institutional neglect and/or its consequences on children's development, see also Chaps. 11, 12, 14, 15, 16, and 19.

5.2 *Emotional Abuse in Institutional Settings*

Another form of child maltreatment is emotional abuse which

> *Includes the failure to provide a developmentally appropriate, supportive environment, including the availability of a primary attachment figure, so that the child can develop a stable and full range of emotional and social competencies commensurate with her or his personal potentials and in the context of the society in which the child dwells. There may also be acts towards the child that cause or have a high probability of causing harm to the child's health or physical, mental, spiritual, moral or social development. These acts must be reasonably within the control of the parent or person in a relationship of responsibility, trust or power. Acts include restriction of movement, patterns of belittling, denigrating, scapegoating, threatening, scaring, discriminating, ridiculing or other non-physical forms of hostile or rejecting treatment.* (WHO, 1999, p. 15)

Furthermore, the American Professional Society on the Abuse of Children (APSAC, 1995) has described psychological (emotional) abuse as a "*repeated pattern of caregiver behavior or extreme incident(s) that convey to children that they are worthless, flawed, unloved, unwanted, endangered, or of value only in meeting another's needs*." They further list six types of psychological maltreatment, including (a) spurning (verbal and nonverbal hostile rejecting/degrading), (b) terrorizing (behavior that threatens or is likely to harm the child physically or place the child or the child's loved objects in danger), (c) exploiting/corrupting (encouraging the child to develop inappropriate behaviors), (d) denying emotional responsiveness (ignoring child's needs to interact, failing to express positive affect to the child, showing no emotion in interactions with the child), (e) isolating (denying child opportunities for interacting/communicating with peers or adults); and (f) mental, health, medical, and educational neglect (ignoring or failing to ensure provision for the child's needs). In sum, all forms of abuse, whether or not they include physical contact, can lead to significant adverse consequences for children as well as long-term consequences into adulthood.

Another definition of emotional abuse was proposed by Glaser (2011), who highlighted five categories and their descriptions, commonly known in Europe as the Framework for the Recognition and Management of Emotional Abuse and Neglect (FRAMEA):

1. Emotional unavailability, unresponsiveness, and neglect. This category reflects the violation of the child's basic need and right to have her/his existence acknowledged.
2. Interacting with the child with hostility, blame, denigration, rejection, or scapegoating. This interaction is usually directed at a particular child and is often based on the belief that the child deserves this response due to basic negative attributions to the child. This category reflects the violation of the child's basic need and right to be valued and loved for what he/she is.
3. Developmentally inappropriate or inconsistent interactions with the child. These include expectations beyond or below the child's developmental capacity, harsh and inconsistent discipline, and exposure to confusing or traumatic events and interactions, in particular domestic violence. This category reflects the violation of the child's basic need and right to be considered at their particular age/developmental stage.
4. Failure to recognize or acknowledge the child's individuality and psychological boundary between the parent and the child. There is inability to distinguish between the child's reality and the adult's beliefs and wishes; the child is used for the fulfillment of the parents' needs as a virtual extension of the parent (e.g., involving children in parental disputes, fabricated or induced illness [Munchausen by Proxy]). This category reflects the violation of the child's basic need and right to be recognized or acknowledged as a unique individual with their own feelings and perceptions.
5. Failing to promote the child's socialization. Includes active mis-socialization or corruption (e.g., isolation, failure to provide adequate stimulation and opportunities for learning). This category reflects the violation of the child's basic need and right to be able to function progressively outside the family.

Reports of emotional abuse of institutionalized children include staff personnel, caregivers, and others depriving children of authentic emotional relationships (by not talking to them); keeping them in a permanent state of insecurity and uncertainty (by using blackmail and threats); punishing them for behaviors that are normal behaviors for their age; setting unreasonable rules and requirements; using ridicule and humiliation (including when the child has enuresis); ignoring children's performances; making them wear inappropriate clothes for their age; denial of leaves, family visits, recreational activities, or trips; denying children of their favorite toys; and/or not providing opportunities for children to make their own choices and decisions (Rus et al., 2013; Stativa et al., 2002). Similar behaviors have been reported in many other institutional settings across the globe including Botswana (Morantz & Heymann, 2010) and Israel (Attar-Schwartz, 2011) and include verbal humiliation, insults, ridicule, and being cursed at by staff. For more information about emotional abuse on institutionalized children, see also Chaps. 3 and 13.

5.3 *Physical Abuse in Institutional Settings*

The World Health Organization has described physical abuse of a child as "*that which results in actual or potential physical harm from an interaction or lack of an interaction, which is reasonably within the control of a parent or person in a position of responsibility, power or trust. There may be a single or repeated incidents*" (WHO, 1999, p. 15).

Child physical abuse in institutional settings is characterized by moderate to severe behaviors directed at residents by staff. Moderate behaviors can include grabbing, pushing, pinching, spanking, kicks, punches, and/or ear or hair pulling, and severe abuse includes the use of instruments to physically punish children (Attar-Schwartz, 2011; Haarr, 2011; Rus et al., 2013; Stativa et al., 2002). These actions can lead to serious physical consequences including head injuries, internal injuries, broken bones, broken teeth, and black eyes (Haarr, 2011). In a review of existing research, Malinosky-Rummell and Hansen (1993) report that one long-term consequence of physical abuse is violence and aggression in adolescence and adulthood. Specifically, research indicates that victims of physical abuse are at risk for perpetrating violence toward family members and nonfamily members. Childhood physical abuse also increases the risk of arrest for violent and nonviolent crimes and negatively impacts school performance and job success (Lansford et al., 2007). For more information about physical abuse on institutionalized children, see also Chaps. 3 and 13.

5.4 *Sexual Abuse in Institutional Settings*

Sexual abuse, as defined by the World Health Organization, is

> *The involvement of a child in sexual activity that he or she does not fully comprehend, is unable to give informed consent to, or for which the child is not developmentally prepared and cannot give consent, or that violate the laws or social taboos of society. Child sexual*

> *abuse is evidenced by this activity between a child and an adult or another child who by age or development is in a relationship of responsibility, trust or power, the activity being intended to gratify or satisfy the needs of the other person. This may include but is not limited to: The inducement or coercion of a child to engage in any unlawful sexual activity; The exploitative use of child in prostitution or other unlawful sexual practices; The exploitative use of children in pornographic performances and materials.* (WHO, 1999, pp. 15–16)

Thus, child sexual abuse can occur under certain conditions, which include a maturational or age difference, when the adult caregiver is in a position of authority, and/or when the child is tricked or violence is used (Finkelhor, 1999). Importantly, though sexual abuse is often thought of as sexual behavior that involves contact, the definition includes noncontact behaviors such as exposing a child to pornographic performances and materials. Thus, these behaviors can include exhibitionism and voyeurism (Bode & Goldman, 2012).

In institutional settings, sexual abuse can be perpetrated on children by staff at the facility, by other adults with whom the child has contact, or by their peers (other residents/children) at the institution as documented in various studies (e.g., Attar-Schwartz, 2014; Euser, Alink, Tharner, van IJzendoorn, & Bakermans-Kranenburg, 2013, 2016; Gavrilovici & Groza, 2007). Also, children in institutionalized care may have experienced sexual abuse prior to placement (due to risk factors present before placement), as well as during placement in such settings. Research on the traumatic experiences of children prior to placement in residential facilities indicates that these children have experienced significant trauma before placement (Collin-Vezina, Coleman, Milne, Sell, & Daigneault, 2011). Childhood sexual abuse has an impact throughout the development of an individual. For instance, children and youth who experienced institutionalization as well as sexual abuse have shown a high occurrence of mental health issues, including depression, post-traumatic stress disorder, obsessive compulsive disorder, and anxiety (Spröber et al., 2014). For additional descriptive information about sexual abuse in institutions, see also Chaps. 3, 8, 9, and 13.

5.5 Witnessing Violence in Institutional Settings

As a form of maltreatment, the World Health Organization defines witnessing domestic violence as "*any form of verbal or physical violence between a caregiver and his or her adult partner or ex-partner*" (as cited in Meinck et al., 2016, p. 6). It is obvious that institutionalized children do not have such experiences, but there is evidence that they witness a lot of institutional abuse. Specifically, reports show that 19% of children in Kazakhstan orphanages have witnessed staff using harsh verbal abuse with other children, 16% of children have reported witnessing staff engage in psychological abuse of other children, 22% of children have reported witnessing staff perpetrating moderate physical violence to children, and 22% have reported witnessing perpetration of severe physical violence by staff to other children. Another study (Stativa et al., 2002) showed that institutionalized children had witnessed their peers being forced to do various chores, steal, beg, and give away various personal belongings. Additionally, Gavrilovici and Groza (2007) showed that institutionalized children were witnesses of a large variety of abusive behaviors, including children being threatened; slapped, hit, punched, or pushed; beaten; stabbed or attacked with a knife; or sexually abused. For additional descriptive information about abuse witnessing in institutions, see also Chap. 3.

6 Conclusion

Unfortunately, even though institutional settings should offer care and protection to children, as documented above, children placed in different types of care settings across many countries, with different political, socioeconomic systems and cultures, have experienced either singular or multiple forms of maltreatment perpetrated by staff and/or peers over short or long periods of time.

Bullying is one way to conceptualize the widespread peer victimization in institutions. While specific details among definitions may vary, bullying is considered an aggressive, physically or emotionally abusive behavior (either physical or emotional abuse) perpetrated by peers that violates the victim's rights (Craig & Pepler, 2007). Examples of bullying include ridicule or name-calling; ignoring or exclusion from a group of friends; hitting, kicking, pushing, shoving, or threatening; spreading lies or false rumors; sending mean notes; or doing other hurtful things (Solberg & Olweus, 2003; Solberg, Olweus, & Endresen, 2007). In addition, bullying among adolescents may include threats to take away or destroy another's belongings or do unpleasant things to them, or using derogatory names with sexual or racial meaning (Kyriakides, Kaloyirou, & Lindsay, 2006). Thus, children in institutional settings may be exposed to peers who utilize verbally or physically abusive behaviors to punish, harm, or control them or force them to do various chores, steal, beg, and give away various personal belongings such as money, food, clothing, and school supplies (e.g., Attar-Schwartz & Khoury-Kassabri, 2015; Rus et al., in press; Sekol & Farrington, 2013).

Furthermore, even though we presented each type of maltreatment separately as defined by WHO (1999), in reality many children and youth in residential care have experienced multiple forms of abuse (e.g., Collin-Vézina, Coleman, Milne, Sell, & Daigneault, 2011; Cyr et al., 2012; Gray et al., 2015; Segura, Pereda, Abad, & Guilera, 2015; Van Vugt, Lanctôt, Paquette, Collin-Vézina, & Lemieux, 2014), which has been defined as poly-victimization by Finkelhor and colleagues (Finkelhor, Ormrod, Turner, & Hamby, 2005). Also, because children who experience physical and sexual abuse often experience concurrent emotional abuse and neglect, the latter should not be overlooked even when the other more outwardly severe forms of abuse are present (Spertus et al., 2003). For additional information about bullying, exploitation, or poly-victimization, see Chaps. 3, 7, and 13.

Maltreatment, whether experienced in one or multiple forms, is associated with negative consequences on the well-being of institutionalized children and adolescents (e.g., Collin-Vézina et al., 2011; Gunnar & van Dulmen, 2007; Hermenau, Hecker, Elbert, & Ruf-Leuschner, 2014; Hermenau et al., 2011; Juffer & van IJzendoorn, 2005; Segura, Pereda, Guilera, & Abad, 2016; Whetten, Ostermann, Whetten, O'Donnell, & Thielman, 2011; Zeanah et al., 2009).

6.1 Contributing Factors of Institutional Maltreatment

Many long-term residential centers have shown to have organizational characteristics and culture that facilitate neglect and abuse by staff and peers. Specifically, dysfunctional organizational features that may explain the prevalence of victimization include poor management of hiring, training, scheduling, and supervision of staff; inadequate management and systems of accountability; inadequate cultural and organizational features to support disclosures of abuse; lack of resources (Colton, 2002; Monks et al., 2009; Rus et al., in press); as well as ineffective implementation of policies regarding violence, referrals of residents, capturing children's reports of peer violence, and ensuring appropriate physical characteristics of living spaces (Barter Renold, Cawson, & Berridge, 2004). Additionally, in such settings, vulnerable children are consistently exposed to their perpetrators and are unable to have privacy (Baker, Cunningham, & Male, 2002).

Violence among institutionalized children can be shaped by rules that residents create among themselves, perceptions, justifications, and group dynamics where dominant members exercise control through violence. Such factors can contribute to a peer culture that facilitates aggression, deprivation, stigmatization, and frustration and poor relationships with staff (Barter et al., 2004; Sekol, 2013). It is likely that children in some long-term residential institutions have opportunity to organize gangs with their own hierarchy, rules, norms, and dynamics and that can't be controlled by staff. In addition, lack of educational activities and individualized developmental programs, and inconsistency in caregiving with little interaction between staff and children may also facilitate peer exploitation and bullying (Rus et al., in press).

Another facilitating environmental factor can be the transitional nature of both staff and peers in institutions. The institutional structure often includes staff that work varying shifts and have high turnover. In addition, residents are also moved in and out of various institutions, influencing the consistency of the environment (Euser et al., 2013). Thus, the victimization of children in residential care should be understood as a complex phenomenon related to individual characteristics and institutional factors (e.g., group dynamics, institutional culture, and ineffective staff) (for more information, see Timmerman & Schreuder, 2014). Additionally, societal factors that increase the risk of abuse in institutional settings include the low prioritization of these children when it comes to governmental policy (Pinheiro, 2006) and community attitudes about children placed in residential care (Colton, 2002), or various societal assumptions about the rights of children (Spröber et al., 2014).

7 Summary

There is a growing body of research showing that maltreatment affects development and can have long-term adverse psychological, behavioral, cognitive, and health effects. This is especially true for children living in institutions, who likely experience maltreatment both before and during their institutionalization. To provide improved preventive and intervention practices, there is a need to develop consistent and universally accepted definitions that can become a common language for researchers, policy-makers, and practitioners. While there is currently no universal consensus on specific definitions of maltreatment, there are some common areas of agreement, and some standardization is occurring due to the development of scales that are beginning to be used consistently in research, practice, and policy-making regarding maltreatment of institutionalized children.

Questions for Discussion

1. In what specific ways has the information in this chapter expanded your understanding about how maltreatment is defined in general or applied to institutionalized children? Name three things that stood out for you and explain why.
2. Think about one of the definitions regarding maltreatment of children, with or without a history of institutionalization, described in this chapter and the context in which this definition was derived. What modification to the definition could you recommend and why?
3. Choose two of the definitions of maltreatment, abuse, or neglect in this chapter. How are these definitions the same as and different from each other? Summarize your reasoning for these similarities and differences.

References

American Psychiatric Association. (2013). *Diagnostic and statistical manual of mental disorders* (5th ed.). Washington, DC: Author.

Ames, E. W., & Carter, M. C. (1992, June). *A study of Romanian orphanage children in Canada: Background, sample, and procedure. Development of Romanian Orphanage Children Adopted to Canada.* Symposium presented at the annual convention of the Canadian Psychological Association, Quebec City, QC.

APSAC. (1995). *Psychosocial evaluation of suspected psychological maltreatment in children and adolescents. Practice Guidelines.* Chicago, IL: American Professional Society on the Abuse of Children.

APSAC. (2008). *Challenges in the evaluation of child neglect. Practice Guidelines.* Elmhurst, IL: American Professional Society on the Abuse of Children.

Attar-Schwartz, S. (2011). Maltreatment by staff in residential care facilities: The adolescents' perspectives. *Social Service Review, 85*(4), 635–664. doi:10.1086/664009.

Attar-Schwartz, S. (2014). Experiences of sexual victimization by peers among adolescents in residential care settings. *Social Service Review, 88*(4), 594–629. doi:10.1016/j.childyouth.2012.11.005.

Attar-Schwartz, S., & Khoury-Kassabri, M. (2015). Indirect and verbal victimization by peers among at-risk youth in residential care. *Child Abuse & Neglect, 42*, 84–98. doi:10.1016/j.chiabu.2014.12.007.

Baker, L., Cunningham, A., & Male, C. (2002). *Peer-to-peer aggression in residential settings: Increasing understanding to enhance intervention*. London, ON: Centre for Children and Families in the Justice System of the London Family Court Clinic Incorporated. http://www.lfcc.on.ca/peerviolence.pdf. Accessed 29 Jan 2015.
Banyard, V. L., Williams, L. M., & Siegel, J. A. (2001). The long-term mental health consequences of child sexual abuse: An exploratory study of the impact of multiple traumas in a sample of women. *Journal of Traumatic Stress, 14*, 697–715.
Barnett, D., Manly, J. T., & Cicchetti, D. (1991). Continuing toward an operational definition of psychological maltreatment. *Development and Psychopathology, 3*(1), 19–29.
Barnett, D., Manly, J. T., & Cicchetti, D. (1993). Defining child maltreatment: The interface between policy and research. In D. Cicchetti & S. L. Toth (Eds.), *Child abuse, child development, and social policy: Advances in applied developmental psychology, vol 8* (pp. 7–74). Norwood, NJ: Ablex Publishing.
Barter, C., Renold, E., Cawson, P., & Berridge, D. (2004). *Peer violence in children's residential-care*. Basingstoke, UK: Palgrave MacMillan.
Bejenaru, A., & Tucker, S. (2014). Challenging dominant representations of residential childcare in Romania: An exploration of the views of children and young people living in the care system. *Journal of Youth Studies* (ahead-of-print), 1–14. doi:10.1080/13676261.2014.918250.
Bellis, M. A., Hughes, K., Leckenby, N., Jones, L., Baban, A., Kachaeva, M., … Terzic, N. (2014). Adverse childhood experiences and associations with health-harming behaviours in young adults: Surveys in eight eastern European countries. *Bulletin of the World Health Organization, 92*(9), 641–655. doi:10.2471/BLT.13.129247.
Belsky, J. (1980). Child maltreatment: An ecological integration. *American Psychologist, 35*(4), 320–335. doi:10.1037/0003-066X.35.4.320.
Bernet, C. Z., & Stein, M. B. (1999). Relationship of childhood maltreatment to the onset and course of major depression in adulthood. *Depression and Anxiety, 9*, 169–174.
Bernstein, D.P., Fink, L., Handelsman, L., Foote, J., Lovejoy, M., Wenzel, K.,… Ruggiero, J. (1994). Initial reliability and validity of a new retrospective measure of child abuse and neglect. *The American Journal of Psychiatry, 151*(8), 1132–1136.
Bernstein, D.P., Stein, J.A., Newcomb, M.D., Walker, E., Pogge, D., Ahluvalia, T.,… Zule W. (2003). Development and validation of a brief screening version of the childhood trauma questionnaire. *Child Abuse & Neglect, 27*(2), 169–190.
Bode, A., & Goldman, J. G. (2012). The impact of child sexual abuse on the education of boys in residential care between 1950 and 1975. *Pastoral Care in Education, 30*(4), 331–344.
Carson, D. K., Foster, J. M., & Tripathi, N. (2013). Child sexual abuse in India: Current issues and research. *Psychological Studies, 58*(3), 318–325. doi:10.1007/s12646-013-0198-6.
Castle, J., Groothues, C., Bredenkamp, D., Becket, C., O'Connor, T., Rutter, M., & E.R.A. Study Team. (1999). Effects of qualities of early institutional care on cognitive attainment. *American Journal of Orthopsychiatry, 69*(4), 424–437.
Child Welfare Information Gateway. (2013). *Chronic child neglect*. Washington, DC: U.S. Department of Health and Human Services, Children's Bureau.
Children's Health Care Collaborative Study Group. (1992). Romanian health and social care system for the children and families: Future directions in health care reform. *BJM, 304*, 556–559. doi:10.1136/bmj.304.6826.556.
Cicchetti, D. (1991). Defining psychological maltreatment: Reflections and future directions (editorial). *Development and Psychopathology, 3*, 1–2.
Cicchetti, D., & Rizley, R. (1981). Developmental perspectives on the etiology, intergenerational transmission, and sequelae of child maltreatment. *New Directions for Child and Adolescent Development, 1981*(11), 31–55. doi:10.1002/cd.23219811104.
Cicchetti, D., Toth, S. L., & Maughan, A. (2000). An ecological-transactional model of child maltreatment. In A. J. Sameroff, M. Lewis, & S. M. Miller (Eds.), *Handbook of developmental psychopathology* (pp. 689–722). New York, NY: Springer. Retrieved from http://dx.doi.org/10.1007/978-1-4615-4163-9.

Cicchetti, D., & Valentino, K. (2006). An ecological–transactional perspective on child maltreatment: Failure of the average expectable environment and its influence on child development. In D. Cicchetti & D. J. Cohen (Eds.), *Developmental psychopathology, Risk, disorder and adaptation* (vol. 3, pp. 129–201). Hoboken, NJ: Wiley.

Collin-Vezina, D., Coleman, K., Milne, L., Sell, J., & Daigneault, I. (2011). Trauma experiences, maltreatment-related impairments, and resilience among child welfare youth in residential care. *International Journal of Mental Health & Addiction, 9*(5), 577–589.

Colton, M. (2002). Factors associated with abuse in residential child care institutions. *Children & Society, 16*(1), 33–44.

Craig, W. M., & Pepler, D. J. (2007). Understanding bullying: From research to practice. *Canadian Psychology, 48*(2), 86–93. doi:10.1037/cp2007010.

Crosson-Tower, C. (2002). *Understanding child abuse and neglect* (5th ed.). Boston, MA: Allyn and Bacon.

Cyr, K., Chamberland, C., Lessard, G., Clément, M. È., Wemmers, J. A., Collin-Vézina, D., … Damant, D. (2012). Polyvictimization in a child welfare sample of children and youths. *Psychology of Violence, 2*(4), 385.

Davidson-Arad, B., Dekel, R., & Wozner, Y. (2004). Correspondence in residents' and staff members' assessments of the quality of life of children in residential care facilities. *Social Indicators Research, 68*(1), 77–89.

Deb, S. (2006). *Children in agony: A source book*. New Delhi, India: Concept Pub.

Department of Health, Department for Education and Employment and Home Office. (2000). *Framework for the assessment of children in need and their families*. London, UK: The Stationery Office.

Dobrova-Krol, N. A., van IJzendoorn, M. H., Bakermans-Kranenburg, M. J., & Juffer, F. (2010). Effects of perinatal HIV infection and early institutional rearing on physical and cognitive development of children in Ukraine. *Child Development, 81*(1), 237–251.

Drury, S. S., Theall, K., Gleason, M. M., Smyke, A. T., De Vivo, I., Wong, J. Y., … Nelson, C. A. (2012). Telomere length and early severe social deprivation: Linking early adversity and cellular aging. *Molecular Psychiatry, 17*(7), 719–727. doi:10.1038/mp.2011.53.

Egeland, B., Sroufe, L. A., & Erickson, M. F. (1983). Developmental consequences of different patterns of maltreatment. *Child Abuse and Neglect, 7*, 459–469.

Embleton, L., Ayuku, D., Kamanda, A., Atwoli, L., Ayaya, S., Vreeman, R., … Braitstein, P. (2014). Models of care for orphaned and separated children and upholding children's rights: Cross-sectional evidence from western Kenya. *BMC International Health and Human Rights, 149*. doi:10.1186/1472-698X-14-9

English, D. J., Bangdiwala, S. I., & Runyan, D. K. (2005). The dimensions of maltreatment: Introduction. *Child Abuse & Neglect, 29*(5), 441–460. doi:10.1016/j.chiabu.2003.09.023.

English, D. J., & The LONGSCAN Investigators. (1997). *Modified maltreatment classification system (MMCS)*. Retrieved from http://www.unc.edu/depts/sph/longscan/pages/maltx/mmcs/LONGSCAN%20MMCS%20Coding.pdf

Euser, S., Alink, L. A., Tharner, A., van IJzendoorn, M. H., & Bakermans-Kranenburg, M. J. (2016). The prevalence of child sexual abuse in out-of-home care: Increased risk for children with a mild intellectual disability. *Journal of Applied Research in Intellectual Disabilities, 29*, 83–92. doi:10.1111/jar.12160.

Euser, S., Alink, L. R. A., Tharner, A., van Ijzendoorn, M. H., & Bakermans-Kranenburg, M. J. (2013). The prevalence of child sexual abuse in out-of-home care: A comparison between abuse in residential and in foster care. *Child Maltreatment, 18*(4), 221–231.

Finkelhor, D. (1999). Child sexual abuse. Challenges facing child protection and mental health professionals. In E. Ullmann & W. Hilweg (Eds.), *Childhood and trauma – Separation, abuse, war* (pp. 101–115). Burlington, VT: Ashgate Publishing Company.

Finkelhor, D., & Browne, A. (1985). The traumatic impact of child sexual abuse: A conceptualization. *American Journal of Orthopsychiatry, 55*, 530–541.

Finkelhor, D., Ormrod, R., Turner, H., & Hamby, S. L. (2005). Measuring poly-victimization using the juvenile victimization Questionnaire. *Child Abuse & Neglect, 29*(11), 1297–1312.

Friedrich, W. H., Urquiza, A. Y., & Bilke, R. L. (1986). Behavior problems in sexually abused young children. *Journal of Pediatric Psychology, 11*(1), 47–57.
Fusco, R. A., & Cahalane, H. (2013). Young children in the child welfare system: What factors contribute to trauma symptomology? *Child Welfare, 92*(5), 37–58.
Gavrilovici, O., & Groza, V. (2007). Incidence, prevalence and trauma associated with exposure to violence in Romanian institutionalized children. *International Journal of Child & Family Welfare, 10*(3–4), 125–138.
General Assembly of the United Nations (1989, November 20). *Convention on the rights of the child.* General assembly resolution 44/25. Geneva: Office of the High Commissioner for Human Rights.
Giovanni, J. M., & Becerra, R. M. (1979). *Defining child abuse.* New York, NY: The Free Press.
Glaser, D. (2011). How to deal with emotional abuse and neglect-further development of a conceptual framework (FRAMEA). *Child Abuse and Neglect, 35*, 866–875. doi:10.1016/j.chiabu.2011.08.002.
Goodwin, R. D., & Stein, M. B. (2004). Association between childhood trauma and physical disorders among adults in the United States. *Psychological Medicine, 34*(3), 509–520.
Grassi-Oliveira, R., Ashy, M., & Stein, L. M. (2008). Psychobiology of childhood maltreatment: Effects of allostatic load? *Revista Brasileira de Psiquiatria, 30*(1), 60–68.
Gray, C. L., Pence, B. W., Ostermann, J., Whetten, R. A., O'Donnell, K., Thielman, N. M., & Whetten, K. (2015). Prevalence and incidence of traumatic experiences among orphans in institutional and family-based settings in 5 low- and middle-income countries: A longitudinal study. *Global Health, Science And Practice, 3*(3), 395–404. doi:10.9745/GHSP-D-15-00093.
Greeson, J. P., Briggs, E. C., Kisiel, C. L., Layne, C. M., Ake III, G. S., Ko, S. J., … Fairbank, J.A. (2011). Complex trauma and mental health in children and adolescents placed in foster care: Findings from the National Child Traumatic Stress Network. *Child Welfare, 90*(6), 91–108.
Groark, C. J., McCall, R. B., & Fish, L. (2011). Characteristics of environments, caregivers, and children in three central American orphanages. *Infant Mental Health Journal, 32*(2), 232–250. doi:10.1002/imhj.20292.
Groze, V., & Ileana, D. (1996). A follow-up study of adopted children from Romania. *Child & Adolescent Social Work Journal, 13*(6), 541–565.
Gunnar, M. R. (2001). Effects of early deprivation: Findings from orphanage-reared infants and children. In C. A. Nelson & M. Luciana (Eds.), *Handbook of developmental cognitive neuroscience* (pp. 617–629). Cambridge, MA: MIT Press.
Gunnar, M. R., & van Dulmen, M. M. (2007). Behavior problems in post institutionalized internationally adopted children. *Development and Psychopathology, 19*, 129–148. doi:10.1017/S0954579407070071.
Haarr, R. N. (2011). *Violence against children in state-run residential institutions in Kazakhstan: An assessment.* Astana, Kazakhstan: United Nations Children's Fund. Retrieved September 20, 2016, from http://www.ceecis.org/ccc/publications/Violence_against_children_in_state-run_residential_institutions_in Kazakhstan_2011_ENG.pdf
Hamarman, S., & Bernet, W. (2000). Evaluating and reporting emotional abuse in children: Parent-based, action-based focus aids in clinical decision-making. *Journal of the American Academy of Child & Adolescent Psychiatry, 39*(7), 928–930.
Hardt, J., Sidor, A., Nickel, R., Kappis, B., Petrak, P., & Egle, U. T. (2008). Childhood adversities and suicide attempts: A retrospective study. *Journal of Family Violence, 23*, 713–718.
Hart, H., & Rubia, K. (2012). Neuroimaging of child abuse: A critical review. *Frontiers in Human Neuroscience, 652*. doi:10.3389/fnhum.2012.00052.
Hermenau, K., Hecker, T., Elbert, T., & Ruf-Leuschner, M. (2014). Maltreatment and mental health in institutional care–comparing early and late institutionalized children in Tanzania. *Infant Mental Health Journal, 35*(2), 102–110. doi:10.1002/imhj.21440.
Hermenau, K., Hecker, T., Ruf, M., Schauer, E., Elbert, T., & Schauer, M. (2011). Childhood adversity, mental ill-health and aggressive behavior in an African orphanage: Changes in response to trauma-focused therapy and the implementation of a new instructional system. *Child & Adolescent Psychiatry & Mental Health, 5*(1), 29–37. doi:10.1186/1753-2000-5-29.

Herrenkohl, R. C. (2005). The definition of child maltreatment: From case study to construct. *Child Abuse & Neglect, 29*(5), 413–424. doi:10.1016/j.chiabu.2005.04.002.

Hildyard, K., & Wolfe, D. (2002). Child neglect: Developmental issues and outcomes. *Child Abuse & Neglect, 26*, 679–695.

Hoff, L. A. (2009). *Violence and abuse issues: Cross-cultural perspectives for health and social service*. Abingdon, UK; New York, NY: Routledge.

Humphreys, K. L., Esteves, K., Zeanah, C. H., Fox, N. A., Nelson, C. A., & Drury, S. S. (2016). Accelerated telomere shortening: Tracking the lasting impact of early institutional care at the cellular level. *Psychiatry Research, 246*, 95–100. doi:10.1016/j.psychres.2016.09.023.

Institute of Medicine (U.S.), & National Research Council (U.S.). (2013). *New directions in child abuse and neglect research*. Washington, DC: National Academies Press.

Johnson, D. E., Miller, L. C., Iverson, S., Thomas, W., Franchino, B., Dole, K., … Hostetter, M. K. (1992). The health of children adopted from Romania. *Journal of the American Medical Association, 268*(24), 3446–3451.

Juffer, F., & van IJzendoorn, M. H. (2005). Behavior problems and mental health referrals of international adoptees: A meta-analysis. *JAMA: Journal of the American Medical Association, 293*, 2501–2515. doi:10.1001/jama.293.20.2501.

Kolko, D. J., Hurlburt, M. S., Zhang, J., Barth, R. P., Leslie, L. K., & Burns, B. J. (2010). Posttraumatic stress symptoms in children and adolescents referred for child welfare investigation: A national sample of in-home and out-of-home care. *Child Maltreatment, 15*(1), 48–63.

Krastins, A., Francis, A. J. P., Field, A. M., & Carr, S. N. (2014). Childhood predictors of adulthood antisocial personality symptomology. *Australian Psychologist, 49*, 142–150.

Kyriakides, L., Kaloyirou, C., & Lindsay, G. (2006). An analysis of the revised olweus bully/victim questionnaire using the Rasch measurement model. *British Journal of Educational Psychology, 76*(4), 781–801. doi:10.1348/000709905X53499.

Lansford, J. E., Dodge, K. A., Pettit, G. S., Bates, J. E., Crozier, J., & Kaplow, J. (2002). A 12-year prospective study of the long-term effects of early child physical maltreatment on psychological, behavioral, and academic problems in adolescence. *Archives of Pediatrics & Adolescent Medicine, 156*(8), 824–830.

Lansford, J. E., Miller-Johnson, S., Berlin, L. J., Dodge, K. A., Bates, J. E., & Pettit, G. S. (2007). Early physical abuse and later violent delinquency: A prospective longitudinal study. *Child Maltreatment, 12*(3), 233–245.

Lee, S. J., Guterman, N. B., & Lee, Y. (2008). Risk factors for paternal physical child abuse. *Child Abuse & Neglect, 32*(9), 846–858. doi:10.1016/j.chiabu.2007.11.006.

Lind, M. J., Aggen, S. H., Kendler, K. S., York, T. P., & Amstadter, A. B. (2016). An epidemiologic study of childhood sexual abuse and adult sleep disturbances. *Psychological Trauma: Theory, Research, Practice, and Policy, 8*(2), 198–205.

Livingston, R. (1987). Sexually and physically abused children. *Journal of the American Academy of Child and Adolescent Psychiatry, 26*(3), 413–415.

MacKenzie, M. J., Kotch, J. B., & Lee, L. C. (2011). Toward a cumulative ecological risk model for the etiology of child maltreatment. *Children and Youth Services Review, 33*(9), 1638–1647. doi:10.1016/j.childyouth.2011.04.018.

Malinosky-Rummell, R., & Hansen, D. J. (1993). Long-term consequences of childhood physical abuse. *Psychological Bulletin, 114*(1), 68.

Manly, J. T. (2005). Advances in research definitions of child maltreatment. *Child Abuse & Neglect, 29*(5), 425–439. doi:10.1016/j.chiabu.2005.04.001.

McCall, R. B. (2011). IX. Research, practice, and policy perspectives on issues of children without permanent parental care. *Monographs of the Society for Research in Child Development, 76*(4), 223–272.

McCall, R. B., Groark, C. J., & Fish, L. (2010). A caregiver–child socioemotional and relationship rating scale. *Infant Mental Health Journal, 31*(2), 201–219. doi:10.1002/imhj.20252.

McCall, R. B., Groark, C. J., Fish, L., Harkins, D., Serrano, G., & Gordon, K. (2010). A socioemotional intervention in a Latin American orphanage. *Infant Mental Health Journal, 31*(5), 521–542. doi:10.1002/imhj.20270.

McMullan, S J., & Fisher, L. (1992, June). *Developmental progress of Romanian orphanage children in Canada. Development of Romanian orphanage children adopted to Canada.* Symposium presented at the annual convention of the Canadian Psychological Association, Quebec City, QC.

Meinck, F., Steinert, J. I., Sethi, D., Gilbert, R., Bellis, M. A., Mikton, C., … Baban, A. (2016). *Measuring and monitoring national prevalence of child maltreatment: A practical handbook.* Retrieved from http://www.euro.who.int/__data/assets/pdf_file/0003/317505/Measuring-monitoring-national-prevalence-child-maltreatment-practical-handbook.pdf

Misca, G. M. (2003). *Romania's "orphans": Developmental adjustment of adolescents growing up in childcare institutions in Romania* (Doctoral dissertation). Newcastle University, Newcastle upon Tyne, UK.

Mock, S. E., & Arai, S. M. (2011). Childhood trauma and chronic illness in adulthood: Mental health and socioeconomic status as explanatory factors and buffers. *Frontiers in Psychology, 1,* 246. doi:10.3389/fpsyg.2010.00246.

Monks, C. P., Smith, P. K., Naylor, P., Barter, C., Ireland, J. L., & Coyne, I. (2009). Bullying in different contexts: Commonalities, differences and the role of theory. *Aggression and Violent Behavior, 14*(2), 146–156.

Morantz, G., & Heymann, J. (2010). Life in institutional care: The voices of children in a residential facility in Botswana. *AIDS Care, 22*(1), 10–16. doi:10.1080/09540120903012601.

Morrison, L. (2004). Ceausescu's legacy: Family struggles and institutionalization of children in Romania. *Journal of Family History, 29*(2), 168–182. doi:10.1177/0363199004264899.

National Authority for Child Protection and Adoption (NACPA) & UNICEF. (2004). *Child care system reform in Romania.* Bucuresti, Romania: UNICEF Romania.

National Center on Child Abuse and Neglect (NCCAN). (1981). *Study findings: National study of the incidence and severity of child abuse and neglect (DHHS no. OHDS 81–30325).* Washington, DC: Government Printing Office. Retrieved from https://library.childwelfare.gov/cwig/ws/library/docs/gateway/Record;jsessionid=C4142796529589FB6378F074918402CD?w=+NATIVE%28%27IPDET+PH+IS+%27%27nis-1%27%27%27%29&upp=0&order=+NATIVE%28%27year%2Fdescend%27%29&rpp=-10&r=1&m=3&

National Research Council (NRC). (1993). *Understanding child abuse and neglect.* Washington, DC: National Academy Press.

Olson, S., Stroud, C., & National Research Council (U.S.) (Eds.). (2012). *Child maltreatment research, policy, and practice for the next decade: Workshop summary.* Washington, DC: National Academies Press.

Pelzer, D. (1995). *A child called "it".* Deerfield Beach, FL: Health Communication.

Pinheiro, P. S. (2006). *World report on violence against children.* Geneva, Switzerland: The United Nations Study on Violence Against Children.

Raghavan, C., & Kingston, S. (2006). Child sexual abuse and posttraumatic stress disorder: Therole of age at first use of substances and lifetime traumatic events. *Journal of Traumatic Stress, 19,* 269–278.

Romens, S. E., McDonald, J., Svaren, J., & Pollak, S. D. (2015). Associations between early life stress and gene methylation in children. *Child Development, 86*(1), 303–309.

Rosenberg, D. R., Pajer, K., & Rancurello, M. (1992). Neuropsychiatric assessment of orphans in one Romanian orphanage for "unsalvageables". *JAMA, 268*(24), 3489–3490.

Rus, A. V., Stativa, E., Butterfield, M. E., Pennings, J. S., Burcea, G., & Wenyika, R. (2017). Peer exploitation: Findings from a Romanian nationally representative sample of children living in long-term residential centres. *Child Abuse Review.* doi: 10.1002/car.2464.

Rus, A. V., Stativa, E., Pennings, J. S., Cross, D. R., Ekas, N., Purvis, K., & Parris, S. R. (2013). Severe punishment of children by staff in Romanian placement centers for school-aged children: Effects of child and institutional characteristics. *Child Abuse and Neglect, 37*(12), 1152–1162.

Rutter, M., Beckett, C., Castle, J., Colvert, E., Kreppner, J., Mehta, M, … Sonuga-Barke, E. (2007). Effects of profound early institutional deprivation: An overview of findings from a UK longitudinal study of Romanian adoptees. *European Journal of Developmental Psychology, 4*(3), 332–350. doi:10.1080/17405620701401846.

Rutter, M., & The English and Romanian Adoptees (ERA) Study Team. (1998). Developmental catch-up, and deficit, following adoption after severe global early privation. *Journal of Child Psychology and Psychiatry*, *39*(4), 465–476.

Segura, A., Pereda, N., Abad, J., & Guilera, G. (2015). Victimization and polyvictimization among Spanish youth protected by the child welfare system. *Children and Youth Services Review*, *59*, 105–112.

Segura, A., Pereda, N., Guilera, G., & Abad, J. (2016). Poly-victimization and psychopathology among Spanish adolescents in residential care. *Child Abuse & Neglect*, *55*, 40–55.

Sekol, I. (2013). Peer violence in adolescent residential care: A qualitative examination of contextual and peer factors. *Children and Youth Services Review*, *35*(12), 1901–1912. doi:10.1016/j.childyouth.2013.09.006.

Sekol, I., & Farrington, D. P. (2013). The reliability and validity of self, peer and staff reports of bullying and victimisation in correctional and care institutions. *Psychology, Crime & Law*, *19*(4), 329–344. doi:10.1080/1068316X.2011.631541.

Shaughnessy, J. M. (2014). An essay on poverty and child neglect: New interventions. *Washington and Lee Journal of Civil Rights and Social Justice*, *21*(1), 4–15.

Shetty, P. (2014). Slow progress in ending female genital mutilation. *Bulletin of the World Health Organization*, *92*(1), 6–7. doi:10.2471/BLT.14.020114.

Slep, A. S., Heyman, R. E., & Foran, H. M. (2015). Child maltreatment in DSM-5 and ICD-11. *Family Process*, *54*(1), 17–32. doi:10.1111/famp.12131.

Smith, M. G., & Fong, R. (2004). *The children of neglect: When no one cares*. New York, NY: Brunner-Routledge.

Smyke, A. T., Koga, S. F., Johnson, D. E., Fox, N. A., Marshall, P. J., Nelson, C. A., & Zeanah, C. H. (2007). The caregiving context in institution-reared and family-reared infants and toddlers in Romania. *Journal of Child Psychology & Psychiatry*, *48*(2), 210–218. doi:10.1111/j.1469-7610.2006.01694.x.

Smyke, A. T., Zeanah, C. J., Fox, N. A., & Nelson, C. (2009). A new model of foster care for young children: The Bucharest early intervention project. *Child and Adolescent Psychiatric Clinics of North America*, *18*(3), 721–734.

Solberg, M., Olweus, D., & Endresen, I. (2007). Bullies and victims at school: Are they the same pupils? *The British Journal of Educational Psychology*, *77*(2), 441–464. doi:10.1348/000709906X105689.

Solberg, M. E., & Olweus, D. (2003). Prevalence estimation of school bullying with the olweus bully/victim questionnaire. *Aggressive Behavior*, *29*(3), 239–268. doi:10.1002/ab.10047.

Spertus, I. L., Yehuda, R., Wong, C. M., Halligan, S., & Seremetis, S. V. (2003). Childhood emotional abuse and neglect as predictors of psychological and physical symptoms in women presenting to a primary care practice. *Child Abuse and Neglect*, *27*(11), 1247–1258.

Spröber, N., Schneider, T., Rassenhofer, M., Seitz, A., Liebhardt, H., König, L., & Fegert, J. M. (2014). Child sexual abuse in religiously affiliated and secular institutions: A retrospective descriptive analysis of data provided by victims in a government-sponsored reappraisal program in Germany. *BMC Public Health*, *14*(1), 282–293. doi:10.1186/1471-2458-14-282.

St. Petersburg-USA Orphanage Research Team. (2005). Characteristics of children, caregivers, and orphanages for young children in St. Petersburg, Russian Federation. *Journal of Applied Developmental Psychology*, *26*, 477–506.

St. Petersburg-USA Orphanage Research Team. (2008). The effects of early social-emotional and relationship experience on the development of young orphanage children. *Monographs of the Society for Research in Child Development*, *73*(3), vii. doi:10.1111/j.1540-5834.2008.00483.x.

Stativa, E., Anghelescu, C., Palicari, G., Stanescu, A., & Nanu, R. (2002). *Child abuse in residential care institutions in Romania*. Bucharest, Romania: Extrem Group.

Stephenson, P., Anghelescu, C., Fumarel, S., Georgescu, A., Iorgulescu, D. McCreery, R., … Stativa, E. (1993). Training needs of staff in Romanian institutions for young children. *Child: Care, Health and Development*, *19*, 221–234. doi: 10.1111/j.1365-2214.1993.tb00728.x.

Suglia, S. F., Clark, C. J., Boynton-Jarrett, R., Kressin, N. R., & Koenen, K. C. (2014). Child maltreatment and hypertension in young adulthood. *BMC Public Health*, *14*(1), 1149.

Timmerman, M. C., & Schreuder, P. R. (2014). Sexual abuse of children and youth in residential care: An international review. *Aggression & Violent Behavior, 19*(6), 715–720. doi:10.1016/j.avb.2014.09.001.
Tirella, L. G., Chan, W., Cermak, S. A., Litvinova, A., Salas, K. C., & Miller, L. C. (2008). Time use in Russian baby homes. *Child: Care, Health and Development, 34*(1), 77–86. doi:10.1111/j.1365-2214.2007.00766.x.
Twardosz, S., & Lutzker, J. R. (2010). Child maltreatment and the developing brain: A review of neuroscience perspectives. *Aggression & Violent Behavior, 15*(1), 59–68. doi:10.1016/j.avb.2009.08.003.
Universitatea Babes-Bolyai, Facultatea de Psychologie si Stiinte ale Educatiei. (n.d.). *Scurt istoric al facultatii de Psihologie si Stiinte ale Educatiei* [*Brief history of the faculty of psychology and educational sciences*]. Retrieved July 15, 2016 from http://psiedu.ubbcluj.ro/index.php?id=11-istoric-psihologie
Universitatea Bucuresti, Facultatea de Sociologie si Asistenta Sociala. (n.d.). *Trecut* [*Past*]. Retrieved July 15, 2016 from http://sas.unibuc.ro/trecut_ro
van IJzendoorn, M. H., Palacios, J., Sonuga-Barke, E. S., Gunnar, M. R., Vorria, P., McCall, R. B., … Juffer, F. (2011). Children without permanent parents: Research, practice, and policy: I. Children in institutional care: Delayed development and resilience. *Monographs of the Society for Research in Child Development, 76*(4), 8–30. doi:10.1111/j.1540-5834.2011.00626.x.
Van Vugt, E., Lanctôt, N., Paquette, G., Collin-Vézina, D., & Lemieux, A. (2014). Girls in residential care: From child maltreatment to trauma-related symptoms in emerging adulthood. *Child Abuse & Neglect, 38*, 114–122. doi:10.1016/j.chiabu.2013.10.015.
Vorria, P., Papaligoura, Z., Dunn, J., van IJzendoorn, M. H., Steele, H., Kontopoulou, A., & Sarafidou, Y. (2003). Early experiences and attachment relationships of Greek infants raised in residential group care. *Journal of Child Psychology & Psychiatry & Allied Disciplines, 44*(8), 1208–1220. doi:10.1111/1469-7610.00202.
Vrshek-Schallhorn, S., Wolitzky-Taylor, K., Doane, L.D., Epstein, A., Sumner, J.A., Mineka, S., … Adam, E.K. (2014). Validating new summary indices for the childhood trauma interview: Associations with first onsets of major depressive disorder and anxiety disorders. *Psychological Assessment, 26*(3), 730–740.
Wegman, H. L., & Stetler, C. (2009). A meta-analytic review of the effects of childhood abuse on medical outcomes in adulthood. *Psychosomatic Medicine, 71*(8), 805–812. doi:10.1097/PSY.0b013e3181bb2b46.
Whetten, K., Ostermann, J., Whetten, R., O'Donnell, K., & Thielman, N. (2011). More than the loss of a parent: Potentially traumatic events among orphaned and abandoned children. *Journal of Traumatic Stress, 24*(2), 174–182. doi:10.1002/jts.20625.
Williams, C. J. (1990, December 10). The unwanted children: Casualties left by a tyrant. *Los Angeles Times*, pp. A1(Col. 5)-A17.
World Health Organization (WHO). (1999). *Report of the consultation on child abuse prevention, 29–31 March 1999*. Geneva, Switzerland: WHO.
World Health Organization (WHO). (2009). *Changing cultural and social norms that support violence [electronic resource]*. Geneva, Switzerland: WHO.
Yuce, M., Karabekiroglu, K., Yildirim, Z., Sahin, S., Sapmaz, D., Babadagi, Z., … Aydin, B. (2015). The psychiatric consequences of child and adolescent sexual abuse. *Archives of Neuropsychiatry, 52*(4), 393–399.
Zeanah, C. H., Egger, H. L., Smyke, A. T., Nelson, C. A., Fox, N. A., Marshall, P., & Guthrie, D. (2009). Institutional rearing and psychiatric disorders in Romanian preschool children. *American Journal of Psychiatry, 166*, 777–785.
Zeanah, C. H., Nelson, C. A., Fox, N. A., Smyke, A. T., Marshall, P., Parker, S. W., & Koga, S. (2003). Designing research to study the effects of institutionalization on brain and behavioral development: The Bucharest early intervention project. *Development and Psychopathology, 15*(4), 885–907. doi:10.1017/S095457940300045.
Zuravin, S. J. (1991). Research definitions of child physical abuse and neglect: Current problems. In R. H. Starr & D. A. Wolfe (Eds.), *The effects of child abuse and neglect: Issues and research* (pp. 100–128). London, UK: Guilford Press.

Chapter 2
Institutional Neglect in Romania's Long-Term Residential Centers in the 1990s from the Perspective of Children's Rights

Ecaterina Stativa, Adrian V. Rus, Sheri R. Parris, Jacquelyn S. Pennings, and Oana Clocotici

In determining the scope of children's rights, ultimately, there are just two questions. First, are children persons deserving of respect? The answer to this question is unequivocally yes … Second, what interests must be protected for a child to be (as a child) and become (as an adult) a meaningful participant in community life and, in so doing, to develop and express her or his unique personality?

Melton (2008), pp. 913–914)

E. Stativa (✉)
Social Pediatrics and Obstetrics Research Department, National Institute for Mother and Child Health "Alessandrescu-Rusescu",
B-dul Lacul Tei 120, cod 0209395 Bucharest, Romania
e-mail: ecaterina.stativa@gmail.com

A.V. Rus
Department of Social and Behavioral Science, Southwestern Christian University, Bethany, OK, USA
e-mail: adrian.rus@swcu.edu

S.R. Parris
Texas Christian University, Fort Worth, TX, USA
e-mail: sheri.parris@gmail.com

J.S. Pennings
Elite Research, LLC, Irving, TX 75063, USA
e-mail: jacspen@gmail.com

O. Clocotici
National Institute for Mother and Child Health "Alessandrescu-Rusescu", Bucharest, Romania
e-mail: mariaoana@yahoo.com

A.V. Rus et al. (eds.), *Child Maltreatment in Residential Care*,
DOI 10.1007/978-3-319-57990-0_2

1 Introduction

The World Health Organization (WHO, 1999) adopted a comprehensive definition of neglect, describing it as "*the failure to provide for the development of the child in all spheres: health, education, emotional development, nutrition, shelter, and safe living conditions, in the context of resources reasonably available to the family or caretakers and causes or has a high probability of causing harm to the child's health or physical, mental, spiritual, moral, or social development. This includes the failure to properly supervise and protect children from harm as much as is feasible*" (p. 15). It is not uncommon to see the terms *neglect*, *privation*, and/or *deprivation* used interchangeably without any delineation as to differences that may or may not be inferred by the use of these terms. Neglect is considered chronic if one or more needs basic to a child's healthy development are not met, it is perpetrated by a parent or caregiver, or it happens on a recurring or enduring basis (Child Welfare Information Gateway, 2013).

Institutional structural neglect has been described as a very harsh living condition that "*includes minimum physical resources, unfavourable and unstable staffing patterns, and socially and emotionally inadequate caregiver-child interactions*" (van IJzendoorn et al., 2011, p. 8). In the same vein, Gunnar (2001) proposed four categories of developmental needs and four levels of neglect that correspond with how these needs are, or are not, met in institutional settings: (1) health and nutrition; (2) physical and mental stimulation which support sensorimotor, cognitive, and language development; (3) adult-child and child-child social stimulation; and (4) stable and consistent relationships in which emotional attachments could form (adequate physical and mental stimulation cannot take place without social stimulation or consistent relationships). Subsequently, three levels of privation were delineated within institutions. First, *global privation/deprivation* occurred in institutions when the entire range of needs were not met (Gunnar, 2001; Rutter & the ERA Study Team, 1998). Second, most of the institutions presented in published literature (*psychologically depriving institutions*) provided acceptable health, nutrition, safety, and toys, but failed to provide stimulation. Third, some institutions met all of the children's developmental needs except for the need for long-term relationships with consistent caregivers (Gunnar, 2001). Regarding such relationships, it was proposed that *quality institutions* could provide stable and consistent caregiving, yet there would still be deprivation of a regular family life embedded in a regular social environment (van IJzendoorn et al., 2011). Even though Gunnar's model of the developmental needs of institutionalized children and, subsequently, the three levels of institutional privation have merit, they do not present all needs or challenges experienced by institutionalized children. Additionally, Gil (1982) expands the origins of the institutional maltreatment of children to the social system in its entirety and defines it "*as involving … any system, programme, policy or procedure or individual interaction with a child in placement that abuses, neglects or is detrimental to the child's health, safety or emotional and physical well-being, or in any way exploits or violates the child's basic rights*" (p. 458).

In the 1990s, Romania had a negative reputation abroad for how children were cared for in long-term residential institutions, and shocking images presented in the media highlighted serious neglect of their needs. The consequences of neglect on children's development were highlighted in scientific literature as well, especially through the study of children adopted from Romanian care institutions in the early 1990s (Ames & Carter, 1992; Groze & Ileana, 1996; Johnson et al., 1992). However, by 1999 there were not any empirical studies that measured children's quality of life in Romanian institutions. Consequently, in this chapter we present:

1. Relatively recent studies of international institutional neglect
2. Background about the caregiving context in Romania
3. Data collected during the cross-sectional Survey on Child Abuse in Residential Care Institutions in Romania (SCARCIR; Stativa, Anghelescu, Palicari, Stanescu, & Nanu, 2002), which helped to design a scale to evaluate institutionalized children's rearing conditions in accordance with the United Nations Convention on the Rights of the Child (UNCRC; UN General Assembly, 1989)
4. The extent of how well children's rights were upheld within four types of Romanian long-term residential centers in late 1990s (i.e., nurseries, centers for preschool, school-aged, and severely handicapped/disabled children)

1.1 Institutional Neglect

1.1.1 International Empirical Assessments of the Quality of Institutional Care

Even though various studies have tried to provide a description of children's life in residential care institutions, as a heterogeneous phenomenon, institutional neglect incorporates different facets making it quite difficult to define conceptually and to measure. However, relatively recent attempts were made to empirically measure institutional rearing conditions, following different theoretical approaches in various places and showing variability in the quality of institutional settings when compared with family environments.

As anticipated, some relatively recent empirical assessments of children's rearing, including their physical and relational environment, showed that institutions had lower-quality conditions than family settings in countries like Romania, Greece, and Ukraine (Dobrova-Krol, van IJzendoorn, Bakermans-Kranenburg, & Juffer, 2010; Smyke et al., 2007; Vorria et al., 2003). A similar picture was offered by Groark and colleagues (Groark, McCall, & Fish, 2011) who studied the characteristics of three Central American orphanages and found them to be sparse (very limited amount of furniture and toys), with specified playtimes and a limited amount of organized activities beyond routine care. While caregivers talked and listened to children, with occasional displays of warmth and affection, this occurred mainly during routine caregiving activities. At other times, caregivers' behavior toward children demonstrated lack of availability, responsiveness, support, and empathy. In short, children experienced very little warm, sensitive, responsive, and contingent caregiver-child interaction (Groark et al., 2011).

Alternatively, other studies found that institutional settings had better quality care when compared with family care. In Kenya, Embleton et al. (2014) compared different models of care (i.e., institutional care, family-based care, community-based care, and self-care) with respect to their ability to uphold children's rights (according to the United Nations Convention on the Rights of the Child framework) and provide basic material needs. The authors found that children in institutional care had more of their basic material needs met (provided an adequate standard of living) in comparison to those in family-based care. In Israel's residential care facilities, children's quality of life was assessed (Davidson-Arad, Dekel, & Wozner, 2004) by residents and staff from the perspective of the systemic life quality model (Shye, 1989). Even though some similarities of perception of quality of life between residents and staff were found (e.g., residents' compatibility with the cultural expectations of the facility, their integrity and values, and possession of cultural roots, ability to get along with the staff and their sense of belonging, ability to organize their physical environment as they wished), this study showed that resident's perceptions of their quality of life were higher with respect to their cultural (e.g., such as writing, music, and art) and social expressiveness (e.g., social influence and status and to their having close friends), physical conditions (e.g., food, clothing, living quarters), sense of physical health, and their sense of security from physical harm. As reported by the authors (Davidson-Arad et al., 2004), the higher evaluation of residents' quality of life may be attributed to the fact that children came from lower socioeconomic backgrounds, and, therefore, their lives in residential care were significantly improved regarding these features. Similarly, orphanages in the Russian Federation were shown (St. Petersburg–USA Orphanage Research Team, 2005, 2008) to have good physical environments, toys, and equipment as well as acceptable medical care, sanitation, and nutrition. However, these settings were of lesser quality than US early care and education environments.

Comparing the quality of children's life placed in institutional settings across the globe with a different socioeconomic, politic, cultural, or religious background can be difficult because of different criteria for defining the quality of life or various methodologies for measuring it.

1.1.2 Caregiving Context in Romanian Long-Term Residential Centers in the 1990s

Until 1966, Romania did not face the problem of the unwanted abandoned child as abortion and birth control methods were liberalized so that every woman/family could decide on the size of their family as they wished. Abortion was practiced on a large scale and was most important means of fertility control. After the implementation of the 1966 pronatalist decree (770/1966), children began to be abandoned in maternities and pediatric hospitals. Since the old system for the protection of minors was regulated under the Government Decision no. 809/1954 on the protection of children without parents or lacking the possibility to be raised by the family and could not cover the new issues that appeared following the pronatalist decree, in 1970, the government passed Law 3 on the protection of certain categories of minors. This law allowed parents to leave their children in state care without any sanctions for such abandonment, if the parents decided that they could not provide proper conditions to raise them at home.

During this period of the communist regime, 1966–1989, very little was known to the general public about institutionalized children, including the number or children's quality of life in those long-term residential centers (or orphanages). Professionals working within the health system (maternities wards and pediatric hospitals) were in part aware of the phenomenon of abandonment of children at their birth or in their infancy, and the abandonment was blamed on the extremely unpopular pronatalist policies of Ceausescu's communist regime (for more information about this, see Chap. 5). This policy created a situation in which many unwanted children were abandoned and left in the care of the state, especially if they were born with low weight or had health problems. Thus, since there were no social services available, because the communist state denied the existence of the social problems and implicitly the necessity of such social services, the maternity wards and pediatric hospitals took the responsibility of taking care of newborn abandoned children. The medical staff of these health units facilitated the placement of abandoned children in residential institutions created under Law 3/1970. During this time, Romania gathered in its institutions thousands of very young children without anyone considering the major risks to which children were exposed by early institutionalization.

For abandoned children under 3 years of age, who were placed within *nurseries*, which were subordinated to the Health Ministry, the standards of care were only related to food support (quantity and quality) and hygiene rules to prevent disease outbreaks that would lead to any deaths. Infant mortality was very closely monitored from the perspective of attaining the targets of pronatalist policy. Nurseries were identical to pediatric hospitals not only in terms of the physical appearance but also in terms of the routine activities. The children in the nurseries were medically examined every day even if they were healthy, but they did not enjoy nurturing interactions that were vital for their cognitive or emotional development. These children were simple objects of work for the employed staff made up of physicians, nurses, and medical support personal. In 1997, there were 58 nurseries in the Romanian child protection system which housed 9309 children (DPC & EU/PHARE, 1997).

For older children placed in long-term residential institutions for *preschool-* and *school-aged* children ("case de copii"), the care standards highlighted the importance of food safety regulations and children's enrollment in various forms of mass and special education (i.e., kindergarten and school). That is why there was no difference between a school boarding house and a residential institution for school-aged children. In 1997, a large number of children over 3 years of age (35,165) lived in 267 long-term residential institutions (DPC & EU/PHARE, 1997). The personnel of these institutions were made up of teachers as these institutions were subordinated to the Ministry of Education and the school inspectorates, and just like the medical personnel in the nurseries, they had no special training to deal with the emotional need of the institutionalized children. Thus, these children lived their lives without security and affection in an institutional culture dominated by violence and abuses administered by peers and caregivers. This organizational culture was facilitated by the abolishment of social work (1969), sociology, psychology, and pedagogy (1977) as academic disciplines across all Romanian universities by the communist regime due to political and ideological reasons until 1989 (Universitatea Bucuresti, Facultatea de Sociologie si Asistenta Sociala, n.d.; Universitatea Babes-Bolyai, Facultatea de Psychologie si Stiinte ale Educatiei, n.d.).

Residential institutions for children with *disabilities* were units for the protection of children 3 years of age and up with chronic diseases and severe "irrecoverable" handicaps (which functioned under the Law 3/1970). In 1997, there were 33 such centers accommodating 4473 children (DPC & EU/PHARE, 1997). The staff was made of physicians, nurses, and medical support personnel.

As specified above, the Romanian public knew very little about the institutionalized children during the communist regime and shortly after. A proof of that is also the fact that although the abolition of the pronatalist decree was the second legislative measure adopted by the revolutionary government after the fall of Ceausescu's regime in December 1989, the population was not informed about the large number of unwanted children placed in institutions, but people learned about the approximately 10,000 women who died following a clandestine abortion (Stephenson, Wagner, Badea, & Serbanescu, 1992). Shedding light on the image and the life conditions of these institutionalized children, even after 1990, cannot be fully understood because the historical information is incomplete. The December 1989 revolution in Romania was broadcast "live" to the whole world via television. The wave of sympathy Romania enjoyed from countries in different parts of the world garnered immediate material and humanitarian support. During the very first days of the revolution, numerous convoys brought food, medicines, and other strictly necessary products which had been scarce in the country for a long time. The Romanian authorities guided most of these goods to the pediatric hospitals and residential institutions where children lived, especially to the centers for children with severe disabilities and chronic diseases. The foreigners accompanying such convoys entered these institutions and were shocked by the conditions in which children were living, and so they widely publicized them. Touching images came from the settings where children with chronic diseases and severe handicaps labeled as "irrecoverable" in the communist years lived. Mention must be made of the fact that the images of children in these residential settings were incorrectly projected and generalized for all the children in all types of long-term residential institutions in Romania where, although children had modest life conditions, these could not be compared to the deeply inhuman conditions of those placed in institutions for severe chronic diseases and handicaps.

Given the fact that these children were presented as abandoned in the foreign media, a great interest for their adoption emerged. The national legislation on international adoption was unclear after the fall of the communist regime, and the state authority exercised via its institutions was weak because it was still attributed to a provisional government. Consequently, children could be easily adopted as illegal Romanian, and foreign networks for adoption had already developed within a couple of weeks after the collapse of the communist regime. There was no control of the adoption process, and there was nobody to protect children's interests (Zugravescu & Sandell, 1991). The first law regulating adoption after 1989 was Law 11 of June 30, 1990. This law provided that adoption must be made in the child's interest and that it must be decided in the court in the presence of two judges and one prosecutor. The Law 11/1990 emerged after a wave of international adoptions had already been performed without much regulation and without observing some relevant international conventions. In 1990, about 3000 Romanian children were adopted, and in the first 2 months of 1991, about 1300 more children were adopted (Denechere & Scutaru, 2010). In the first quarter of 1991, a total of 2000 children left the country for adoption purposes. This figure represents more than a third of the global number of all international adoptions for that period (Jaffe, 1995). In this context, we must mention the idea that, although the dramatic images of the institutionalized children were real, there was also the hunch that this excessive publicity sometimes served to manipulate sentiment through images and facilitate public pressure for promoting international adoptions. In Romania, hundreds of organizations dealing with international adoptions were set up, and there was always the suspicion that many of these are performed without respecting international agreements. This idea was also reiterated by the baroness Emma Nicholson, Special Rapporteur for Romania's EU accession 1999–2004, who recommended that the Romanian government institute a moratorium on international adoptions, which was implemented on October 2001 (Iusmen, 2014).

Under the same auspices of doubt, many persons who knew the situation of Romanian institutionalized children wondered why only the Romanian children had been so publicized, whereas the institutionalized children of Ukraine, Belarus, or Russia were in very similar if not identical situations. The images of the Romanian institutionalized children impressed the entire world by focusing on the precariousness of the material conditions in which children were living. There were also other numerous aspects less "spectacular" but with very serious consequences for all the children in the protection residential system. One of the serious issues was the very protection system that allowed the placement of young children in residential institutions for unlimited period of times. As statistics show, 80% of the children placed in nurseries came from among the children abandoned upon birth in maternities (DPC & EU/PHARE, 1997), and their development was compromised by the total lack of caregiver-child interaction. In fact, these were the most serious problems of the Romanian protection system, and their importance exceeded the precariousness of material conditions. They also proved to be difficult to solve; successive waves of reforms were necessary to create new institutions, services, laws, procedures, and standards so that these conditions could be changed fundamentally. Despite all that, while conditions are much better, they are still not perfect today.

Early institutionalization and inadequate models of care, especially in terms of caregiver-child interaction, deeply affected the development of these children. The first who identified this problem were the parents from different foreign countries who adopted children. They encountered "unexpected" mental and behavioral problems among the children and resorted to specialists in order to understand them. This spurred an interest for taking a scientific approach to problems related to chronic neglect at early ages, especially regarding Romanian institutionalized children. Following their studies, researchers had evidence that early institutionalization had extremely serious consequences on children's development (Nelson, Fox, & Zeanah, 2014). Studies on the causes of children's institutionalization were conducted in 1991 and 1996 in Romania as well, focusing on the problems of children from the perspective of finding solutions that would facilitate the removal of children from the residential system and prevent the perpetuation of long-term institutionalization from an early age (Ministry of Health, Institute for Mother and Child Care & UNICEF, 1991; Stephenson, Anghelescu, Stativa, & Pasti, 1997).

The signing of the UN Convention on children's rights had a special importance for the improvement of life of the Romanian children because it was the first step toward later efforts to progressively implement all the provisions of the convention into the national legislation and to observe children's rights. The rights strictly pertaining to institutionalized children referred to the protection against abuses and neglect. But changes did not occur immediately. The UNICEF representative in Romania, USAID, the European Union Funds (Phare technical assistance for the Romanian government for the institutional reform in the field of protection of children's rights 1993–1997), and nongovernmental organizations invested many resources so that the Romanian state might, through the ratification of the Convention, take steps for the improvement of the condition of institutionalized children. Thus, ever since the beginning of the 1990s, important resources have been allocated for the training of the personnel working in the protection institutions.

The basic concepts defining quality of care had to be turned into practices and implemented by care workers. In addition, generally accepted practices in the social services fields for meeting children's developmental needs were almost unknown to the Romanian protection institutions' personnel. That is why institutional staff did not perceive the need for such training. For instance, a study conducted in 1992 in nurseries, in relation to the training needs of nursery personnel, found that most professionals wanted to train in the medical field and less perceived the need to train in domains focusing on the care and development of institutionalized children (Stephenson et al., 1993).

Despite the fact that the communist regime was abolished in 1989 and that Romania had ratified the UN Convention on children's rights (1989), the quality of children's life had changed very little due to the Romanian state ignoring and even denying the extremely serious problems of the children living in its protection institutions and preserving them under the Law 3/1970. An essential legislative regulation portraying in spirit the rights of children as provided in the UN Convention emerged for the first time 7 years after the fall of communism and the ratification of the Convention. These are the Emergency Ordinances 25 and 26/1997. Their implementation represented the first profound structural reform in the field of protection of children's rights. This regulation repealed Law 3/1970 on the protection of certain categories of minors. Two years after the beginning of the structural reform in the field of protection of children's rights, the life quality of institutionalized children was still in deficit from the perspective of child's rights even if some things had changed, especially at the level of infrastructure of the protection institutions. Most children were still living in the same conditions in terms of the relationships with their caregivers and peers as there were not any internal mechanisms or mechanisms at the level of competent authorities by which neglect or abuses might have been identified and sanctioned. These conditions were affirmed by the two country reports that Romania had to send to the UN Committee for the period 1992–1997 as a signatory state of the Convention, as well as by the Committee recommendations and by the numerous inquiries of some NGO and foreign press agencies (NACPA & UNICEF, 2004).

1.2 Background and Objectives of the Current Study

The data for the present study were collected in 1999 (see the study Survey on Child Abuse in Residential Care Institutions in Romania; SCARCIR; Stativa et al., 2002), 2 years after the reforms had begun in the field of protection of children's rights in Romania. The study was strongly supported by the government installed in 1996; by the Director of DPC EU/Phare Bridging Programme, 1998–1999; and UNICEF. This is the first Romanian study analyzing institutional neglect and abuses in institutions by using the only authentic and available reference at that moment in Romania, namely, the UN Convention on children's rights.

In this period, following the Government Ordinances 25 and 26/1997, child protection institutions were decentralized, and special legislation was adopted to create alternatives to institutionalization and regulate adoption procedures. Measures were also taken to prevent institutionalization by providing support to families and closing the large institutions (Government Ordinance 25/1997, Government Ordinance 26/1997, Law 108/1998, Law 87/1998). However, despite these reforms, at the time data were collected, long-term residential centers were places where children's physical, psychological, and emotional needs were still not fully addressed and many children continued to experience some form of neglect and abuse (Gavrilovici & Groza, 2007; Rus et al., 2013; Rus et al., in press; Stativa et al., 2002). The delay in obtaining positive results can be explained by the fact that the standards of care in institutions were created only after Law 272/2004 was promulgated. Using as a reference the UN Convention on children's rights (UN General Assembly, 1989), this study is a more thorough analysis of the extent to which children's basic human rights were upheld within Romanian long-term residential centers. Consequently, our research had two objectives, namely, to (1) assess how well the items asked in SCARCIR grouped together and matched up with the UNCRC criteria (UN General

Assembly, 1989) using exploratory factor analysis and (2) measure how well children's rights (i.e., identity, personal history, free expression, information, periodic review, protective measures and legal status, have a family, health, education, personalized care, and quality care) were defended across each of four types of long-term residential centers (i.e., nurseries, residential centers for preschool-aged and school-aged children, and centers for children with severe disabilities).

2 Method

2.1 *Participants*

We performed a secondary analysis of data used for the SCARCIR (Stativa et al., 2002). The data for the sampling base was acquired from the Directorate for Child Protection – EU/Phare – Bridging Programme for 1999 (data for long-term residential centers for preschool- and school-aged children) and the State Secretariat for Persons with Disabilities (SSPH, data for residential institutions for children with disabilities). According to this data, in 1999 there were 267 long-term residential centers for preschool- and school-aged children with 37,000 children and 35 residential institutions for children with disabilities with 3455 children out of 5.6 million children in Romania between 0 and 18 years old.

The original dataset included a national representative sample of 3164 (1701 boys and 1463 girls) children in residential care institutions between 0 and 19 years of age ($M = 9.45$; $SD = 5.39$), representing 7.8% of the entire population of institutionalized Romanian children in 1999. Specifically, 739 (23.4%) children resided in 16 *nurseries* (cradles); 414 (13.1%) children resided in 13 long-term residential centers for *preschool-aged* children; 1703 (53.8%) children resided in 43 long-term residential centers for *school-aged* children; and 308 (9.7%) children resided in 8 residential institutions for children with *disabilities* which were commonly located in isolated places (see Table 2.1). Children in long-term residential centers for preschool- and school-aged children were those determined to be "normal" or without severe neuropsychiatric or physical problems, and residential institutions for children with disabilities housed mainly children with intellectual deficiencies, as well as those with psychiatric, physical, and sensory problems (Stativa et al., 2002) (for a complete description of these types of Romanian institutions and their internal organization, see Rus et al., 2013).

Mean age at child's first placement within an institution was 48.92 months ($SD = 50.85$) which ranged from 0 to 218 months. Children had siblings residing either in the same institution (30.8%) or in another long-term residential center (5.6%), and many reported having at least some contact with their parents (68.6%) during the year when data were collected (see Table 2.1). Most of the children (42.2%) resided in the institution where they were received directly from their biological families, 38.8% were transferred from another long-term residential center, and

Table 2.1 Frequencies and percentages of child and institution characteristics

	Overall		Type of long-term residential center						Disabled	
			Nursery		Preschool aged		School aged			
	N	%	*n*	%	*n*	%	*n*	%	*n*	%
Child level[a]										
Number of children	3164	100	739	23.4	414	13.1	1703	53.8	308	9.7
Gender										
Male	1701	53.8	395	53.5	230	55.6	913	53.6	163	52.9
Female	1463	46.2	344	46.5	184	44.4	790	46.4	145	47.1
Sibling(s)										
Placed in the same center	976	30.8	88	11.9	139	33.6	736	43.2	13	4.2
Placed in another center	177	5.6	40	5.4	23	5.6	104	6.1	10	3.2
No sibling	1537	48.6	423	57.2	203	49.0	698	41.0	213	69.2
No information	474	15.0	188	25.4	49	11.8	165	9.7	72	23.4
Visited by parents this year										
Yes	1972	68.6	376	56.0	265	70.7	1173	75.4	158	57.5
No	904	31.4	295	44.0	110	29.3	382	24.6	117	42.5
Provenience of the child										
From family	1343	42.4	202	27.3	183	44.2	885	52.0	73	23.7
From a different center	1228	38.8	43	5.8	197	47.6	779	45.7	209	67.9
From a center for disabled	33	1.0	10	1.4	6	1.4	1	0.1	16	5.2
From a medical institution	518	16.4	470	63.6	18	4.3	22	1.3	8	2.6
From street	17	0.5	6	0.8	5	1.2	5	0.3	1	0.3
Other	5	0.2	4	0.5	1	0.2	0	0	0	0
Unknown	20	0.6	4	0.5	4	1.0	11	0.6	1	0.3
Institution size										
Small (1–100 children)	637	20.1	126	17.1	164	39.6	300	17.6	47	15.3
Medium (101–200 children)	1476	46.6	409	55.3	78	18.8	788	46.3	201	65.3
Large (201–300 children)	553	17.5	88	11.9	172	41.5	233	13.7	60	19.5
Very large (301–400 and more children)	498	15.7	116	15.7	0	0	384	22.4	0	0
Institution level[b]										
Number of residential centers	80	100	16	20.0	13	16.2	43	53.8	8	10

[a]Child level shows the number of children in each type of institution
[b]Institution level shows the number of long-term residential centers corresponding to the type of institution

16.4% were received from a medical institution (see Table 2.1). The ratio of children for each caregiver during the daytime ranged from 3 to 32 children ($M = 9.89$, $SD = 4.81$). Institutions (see Table 2.1) were grouped as (a) small (up to 100 children, 20.1% of children), (b) medium (101–200 children, 46.6% of children), (c) large (201–300 children, 17.5% of children), and very large (301 to over 400 children, 15.7% of children). Further descriptions of the purpose of SCARCIR, as well as the sampling methods, data collection procedure, participants, and the characteristics of the resultant dataset, are presented elsewhere (for a complete review, see Rus et al., 2013; Stativa et al., 2002).

2.2 Procedures

Data for the SCARCIR study was collected in October and November of 1999, approximately 2 years after the national child protection system began reforms. The sample was designed and stratified with independent samples for the eight regions of Romania. The distribution of the samples by region was calculated by weighting the number of institutionalized children in a particular region against the total sample size. These numbers were structured by the types of institutions in each region. The total sample, weighted by region and type of institution, was also structured and distributed according to age groups and gender within the sample. Consequently, each regional group, or type of institution, was weighted by age group and gender within each age group. An institution's size determined whether one or several institutions of the same type were included in the sample. All of these factors were considered in the construction of an appropriately structured total sample.

Fourteen researchers collected data for this study. All researchers had extensive experience collecting data and interviewing children in residential care institutions. For the purpose of the SCARCIR study, the researchers received an additional 4 days of training. To produce a sample appropriately weighted by age group and gender, two researchers per institution made random selections from the personal files that were kept for all institutionalized children. All files were arranged alphabetically and kept within locked cabinets at each institution. The researchers chose randomly from these files until they had obtained the appropriate structure of the sample for that particular institution. Data was then extracted from the documents in each file, and interviews were conducted with the children whose files were selected.

2.3 Measures

All quantitative data were collected through an original instrument created by one of the authors (Stativa et al., 2002) after visiting numerous long-term residential centers where maltreatment was noticed. Consequently, the measure of maltreatment became not only important for revealing the magnitude of abuse and neglect across residential care institutions but also as a tool for policy-makers in their effort to prevent and reduce these incidences. At the time (late 1990s), Romanian centers lacked standards, regulations, or specific laws that could ensure quality care for children (e.g., institutional guidelines did not specifically require that caregivers interact with children or provide an enriched environment for them). Because there was no instrument to measure maltreatment (i.e., abuse and neglect) of institutionalized children, the benchmark used to assess maltreatment in Romanian long-term residential centers was the UNCRC (UN General Assembly, 1989). As noted earlier, the Romanian government had agreed to abide by these rights, and they became the foundation for many changes in the Romanian child welfare system. Thus, the SCARCIR consisted of two sections that captured information about the life experiences of institutionalized Romanian children. The second section consisted of survey questions for children over 7 years of age, about their experiences regarding acts of neglect and physical, emotional, and sexual abuse in institutions (this information was not assessed for the present study). Most importantly, the first section was designed to collect information about respect for children's rights. Thus, articles from the UNCRC (UN General Assembly, 1989) were considered meaningful within the context of institutionalized children and were adapted into various rights and items in order to quantify how well they were respected within the institutional care system.

2.3.1 The Right to Legal Identity

This right was adopted by considering Article 7 of the UN Convention, stating "*the child shall be registered immediately after birth and shall have the right from birth to a name...*" (UN General Assembly, 1989, p. 3) and was measured by the absence or presence (no vs. yes) of a valid identification document such as a birth certificate or identity card (for children over 14) within the child's files (see Table 2.2). Ensuring this right became a priority of the authorities in the late 1990s after a high number of abandoned children were found to have no identification documents in the early 1990s. A common reason for this often stemmed from the difficult and sometimes impossible task of identifying or locating the children's parents.

2.3.2 The Right to Personal History

This right (see Table 2.2) was measured by an item that assessed the possibility of retracing the child's personal history (where child lived from birth until data were collected) and is linked with Article 8 stating "*...the right of the child to preserve his or her identity...*" (UN General Assembly, p. 3). The possibility (no vs. yes) of retracing each child's personal history was evaluated in our survey through analysis of the documents in their personal file (e.g., identity documents, medical records, a summary social investigation record concerning the living conditions of the family,

Table 2.2 Factor loadings and Cronbach's alpha for the items indicating children's rights

UN rights of the child[a]	The name of the right and the item(s) associated with it	*N* Total	*n* Yes	%	Factor loading	Cronbach's alpha
Article 7	**The right to legal identity**					
	The child's identification document	3164	3084	97.5	(na)	(na)
Article 8	**The right to personal history**					
	The possibility of retracing the child's personal history (where child lived from birth until when data were collected)	3164	1771	56.0	(na)	(na)
Article 12	**The right to free expression of opinions**[b]					
	The child's opinion on the protective measure was recorded	1453	95	6.5	(na)	(na)
Article 17	**The right for information**[b]					
	The child received a written text about his protection measure	1395	294	17.3	(na)	(na)
Article 25	**The right for a periodic review of the protective measure**					
	The child received a reevaluation during the current year	3164	872	27.6	(na)	(na)
Article 8, 20	**The right for protective measure and legal status**					**0.797**
	The child currently has protective measure	3164	3110	98.3	0.834	
	The child had protective measure when placed in institution	3164	3108	98.2	0.814	
	The child currently has legal status	3164	3097	97.9	0.793	
	The child had legal status when placed in institution	3164	3069	97.0	0.737	
Article 8 & 9	**The right to have a family**					**0.617**
	In this institution, there are records of relatives' visits	3121	2945	94.4	0.654	
	There is an accommodation space for parents during nighttime	3120	941	30.2	0.606	
	In this institution, there are records of correspondence between parent/institution	3118	950	30.5	0.596	
	In this institution, there is an accommodation space for parents during daytime	3122	2308	73.9	0.587	
	In this institution, there are records of parents' visits	3122	3025	96.9	0.564	
	In this institution, there are records of phone calls between parent/institution	3050	659	21.6	0.552	

(continued)

Table 2.2 (continued)

UN rights of the child[a]	The name of the right and the item(s) associated with it	N Total	n Yes	%	Factor loading	Cronbach's alpha
Article 24	**The right to health**					**0.610**
	The treatment and rehabilitation needs are written in child's medical file	1363	1141	83.7	0.738	
	The child receives general medical assistance	3069	2993	97.5	0.699	
	The child's record showed that a general medical examination was done	2900	1506	51.9	0.611	
	The child receives the treatment written in his/her medical file	1300	941	72.4	0.606	
	The child had the anthropometric measurements done	2909	1934	66.5	0.591	
Article 28	**The right to education**					**0.592**
	The child has free access to the library	2833	1394	49.2	0.841	
	The child has personal space for doing homework/study	3062	1850	60.4	0.831	
	The child is included in a form of education	2248	2081	92.6	0.515	

[a]This column shows the United Nations Convention on the Rights of the Child (UN General Assembly, 1989) which can be related with the items constructed in this study
[b]Only school-aged children's information was reported

decisions by authorities concerning protective measures implemented, etc.). Previous studies (Ministry of Health, Institute for Mother and Child Care & UNICEF, 1991; Stephenson et al., 1997) highlighted the lack of documentation in children's personal files; thus, retracing children's origins, their life along with biological parents, or their routes through child protection services were very difficult tasks. This situation was worsened by the fact that when children were transferred to a different center, the child's file (or a copy of it) was not transferred to the new institution; thus, many of institutionalized children grew up not knowing their personal history. Later, this issue was addressed by two laws (Governmental Ordinances 69/2004 and 288/2006) which established minimum standards regarding case management in the child protection system.

2.3.3 The Right to Free Expression of Opinions

In order to evaluate the observance of this right (see Table 2.2), we checked whether (no vs. yes) the opinions of children ages 7 years and older were recorded in the report on their protective measure. This is linked with Article 12 stating that the child "...*is capable of forming his or her own views and the right to express those views freely in all matters affecting the child...*" (UN General Assembly, p. 4).

2.3.4 The Right for Information

Children over 10 years old had the right to be informed (see Table 2.2) in written form about the protection measure concerning their own person that was implemented (no vs. yes) by the Committee for Child Protection, and the observance of this right was mandatory. It is linked with Article 17 stating that "...*the child has access to information and material from a diversity of national and international sources, especially those aimed at the promotion of his or her social, spiritual and moral well-being and physical and mental health*" (UN General Assembly, p. 5).

2.3.5 The Right to Periodic Review of the Protective Measure

This measure is linked with Article 25 of the UNCRC which recognizes the right of a child "... *to a periodic review of the treatment provided to the child and all other circumstances relevant to his or her placement*" (UN General Assembly, 1989, p. 8), and it was measured by an item regarding whether the child received (no vs. yes) a reevaluation during the year when the study was conducted (see Table 2.2). The obligation to review the protection measures concerning children in difficulty was first introduced in Romania by Emergency Ordinance no. 26/1997. According to the provisions in that ordinance, the protection measures need to be reviewed at least every 3 months, and they had to either be revoked or replaced in order to serve the best interests of each child. The protective measure review was done by an interdisciplinary team. Children may have benefited from the review, for example, by a change in placement to an extended or different family or improved access to medical or educational services. Reviewing is one of the key elements of the reform initiated in 1997, because its implementation triggered significant changes in the child protection system, including a reduction of the number of children in residential care institutions, as well as the time spent by the children in those institutions.

2.3.6 The Right of the Protective Measure and Legal Status

This right is linked with Articles 8 and 20 of the UNCRC and was measured by four items (see Table 2.2). Two items assessed whether (no vs. yes) there was a protection measure (e.g., placement, custody, educational measure, emergency placement, placement with termination of parental rights, etc.) decided by a governmental authority regarding admission of the child to the institution. The other two items assessed whether (no vs. yes) the child had a legal status (e.g., child having parent/s, guardians, etc.). Importantly, the protection measure and legal status were measured both at the time of placement within the institution and when data were collected because the SCARCIR study sought to evaluate whether the interest of the child was addressed by the child's protective measure.

2.3.7 The Right to Have a Family

In order to evaluate how institutional settings respected this right, six items (see Table 2.2) measured whether or not institutions had records of relatives and parents' visits, accommodation space for parents during night- and daytime visits, and records of written correspondence and phone calls between parents and the institution. This right is linked with Articles 8 and 9 of the UNCRC stating that the child has the right to preserve his/her relationship with the family on a regular basis (UN General Assembly, 1989 p. 3).

2.3.8 The Right to Health

This measure is linked with Article 24 of the UNCRC which recognizes"... *the right of the child to the enjoyment of the highest attainable standard of health and to facilities for the treatment of illness and rehabilitation of health...*" (UN General Assembly, 1989, p. 7), and as shown in Table 2.2, it was measured by five related items measuring whether or not the child (a) had treatment and rehabilitation needs recorded in his/her medical file, (b) received general medical assistance, (c) had records of general medical examinations, (d) received the treatment written in medical file, and (e) had anthropometric measures (i.e., height and weight) completed.

2.3.9 The Right to Education

This measure is linked with Article 28 of the UNCRC (UN General Assembly, 1989) and was measured by three items (see Table 2.2) to determine whether or not the child had free access to the library, personal space for doing homework or study, and was included in an age-appropriate form of education.

2.3.10 The Right to Personalized Care

This measure is linked with Articles 20, 23, 25, and 39 of the UNCRC (UN General Assembly, 1989) and was measured by five items (see Table 2.3) assessing whether or not the child had a written personalized plan and whether or not the plan contained information about the institution/s where the child lived, a personalized education/socialization program, a personalized development program, and information about time spent in the current institution.

2.3.11 The Right to Quality Care

This measure (see Table 2.3) is linked with article 27 of the UNCRC, "... *the right of every child to a standard of living adequate for the child's physical, mental, spiritual, moral and social development...*" (UN General Assembly, 1989, p. 8) and was

Table 2.3 Factor loadings and Cronbach's alpha for the items indicating children's rights (continued)

UN rights of the child[a]	The name of the right and the item(s) associated with it	*N* Total	*n* Yes	%	Factor loading	Cronbach's alpha
Article 20, 23, 25, and 39	**The right for personalized care**					**0.761**
	The personalized plan contains information about other institution(s) where child has resided	3164	219	6.9	0.747	
	There is a written personalized drafted plan for the child	3164	634	20.0	0.747	
	The personalized plan contains a personalized educational/socialization program	3164	1154	36.5	0.723	
	The personalized plan contains a personalized development program	3164	1136	35.9	0.714	
	The personalized plan contains information about time spent in the current institution	3164	454	14.3	0.696	
Article 27	**The right for quality care**					
	(a) Child appearance					**0.596**
	The child is unkempt/sloppy	3029	320	10.6	0.633	
	The child is dirty	3026	186	6.1	0.625	
	The child's hair is shaved/closely cut (lack of individualization)	3025	26	0.9	0.625	
	The child is barefoot	3028	44	1.5	0.619	
	The child does not have appropriate clothing according to his/her gender	3012	241	8.0	0.543	
	Difficult to distinguish child's gender by his/her physiognomy (lack of individualization)	2993	226	7.6	0.538	
	(b) Child personal items					**0.633**
	The child has his/her own cabinet	3087	2008	65.0	0.861	
	The child has his/her own personal items	3085	2633	85.3	0.861	
	(c) Child hygiene					**0.701**
	The child uses fully functional toilets[b]	3015	796	26.4	0.880	
	The child uses unsanitary toilets	2972	483	16.3	0.880	
	(d) Child recreation					**0.678**
	The child has free access to the club/playroom	2987	2376	79.5	0.882	

(continued)

Table 2.3 (continued)

UN rights of the child[a]	The name of the right and the item(s) associated with it	*N* Total	*n* Yes	%	Factor loading	Cronbach's alpha
	The child has free access to the gym/playground	2995	2041	68.1	0.842	
	The child has a personal space for play and/or recreation in dormitory	3087	1898	61.5	0.623	
	(e) Child relationships					**0.746**
	The children are placed in the same room according to personal affinity	3036	1208	39.8	0.869	
	The children are placed in the same room according to their age[c]	3018	1301	43.1	0.813	
	The children are placed in the same room with siblings (brothers together, sisters together)	3048	2156	70.7	0.758	
	(f) Optimal child-staff ratio					**0.689**
	The optimal child-staff ratio is met during morning	3164	1768	55.9	0.872	
	The optimal child-staff ratio is met during daytime	3164	1901	60.1	0.870	
	The optimal child-staff ratio is met during night	3164	410	13.0	0.577	

[a]This column shows the United Nations Convention on the Rights of the Child (UN General Assembly, 1989) which can be related with the items constructed in this study
[b,c]The items were reverse coded

measured by six subscales, each containing a couple of items (see Table 2.3). Specifically, the quality of care was measured through items that were related with:

(a) Child's appearance (i.e., six items measured whether or not at the time of assessment the child was found unkempt/sloppy, dirty, having his/her hair shaved/closely cut as expression of the lack of individualization, barefooted, and not having appropriate clothing according to his/her gender and whether or not the evaluator had difficulties distinguishing child's gender by his/her physiognomy which showed a lack of individualization)
(b) Possessions of personal items (i.e., two items measuring whether the child did or did not have a cabinet and/or personal items such as clothes, books, or personal hygiene items)
(c) Child's hygiene (i.e., two items measuring whether the child had access to fully functional and/or unsanitary toilets)
(d) Child's recreation (i.e., three items measuring whether or not the child had free access to the club/playroom, gym/playground, and a personal space for play and/or recreation within dormitory)

(e) Child's relationships (i.e., three items measuring whether or not children were placed in the same room according to personal affinity, their age, or with their siblings)
(f) Child-staff ratio (i.e., three items determining whether or not the optimal child-staff ratio was met during morning, daytime, and nighttime). For more information about these standards, see AAP, APHA, and NRCHSCCEE, 2011.

To complete this section, information was obtained from children's social files, medical records, and other records available in the institutions or made available by either the management or the educational, social, and medical personnel. The instrument was piloted with a sample of 120 children in five institutions within three Romanian counties. The final version was completed based on information gathered during the pilot study. Children included in the pilot study were not included in the SCARCIR sample. In addition to the quantitative data collected through this instrument, qualitative data were collected from 18 case studies, 9 focus group sessions with institutional staff (totaling 66 educational staff and caregivers), 5 interviews with managers of the specialized public services, and 7 focus group sessions with children in residential care (totaling 48 children). However, the information obtained from case studies, interviews, and focus groups were not analyzed for the current study. Importantly, the measurement of all items related with children's rights had a binary distribution (*no* = *0* versus *yes* = *1*).

2.4 Data Analysis Plan

Data were analyzed using IBM SPSS version 19 (IBM, 2010). Items that were considered for analysis were from children's records. No data from children's interviews were used in the current analysis. All item responses were in a yes or no format. Some records contained missing items and analysis was done on available data. Scores were computed using person-mean imputation (Bono, Ried, Kimberlin, & Vogel, 2007; Downey & King, 1998). Statistical analysis included principal exploratory factor analysis, reliability analysis, descriptive analysis in the form of frequencies and percentages, and cross tabulations.

3 Results

3.1 Exploratory Factor Analyses

A series of exploratory factor analyses were conducted separately on each set of items identified to represent the various rights of children. For each factor analysis, items with factor loadings below 0.50 were removed, one at a time, with the item with the lowest loading removed first. Items were removed one at a time to allow for the adjustment of item loading values with the reduced number of items. Once a set of items with loadings above 0.50 was identified for each right, the reliability coefficient was computed for each right. The factor loadings and Cronbach's alphas are presented in Tables 2.2 and 2.3. The reliability coefficients range from 0.592 to 0.797. All items were measured on a yes or no scale. Due to the dichotomous nature of each of the individual items, the reliability coefficients were deemed acceptable (Cortina, 1993). The total number of responses, number of yes responses, and percent of yes responses are shown for each of the items in each factor.

3.2 *Children's Rights Across Institutional Settings*

Next, sum scores were computed for each right. Prior to the sum computation, recoding was conducted as needed so that items within the same factor were positively correlated. An examination of the distribution of the sum scores indicated severe skewness of most of the rights. Thus, scores for each of the rights were dichotomized into low vs. high scores. Missingness was addressed using person-mean imputation such that scores were given if children had at least half of the items making up the scale score. Thus, if the child had at least half of the items, the mean of the items was computed and then multiplied by the total number of items in the scale to derive a sum score (Bono et al., 2007; Downey & King, 1998).

The first two columns of Table 2.4 show the frequencies and percentages of children with high and low scores for each of the rights. The remaining columns show the results of a series of cross tabulations of children's rights.

3.2.1 Nurseries

The descriptive analysis (see Table 2.4) revealed that 99.5% of children placed in nurseries had their right to identity respected. The same very high percentage was observed regarding the rights to protective measure (97.2%) and health (94.2%). Additionally, a high percentage of children (67%) had their right to quality care/recreation respected. Furthermore, a relatively high proportion of children had their rights upheld (institution respected more their rights) regarding personalized care (47.4%), personal history (45.7%), personal items (36.8%), have a family (30.7%), and periodic review (27.6%). A relatively small percentage of children had their rights regarding quality care respected in nurseries, such as relationships (16.5%), appearance (14%), child-staff ratio (11.5%), and hygiene (10.8%), and a very low proportion of children had their right to education (2.8%) respected.

Table 2.4 Frequencies and percentages of children's rights by type of institution

	Overall		Type of institutional organization						Disabled	
			Nursery		Preschool aged		School aged			
The right to	*N*	%	*n*	%	*n*	%	*n*	%	*n*	%
Legal identity										
No (0)	80	2.5	4	0.5	21	5.1	53	3.1	2	0.6
Yes (1)	3084	97.5	735	99.5	393	94.9	1650	96.9	306	99.4
Personal history										
No (0)	1393	44.0	401	54.3	142	34.3	696	40.9	154	50
Yes (1)	1771	56.0	338	45.7	272	65.7	1007	59.1	154	50
Periodic review										
No (0)	2292	72.4	535	72.4	252	60.9	1205	70.8	300	97.4
Yes (1)	872	27.6	204	27.6	162	39.1	498	29.2	8	2.6
Protective measures										
Low (0–3)	141	4.5	21	2.8	25	6.0	71	4.2	24	7.8
High (4)	3023	95.5	718	97.2	389	94.0	1632	95.8	284	92.2
Have a family										
Low (0–3)	1754	55.8	512	69.3	129	31.2	806	47.8	307	99.7
High (4–6)	1392	44.2	227	30.7	285	68.8	879	52.2	1	0.3
Health										
Low (0–3)	1071	37.1	43	5.8	181	49.6	722	49.0	125	40.6
High (4–5)	1812	62.9	694	94.2	184	50.4	751	51.0	183	59.4
Education										
Low (0–1)	1311	43.1	706	97.2	133	32.3	217	13.5	255	86.4
High (2–3)	1728	56.9	20	2.8	279	67.7	1389	86.5	40	13.6
Personalized care										
Low (0)	1739	55.0	389	52.6	254	61.4	828	48.6	268	87.0
High (1–5)	1425	45.0	350	47.4	160	38.6	875	51.4	40	13.0
Appearance										
Low (0)	2412	79.7	635	86.0	272	66.7	1305	82.3	200	67.6
High (1–6)	616	20.3	103	14.0	136	33.3	281	17.7	96	32.4
Personal items										
Low (0)	1122	36.3	467	63.2	186	45.0	312	19.1	157	51.3
High (1–2)	1967	63.7	272	36.8	227	55.0	1319	80.9	149	48.7
Hygiene										
Low (0)	2138	70.7	659	89.2	372	83.8	946	59.5	206	67.1
High (1–2)	887	29.3	80	10.8	63	16.2	643	40.5	101	32.9
Recreation										
Low (0–1)	808	26.5	244	33.0	28	6.8	367	22.8	169	58.1
High (2–3)	2245	73.5	495	67.0	385	93.2	1243	77.2	122	41.9
Relationships										
Low (0–1)	1582	51.9	617	83.5	137	33.2	650	40.4	178	61.6
High (2–3)	1466	48.1	122	16.5	276	66.8	957	59.6	111	38.4
Optimal child-staff ratio										
Low (0–1)	1548	48.9	654	88.5	138	33.3	645	37.9	111	36.0
High (2–3)	1616	51.1	85	11.5	276	66.7	1058	62.1	197	64.0

Notes: Because of how missing was dealt with, decimals were possible. Everything 0.5 and lower was rounded down. Above 0.5 was rounded up

3.2.2 Centers for Preschool-Aged Children

As shown in Table 2.4, more than 93% of children placed in long-term residential centers for preschool-aged children had their rights to identity, protective measure, and quality care/recreation respected. Additionally, regarding the rights to personal history, have a family, health, education, and some quality care subscale items (i.e., personal items, relationships, and child-staff ratio), more than 50% of children had these rights respected or had high scores for these rights (institution respected more their rights). Less than 50% of children had their rights to periodic review, personalized care, and some quality care subscale items (i.e., appearance and hygiene) respected.

3.2.3 Centers for School-Aged Children

Regarding the children placed in long-term residential centers for school-aged children, the results (see Table 2.4) showed that more than 80% had their right to identity, protective measures, education, and quality care (i.e., personal items) respected or had high scores for these rights (institution respected more their rights). Additionally, between 51% and 77.2% of children had their right to personal history, have a family, health, personalized care, and quality care (i.e., recreation, relationships, and child-staff ratio) respected or had high scores for these rights. For two aspects of the right to quality care (i.e., appearance and hygiene), only 17.7% and 40.5% of children had high scores for these rights. Finally, 29.2% percent of children had their right for periodic review respected.

3.2.4 Centers for Disabled Children

As shown in Table 2.4, 92.2% and 99.4% of children placed in long-term residential centers for children with disabilities had their rights to identity and protective measures respected. Furthermore, between 50% and 64% of children had their rights to personal history, health, and quality care (i.e., child staff ratio) respected. Additionally, a relatively high proportion of children had their rights upheld or had high scores for these rights regarding personal items (48.7%), recreation (41.9%), hygiene (32.9%), appearance (32.4%), and relationships (38.4%). A low or very low percentage of children had their rights to education (13.6%), personalized care (13%), periodic review (2.6%), and have a family (0.3%) respected or had high scores for these rights.

The rights to free expression of opinions and for information were not included in Table 2.4 because they measured only older children (placed mainly in centers for school aged).

4 Discussion

The results (see Table 2.4) were mixed showing that each type of institution respected children's rights, with some rights being better respected, meaning that these rights covered a larger number of children. Each type of institution (i.e., nurseries, centers for preschool- and school-aged and disabled children) had its own strengths and weaknesses that manifested in how well they respected the most basic human rights of institutionalized children. Many of these differences within each type of institution could be attributed to characteristics of children (e.g., age, provenience, closeness of biological parents, etc.) and institutions (e.g., organizational structure, staff qualification, size, location, etc.). Thus, the outcomes should be interpreted taking in account institutions' structural differences which focused on taking care of a specific demographic section of institutionalized children and, consequently, had specific challenges when data was collected. Hence, future studies could investigate the effects of individual and institutional characteristics on the extent and types of respect given to children's basic human rights in each of these types of institutions. Instead of testing the differences within each across all four types of institutions using the z-test of proportions, we chose only to report the percentage of respect for children's rights in each type of institution as seen below.

4.1 Right to Legal Identity

In the 1990s there had been much talk about the fact that in Romania many abandoned children did not have any identity documents. This was true, but it did not refer only to the children in residential centers but also to those abandoned in maternities and pediatric hospitals. The lack of identity documents for these children was also the reason they spent much time in these hospitals before being placed in protection residential centers. The Law 119/1996 facilitated the drawing up of civil status documents making direct reference to the children abandoned in maternities and the procedures and terms that had to be observed in such cases. Even under Law 3/1970, no child could be admitted to a protection residential center without having a birth certificate. Institutionalized children not having identity documents were generally those placed in residential centers following a judgment delivered as a matter of urgency, due to their risk of being abused in their biological families or because they were abandoned. However, child's legal identity documentation had to be clarified in about 30 days after the initial emergency placement. In the case of children over 14, having identity documents also meant to have an identity card besides the birth certificate. In some cases, the issuing of the identity card was postponed as being conditioned on finding the child's parents and their domicile without which the law in force at that time did not allow the issuing of an identity card. Mention must be made of the fact that the residential centers did not have any authority in facilitating or procuring children's identity documents (birth certificates or identity cards). This authority belonged to the county directorates for child protection.

4.2 Right to Personal History

The right to personal history was one of the most ignored rights of institutionalized children. The percentage of children for whom personal history was impossible to retrace based on documents existing in their files was very high in all types of institutions. For example, we found that for many children in our sample, the place where the child came from was not mentioned in their files. As for children in nurseries, about 80% came from maternities and hospitals. This was rarely mentioned in their files, although the time spent in hospitals was often weeks or even months (Stephenson et al., 1997). According to a study carried out in 2003–2004, more than 50% of the children abandoned in maternities spent more than 50 days in such units until the first protective measure was taken (Stativa, Anghelescu, Mitulescu, Nanu, & Stanciu, 2005). Another aspect contributing to the impossibility to retrace personal history is the manner in which children were transferred from one unit to another. Each transfer was made following a decision of the Commission for the Protection of Child Rights, and this document was sufficient for the child to be admitted to a particular institution. These documents typically remained in the institution and were subsequently archived. There were no procedures for the transfer of documents, leading to institutions determining individually how to proceed. For this reason and as it has already been specified in other studies, it is very difficult to retrace children's pathways from documents (Stephenson et al., 1997).

4.3 The Right to Periodic Review

This right began to be respected in 1997, after Government Ordinance 26/1997 was approved. The observance of this right was crucial in order to give institutionalized children the chance for normal development. After approval of this ordinance, any protective measure established for a child had to be reviewed at least once every 3 months. This review was made on the basis of a complex assessment of the child by a multidisciplinary committee. If they noticed that the protective measure was not in favor of the child, it had to be changed. At least this is what the law specified. In practice, the protective measure was reevaluated, but in order to change the protective measure, it was necessary to create alternatives to the protective measures. This process started only after 2004, following the Law 272/2004 on the protection and promotion of child rights.

4.4 The Right to Protective Measure

The right to protective measure was observed in all types of institutions. The few exceptions were probably due to an administrative issue related to the process of institution takeover in which they were transferred from the ministries to the new county authorities. On this occasion, the protective measures taken under the Law 3/1970 were canceled, and the new decisional bodies enacted protective measures bearing other names.

4.5 The Right to Family

The right to family represents one of the fundamental rights providing the child with the environment considered to be the best for their normal development. Ever since the early 1990s, it was considered that the breaking of relationships between children and their biological parents was the result of administrative deficiencies that did not encourage parents' visits to institutions. Thus, the absence of an arranged space for such meetings or the possibility to accommodate parents overnight and the lack of procedures for the recording of visits, telephone calls, or mail discouraged the relationships between parents and children. The most dramatic situation was in residential institutions for children with disabilities because parents were told for decades that their children were irrecoverable, and they were not told that such children had the same needs as all human beings.

Before Government Ordinance 26/1997 came into effect, many institutions took steps to arrange such spaces. Thus, 80% of nurseries, 60% of residential institutions for children with disabilities, and 57% of residential institutions for preschool and school children had such spaces in place at the beginning of 1997. According to the 1997 Census data, 50% of the children in nurseries, 26% of the children in residential institutions for preschool and school children, and 25% of the children in residential institutions for children with disabilities were visited by their parents at least once every 6 months (DPC & EU/PHARE, 1997). Mention must also be made of the fact that most of the children in these residential institutions had parents who were alive and enjoying their full parental rights. In nurseries, 8% of children had only one parent and 0.9% lost both their parents. In residential institutions for preschool and school children, 20% of children had only one parent, and 0.2% lost both their parents. In the in residential institutions for children with disabilities, 14% of children had only one parent and 3% lost their both parents (DPC & EU/PHARE, 1997).

4.6 The Right to Health

The right to health was differentiated for children according to the type of institution. In nurseries, almost all children had the right to health observed at several levels. This may be due to the medical character of the nurseries through its long appurtenance to the Ministry of Health. On the other hand, the situation with the residential institutions for children with disabilities was precarious, although the health needs were high. Following the reforms that began in 1997, the development of some needed rehabilitation treatments and procedures in these institutions took place. But this happened slowly due to the absence of financing and personnel, as well as the absence of the mentality that these children had rehabilitation potential. Undoubtedly, the right to health could have also been measured by other indicators that may have provided other interpretations for this right in the institutional context. Specifically, we refer to healthcare quality indicators with measurable impact on children's development. These would have been useful to capture those models of care/recovery of which have been profoundly wrong or deficient and that probably caused a very high prevalence of growth disorders, emotional, or cognitive in children (e.g., see Chap. 5) or even the policies that led to such models of care. We refer to those policies that allowed young children to be indefinitely institutionalized in long-term residential centers, which decisively contributed to worsening or altering their health. Solid scientific evidence has revealed that only an early exit from the institutional environment can give young children a chance to a recover from their delayed development; otherwise, recovery may be almost impossible despite subsequent recovery strategies (Johnson et al., 2010).

4.7 The Right to Education

Children were included very successfully in different forms of education. This was a big gain mainly for children over the age of 2 from nurseries and for those in residential institutions for children with disabilities, as their inclusion in a form of education before the 1997 reform was difficult to conceive for the authorities managing those institutions. But in this case, as in the case of the right to health, despite the fact that most children were enrolled in various forms of education, their later social and professional integration was problematic after leaving the institutions. Their schooling did not address real-life demands, and consequently in reality their right to education was not fulfilled adequately. Lack of concern for developing the life skills of institutionalized children made their socio-professional integration and the ability to have an independent, productive life extremely difficult (Hope and Homes for Children & Organizatia "Salvati Copiii", 2006; Mitulescu, Mitulescu, & Stativa, 2005; Onica-Chipea, Baltatescu, Chipea, & Oprea, 2008).

4.8 The Right to Personalized Care

The right to personalized care was a new concept introduced by the legislation of the 1997 reform. This is a fundamental right of the institutionalized child especially in a system that was recently separated from a protection system conceived to be rough, uniform, and impersonal and which did not take into account the needs of every child. The percentage of children who enjoyed customized care in 1999 was relatively decent, except for residential institutions for children with disabilities. Personalized care relied on a customized plan. It was a new instrument in the culture of institutional care, and even if the highest percentage of beneficiaries of such care barely exceeded 50% (in the residential institutions for school-aged children), it must be considered as a glass half full. Despite that, the percentage of children who enjoyed this right in nurseries was surprisingly low. It must be said that orphanage managers and personnel received the most training courses during the ninth decade of the past century, including issues such as the customized plan and care.

4.9 The Right to Quality Care

The right to quality care was assessed in this study by a couple of items (see Tables 2.3 and 2.4). These describe elementary aspects of a normal life that most children could not enjoy until 1999 in Romanian care settings. The practice of cutting children's hair very short for fear of parasites or of not taking into account their clothing preferences was not related to material resources but to the lack of respect toward these children. The high percentages of children who did not have this right respected across institutions confirmed the lack of interest of institutional staff for children's wishes. The same is true for the observance of their right to have or to keep personal items. It was a big gain for children to have personal lockers, and 81% of school-aged children had this need met.

The right to recreational activities for institutionalized children meant having the opportunity to enter their rooms to relax at any time. Most of the institutions had the custom that children were allowed to go to their rooms only after dinner. They would enter the room in an orderly line, and they would go out of the room in the same way without being allowed to freely use the dormitory. In the 1990s, many institutions set up clubs where children could meet and play games or indoor activities. Our study revealed that this right was protected especially for children in nurseries and long-term residential centers for preschool- and school-aged children and less for children in residential centers for the disabled.

As for hygiene, the situation was precarious in almost all protection institutions. Very few restrooms were fully functional. Investments had not been made in their maintenance, and most institutions had more than a hundred children.

In addition, the quality of care depended a lot on the child-staff ratio. The worst situation was that of nurseries where hospital care standards were still being used, and these settings also put little importance on child-caregiver interaction, especially for the young children. The results showed that most of the children, except for those placed in nurseries, had this right respected. Overall, the ratio was better during the daytime, whereas during the nighttime, institutions lacked enough personnel to take care of children. During nighttime shifts, usually, children released their frustrations accumulated during the day and could become aggressive toward others. During this shift, children were supervised by the night guards and supervisors. Most often, these institutional personnel had a low educational attainment (e.g., primary school) and lacked any psycho-pedagogical training. In general, each supervisor had in their care as many bedrooms as were on one floor of a building. In order to manage a large number of bedrooms in institutions for school-aged children, supervisors "delegated" some of their tasks and responsibilities to the older children, a context in which the later used this power to abuse and exploit younger children. This practice seemed to be very generalized across Romanian institutional settings. Within nurseries the child-staff ratios were determined by the requirements of hospitals and taking into account the rhythms of feeding, hygiene, and care of young children, whereas ratios in centers for school-aged children were specific for school systems. School-aged children, after attending school in the morning or afternoon, were supervised and helped with their homework by teachers. We highlight that the child-staff ratio can be seen as a true indicator of quality care only if the caregivers are able to understand and meet institutionalized children's needs.

In conclusion, the goal of defending children's basic rights was ultimately to respect children's human dignity and, consequently, to reduce the disadvantages institutionalized children experienced outside of their biological families. Romania has gradually reformed the whole child protection system, trying to change or abolish the laws and practices that have proved devastating to children's development. These include the prohibition of placing children under 3 years of age in long-term residential institutions, with the alternative being foster families.

Also, preventing children's institutionalization for economic reasons stood central in the protection policies, and social services were set up in all administrative-territorial units (communes, towns). More details about care reform are found in Chap. 5. However, the media in Romania, following journalistic investigations, reveals from time to time abuses to which children are exposed in currently existing residential centers, especially from the staff. This suggests that it is still difficult to prevent abuses even though the reformed child protection system has in place various institutions and mechanisms designed to deal with this phenomenon. Therefore, in our opinion, especially for a country like Romania, which is currently classified as an upper middle-income country (World Bank, 2017), the best residential institution will be one that no longer exists.

5 Strengths and Limitations

Our study is the only comprehensive investigation of institutional neglect experienced by Romanian children placed in long-term residential centers, and it expands the measurement of institutional neglect by highlighting specific areas where children were vulnerable according to the United Nations Convention on the Rights of the Child (UN General Assembly, 1989). By using a nationally representative sample of children and institutions across all eight developmental regions of Romania in rural and urban areas, this study offered a fairly accurate image of the extent of adherence to children's basic rights by residential care institutions. Additionally, for the first time in Romania, children's rights were measured using an empirical tool grounded on the United Nations Convention on the Rights of the Child (UN General Assembly, 1989).

Still, the present study has some limitations. First, we admit that this study examined only 14 different facets of children's rights placed within institutional settings, but the list could be much longer (e.g., nutritional, cultural, or other facets of neglect were not analyzed in this study). Second, our data only allowed us to examine the association between basic human rights of children across various types of institutions (i.e., nurseries, centers for preschool- and school-aged and disabled children), and, therefore, the cross-sectional design does not allow us to infer a causal relationship between these variables. Third, the yes/no nature of the items was also a statistical limitation. Greater variance in the item responses would allow for more precise grouping of the items in the exploratory factor analysis and more precise reliability assessment. However, the collection of more detailed information regarding the children was not possible due to the constraints of the original study. Thus, analysis was conducted using the available data, and descriptive statistics of each item are presented to provide additional detail.

6 Implications for Improving Children's Care

It is important to realize that the data reported here were collected after an extensive governmental effort to scientifically measure the prevalence and forms of maltreatment (i.e., abuse and neglect) within institutions. The first governmental measurement of children's rights was approved in 1997 (approximately 7 years after the collapse of the communist regime that triggered massive social, political, and economic changes) and covered the period 1997–2000 although Romania ratified the UNCRC (UN General Assembly, 1989) in September 1990 and adopted its own national plan of action regarding child protection based on the World Summit for Children (UNICEF, 1990) in the mid-1990s. The implementation of this governmental measurement in 1997 marked the beginning of the major reform of the Romanian child protection system. Specifically, it triggered the first steps in the direction of reform of the regulatory framework regarding child protection, restructuring and diversification of child care institutions, development of an alternative type of care (i.e., familial) from the traditional residential care (typical orphanages), as well as prevention of child abandonment ("Protecția drepturilor copilului – experiența României," n.d.). Fortunately, the effort to improve the quality of institutional care continued after the study was done, and the Romanian child protection system has been drastically changed to include smaller public and residential care facilities and new standards of care and safety (Bejenaru & Tucker, 2014).

We hope that this snapshot of children's quality of life in Romanian institutions, taken during a period when institutions were undergoing immense changes, will help other authorities across the globe responsible for the residential care of children to identify the most basic human rights and build good quality and efficient standards of care for abandoned or orphaned children.

7 Summary

Romanian institutionalized children experienced one of the most severe forms of institutional structural neglect during the communist era, but such conditions continued even after the collapse of the communist regime in December 1989. After ratifying the United Nations Convention on the Rights of the Child and adoption of its own national plan of action regarding child protection, Romanian authorities implemented a massive change of its child protection system, and new standards of care were put in place over a period of many years. These reforms gradually improved the quality of life as fundamental children's rights began to be upheld by long-term residential centers. However, at the end of 1999 when our data was collected, it was clear that the change was not homogenous, and there was variability in the extent of how well children's needs and basic rights were met.

Questions for Discussion

1. Read the United Nations Convention on the Rights of the Child (UNCRC; UN General Assembly, 1989) by accessing the following web link http://www.ohchr.org/Documents/ProfessionalInterest/crc.pdf, and delineate how children's rights could be measured within long-term residential centers in your region or country taking into account the socioeconomic, historical, political, and cultural characteristics.
2. The quote at the beginning of this chapter comes from an article by Gary Melton (2008) titled "Beyond Balancing: Toward an Integrated Approach to Children's Rights." On page 917 of this article, Melton asks, "Under what circumstances do children feel like people? When do they feel that they are meaningful participants in settings of which they are a part?" Provide your own response to these questions within the context of institutionalization.
3. Name two areas of concern that make, or may make, implementation of rights for children more difficult than rights granted to adults. What measures can be taken to ensure that these areas of concern are addressed so that implementation of children's rights is not impeded?

References

American Academy of Pediatrics (AAP), American Public Health Association (APHA), & National Resource Center for Health and Safety in Child Care and Early Education (NRCHSCCEE). (2011). *Caring for our children: National health and safety performance standards; Guidelines for early care and education programs* (3rd ed.). Elk Grove Village, IL/Washington, DC: American Academy of Pediatrics/American Public Health Association.

Ames, E. W., & Carter, M. C. (1992, June). A study of Romanian orphanage children in Canada: Background, sample, and procedure. In *Development of Romanian orphanage children adopted to Canada*. Symposium presented at the Annual Convention of the Canadian Psychological Association, Quebec City, QC.
Bejenaru, A., & Tucker, S. (2014). Challenging dominant representations of residential childcare in Romania: An exploration of the views of children and young people living in the care system. *Journal of Youth Studies*, 1–14. doi:10.1080/13676261.2014.918250. (ahead-of-print).
Bono, C., Ried, L. D., Kimberlin, C., & Vogel, B. (2007). Missing data on the Center for Epidemiologic Studies Depression Scale: A comparison of 4 imputation techniques. *Research in Social and Administrative Pharmacy*, *3*(1), 1–27.
Child Welfare Information Gateway. (2013). *Chronic child neglect*. Washington, DC: U.S. Department of Health and Human Services, Children's Bureau.
Cortina, J. M. (1993). What is coefficient Alpha? An examination of theory and applications. *Journal of Applied Psychology*, *78*(1), 98–104.
Davidson-Arad, B., Dekel, R., & Wozner, Y. (2004). Correspondence in residents' and staff members' assessments of the quality of life of children in residential care facilities. *Social Indicators Research*, *68*(1), 77–89.
Denechere, Y., & Scutaru, B. (2010). International adoption of Romanian children and Romania's admission to the European Union (1990–2007). *Eastern Journal of European Studies*, *1*(1), 135–151.
Department of Child Protection (DPC) & EU/PHARE. (1997). *Recensamantul copiilor/tinerilor plasati in institutiile de ocrotire din Romania* [Census of children/youth placed in child protection institutions in Romania] (Vol. 1–3). Bucharest, Romania: Childhood Protection Program Technical Assistance Unit.
Dobrova-Krol, N. A., van IJzendoorn, M. H., Bakermans-Kranenburg, M. J., & Juffer, F. (2010). Effects of perinatal HIV infection and early institutional rearing on physical and cognitive development of children in Ukraine. *Child Development*, *81*(1), 237–251.
Downey, R. G., & King, C. V. (1998). Missing data in Likert ratings: A comparison of replacement methods. *Journal of General Psychology*, *125*, 175–191.
Embleton, L., Ayuku, D., Kamanda, A., Atwoli, L., Ayaya, S., Vreeman, R., … Braitstein, P. (2014). Models of care for orphaned and separated children and upholding children's rights: Cross-sectional evidence from western Kenya. *BMC International Health and Human Rights*, *149*. doi:10.1186/1472-698X-14-9.
Gavrilovici, O., & Groza, V. (2007). Incidence, prevalence and trauma associated with exposure to violence in Romanian institutionalized children. *International Journal of Child & Family Welfare*, *10*(3–4), 125–138.
Gil, E. (1982). Institutional abuse of children in out-of-home care. In R. Hanson (Ed.), *Institutional abuse of children and youth*. New York, NY: Haworth Press. apud *Jonathan Evans* Institutional abuse and children's home, p. 458.
Groark, C. J., McCall, R. B., & Fish, L. (2011). Characteristics of environments, caregivers, and children in three Central American orphanages. *Infant Mental Health Journal*, *32*(2), 232–250. doi:10.1002/imhj.20292.
Groze, V., & Ileana, D. (1996). A follow-up study of adopted children from Romania. *Child & Adolescent Social Work Journal*, *13*(6), 541–565.
Gunnar, M. R. (2001). Effects of early deprivation: Findings from orphanage-reared infants and children. In C. A. Nelson & M. Luciana (Eds.), *Handbook of developmental cognitive neuroscience* (pp. 617–629). Cambridge, MA: MIT Press.
Hope and Homes for Children & Organizatia "Salvati Copiii". (2006). *Manual de proceduri privind insertia socio-profesionala a tinerilor care parasesc sistemul de protectia a copilului* [Manual procedures for insertion of socio-professional care for youth leaving the child protection system]. Bucuresti, Romania: Europrint.
IBM Corp. Released 2010. *IBM SPSS statistics for Windows, version 19.0*. Armonk, NY: Author.
Iusmen, I. (2014). *Children's rights Eastern enlargement and the EU human right regime*. Manchester, UK/New York, NY: Manchester University Press.

Jaffe, E. D. (1995). *Intercountry adoptions: Laws and perspectives of "sending" countries*. Dordrecht, The Netherlands: Martinus Nijhoff Publishers.

Johnson, D. E., Guthrie, D., Smyke, A. T., Koga, S. F., Fox, N. A., Zeanah, C. H., & Nelson, C. (2010). Growth and associations between auxology, caregiving environment, and cognition in socially deprived Romanian children randomized to foster vs ongoing institutional care. *Archives of Pediatrics & Adolescent Medicine*, *164*(6), 507–516. doi:10.1001/archpediatrics.2010.56.

Johnson, D. E., Miller, L. C., Iverson, S., Thomas, W., Franchino, B., Dole, K., ... Hostetter, M. K. (1992). The health of children adopted from Romania. *Journal of the American Medical Association*, *268*(24), 3446–3451.

Melton, G. B. (2008). Beyond balancing: Toward an integrated approach to children's rights. *Journal of Social Issues*, *64*(4), 903–920.

Ministry of Health, Institute for Mother and Child Care, & UNICEF. (1991). *Cauze ale institutionalizarii copiilor in leagane si sectii de distrofici in Romania* [Causes of children's institutionalization in "leagane" and dystrophic centers in Romania]. Retrieved from http://iomc.ro/uploads/documents/Cauzele_institutionalizarii_1991.pdf

Mitulescu, S., Mitulescu, R., & Stativa, E. (2005). Long-term effects of institutionalization. Pilot study in Prahova County. *Social Work Review, Nr.1-2*/2005, Editura Polirom.

National Authority for Child Protection and Adoption (NACPA), & UNICEF. (2004). *Child care system reform in Romania*. Bucharest, Romania: UNICEF.

Nelson, C. A., Fox, N. A., & Zeanah, C. H. (2014). *Romania's abandoned children deprivation, brain development, and the struggle for recovery*. Cambridge, MA: Harvard University Press.

Onica-Chipea, L., Baltatescu, S., Chipea, F., & Oprea, I. (2008). *Studiu privind modul de integrare în societate a tinerilor care au fost socializați în instituțiile de protecția copilului în județul Bihor* [Study on how to integrate into society the young people who have been socialized in childcare institutions in Bihor County]. Universitatea din Oradea: Facultatea de Stiinte Socio-Umane.

Protecția drepturilor copilului – experiența României. (n.d.). Retrieved October 16, 2016, from http://www.drepturilecopiilor.ro/downloads/conference/Bogdan%20Adrian%20Panait%20-%20RO.pdf

Rus, A. V., Stativa, E., Butterfield, M. E., Pennings, J. S., Parris, S. R., Burcea, G., & Wenyika, R. (2016). Peer exploitation: Findings from a Romanian nationally representative sample of children living in long-term residential centres. Child Abuse Review. Published online in Wiley Online Library (wileyonlinelibrary.com). doi:10.1002/car.2464"10.1002/car.2464

Rus, A. V., Stativa, E., Pennings, J. S., Cross, D. R., Ekas, N., Purvis, K. B., & Parris, S. R. (2013). Severe punishment of children by staff in Romanian placement centers for school-aged children: Effects of child and institutional characteristics. *Child Abuse & Neglect*, *37*(12), 1152–1162. doi:10.1016/j.chiabu.2013.07.003.

Rutter, M., & The English and Romanian Adoptees (ERA) Study Team. (1998). Developmental catch-up, and deficit, following adoption after severe global early privation. *Journal of Child Psychology and Psychiatry*, *39*(4), 465–476.

Shye, S. (1989). The systemic life quality model: A basis for urban renewal evaluation. *Social Indicators Research*, *21*(4), 343–378. doi:10.1007/BF00303952.

Smyke, A. T., Koga, S. F., Johnson, D. E., Fox, N. A., Marshall, P. J., Nelson, C. A., & Zeanah, C. H. (2007). The caregiving context in institution-reared and family-reared infants and toddlers in Romania. *Journal of Child Psychology & Psychiatry*, *48*(2), 210–218. doi:10.1111/j.1469-7610.2006.01694.x.

St. Petersburg–USA Orphanage Research Team. (2005). Characteristics of children, caregivers, and orphanages for young children in St. Petersburg, Russian Federation. *Journal of Applied Developmental Psychology*, *26*, 477–506.

St. Petersburg–USA Orphanage Research Team. (2008). The effects of early social-emotional and relationship experience on the development of young orphanage children. *Monographs of the Society for Research in Child Development*, *73*(3, Serial No. 291), 1–262.

Stativa, E., Anghelescu, C., Mitulescu, R., Nanu, M., & Stanciu, N. (2005). The situation of child abandonment in Romania. *UNICEF Romania*. Retrieved from https://www.unicef.org/ceecis/GDD_2005_Romania_Child_abandonment.pdf

Stativa, E., Anghelescu, C., Palicari, G., Stanescu, A., & Nanu, R. (2002). *Child abuse in residential care institutions in Romania*. Bucharest, Romania: Extrem Group.

Stephenson, P., Anghelescu, C., Fumarel, S., Georgescu, A., Iorgulescu, D., McCreery, R., … Stativa, E. (1993). Training needs of staff in Romanian institutions for young children. *Child: Care, Health and Development, 19*, 221–234. doi:10.1111/j.1365-2214.1993.tb00728.x.

Stephenson, P., Anghelescu, C., Stativa, E., & Pasti, S. (1997). *Cauzele instituționalizării copiilor din România* [The causes of children institutionalization in Romania]. Bucharest, Romania: UNICEF/International Foundation for Children and Families.

Stephenson, P., Wagner, M., Badea, M., & Serbanescu, F. (1992). Commentary: The public health consequences of restricted induced abortion – Lessons from Romania. *American Journal of Public Health, 82*(10), 1328–1331.

UN General Assembly. (1989, November 20). *Convention on the rights of the child* (United Nations, Treaty Series, Vol. 1577, p. 3). Retrieved from http://www.ohchr.org/Documents/ProfessionalInterest/crc.pdf

UNICEF. (1990). *A promise to children*. Retrieved from https://www.unicef.org/wsc/

Universitatea Babes-Bolyai, Facultatea de Psychologie si Stiinte ale Educatiei. (n.d.). *Scurtistoric al facultatii de Psihologie si Stiinte ale Educatiei* [Brief history of the Faculty of Psychology and Educational Sciences]. Retrieved from http://psiedu.ubbcluj.ro/index.php?id=11-istoric-psihologie

Universitatea Bucuresti, Facultatea de Sociologie si Asistenta Sociala. (n.d.). *Trecut* [Past]. Retrieved from http://sas.unibuc.ro/trecut_ro

van IJzendoorn, M. H., Palacios, J., Sonuga-Barke, E. S., Gunnar, M. R., Vorria, P., McCall, R. B., … Juffer, F. (2011). Children without permanent parents: Research, practice, and policy: I. Children in institutional care: Delayed development and resilience. *Monographs of the Society for Research in Child Development, 76*(4), 8–30. doi:10.1111/j.1540-5834.2011.00626.x.

Vorria, P., Papaligoura, Z., Dunn, J., van IJzendoorn, M. H., Steele, H., Kontopoulou, A., & Sarafidou, Y. (2003). Early experiences and attachment relationships of Greek infants raised in residential group care. *Journal of Child Psychology & Psychiatry & Allied Disciplines, 44*(8), 1208–1220. doi:10.1111/1469-7610.00202.

World Bank. (2017). *Data for upper middle income, Romania*. Retrieved from http://data.worldbank.org/?locations=XT-RO

World Health Organization (WHO). (1999, March 29–31). *Report of the consultation on child abuse prevention*. Geneva, Switzerland: Author.

Zugravescu A., & Sandell A. (1991, September). Adoption in Romania. The care of Romanian children. *Newsletter*.

Chapter 3
Punishment, Peer Exploitation, and Sexual Abuse in Long-Term Romanian Residential Centers: Findings from a Nationally Representative Sample of Institutionalized Children

Adrian V. Rus, Ecaterina Stativa, Sheri R. Parris, Jacquelyn S. Pennings, Max E. Butterfield, Wesley C. Lee, and Ovidiu Gavrilovici

> *The true nature of a nation's standing is how well it attends to its children …When we work together to end violence in their lives, we rise to the best in ourselves, we help children reach their full potential, and we promote a future of peace and dignity for the next generation.*
>
> World Health Organization (2016, p. 11)

A.V. Rus (✉)
Department of Social and Behavioral Sciences, Southwestern Christian University, 7210 NW 39th Expressway, Bethany, OK 73008-0340, USA
e-mail: adrian.rus@swcu.edu; aadrianrus@gmail.com

E. Stativa
Social Pediatrics and Obstetrics Research Department, The National Institute for Mother and Child Health "Alessandrescu-Rusescu", Bucharest, Romania
e-mail: ecaterina.stativa@gmail.com

S.R. Parris
Texas Christian University, Fort Worth, TX, USA
e-mail: sheri.parris@gmail.com

J.S. Pennings
Elite Research, LLC, Irving, TX 75063, USA
e-mail: jacspen@gmail.com

M.E. Butterfield
Point Loma Nazarene University, San Diego, CA, USA
e-mail: mbutter@pointloma.edu

W.C. Lee
Southern Nazarene University, Bethany, OK, USA
e-mail: wlee@snu.edu

O. Gavrilovici
"Alexandru Ioan Cuza" University of Iaşi, Iaşi, Romania
e-mail: gavrilov@uaic.ro

A.V. Rus et al. (eds.), *Child Maltreatment in Residential Care*,
DOI 10.1007/978-3-319-57990-0_3

1 Introduction

Despite the responsibility of residential institutions to provide care and protection for children, many have harbored conditions where children have become victims or witnesses of many types of abuse. This phenomenon is not restricted to geography or a country's level of development, as various types of institutional abuse have relatively recently been reported in European countries such as Romania (Gavrilovici & Groza, 2007a; Rus et al., 2013; Stativa, Anghelescu, Palicari, Stanescu, & Nanu, 2002), Spain (Segura, Pereda, Abad, & Guilera, 2015; Segura, Pereda, Guilera, & Abad, 2016), the Netherlands (Euser, Alink, Tharner, van IJzendoorn, & Bakermans-Kranenburg, 2013; Euser, Alink, Tharner, van IJzendoorn, & Bakermans-Kranenburg, 2014; Euser, Alink, Tharner, van IJzendoorn, & Bakermans-Kranenburg, 2016), Germany (Spröber et al., 2014), and Croatia (Sekol, 2013; Sekol & Farrington, 2009, 2013); Middle East countries such as Israel (Attar-Schwartz, 2011, 2013, 2014; Attar-Schwartz & Khoury-Kassabri, 2015; Khoury-Kassabri & Attar-Schwartz, 2014; Pinchover & Attar-Schwartz, 2014); former Soviet Union countries, such as Kazakhstan (Haarr, 2011); the United States (Rosenthal, Motz, Edmonson, & Groze, 1991); South American countries (Luna, Luna, & Brizuela, 2011); and African and Asian countries such as Cambodia, Ethiopia, India, Kenya, Tanzania, and Botswana (Gray et al., 2015; Hermenau, Eggert, Landolt, & Hecker, 2015; Hermenau, Hecker, Elbert, & Ruf-Leuschner, 2014; Morantz & Heymann, 2010). Understanding and preventing this widespread phenomenon are important because trauma experienced by institutionalized children has significant negative consequences on their well-being (e.g., Escueta, Whetten, Ostermann, & O'Donnell, 2014; Hermenau et al., 2011, 2014; Segura et al., 2016; Whetten, Ostermann, Whetten, O'Donnell, & Thielman, 2011). Previous studies have found that many factors contribute to institutional child abuse, including substandard training, supervision, and selection of staff; poor management; inappropriate organizational cultures; failure to identify abusive staff; and lack of responsiveness regarding child-on-child abuse (Colton, 2002). Additionally, there is evidence that governments show a relatively low priority to children in residential care, and they usually change existing policies only when extreme problems are exposed and institutions have insufficient staffing, monitoring, and oversight or fail to segregate vulnerable children (due to age, size, sex, etc.) from dangerous peers (Pinheiro, 2006).

In this chapter, we intend to investigate the prevalence of abuse (i.e., emotional, physical, and sexual) by staff and peers experienced by Romanian children in institutional care (note: the terms orphanage, care institution, institutional care facility, and long-term residential center are used interchangeably in this chapter). Specifically, we will (1) define the concepts of punishments administered by staff, including administrative personnel, educational/care staff, and night attendants (for convenience henceforth referred to as staff), bullying and peer exploitation within the institutional context taking into account various conceptual and research-based frameworks, and sexual abuse by staff and/or other adults or peers and (2) investigate the prevalence of punishments, peer exploitation, and sexual abuse by staff and/or other adults or peers that children were victims of or aware of in institutional settings.

2 Punishment by Institutional Staff

In Romanian residential care institutions, children experienced a variety of severe punishments from institutional staff, including administrative, educational/care staff, and night attendants (Rus et al., 2013; Stativa et al., 2002). Specifically, these punishments included emotional and/or psychological abuse such as deprivation of nurturing relationships (by ignoring the child); promoting insecurity and uncertainty (through blackmail and threats); punishment for behaviors typical for the child's age; setting unreasonable rules and requirements; using ridicule and humiliation (including for bedwetting); ignoring children's performances; making them wear inappropriate clothing for their age; delay or cancelation of leaves, family visits, recreational activities, or camping trips; denial of favorite toys; and/or not allowing children to make their own choices and decisions. Physical abuse by staff included moderate (spankings, punches, kicks, or ear and hair pulling) and severe physical beatings (including with a plank or a wet rope), washing the child's face with excessive amounts of water and soap, withholding meals or desserts, physical isolation (making the child stand in a corner or sit on a chair or isolation from other children during playtime), and/or forcing the child to complete humiliating tasks such as mopping floors, cleaning toilets and shower rooms, sweeping the dormitory and courtyards, watering the flowers, or canteen duty. Some of these activities could be seen as normal chores in other situational contexts, but most likely institutionalized children were forced to do them. It is important to note also that many of the punishments children experienced included emotional and/or psychological abuse that could escalate to physical abuse.

A similar study (Haarr, 2011) of institutionalized children and youth in Kazakhstan showed that 9% of them declared they were physically attacked and hurt by staff, experiencing small and large bruises, scrapes, and cuts, black eyes, sprains, broken bones, broken teeth, internal injuries, being knocked out or hit unconscious, and head, eye, and ear injuries. Also, Attar-Schwartz (2011) found that overall 25% of Israeli institutionalized adolescents reported being maltreated (moderately severe violent acts) by staff during the month prior to the survey (19% were grabbed or pushed, 16% were pinched, 12% were slapped, and 11% were kicked or punched [some experienced more than one type during the month]). Additionally, this study showed that overall approximately 30% of adolescents reported being victims of verbal abuse by staff (30% were verbally humiliated, insulted, or ridiculed; 15% were cursed at [some experienced both types during the month]). In another study, 25% of children assessed in Botswana reported experiencing both verbal and physical punishments by their caregivers (Morantz & Heymann, 2010).

The present study also focused on a subject rarely studied within long-term residential centers, namely, children witnessing staff using violence against other children. A recent report (Haarr, 2011) revealed that 19% of children in Kazakhstan orphanages reported witnessing staff using harsh verbal abuse on children/youth (i.e., swearing or cursing at children; calling them names such as idiot, stupid, and bastard; and using language with the intent to hurt or frighten). Additionally, 16% of children reported witnessing psychological abuse of other children by staff (i.e., restricting access to the toilet; destruction of children's property, e.g., clothes, toys, and personal things; acting in a threatening manner to create fear of physical harm; locking children in an isolated room/small space for a long time; tying children up; or chaining them to something). Furthermore, the report (Haarr, 2011) also showed that almost 22% of children witnessed staff administering moderate physical violence to children (i.e., pinching, twisting ears and arms), and 22% of children witnessed staff administering severe physical violence to children (i.e., shaking; slapping in the face or on the head; slapping on the buttocks, back, leg, and arm; grabbing, pushing, or knocking children down; hitting or kicking children; hitting children with a hard object or weapon, e.g., stick, belt, whip, and ruler; hitting children hard enough to leave marks or injuries; burning children with cigarettes or other hot items).

3 Exploitation by Peers

Bullying and aggression among peers has shown to be a widespread problem among juveniles in school settings (Burger, Strohmeier, Spröber, Bauman, & Rigby, 2015; Chester et al., 2015; Elgar et al., 2015; Harel-Fisch et al., 2011; Smith, Pepler, & Rigby, 2004), inmates in prisons (Ireland, 1999; Ireland & Ireland, 2003), patients in secure hospitals (Ireland & Snowden, 2002), and adolescents in residential institutions (Attar-Schwartz & Khoury-Kassabri, 2015; Sekol, 2013; Sekol & Farrington, 2009, 2013). Yet, little research has focused on peer-on-peer violence in residential child care settings (Monks et al., 2009).

Bullying is a complex behavior that can be viewed through multiple theoretical frameworks (e.g., ethological, ecological and socioecological, cognitive and social-cognitive, genetic and other biologic theories), and describing it becomes more complex due to variations in definitions among different languages (Smith, Cowie, Olafsson, & Liefooghe, 2002). However, there are three common criteria used to define bullying in schools, namely, that it is (1) an intentional aggressive behavior, (2) carried out repeatedly and over time, and (3) enacted within an interpersonal relationship characterized by an imbalance of power where the victim has difficulties defending himself or herself (Olweus, 2011). Consequently, regardless of the variation in definitions, bullying is considered a form of aggressive behavior or abuse by peers that infringes on the victim's rights (Craig & Pepler, 2007; Olweus, 2011). Examples of bullying may include ridicule or name-calling; ignoring or exclusion from a group of friends; hitting, kicking, pushing, shoving, or threatening; spreading lies or false rumors; sending mean notes; or doing other hurtful things (Solberg & Olweus, 2003; Solberg, Olweus, & Endresen, 2007). In addition, bullying among adolescents may include remarks about money or other items that may be taken away or destroyed, threats to do unpleasant things, or using derogatory names with sexual or racial meaning (Kyriakides, Kaloyirou, & Lindsay, 2006).

The socioecological perspective (Swearer et al., 2006) can help us understand bullying and exploitation by highlighting the importance of certain characteristics of individuals and their surroundings. In addition, institutional settings had (and may still have in some places) context-specific characteristics that also need to be considered. For instance, long-term residential centers in Romania were considered a "closed system" that lacked accountability to an external controlling and auditing authority. They also lacked resources to assess child abuse or the extent to which it occurred, and therefore it was not addressed appropriately. Additionally, many of these residential care facilities had an organizational structure and culture that facilitated violence (Gavrilovici & Groza, 2007a; Rus et al., 2013; Stativa et al., 2002), and the aggressive behaviors were an integral part of a "clan-like" living situation (Baker, Cunningham, & Male, 2002), where children were continuously and inescapably victims of their aggressors. Additionally, institutionalized children may also have experienced an invasion of their personal space, been placed within the same residential settings with peers from different backgrounds, experienced detachment from external support networks, and been part of an institutional culture of nondisclosure of bullying or attacks at night, all of which could increase the impact of bullying (Monks et al., 2009).

As prison studies have shown (Ireland & Ireland, 2003), bullying behavior among prisoners can be explained by (a) fear of future victimization, (b) "baroning" (when the bully and victim enter this relationship voluntarily), (c) a need to achieve status among peers, or (d) a need to obtain material goods. Additionally, bullying in prison can include behaviors such as shouting at victims during the night or when in their cell, stealing property, forcing the victim to swap property or buy canteen for another, or taxation of property (Ireland & Ireland, 2003), and some of these practices may have also been common among Romanian children placed in institutions.

This study provides a report on whether Romanian institutionalized children were witness to or forced to do various chores, steal, beg, and/or give away various personal belongings for the benefit of their older peers. Throughout this chapter, we refer to these four aggressive behaviors as *exploitation* because they cannot be fully described or explained by current theories that are solely used to measure peer-to-peer aggression or juvenile bullying in schools.

4 Sexual Abuse

As very well documented, children in residential care also experienced sexual abuse. Specifically, in a study of 448 Romanian institutionalized children (ages 8–17), Gavrilovici and Groza (2007a) found that 31.2% of males and 27% of females reported being sexually abused in the past year. In addition, 44.9% of males and 52.8% of females witnessed their peers being sexually abused in the past year. However, this study did not identify whether these children were exposed to violence from their caregivers, educators, teachers, peers, or other individuals.

A high rate of moderately severe sexual violence in residential care settings for at-risk children was also found by Attar-Schwartz (2014) in Israel. In this study, 40% of the adolescents were victims of at least one act of peer sexual violent behavior in the month prior to the survey, with similar rates for girls and boys, as well as Arab and Jewish children. These results are explained by adolescents' individual characteristics (i.e., adjustment difficulties; self-reported experiences of physical abuse by staff, or perception of the antiviolence policy of the care setting) and by the social context of the institutional care settings' characteristics (i.e., percentage of males in the institution, average level of adjustment difficulties in the institution, and structure of the care setting – group settings or settings with familial elements).

Furthermore, studying the prevalence of child sexual abuse in out-of-home care in 2010, Euser and colleagues (2013) found that children in residential care experience sexual abuse more frequently than children in the general Dutch population. Professionals working in residential centers reported a prevalence of 5 per 1000 sexual abuse cases. However, children with mild intellectual disabilities and placed in out-of-home care were more vulnerable to sexual abuse, with a prevalence of 9.7 per 1000 children. Children in residential care self-reported a much higher prevalence at 280 sexual abuse cases per 1000 children (Euser et al., 2016).

The consequences of sexual abuse are dramatic as shown by a retrospective descriptive analysis study (Spröber et al., 2014) that measured the magnitude and the effects of child sexual abuse occurring between 1950 and 1980 in German religiously affiliated and secular care institutions. Specifically, out of 1050 victims of abuse, the majority of participants in this study (with an average age of 52 years) reported at least one psychiatric problem (the most common diagnoses reported were depressive episodes, post-traumatic stress syndrome, and anxiety or obsessive-compulsive disorder).

Thus, the sexual abuse of children in residential care should be understood as a complex phenomenon related to individual characteristics (e.g., histories of sexual abuse prior to placement or gender) and institutional factors (e.g., group dynamics, institutional culture, and unpreparedness of professionals to deal with issues of sexuality) (for more information, see Timmerman & Schreuder, 2014) or to societal assumptions about the rights of children (Spröber et al., 2014).

5 Purpose and Research Question of the Current Study

Data for this chapter were collected in 1999 during a third phase of reforms within the Romanian child welfare system. This third phase occurred between 1997 and 2000 and sought to reduce the maltreatment of children that had brought negative international attention to Romania (for a review, see Rus, Parris, Cross, Purvis, & Drăghici, 2011). The reform efforts began in 1990, when the Romanian government signed the United Nations Convention on the Rights of the Child (UN General Assembly, 1989) and thus undertook the responsibility to comply with these rights. Beginning in 1996, children in most institutions were informed of their rights, which included a ban on all types of physical and emotional abuse by staff or peers. Also during this period, legislation was enacted to create alternatives to institutional settings and to regulate adoptions, provide support for families to prevent children from entering residential care settings, and decentralize or close institutions. After closing the large institutions, children were placed in more child-friendly settings, such as centers with a family-type organization. Because reforms happened over a period of years, when our data was collected in 1999, some traditional-type institutions were still in operation as the newer family-type centers were emerging. The *traditional* long-term residential centers or orphanages were eventually eliminated. These traditional-type institutions housed large numbers of children in large buildings with each floor containing 14–20 bedrooms with about 8–10 beds each and no personal space. There was also an inconsistency in caregivers, who lacked psychological investment in the children, and high levels of abuse (for more information about this type of center, see Chap. 2). On the other hand, *family-type* centers housed fewer children in small houses or apartments or in larger buildings organized into autonomous subunits of up to 50 children and further divided into modules of up to 10 children. The rooms and daily activities were organized to resemble a family model and to provide individualized care (Stativa et al., 2002). In addition to the traditional and family-type long-term residential settings, a third type of setting was also in operation at the time of our data collection. These were *mixed-type* centers where traditional and family-type settings coexisted within one building, in varying proportions. In a typical two-story mixed-type center, one floor contained a family-type setting, and another floor contained a traditional-style placement center (Stativa et al., 2002).

Data for this study was derived from the cross-sectional Survey on Child Abuse in Residential Care Institutions in Romania (SCARCIR; Stativa et al., 2002) that sought information about various types of abuse, including staff and peer victimization and awareness of exploitation. Subsequently, our analysis of the data sought to determine the magnitude of (1) experience and awareness of 12 types of punishments administered by the institutional staff (for a complete list, see Sect. 5.1.5); (2) exploitation expressed through four specific behaviors where institutionalized children or/and teenagers forced the younger ones to (a) do various chores, (b) steal, (c) beg, and (d) give them various personal belongings (i.e., money, food, clothing, and school supplies) or they witnessed (were aware of) such exploitative situations; and (3) experience and awareness of sexual abuse perpetrated by institutional staff and/or peers. Additionally, (4) we wanted to assess the extent of children's awareness of and victimization through punishments by staff, sexual abuse, and peer exploitation across the three different types of residential settings (i.e., traditional, familial, and mixed).

5.1 *Method*

5.1.1 Survey on Child Abuse in Residential Care Institutions in Romania (SCARCIR)

We performed a secondary analysis of data from the Survey on Child Abuse in Residential Care Institutions in Romania (SCARCIR) (for a complete review of the SCARCIR, including methodology, see Rus et al., 2013; Stativa et al., 2002).

5.1.2 Participants in the Current Study

The original data set included a national representative sample of 3164 children (1701 boys and 1463 girls) in residential care institutions with ages between 0 and 19 years ($M = 9.45$; $SD = 5.39$), representing 7.8% of the entire population of institutionalized Romanian children in 1999. Three criteria were used to include children from the original study in the current secondary analysis. First, because the SCARCIR survey on punishments was only applied to children (a) over 7 years of age and (b) who resided in placement centers for school-aged children (children residing in cradles, placement centers for preschool children, and cămine spital were excluded from the survey on punishments; in total $N = 1461$), all participants in the current study were limited to these two criteria ($N = 1703$). Furthermore, the third criterion was a requirement that the children must have both the first part of the survey (files – information was obtained from a variety of documents, such as the children's social files, medical records, and other records available in the institutions or made available by either the management or the educational, social, and medical personnel) and the second part of the survey (interview referring to acts of neglect and abuse in institutions). Consequently, 192 children were excluded from the final sample due to the lack of these data. Therefore, participants from the original SCARCIR data set who did not meet the three abovementioned criteria were excluded, resulting in a final sample for the current study of 1511 children (802 boys and 709 girls) with ages between 7 and 19 years ($M = 12.67$; $SD = 2.84$) and living in 53 long-term residential centers, representing 47.8% of the SCARCIR initial sample. Notably, the sample for the current study ($N = 1511$) represents 88.7% of the original SCARCIR national representative sample of children residing in placement centers for school-aged children ($N = 1703$). Further descriptions of the purpose of SCARCIR and research methodology are presented elsewhere (for a complete review, see Rus et al., 2013; Rus et al., in press; Stativa et al., 2002; Chap. 2).

5.1.3 Measures

One of the coauthors of the present study (Stativa) is an expert who participated in the reforms of the Romanian child protection system in the 1990s. She formed the idea to measure abuse after extensive discussions with institutionalized children and youth and their caregivers. These discussions revealed a variety of abusive experiences endured by institutionalized children from staff and peers. Consequently, a preliminary questionnaire was created and then piloted four times on 20–25 children from various institutions to check the acceptability of questions by the children, the rate of nonresponses, and the length of the interview. During this process, the researchers indeed found that punishments by institutional staff and peer exploitation were real issues and were generalized across institutional settings. This finding encouraged the researchers to include questions to capture these behaviors. From the beginning, the survey sought to measure atypical abusive or exploitative behaviors never before reported in institutional settings. Later, in addition to the quantitative data collected by means of the SCARCIR survey, focus groups held with children and staff also confirmed the presence of these behaviors.

5.1.4 Experience and Awareness of Punishments, Exploitation, and Sexual Abuse

Assuming that children could underreport the abuse (i.e., punishments, exploitation, and sexual abuse) they witnessed or experienced due to fear of negative consequences and, therefore, be reluctant to disclose such sensitive information, they were first asked if they had knowledge of, or were aware of, abuse in the long-term residential center where they lived. Then, specific questions were asked that inquired whether they experienced various forms of abuse.

5.1.5 Experience and Awareness of Punishments

Specifically, children were first asked the following question: "In this institution, are there children who are severely punished (including beaten) by the institutional staff?" The measurement of this item had a binary distribution (no versus yes). Next, children were asked: "Have you happened to be severely punished (beaten) by the staff?" The measurement of this item had a binary distribution (no versus yes). If yes, they were asked: "If yes (you happened to be severely punished), what was the punishment?" Children were given 12 possible responses from which to choose including (1) *humiliation (humiliating language, attitudes, and gestures)*, (2) *threatening (blackmail)*, (3) *prohibition of family visits*, (4) *prohibition of recreation activities*, (5) *prohibition of meals*, (6) *prohibition of leaves*, (7) *obligatory chores*, (8) *mild corporal punishments (including spankings, punches, kicks, or ear and hair pulling)*, (9) *severe corporal punishments (including with a plank or a wet rope)*, (10) *physical isolation (making the child stand in a corner)*, (11) *isolation from group (isolating the child from other children when they were playing)*, and (12) *other punishments (not defined in this study)*. The measurement of these 12 forms of punishments had a binary distribution (no versus yes). Children who answered "yes" to any of these items were coded as having been punished by staff. Those who answered "no" to all items were coded as not having been punished by the staff. Based on these 12 responses, a composite variable was created (i.e., child experience of being punished by staff) summing up the responses (no versus yes).

5.1.6 Experiences and Awareness of Peer Exploitation

The data from structured interviews contained children's answers to four sets of questions related to their experiences of exploitation by older children and exploitation awareness. This outcome was captured by the following question: "Do older children/teenagers in this center exploit the younger ones by forcing them to (1) do various chores, (2) steal, (3) beg, and (4) give them various personal belongings (i.e., money, food, clothing, and school supplies)?" Next, children were asked if they personally experienced exploitation by asking: "Have you been forced to (1) do various chores, (2) steal, (3) beg, and (4) give them various personal belongings (i.e., money, food, clothing, and school supplies)?" Those who answered "yes" to any of these items were coded as having been exploited by older children or having awareness of exploitation in the institution where they lived. Those who answered "no" to all items were coded as not having been exploited or not being aware of exploitation. Thus, the outcome variables, namely, (a) the awareness of exploitation and (b) the experience of exploitation had a binary distribution (*no* versus *yes*).

5.1.7 Experience and Awareness of Sexual Abuse

Children were also subjected to sexual abuse by staff and/or other adults or peers who were or were not in contact with them through the institution (for more information, see Stativa et al., 2002). This outcome was captured by two questions, namely, "In this center, are there children forced (blackmailed) to have sexual relationships?" and "Has it ever happened to you to be forced by anyone to have such a relationship?" The responses to these two questions had a binary distribution (*no* versus *yes*).

5.2 *Analysis Plan*

Data from children's interviews were used in the current analysis. Data were analyzed using IBM SPSS (Version 23, 2015). All item responses were in a yes-or-no format. Some responses contained missing items and analysis was done on available data. Statistical analysis included descriptive analysis in the form of frequencies and percentages. Also, a series of cross tabulations with chi square tests of association were performed to examine differences in children's experience and awareness of various forms of abuse between traditional-type institutions and family-type and mixed-type (traditional and family-type) facilities. Cramer's V statistics are reported as a measure of effect size.

5.3 *Results*

5.3.1 Descriptive Analysis

The average time children were institutionalized was 5.71 years ($SD = 3.98$; $Mdn = 6.0$), ranging from 0 to 18 years. The mean age at the first placement was 72.34 months ($SD = 48.09$; $Mdn = 79.0$), ranging from 0 to 218 months. The ratio of

Table 3.1 Frequencies and percentages of child characteristics

	Overall		Type of institutional organization					
			Traditional		Family type		Mixed	
	N	%	*n*	%	*n*	%	*n*	%
Child level								
Number of children	1511	100	906	60.0	116	7.7	489	32.4
Gender								
Male	802	53.1	460	52.3	70	56.5	272	53.5
Female	709	46.9	419	47.7	55	43.5	236	46.5
Siblings in institution(s)								
No	594	42.7	361	42.8	56	51.4	177	40.5
Yes, in this center	696	50.1	430	50.9	42	38.5	224	51.3
Yes, in another center	100	7.2	53	6.3	11	10.1	36	8.2
Visited by parents this year								
No	333	23.8	191	22.8	25	22.9	117	25.7
Yes	1067	76.2	645	77.2	84	77.1	338	74.3
Institution size								
Small (1–100 children)	284	18.8	225	24.8	5	4.3	54	11.0
Medium (101–200 children)	657	43.5	338	37.3	79	68.1	240	49.1
Large (201–300 children)	306	20.3	79	8.7	32	27.6	195	39.9
Very large (301–400 children)	264	17.5	264	29.1	0	0	0	0
Institution level								
Number of residential centers	53	100	34	66.7	5	7.8	14	25.5
Institution location								
Rural	17	32.1	10	28.6	4	80	3	23.1
Urban	36	67.9	25	71.4	1	20	10	76.9

Note: Descriptive percentages not summing to 100% reflect missing data

children for each caregiver during the day ranged from 3 to 32 ($M = 9.76$; $Mdn = 9.0$; $SD = 5.37$). As seen in Table 3.1, a slight majority of children had siblings residing in the same institution (50.1%), and many reported being visited by their parents during the year when data were collected (76.2%). For the purpose of the current study, these institutions were grouped as (a) small institutions with up to 100 children (18.8% of children), (b) medium institutions with 101 to 200 children (43.5% of children), (c) large institutions with 201 to 300 (20.3% of children), and (d) very large institutions with 301 to 400 children (17.5% of children). Out of 1511 institutionalized children, 60% were placed within 34 institutions that had a traditional type of organization, 7.7% were placed within 5 institutions that had a familial type of organization, and 32.4% were placed in 14 institutions with a mixed-type model of organization. Mixed-type organizations were institutions in which the two previous models (traditional and familial) coexisted in varying proportions. Out of 53 institutions, 36 were located in urban areas, comprising 70.2% of the institutions in our sample.

Table 3.2 Frequencies and percentages of experience and awareness of various forms of abuse in the institution

	N	No	%	Yes	%
Child experience of punishment, exploitation, and abuse					
Child experience of being punished by staff (*types of punishments*)	**1457**	**807**	**55.4**	**650**	**44.6**
Mild corporal punishments	1462	954	65.3	508	34.7
Severe corporal punishments	1462	1202	82.2	260	17.8
Prohibition of recreation activities	1462	1312	89.7	150	10.3
Obligatory chores	1462	1339	91.6	123	8.4
Prohibition of meals	1462	1342	91.8	120	8.2
Humiliation	1461	1370	93.8	91	6.2
Prohibition of leaves	1462	1371	93.8	91	6.2
Threatening	1462	1375	94.0	87	6.0
Prohibition of family visits	1462	1424	97.4	38	2.6
Isolation from group	1462	1432	97.9	30	2.1
Physical isolation	1462	1440	98.5	22	1.5
Other punishments	1458	1445	99.1	13	0.9
Child experiences of exploitation by peers (*types of exploitation situations*)	**1415**	**1000**	**70.7**	**415**	**29.3**
Various chores (odd jobs)	1427	1115	78.1	312	21.9
Steal	1430	1314	91.9	116	8.1
Beg	1429	1342	93.9	87	6.1
Give away belongings	1428	1118	78.3	310	21.7
Child experience of being forced to have sex	**1259**	**1199**	**95.2**	**60**	**4.8**
Child awareness of punishments, exploitation, and abuse					
Child awareness of peers being severely punished by staff in institution	**1451**	**729**	**50.2**	**722**	**49.8**
Child awareness of peer exploitation (*types of exploitation situations*)	**1386**	**819**	**59.1**	**567**	**40.9**
Various chores (odd jobs)	1434	925	64.5	472	32.9
Steal	1429	1155	80.8	237	16.6
Beg	1428	1204	84.3	187	13.1
Give away belongings	1486	1017	68.4	431	29.0
Child awareness of peers being forced to have sex	**1163**	**892**	**76.7**	**271**	**23.3**

Note: Descriptive percentages not summing to 100% reflect missing data and/or children choosing not to respond to the question

5.3.2 Experiences of Punishments, Exploitation, and Sexual Abuse

Overall, as shown in Table 3.2, 44.6% of children reported being victims of at least one of the twelve forms of punishments administered by staff listed in the survey. Specifically, most of the children reported receiving moderate (34.7%) and severe (17.8%) corporal punishments and/or prohibition of recreational activities (10.3%). Additionally, they were forced to do chores (8.4%), denied meals (8.2%), humiliated

(6.2%), denied leaves (6.2%), threatened (6%), prohibited from family visits (2.6%), isolated from the group (2.1%), physically isolated (1.5%), or experiencing other types of punishments (0.9%). Furthermore, almost 30% of children reported experiencing at least one of the four forms of peer exploitation. Specifically, 21.9% were forced to do various chores (odd jobs) for older peers, 8.1% were forced to steal, 6.1% were forced to beg, and 21.7% were forced to give up personal belongings. In addition, 4.8% of children reported experiencing sexual abuse by staff and/or other adults or peers.

The results also (see Table 3.3) reveal that a significantly higher proportion of children in traditional and family-type institutions (49.9% and 53.7%) reported experiencing punishments compared to those in mixed-type institutions (33.2%). Additionally, a significantly higher proportion of children in traditional and family-type institutions (37.1% and 28.5%) reported experiencing peer exploitation compared to those in mixed-type institutions (15.4%). Finally, a significantly greater proportion of children in family-type institutions reported being forced to have sex (11.4%) compared to children in traditional and mixed-type institutions (4.8% and 2.7%) by staff and/or other adults or peers who were or were not in contact with them through the institution.

5.3.3 Awareness of Punishments, Exploitation, and Sexual Abuse

As seen in Table 3.2, children also were aware that their peers were severely punished by staff (49.8%), and 40.9% were aware of peers being exploited by older peers. Specifically, 32.9% were aware of others being forced to do various chores (odd jobs) for older peers, 16.6% were aware of peers being forced to steal, 13.1% were aware of peers being forced to beg, and 29% were aware of peers being forced to give up personal belongings. Moreover, 23.3% of children reported awareness of peers being sexually abused. The results also (see Table 3.3) showed that a significantly lower proportion of children in mixed-type institutions (34.3%) reported awareness of peers being punished by staff compared to those in traditional and family-type institutions (58.2% and 55%). Additionally, a significantly higher proportion of children in traditional and family-type institutions (51% and 43.4%) reported awareness of children being exploited by their peers compared to the proportion of children in mixed-type institutions (21.2%). Finally, a significantly higher proportion of children in family-type institutions (50%) reported awareness of children being forced to have sexual relationships by staff and/or other adults or peers (who were or were not in contact with them through the institution) compared to the proportion of children in traditional and mixed-type institutions (22.3% and 16.6%).

6 Discussion

Using a Romanian nationally representative sample of institutionalized children, out of 1511 children placed in 53 long-term residential centers for school-aged children that represented three different organizational types (i.e., traditional, familial,

Table 3.3 Frequencies and percentages of children's experience and awareness of abuse by the type of institutional organization

			Type of institutional organization								
	Overall		Traditional		Family type		Mixed				
	N	%	*n*	%	*n*	%	*n*	%	$\chi 2$	*Cramer's V*	*p*
Experience of punishments									**39.33**	**.164**	**< .001**
No	807	55.4	425[a]	50.1	56[a]	46.3	326[b]	66.8			
Yes	650	44.6	423[a]	49.9	65[a]	53.7	162[b]	33.2			
Experiences of exploitation									**67.27**	**.218**	**< .001**
No	1000	70.7	526[a]	62.9	88[a]	71.5	386[b]	84.6			
Yes	415	29.3	310[a]	37.1	35[a]	28.5	70[b]	15.4			
Experience of forced sex relationships									**14.73**	**.108**	**.001**
No	1199	95.2	707[a]	95.2	101[b]	88.6	391[a]	97.3			
Yes	60	4.8	36[a]	4.8	13[b]	11.4	11[a]	2.7			
Awareness of punishments									**72.71**	**.224**	**< .001**
No	729	50.2	349[a]	41.8	54[a]	45.0	326[b]	65.7			
Yes	722	49.8	486[a]	58.2	66[a]	55.0	170[b]	34.3			
Awareness of exploitation									**105.94**	**.276**	**< .001**
No	819	59.1	404[a]	49.0	69[a]	56.6	346[b]	78.8			
Yes	567	40.9	421[a]	51.0	53[a]	43.4	93[b]	21.2			
Awareness of forced sex relationships									**54.69**	**.217**	**< .001**
No	892	76.7	539[a]	77.7	57[b]	50.0	296[a]	83.4			
Yes	271	23.3	155[a]	22.3	57[b]	50.0	59[a]	16.6			

Note: Differences are tested within demographic item using *z*-test of proportions. Across rows, proportions with different superscripts within the same block (e.g., child experience of being punished by staff) are significantly different ($p < 0.05$). Differences are tested within item using *z*-test of proportions with Bonferroni corrections and mixed), nearly five in ten reported experiencing or being aware (45% and 50%) of punishments administered by institutional staff (see Table 3.2).

Additionally, nearly three in ten (29%) and four in ten (41%) reported experiencing and/or being aware of exploitation practices. Nearly five in one hundred (4.8%) declared that they experienced being forced to have sex, but nearly twenty in one hundred (23%) declared that they were aware of children being sexually abused.

These results are in agreement with previous reports highlighting an increased level of violence (i.e., abuse, bullying, or exploitation) children experienced or witnessed within long-term residential centers. Specifically, Gavrilovici and Groza (2007a) is one of the only studies we are aware of that measured the magnitude of violence perpetrated on Romanian institutionalized youth ($N = 448$; ages 8–17) in Romania (data collected in 2001 from six institutions located in rural, urban, and semi-urban settings within Iasi County). The authors found that children residing in institutions self-reported being threatened in the past year (68.8% of males and 63.9% of females), slapped/hit/punched/pushed in the institution (73% of males and 68.2% of females), beaten up in the institution (45.1% of males and 37.3% of females), attacked/stabbed with a knife (12.1% of males and 6% of females), and/or sexually abused (31.2% of males and 27% of females). Additionally, children witnessed their peers being threatened (71.6% of males and 69.5% of females), slapped/hit/punched/pushed in the institution (81.4% of males and 82.4% of females), beaten up in the institution (72.6% of males and 72.1% of females), attacked/stabbed with a knife (26.5% of males and 23.4% of females), and/or sexually abused (44.9% of males and 52.8% of females). In another study, Sekol and Farrington (2009) measured 601 young (11–21 years of age) people residing in 22 residential institutions in Croatia and found that 66.8% of children placed in children's homes and 56.3% placed in correctional homes were victims of bullying.

The analyses showed that children in traditional and, surprisingly, family-type institutions reported experiencing and awareness of punishments and exploitations in a higher proportion than those in mixed-type institutions. Additionally, a significantly higher proportion of children in traditional and, again unpredictably, family-type institutions reported experience and awareness of children being exploited by their peers compared to the proportion of children in mixed-type institutions. Finally, a completely unexpected result showed a significantly greater proportion of children in family-type institutions reported experiencing and/or awareness of children being forced to have sex compared to children in traditional and mixed-type institutions.

Overall, these results do not support the assumption that the reforms designed to diminish abuse within the long-term residential system improved children's living conditions by decreasing the level of abuse. Unpredictably, children placed within family-type long-term residential settings reported abuse as much as children in traditional residential settings.

6.1 Why Did Children in Traditional-Type Settings Report More Abuse?

Because traditional-type institutions had adverse living conditions and organizational structures (see Rus et al., 2013; Stativa et al., 2002), individualized care of children could not be provided. The ill-suited organizational features also facilitated staff and peer-to-peer aggression, and the lack of privacy allowed for many children to witness aggressive behaviors. As previously shown, these situations could have been exacerbated by inadequate management and systems of accountability and staff recruitment, training, and supervision (Colton, 2002; Monks et al., 2009); failure to segregate vulnerable children according to their age, size, or sex, from dangerous peers (Pinheiro, 2006); physical structure and size of residential settings; lack of clear placement goals, use of emergency placements, and lack of external professional assistance (Monks et al., 2009); and/or inappropriate staff conduct (Freundlich, Avery, & Padgett, 2007).

In addition, there was inconsistency in caregiving and little interaction between staff and children (Smyke, Zeanah, Fox, & Nelson, 2009), lack of educational activities (Rutter et al., 2007), and lack of individualized developmental programs for children (Children's Health Care Collaborative Study Group, 1994) that might have contributed to the violence children experienced or witnessed within long-term residential centers. In addition, peer group cultural norms in residential centers (Barter, Renold, Berridge, & Cawson, 2004; Sekol, 2013) may have also contributed to awareness of exploitation, facilitated by many factors such as deprivation, stigmatization, frustration, and poor relationships with staff (Barter et al., 2004; Sekol, 2013). Violence among peers was shaped by residents' own rules, perceptions, justifications, and group dynamics where dominant members used violence to exercise control. Due to lack of supervision, children in traditional-type institutions likely had greater opportunity to organize gangs with their own hierarchy, rules, norms, and dynamics, which could not be controlled by staff.

The culture of violence that permeated these institutions may have contributed to their status as closed institutions. Thus, without accountability to an effective external controlling authority, and without resources to enable the detection and measurement of child abuse, the extent of the abuse by staff and peers could not be determined and, consequently, was not addressed. Considering the sociological concept of "total institutions," Goffman (1961) described how power is constructed and performed. He maintained that within total institutions there are two types of segregation: (a) between the "managed" group (inmates, in a prison; children, in an orphanage) and the "supervisory" staff and (b) spatially (with both inmates in prison and children in traditional-type institutions living in restricted areas with limited contact to the outer world). For children, all aspects of life (work, play, education, sleep) were carried out in the residential institution and often in groups under firm scheduling. This regulated system of living helped staff to maintain authority and wield control by various means such as restricting opportunities to affirm or exercise agency or personal choices (for more information about total institutions in the

Romanian context, see Gavrilovici, 2007b). Consequently, these institutional characteristics might have contributed to the perpetuation of abuse.

Furthermore, the lack of specialists within institutions (psychologists, physical therapists, teachers, or social workers) and lack of professional training for staff (Stephenson et al., 1993) might have facilitated the culture of abuse. The few specialists who did work in these institutions lacked special training and thus were unable to detect or appropriately address this issue.

As shown by research on violence among prison inmates (Ireland & Ireland, 2003), the exploitation of children in residential centers can also be explained by a mutual relationship between bully and victim ("baroning") where both enter the abusive relationship with different expectations. For instance, the bully may want material goods (i.e., money, food, clothing, school supplies) or high status, whereas the victim may want protection from other peers.

Given the widespread awareness among the institutionalized children of abuse that occurred at the hands of staff members, an open question is how the awareness itself affected children's behavior. One common lay belief is that punishment, especially of the severe variety, would deter poor behavior among both punished children and children who merely observed it. In other words, staff members may believe that beating one child for a behavior could deter all the others from doing the same thing in the future. A variety of previous research has demonstrated that these observations of violence – what we have called "awareness" in the present investigation – typically result in negative behavioral and emotional outcomes for the child observers. For instance, children in families where domestic abuse occurs are often present to observe violence in their environments that they may not be directly involved in (e.g., Blair, McFarlane, Nava, Gilroy, & Maddoux, 2015; Hamby, Finkelhor, Turner, & Ormrod, 2011), and as a result, they appear to be more at risk for a variety of negative mental health outcomes, as well as behavioral problems at home and in school (Kitzmann, Gaylord, Holt, & Kenny, 2003; Lemmey et al., 2001; McFarlane, Grof, O'Brian, & Watson, 2003).

In addition to this empirical research evidence, one prominent theoretical perspective, Social Learning Theory, would also suggest that punishments (and awareness of them) may have contributed to one of the problems under study in the present investigation: exploitation/peer to peer violence. Because children who observe violent adults tend to be violent themselves, whether this violence has been committed against the children or against someone else (Bandura, 1972; Bandura & Walters, 1963; Gershoff & Grogan-Kaylor, 2016), observing harsh punishments by staff members may actually legitimize peer abuse and encourage violence and misbehavior. Some theorists have even gone so far as to suggest that observation of violence may give ideas to future perpetrators of ways to maximize the impact of the violence while at the same time minimizing the likelihood of detection. In this way, social learning may be an important trigger of future criminality as well (Burgess & Akers, 1966; Pfohl, 1994; Sutherland, 2009). Rather than curbing poor behavior, then, abuse by adult staff members may create conditions conducive to a worsening cycle of violence, negative mental health outcomes, and behavioral problems. In all, this suggests that both victimhood and awareness of abuse may be important predictors of a variety of key outcomes, and they may each be deserving of further study and consideration in the research literature.

Additionally, the punishment of children in Romanian long-term residential centers should be considered within the general context of the cultural norms, beliefs, and practices regarding parenting in Romanian society at that time. Discipline methods in institutions were likely reflective, to some extent, of discipline practices used among Romanian parents raising their own children (Browne et al., 2002; Iliescu, Preda, Stativa, Vitcu, & Ovedenie, 2007) which often included physical punishments (e.g., beating, slapping, ear and hair pulling, and shaking). Importantly for the current study, little is known about bullying or exploitation in the general population of noninstitutionalized children during the period when the data of the present study were collected. However, recently findings showed that more than 50% (Asociatia Telefonul Copilului, 2014; Filipeanu, 2012) of children or teenagers interviewed reported that they were victims of bullying in school settings, suggesting also that this phenomenon might have been present when data of this study was collected.

6.2 Why Did Children in Family-Type Settings Report More Abuse?

Undoubtedly, the new types of placement centers (i.e., family-type organization) provided more appropriate living conditions for children, knowing that they enjoyed individualized care that resembled the family model and lived within modules with up to ten children. Specifically, some of those large barracks were transformed into smaller and friendly spaces with a smaller number of children in the room, having furniture that allowed for personalization of the rooms (e.g., tables or couches), common spaces for recreation with TV, library, and club activities, and sometimes these units had their own kitchens and bathrooms. However, unexpected results in this study showed that these children reported as much or more abuse as those placed in traditional-type institutions. In comparison to children in traditional and mixed-type centers, those in family-type centers reported the highest rate of punishments and awareness of punishments as well as sexual abuse and awareness of sexual abuse. Regarding peer exploitation and awareness of peer exploitation, they reported a rate lower than traditional-type institutions but higher than mixed-type centers. These results suggest that policies prohibiting abuse in residential settings in the early 1990s most probably failed and children were exposed to high levels of abuse.

Due to the nonexperimental research design, this finding allows us only to speculate some possible explanations. Thus, one explanation could be that the privacy within the family-type institutions could have been greater than the privacy in traditional type; therefore, the opportunity to offend was possibly greater. Another possible explanation, children could seek out the caretakers who were less abusive within the traditional system, whereas children in a familial institution were not afforded this opportunity. Consequently, the latter might have been under greater duress than the former; therefore, the latter reported a higher magnitude of abuse. Furthermore, it should be highlighted that, typically, older children were placed in such family-type settings and they might have been more likely to experience abuse and open to disclose their experience and awareness of the abuse.

However, these results should be interpreted cautiously knowing that the group of children placed in family-type settings was much smaller than the other two groups (i.e., traditional and mixed type of institutions) representing only about 8% of the total number of children studied. Additionally, children were placed in these institutions only about 1 year before they were interviewed, and consequently, the reforms of the child welfare system were still ongoing and unlikely to show anticipated outcomes (reduction of the magnitude of abuse) based on what might be anticipated after reforms were fully completed.

6.3 Why Did Children in Mixed-Type Settings Report Less Abuse?

Surprisingly, children placed in mixed-type residential centers showed better results (less abuse) compared with children in traditional or family-type institutions. It is important to note that in mixed-type centers, both traditional and family-type settings coexisted within one building in varying proportions, with some children placed in the traditional setting and others in the family-type setting. One possible explanation for these results could be that in these mixed-type centers, the administrative and staff personnel were more motivated to curb the abuse of the children or children felt more secure (i.e., decreased fear of retaliation) when reporting abuse. Alternatively, some institutional characteristics could have influenced the magnitude of abuse, such as our finding reported in another study that the number of the children in dorms was associated with peer exploitation victimization (Rus et al., 2017). Future multilevel analyses, where both personal and institutional characteristics are analyzed simultaneously, could offer a better perspective of protective and risk factors regarding each form of abuse (experienced or witnessed).

7 Strengths and Limitations

Our study is the most comprehensive investigation to measure physical, emotional, and sexual abuse within Romanian residential institutions. We used a nationally representative sample of children residing in 51 institutions of varying organization types. Additionally, the design for the measurement of punishment and exploitation was based on children's feedback provided in focus group discussions, helping us to measure several abusive behaviors not previously identified and which are more specific to closed institutional systems and could be further explored in future research.

However, there are several limitations with this study. First, we only examined a particular subset of staff and peer abuse. Other types of abuse may have occurred in this population (perpetrated by both peers and adults). This includes our inability to examine in detail children who exploited other children and how exploited children may have also exploited others (learned violence). Second, our data only allowed us to examine lifetime reports of exploitation and not frequency or trends over time. Third, we were limited in our examination of the prevalence of reported abuse. In general, both under- and over-reporting are a concern with self-report data, and corroboration of these cases by a staff member would have been preferable. However, if these prevalence rates are biased in some way, the most probable direction for such bias would be gross underreporting due to fear of reprisal or retribution by peers or staff. Underreporting could also be due to a phenomenon in which abused children are transformed into abusers over time (especially for those ages 16 and older) and are thus motivated to hide their own abusive behavior (Stativa et al., 2002). In either case, self-reported data from institutionalized youth have shown acceptable reliability in the past (Sekol & Farrington, 2013). Additionally, the survey questions left open the option to report past or present experiences or some combination of these. Although types of organization (i.e., traditional, familial, and mixed) may appear to have a causal relationship with children's exploitation, the cross-sectional design does not allow such inferences to be made. Furthermore, the wording of the questions regarding especially the experience of punishments, exploitation, and sexual abuse could infer that these experiences happened in another institution where the child might have been institutionalized prior.

8 Implications for Improving Children's Care

Even though our data were collected in late 1999, this investigation of staff punishments, peer exploitation, and sexual abuse victimization and awareness has a historical value due to a lack of published research in this area. This information adds to our knowledge of the developmental environment for children in Romanian institutions in that time period. Additionally, our results may be of importance to researchers studying the anthropology of violence or vulnerable children at increased risk for staff and peer abuse and exploitation in short- or long-term institutional settings across the globe or other at-risk groups such as foster or street children.

Even though Romanian authorities had enacted policies prohibiting abuse in residential settings in the early 1990s, we found that a significant number of children still experienced abusive punishment by their caregivers, were victims of or had awareness of exploitation by peers, and/or were sexually abused. These abuses could be hidden because an older law (Law 3/1970) lacking a requirement for periodic psychological evaluation of the children by a specialist remained in place after the establishment of the new protective measure. Without an evaluation to provide a baseline and history of children's status before the new law was enacted, or ongoing issues, it was practically impossible to identify or measure abuse in institutions.

However, an evaluation requirement was later introduced into the new legal framework (see Ordinance 26/1996), and consequently, children were psychologically assessed every 3 months. Today, the child protection system has been reformed, and large state-run residential institutions have been closed or transformed into smaller facilities which coexist along with private residential homes, both having adequate quality standards of care (Bejenaru & Tucker, 2014). In the future, researchers investigating Romanian institutionalized children may want to consider whether the abusive behaviors identified in the present study have decreased since the reformation of the child protection care system.

9 Summary

By investigating the prevalence of victimization and awareness of punishments, exploitation, and sexual abuse, we found that children and adolescents experienced a profound endemic institutional betrayal (Smith & Freyd, 2014). Sadly, these vulnerable children and adolescents were not adequately protected at that time by a system that likely perpetuated a violent institutional culture that, perhaps, may also have been a reflection of the larger Romanian society at the time. In addition, we know that institutional rearing has profound consequences on children's development. Our study highlighted various harmful inputs (Humphreys & Zeanah, 2015) and further demonstrated the complex milieu that comprised life in institutional settings, including awareness and experiences of physical abuse by staff, sexual abuse, and exploitation.

Questions for Discussion

1. Choose one of the types of violence described in this study. Reflect on how this type of violence might affect a child in various domains (e.g., social, emotional, physical, developmental, academic/cognitive, communication, values/beliefs, etc.). Describe in as much detail as possible how this type of violence might affect the child in at least two of these domains, including possible long-term effects.
2. Considering the current state of children's residential settings in your own country or region, what policies and practices are currently in place to prevent violence upon children?
3. Reflecting on your response to the second question, what additional (or different) policies would you recommend to improve upon current policies? Explain the reasoning for your response.

References

Asociatia Telefonul Copilului. (2014). *Impreună pentru tot mai mulţi copii: Raport Anual 2014* [Together for more children: Annual Report 2014]. Retrieved December 14, 2015, from http://www.telefonulcopilului.ro/raport-anual-2014

Attar-Schwartz, S. (2011). Maltreatment by staff in residential care facilities: The adolescents' perspectives. *Social Service Review, 85*(4), 635–664. doi:10.1086/664009.

Attar-Schwartz, S. (2013). Runaway behavior among adolescents in residential care: The role of personal characteristics, victimization experiences while in care, social climate, and institutional factors. *Children & Youth Services Review, 35*(2), 258–267.

Attar-Schwartz, S. (2014). Experiences of sexual victimization by peers among adolescents in residential care settings. *Social Service Review, 88*(4), 594–629. doi:10.1016/j.childyouth.2012.11.005.

Attar-Schwartz, S., & Khoury-Kassabri, M. (2015). Indirect and verbal victimization by peers among at-risk youth in residential care. *Child Abuse & Neglect, 42*, 84–98. doi:10.1016/j.chiabu.2014.12.007.

Baker, L., Cunningham, A., & Male, C. (2002). *Peer-to-peer aggression in residential settings: Increasing understanding to enhance intervention*. London, ON: Centre for Children and Families in the Justice System of the London Family Court Clinic Incorporated.

Bandura, A. (1972). Modeling theory: Some traditions, trends, and disputes. In R. D. Parke (Ed.), *Recent trends in social learning theory* (pp. 35–59). New York, NY: Academic Press, Inc..

Bandura, A., & Walters, R. H. (1963). *Social learning and personality development*. New York, NY: Holt, Rinehart, and Winston.

Barter, C., Renold, E., Berridge, D., & Cawson, P. (2004). *Peer violence in children's residential care*. Palgrave MacMillan. Retrieved September 12, 2016, from http://www.palgraveconnect.com/pc/doifinder/view/10.1057/9780230005617

Bejenaru, A., & Tucker, S. (2014). Challenging dominant representations of residential childcare in Romania: An exploration of the views of children and young people living in the care system. *Journal of Youth Studies*, (ahead-of-print), 1–14. doi:10.1080/13676261.2014.918250.

Blair, F., McFarlane, J., Nava, A., Gilroy, H., & Maddoux, J. (2015). Child witness to domestic abuse: Baseline data analysis for a seven-year prospective study. *Pediatric Nursing, 41*(1), 23–29.

Browne, K., Cârtână, C., Momeu, L., Păunescu, G., Petre, N., & Tokay, R. (2002). *Child abuse and neglect in Romanian families: A national prevalence study 2000*. Bucharest, Romania: Romanian Government National Authority for Child Protection.

Burger, C., Strohmeier, D., Spröber, N., Bauman, S., & Rigby, K. (2015). How teachers respond to school bullying: An examination of self-reported intervention strategy use, moderator effects, and concurrent use of multiple strategies. *Teaching & Teacher Education, 51*, 191–202. doi:10.1016/j.tate.2015.07.004.

Burgess, R., & Akers, R. (1966). A differential association-reinforcement theory of criminal behavior. *Social Problems, 14*(2), 128–147. doi:10.2307/798612.

Chester, K. L., Callaghan, M., Cosma, A., Donnelly, P., Craig, W., Walsh, S., & Molcho, M. (2015). Cross-national time trends in bullying victimization in 33 countries among children aged 11, 13 and 15 from 2002 to 2010. *European Journal of Public Health, 25*, 261–264. doi:10.1093/eurpub/ckv029.

Children's Health Care Collaborative Study Group. (1994). The causes of children's institutionalization in Romania. *Child: Care, Health and Development, 20*, 77–88.

Colton, M. (2002). Factors associated with abuse in residential child care institutions. *Children & Society, 16*, 33–44. doi:10.1002/chi.683.

Craig, W. M., & Pepler, D. J. (2007). Understanding bullying: From research to practice. *Canadian Psychology, 48*(2), 86–93. doi:10.1037/cp2007010.

Elgar, F. J., McKinnon, B., Walsh, S. D., Freeman, J., Donnelly, P. D., de Matos, M. G., … Currie, C. (2015). Structural determinants of youth bullying and fighting in 79 countries. *The Journal of Adolescent Health, 57*(6), 643–650. doi:10.1016/j.jadohealth.2015.08.007.

Escueta, M., Whetten, K., Ostermann, J., & O'Donnell, K. (2014). Adverse childhood experiences, psychosocial well-being and cognitive development among orphans and abandoned children in five low income countries. *BMC International Health & Human Rights, 14*(1), 1–13. doi:10.1186/1472-698X-14-6.

Euser, S., Alink, L. R. A., Tharner, A., van IJzendoorn, M. H., & Bakermans-Kranenburg, M. J. (2013). The prevalence of child sexual abuse in out-of-home care: A compari-

son between abuse in residential and in foster care. *Child Maltreatment*, *18*(4), 221–231. doi:10.1177/1077559513489848.
Euser, S., Alink, L. R. A., Tharner, A., van IJzendoorn, M. H., & Bakermans-Kranenburg, M. J. (2014). Out of home placement to promote safety? The prevalence of physical abuse in residential and foster care. *Children and Youth Services Review*, *37*, 3764–3770. doi:10.1016/j.childyouth.2013.12.002.
Euser, S., Alink, L. R. A., Tharner, A., van IJzendoorn, M. H., & Bakermans-Kranenburg, M. J. (2016). The prevalence of child sexual abuse in out-of-home care: Increased risk for children with a mild intellectual disability. *Journal of Applied Research in Intellectual Disabilities*, *29*, 83–92. doi:10.1111/jar.12160.
Filipeanu, I. (2012). *Fenomenul "bullying" la adolescent* [Bully phenomenon among teenagers] (Unpublished dissertation). Bucharest University, Faculty of Psychology and Educational Sciences, Bucharest, Romania.
Freundlich, M., Avery, R. J., & Padgett, D. (2007). Care or scare: The safety of youth in congregate care in New York City. *Child Abuse & Neglect*, *31*(2), 173–186.
Gavrilovici, O. (2007). *Past and present of total institutions. Romania as a case-study*. The International Conference "An agenda for children. Local, national and European programmes to combat social exclusion", 3–5 May. Florence, Italy: Istituto degli Innocenti.
Gavrilovici, O., & Groza, V. (2007). Incidence, prevalence and trauma associated with exposure to violence in Romanian institutionalized children. *International Journal of Child & Family Welfare*, *10*(3–4), 125–138.
Gershoff, G. T., & Grogan-Kaylor, A. (2016). Spanking and child outcomes: Old controversies and new meta-analyses. *Journal of Family Psychology*, *30*. doi:10.1037/fam0000191.
Goffman, E. (1961). *Asylums: Essays on the social situation of mental patients and other inmates*. New York, NY: Anchor Books.
Gray, C. L., Pence, B. W., Ostermann, J., Whetten, R. A., O'Donnell, K., Thielman, N. M., & Whetten, K. (2015). Prevalence and incidence of traumatic experiences among orphans in institutional and family-based settings in 5 low- and middle-income countries: A longitudinal study. *Global Health, Science and Practice*, *3*(3), 395–404. doi:10.9745/GHSP-D-15-00093.
Haarr, R. N. (2011). *Violence against children in state-run residential institutions in Kazakhstan: An assessment*. Astana, Kazakhstan: United Nations Children's Fund. Retrieved September 20, 2016, from http://www.ceecis.org/ccc/publications/Violence_against_children_in_state-run_residential_institutions_in_Kazakhstan_2011_ENG.pdf
Hamby, S., Finkelhor, D., Turner, H., & Ormrod, R. (2011). Children's exposure to intimate partner violence and other family violence (pp. 1–12). *Juvenile Justice Bulletin – NCJ 232272*. Washington, DC: U.S. Government Printing Office (CV197).
Harel-Fisch, Y., Walsh, S. D., Fogel-Grinvald, H., Amitai, G., Pickett, W., Molcho, M., … Craig, W. (2011). Negative school perceptions and involvement in school bullying: A universal relationship across 40 countries. *Journal of Adolescence*, *34*(4), 639–652. doi:10.1016/j.adolescence.2010.09.008.
Hermenau, K., Eggert, I., Landolt, M. A., & Hecker, T. (2015). Neglect and perceived stigmatization impact psychological distress of orphans in Tanzania. *European Journal of Psychotraumatology*, *6*, 28617. doi:10.3402/ejpt.v6.28617.
Hermenau, K., Hecker, T., Elbert, T., & Ruf-Leuschner, M. (2014). Maltreatment and mental health in institutional care – Comparing early and late institutionalized children in Tanzania. *Infant Mental Health Journal*, *35*(2), 102–110. doi:10.1002/imhj.21440.
Hermenau, K., Hecker, T., Ruf, M., Schauer, E., Elbert, T., & Schauer, M. (2011). Childhood adversity, mental ill-health and aggressive behavior in an African orphanage: Changes in response to trauma-focused therapy and the implementation of a new instructional system. *Child & Adolescent Psychiatry & Mental Health*, *5*(1), 29–37. doi:10.1186/1753-2000-5-29.
Humphreys, K. L., & Zeanah, C. H. (2015). Deviations from the expectable environment in early childhood and emerging psychopathology. *Neuropsychopharmacology*, *40*(1), 154–170. http://doi.org/10.1038/npp.2014.165.

IBM Corp. Released 2015. *IBM SPSS statistics for Windows, version 23*. Armonk, NY: Author.

Iliescu, M., Preda, V., Stativa, E., Vitcu, A., & Ovedenie, A. (2007). *Knowledge, attitudes and practices on parenting in Romania. Section II*. Buzau, Romania: Alpha MDN.

Ireland, J. L. (1999). Bullying behaviors among male and female prisoners: A study of adult and young offenders. *Aggressive Behavior*, *25*(3), 161–178. doi:10.1002/(SICI)1098-2337(1999)25:3<161::AID-AB1>3.0.CO;2-.

Ireland, J. L., & Ireland, C. A. (2003). How do offenders define bullying? A study of adult, young and juvenile male offenders. *Legal & Criminological Psychology*, *8*(2), 159–173. doi:10.1348/135532503322362942.

Ireland, J. L., & Snowden, P. (2002). Bullying in secure hospitals. *Journal of Forensic Psychiatry*, *13*(3), 538–554. doi:10.1080/0958518021000019434.

Khoury-Kassabri, M., & Attar-Schwartz, S. (2014). Adolescents' reports of physical violence by peers in residential care settings: An ecological examination. *Journal of Interpersonal Violence*, *29*(4), 659–682. doi:10.1177/0886260513505208.

Kitzmann, D., Gaylord, N., Holt, A., & Kenny, E. (2003). Child witness to domestic violence: A meta-analytic review. *Journal of Consulting and Clinical Psychology*, *71*, 339–352. doi:10.1037/0022-006X.71.2.339.

Kyriakides, L., Kaloyirou, C., & Lindsay, G. (2006). An analysis of the Revised Olweus Bully/Victim Questionnaire using the Rasch measurement model. *British Journal of Educational Psychology*, *76*(4), 781–801. doi:10.1348/000709905X53499.

Lemmey, D., Malecha, A., McFarlane, J., Willson, P., Watson, K., Gist, J., … Schultz, P. (2001). Severity of violence against women correlates with behavioral problems in their children. *Pediatric Nursing*, *27*, 265–270.

Luna, M., Luna, M. T., & Brizuela, M. S. (2011). *Institutionalised childhood and adolescence: Making serious human rights violations visible*. Washington, DC: Mental Disability Rights International.

McFarlane, J., Grof, J., O'Brian, J., & Watson, K. (2003). Behaviors of children who are exposed and not exposed to intimate partner violence: An analysis of 330 Black, White and Hispanic children. *Pediatrics*, *112*, e202–e207.

Monks, C. P., Smith, P. K., Naylor, P., Barter, C., Ireland, J. L., & Coyne, I. (2009). Bullying in different contexts: Commonalities, differences and the role of theory. *Aggression and Violent Behavior*, *14*(2), 146–156. doi:10.1016/j.avb.2009.01.004.

Morantz, G., & Heymann, J. (2010). Life in institutional care: The voices of children in a residential facility in Botswana. *AIDS Care*, *22*(1), 10–16. doi:10.1080/09540120903012601.

Olweus, D. (2011). Bullying at school and later criminality: Findings from three Swedish community samples of males. *Criminal Behaviour and Mental Health*, *21*(2), 151–156. doi:10.1002/cbm.806.

Pfohl, S. J. (1994). *Images of deviance and social control: A sociological history*. New York, NY: McGraw-Hill.

Pinchover, S., & Attar-Schwartz, S. (2014). Institutional social climate and adjustment difficulties of adolescents in residential care: The mediating role of victimization by peers. *Children & Youth Services Review*, 44393–44399. doi:10.1016/j.childyouth.2014.07.005.

Pinheiro, P. S. (2006). *World report on violence against children*. Geneva, Switzerland: United Nations.

Rosenthal, J. A., Motz, J. K., Edmonson, D. A., & Groze, V. (1991). A descriptive study of abuse and neglect in out-of-home-placement. *Child Abuse & Neglect*, *15*(3), 249–260. doi:10.1016/0145-2134(91)90069-P.

Rus, A. V., Parris, S., Cross, D., Purvis, K., & Drăghici, S. (2011). Reforming the Romanian child welfare system: 1990–2010. *Review of Research and Social Intervention*, *34*, 56–72.

Rus, A. V., Stativa, E., Butterfield, M. E., Pennings, J. S., Parris, S. R., Burcea, G., & Wenyika, R. (2017). Peer Exploitation: Findings from a Romanian Nationally Representative Sample of Children Living in Long-Term Residential Centres. *Child Abuse Review*. doi:10.1002/car.2464.

Rus, A. V., Stativa, E., Pennings, J. S., Cross, D. R., Ekas, N., Purvis, K., & Parris, S. R. (2013). Severe punishment of children by staff in Romanian placement centers for school-aged chil-

dren: Effects of child and institutional characteristics. *Child Abuse & Neglect, 37*(12), 1152–1162. doi:10.1016/j.chiabu.2013.07.003.
Rutter, M., Beckett, C., Castle, J., Colvert, E., Kreppner, J., Mehta, M., ... Sonuga-Barke, E. (2007). Effects of profound early institutional deprivation: An overview of findings from a UK longitudinal study of Romanian adoptees. *European Journal of Developmental Psychology, 4*(3), 332–350. doi:10.1080/17405620701401846.
Segura, A., Pereda, N., Abad, J., & Guilera, G. (2015). Victimization and polyvictimization among Spanish youth protected by the child welfare system. *Children and Youth Services Review, 59*, 105–112. doi:10.1016/j.childyouth.2015.10.011.
Segura, A., Pereda, N., Guilera, G., & Abad, J. (2016). Poly-victimization and psychopathology among Spanish adolescents in residential care. *Child Abuse & Neglect, 55*, 40–51. doi:10.1016/j.chiabu.2016.03.009.
Sekol, I. (2013). Peer violence in adolescent residential care: A qualitative examination of contextual and peer factors. *Children and Youth Services Review, 35*(12), 1901–1912. doi:10.1016/j.childyouth.2013.09.006.
Sekol, I., & Farrington, D. P. (2009). The nature and prevalence of bullying among boys and girls in Croatian care institutions: A descriptive analysis of children's homes and correctional homes. *Kriminologija & Socijalna Integracija, 17*(2), 15–34.
Sekol, I., & Farrington, D. P. (2013). The reliability and validity of self, peer and staff reports of bullying and victimisation in correctional and care institutions. *Psychology, Crime & Law, 19*(4), 329–344. doi:10.1080/1068316X.2011.631541.
Smith, C., & Freyd, J. (2014). Institutional betrayal. *The American Psychologist, 69*(6), 575–587. doi:10.1037/a0037564.
Smith, P. K., Cowie, H. H., Olafsson, R. F., & Liefooghe, A. D. (2002). Definitions of bullying: A comparison of terms used, and age and gender differences, in a fourteen–country international comparison. *Child Development, 73*(4), 1119–1133.
Smith, P. K., Pepler, D., & Rigby, K. (2004). *Bullying in schools: How successful can interventions be?* New York, NY: Cambridge University Press. doi:10.1017/CBO9780511584466.
Smyke, A., Zeanah, C., Fox, N., & Nelson, C. (2009). A new model of foster care for young children: The Bucharest Early Intervention Project. *Child and Adolescent Psychiatric Clinics of North America, 18*(3), 721–734. doi:10.1016/j.chc.2009.03.003.
Solberg, M., Olweus, D., & Endresen, I. (2007). Bullies and victims at school: Are they the same pupils? *The British Journal of Educational Psychology, 77*(2), 441–464. doi:10.1348/000709906X105689.
Solberg, M. E., & Olweus, D. (2003). Prevalence estimation of school bullying with the Olweus Bully/Victim Questionnaire. *Aggressive Behavior, 29*(3), 239–268. doi:10.1002/ab.10047.
Spröber, N., Schneider, T., Rassenhofer, M., Seitz, A., Liebhardt, H., König, L., & Fegert, J. M. (2014). Child sexual abuse in religiously affiliated and secular institutions: A retrospective descriptive analysis of data provided by victims in a government-sponsored reappraisal program in Germany. *BMC Public Health, 14*(1), 282–293. doi:10.1186/1471-2458-14-282.
Stativa, E., Anghelescu, C., Palicari, G., Stanescu, A., & Nanu, R. (2002). *Child abuse in residential care institutions in Romania*. Bucharest, Romania: Extrem Group.
Stephenson, P., Anghelescu, C., Fumarel, S., Georgescu, A., Iorgulescu, D., McCreery, R., ... Staviva, E. (1993). Training needs of staff in Romanian institutions for young children. *Child: Care, Health and Development, 19*, 221–234. doi:10.1111/j.1365-2214.1993.tb00728.x.
Sutherland, E. H. (2009). A sociological theory of criminal behavior. In F. R. Scarpitti, A. L. Nielsen, & J. M. Miller (Eds.), *Crime and criminals contemporary and classic readings in criminology* (2nd ed., pp. 211–213). New York, NY: Oxford University Press.
Swearer, S. M., Peugh, J., Espelage, D. L., Siebecker, A. B., Kingsbury, W. L., & Bevins, K. S. (2006). A social-ecological model for bullying prevention and intervention in early adolescence: An exploratory examination. In S. R. Jimerson & M. Furlong (Eds.), *Handbook of school violence and school safety: From research to practice* (pp. 257–273). Mahwah, NJ: Lawrence Erlbaum Associates Publishers.

Timmerman, M. C., & Schreuder, P. R. (2014). Sexual abuse of children and youth in residential care: An international review. *Aggression & Violent Behavior, 19*(6), 715–720. doi:10.1016/j.avb.2014.09.001.

UN General Assembly. (1989, November 20). *Convention on the rights of the child* (United Nations, Treaty Series, Vol. 1577, p. 3). Available at http://www.refworld.org/docid/3ae6b38f0.html

Whetten, K., Ostermann, J., Whetten, R., O'Donnell, K., & Thielman, N. (2011). More than the loss of a parent: Potentially traumatic events among orphaned and abandoned children. *Journal of Traumatic Stress, 24*(2), 174–182. doi:10.1002/jts.20625.

World Health Organization. (2016). *Inspire: Seven strategies for ending violence against children* (Executive Summary, p. 11). Geneva, Switzerland: WHO Press, World Health Organization. Retrieved from http://apps.who.int/iris/bitstream/10665/246212/1/WHO-NMH-NVI-16.7-eng.pdf?ua=1

Chapter 4
Academic Achievement of Romanian Institutionalized Children: A Social–Ecological Approach

Adrian V. Rus, Ecaterina Stativa, Sheri R. Parris, Jacquelyn S. Pennings, Florin Tibu, Reggies Wenyika, and Gabriel Burcea

> *If we want the best academic outcomes, the most efficient and cost-effective route to achieve that is, counterintuitively, not to narrowly focus on academics, but to also address children's social, emotional, and physical development.*
>
> Adele Diamond (2010, p. 780)

A.V. Rus (✉)
Department of Social and Behavioral Sciences, Southwestern Christian University, 7210 NW 39th Expressway, Bethany, OK 73008-0340, USA
e-mail: adrian.rus@swcu.edu; aadrianrus@gmail.com

E. Stativa
Social Pediatrics and Obstetrics Research Department, The National Institute for Mother and Child Health "Alessandrescu-Rusescu", Bucharest, Romania
e-mail: ecaterina.stativa@gmail.com

S.R. Parris
Texas Christian University, Fort Worth, TX, USA
e-mail: sheri.parris@gmail.com

J.S. Pennings
Elite Research, LLC, Irving, TX, USA
e-mail: jacspen@gmail.com

F. Tibu
Institute of Child Development, Bucharest, Romania
e-mail: florin.tibu@idc.ro

R. Wenyika
Southwestern Christian University, Bethany, OK, USA
e-mail: reggies.wenyika@swcu.edu

G. Burcea
Goldsmiths, University of London, London, UK
e-mail: gb.burcea@gmail.com

A.V. Rus et al. (eds.), *Child Maltreatment in Residential Care*,
DOI 10.1007/978-3-319-57990-0_4

1 Introduction

Undoubtedly, a relatively recent large body of evidence has consistently shown that there is a link between maltreatment (i.e., abuse and neglect) of children in their biological families and their subsequent educational achievement. Consequently, many of the children who experience maltreatment on average receive lower ratings of performance from their school teachers, score lower on cognitive assessments and standardized tests of academic achievement, are more likely to get suspended from school and retained in their grade, have lower grade point averages (GPA), have problems completing homework assignments and report less academic engagement, and are less likely to anticipate attending college (Eckenrode & Laird, 1993; Egeland, Sroufe, & Erickson, 1983; Kendall-Tackett & Eckenrode, 1996; Lansford et al., 2002; Rowe & Eckenrode, 1999; Shonk, Cicchetti, Susan, & Dante, 2001; Slade & Wissow, 2007).

In the context of the foregoing, the focus of this chapter is to show that maltreatment is associated with children's academic performance not only in children living in typical communities but also in their institutionalized counterparts. Before we begin, we should note that there are many ways to describe the settings where separated or orphaned children are cared for: orphanages, care institutions, institutional care facilities, residential care facilities, or long-term residential centers (which are preferred in this study). These terms are often used interchangeably in the literature. In the present study we assessed the relationship between maltreatment and academic performance of children living within the system of Romanian institutional care facilities, once considered one of the worst child-protection care systems in the world (see Viacheslav Samoskin, as cited in National Authority for the Protection of Child's Rights & Phare 2003 "Educational Campaign on Child's Rights", 2006). As far as we know, there are no large empirical studies that have systematically measured academic performance in Romanian institutionalized children, and, therefore, in this chapter we are presenting (1) a brief introduction on the topics of maltreatment and educational performance of institutionalized children and (2) an investigation of children's experience of punishments by staff, as well as other individual and institutional risks and protective factors that may be associated with Romanian children's academic performance.

2 Maltreatment and Educational Performance of Institutionalized Children

As shown by a large body of evidence accumulated in recent years, institutionalization in long-term residential centers is often accompanied by the experiencing and/or witnessing of abuse (i.e., emotional, physical, or sexual) by staff and/or peers (Attar-Schwartz & Khoury-Kassabri, 2015; Attar-Schwartz, 2011, 2013, 2014; Euser, Alink, Tharner, van IJzendoorn, & Bakermans-Kranenburg, 2014, Euser,

Alink, Tharner, van IJzendoorn, & Bakermans-Kranenburg, 2016; Gray et al., 2015; Haarr, 2011; Hermenau, Hecker, Elbert, & Ruf-Leuschner, 2014; Hermenau et al., 2011; Rus et al., 2013; Segura, Pereda, Abad, & Guilera, 2015). The associated traumas experienced by institutionalized children subjected to abuse have significant negative consequences on their well-being (e.g., Escueta, Whetten, Ostermann, & O'Donnell, 2014; Hermenau et al., 2011, 2014; Segura, Pereda, Guilera, & Abad, 2016; Whetten, Ostermann, Whetten, O'Donnell, & Thielman, 2011), including poor academic performance and school functioning (Attar-Schwartz, 2009).

Neglect is the most common form of child maltreatment (Kaplan, Schene, DePanfilis, & Gilmore, 2009) and is manifested by depriving the child of some or all of the most basic physical and psychological needs such as shelter and food security, access to health services, and a nurturing environment. Largely, the abandonment and institutionalization of children represent extreme forms of deprivation that put children at risk for various forms of abuse, neglect, and adverse developmental and health outcomes. The deleterious effects of institutionalization are evident in numerous developmental domains, both physical and psychosocial, and can be long-lasting (Rutter et al., 2010), even though some recent studies show that institutionalized children do not have worse health, emotional and cognitive functioning, or physical growth compared to street children and orphans or abandoned children in other types of care (Braitstein et al., 2013; Whetten et al., 2009). Children raised in institutions exhibit deficits in cognitive (e.g., IQ, executive functioning), emotional (e.g., psychopathology), and social functioning (e.g., disrupted peer relationships) with potentially devastating consequences for well-being outcomes during adulthood (Hodges & Tizard, 1989; Nelson, Fox, & Zeanah, 2014; Rutter, Kreppner, O'Connor, & ERA Study Team, 2001).

Cognitive abilities such as intelligence quotient (IQ; Barnett, 1998) and executive functioning (Alloway & Alloway, 2010) are important prerequisites and powerful predictors of academic achievement in both community and disadvantaged populations of children. Intellectual abilities of children reared in institutions have been reported to be markedly diminished, and for some of these children, their cognition remains compromised long after they are removed from the severely deprived environment (Rutter et al., 1998). For example, in the Bucharest Early Intervention Project (BEIP), which is the first randomized controlled study of foster care as an alternative to institutional care, the mean developmental quotient (DQ; a crude measure of IQ) at age 2 years in a sample of 136 children recruited from Romanian orphanages was an astounding 65 compared to 103 in the control group (see Zeanah et al., 2003). Following randomization, the BEIP children who had been placed in a high-quality foster care group had significantly higher IQ scores at ages 42 and 54 months than the children assigned to the care as usual condition (often consisting of continued institutional care), providing experimental evidence that family placement following institutionalization was tremendously beneficial in terms of cognitive development. The children who benefited most from the foster care intervention were those who had been removed from institutions before 18 months of age (Nelson et al., 2007). Other studies with previously institutionalized children, like the English and Romanian Adoptees Study (ERAS; Rutter et al., 2010) and the Minnesota and Wisconsin

International Adoption Studies (Pollak et al., 2010), also found lower IQ scores compared to never institutionalized children (e.g., Beckett et al., 2006; Kumsta et al., 2015; Loman, Wiik, Frenn, Pollak, & Gunnar, 2009); though, these findings suggested that the children who had been exposed to institutionalization but started living in families during infancy showed significant cognitive catch-up compared to those who were removed from the orphanages at later ages (Beckett et al., 2006).

Similarly, executive functions, which are higher-order skills that regulate cognition and behavior, such as inhibition, working memory, set-shifting, and planning (Miyake, Friedman, Rettinger, Shah, & Hegarty, 2001) and deemed essential for academic success, have been found to be impaired following institutionalization (Bos, Fox, Zeanah, & Nelson, 2009; Loman et al., 2009; Pollak et al., 2010), and foster care intervention could not remediate these deficits (Bos et al., 2009; Tibu et al., 2016). Together, these findings on cognitive outcomes point to the conclusion that institutionalization can have very detrimental long-term effects on IQ and other cognitive functions, except when deprivation has ceased during early infancy.

In line with the poor outcomes on cognitive abilities, there is also strong evidence for lower academic performance in previously institutionalized children. For example, in the ERAS, Beckett et al. (2007) found reduced school achievement at age 11 years, and this association was mainly explained by low IQ. Similarly, a study conducted by Vorria, Ntouma, and Rutter (2015) showed reduced, yet not dramatically lower, teacher-reported grades in 13-year-old children adopted after a mean of 2 years spent in a baby home in Athens, Greece, compared to community controls.

In a large study conducted on over 4000 Israeli adolescents who spent an average of 3 years in institutional care (but not necessarily at a young age), Attar-Schwartz (2009) found a high incidence (i.e., 52%) of low school achievement as reported by the children's caregivers and social workers. In a series of longitudinal studies, Tan and colleagues (Tan, 2009; Tan, Rice, & Mahoney, 2015) investigated the effects of early institutional care on academic performance in a sample of adolescent girls who were adopted by families in the United States from Chinese orphanages during their first 2 years of life. In his 2009 study, Tan used child self-reports, in addition to parent reports, to measure how 9- and 11-year-old children were performing in school. The self-report measure was an adaptation of the teacher report section on academic performance in the Social Skills Rating System (SSRS; Gresham & Elliott, 1990). Results showed that between 15% and 18% of the participants encountered severe difficulties in academic achievement. Moreover, overall developmental delay at adoption time predicted school performance at age 11 years, and the link was mediated by attention difficulties at age 9 years. Similarly, at age 14 years, Tan et al. (2015) reported lower self-reported academic performance in the participants with gross motor developmental delay at adoption.

In the BEIP, academic performance at age 8 years (measured through teacher reports) was poorer in the children who remained in institutions compared to community controls (McDermott, Westerlund, Zeanah, Nelson, & Fox, 2012). Interestingly, in the foster care group, only the children with enhanced error-monitoring brain activity had academic results that were comparable to those obtained by children raised in families, which suggests that increased school performance depends not only on positive changes in the environment but also on the recovery of the cerebral substrates of cognitive functioning.

The meta-analysis conducted by van IJzendoorn, Juffer, and Klein Poelhuis (2005) revealed a significant catch-up in school performance for the adopted children compared to those who continued to live in disadvantaged pre-adoption conditions. However, compared to community children, in their new environment the adoptees continued to have poorer academic performance unless they had been adopted before their first birthday. Indeed, for children removed from their deprived environment during the first year of life, the difference in school achievement compared to control children was minimal. That difference reached statistical significance only when those adopted in their second year of life were considered, and the gap increased to even higher levels when adoption took place at age 2 and beyond. Taken together, findings from this meta-analysis and the other studies that we reviewed generally point to lower academic performance in previously institutionalized children, with the lowest achievement found in those who had stayed in orphanages beyond age 1 or 2 years.

3 Context and Research Purposes of the Current Study

The data in the current study were collected in 1999, during a period of reforms that began in 1990 within the Romanian child welfare system (for a review, see Rus et al., 2011). The reforms were undertaken by the Romanian government to comply with the United Nations Convention on the Rights of the Child (UN General Assembly, 1989). Reforms included (a) informing children of their rights and imposing a ban on all types of physical and emotional abuse by staff or peers, (b) the creation of alternatives to institutional settings (such as family-type centers), (c) regulation of adoptions, (d) support for families to prevent children from being placed in residential care settings, and (e) the decentralization or closing of large institutions. While traditional residential institutions were eventually eliminated, some were still in operation when our data was collected in 1999. The *traditional institutions* were large buildings that housed large numbers of children who experienced inconsistency in caregivers (e.g., high rate of caregiver turnover) and high levels of staff and peers abuse. The newer *family-type* centers housed fewer children in small units (e.g., houses or apartments) or utilized large buildings that had been compartmentalized into smaller groups of up to ten children. The rooms and daily activities were organized to resemble a family model and to provide individualized care (Stativa, Anghelescu, Palicari, Stanescu, & Nanu, 2002). *Mixed-type* centers contained both traditional and family-type settings within the same building (Stativa et al., 2002).

The present investigation, based on a prior survey conducted on child neglect and abuse in residential institutions in Romania (Rus et al., 2013; Stativa et al., 2002), sought to expand our knowledge about the impact of these traumatic experiences on children's academic performance, especially by highlighting different facets of children's personal characteristics, experience of punishments administered by staff, and institutional features that can function as risk or protective factors. Subsequently, the main research purposes of this study were to respond to the following questions: (1) How do children in Romanian long-term residential centers perceive their own academic performance? (2) What are the most important demographic (i.e., age, gender, and child's provenance from a different center or biological family), individual experience (e.g., punishments that the child experienced by staff, type of education, knowledge of projected duration of stay in institution, having trusted adults in institutions, and having help with homework), and environmental predictors (i.e., the institution's openness to protect children's right to education and health, optimal night child–staff ratio, and institutional type of organization) that are linked to children's self-reported academic performance?

Even though the data for the present study were collected in the late 1990s, investigating the predictors of institutionalized children's academic performance has a historical value due to a lack of published research in this area. Additionally, it is expected that such an inquiry will help to provide a more comprehensive picture of the individual and ecological factors that could be used to identify especially vulnerable institutionalized children who are at risk for poor academic performance.

4 Method

A secondary analysis was conducted using data collected during the cross-sectional Survey on Child Abuse in Residential Care Institutions in Romania (SCARCIR; Stativa et al., 2002). Further descriptions of the purpose of SCARCIR, as well as the sampling methods, data collection procedure, participants, and the characteristics of the resultant dataset, are presented elsewhere (for a complete review, see Rus et al., 2013; Stativa et al., 2002).

4.1 Participants

The original dataset included a national representative sample of 3164 children (1701 boys and 1463 girls) in residential care institutions with ages between 0 and 19 years ($M = 9.45$; $SD = 5.39$), representing 7.8% of the entire population of institutionalized Romanian children in 1999. Three criteria were used to include children from the original data in the current secondary analysis, namely, to be (a) 7 years of age or older, (b) formally enrolled in an education program, and (c) to have provided a self-assessment of their academic performance. Therefore, participants from the original SCARCIR data set who did not meet the three abovementioned criteria were excluded, resulting in a final sample for the current study of 1479 children (783 boys and 696 girls) with ages between 7 and 19 years (M = 12.69; SD = 2.83; Mdn = 13.00) living in 53 long-term residential centers. The mean total time of institutionalization was 77.14 months (SD = 53.11; Mdn = 70), and this ranged from 0 to 221 months. The mean age of children at their first placement was 72.67 months (SD = 48.03; Mdn = 79.00), with a range from 0 to 218 months. Additionally, the vast majority of children (87.4%) were not diagnosed as having an intellectual disability.

4.2 *Measures*

4.2.1 The Dependent Variable: Self-Reported Academic Achievement

The outcome, self-reported academic achievement was measured by administering the question "How do you learn at school?" (Romanian: "Cum înveți la școală"). This measurement provided four response options for children: *poor, fair, good,* and *very good.* Then, a binomial variable was created by grouping *poor/fair* and *good/ very good* responses together.

4.3 *Predictors*

The data also included several pieces of information that we used as predictors of self-reported academic achievement and were categorized as child-level and institution level measures.

4.3.1 Child-Level Predictors

These included gender (0 = *female*; 1 = *male*), age at assessment (in years) and at first placement (in months), time spent by the child in long-term residential centers (in months), and presence of a documented intellectual disability (0 = *no*; 1 = *yes*). Children with intellectual disability had this diagnosis documented in their file. The experience of being punished by staff is a composite variable derived from combining the responses on 12 different types of punishments. Specifically, children responded whether or not they ever experienced (1) humiliation (humiliating language, attitudes, and gestures), (2) threatening (blackmail), (3) prohibition of family visits, (4) prohibition of recreation activities, (5) prohibition of meals, (6) prohibition of leaves, (7) obligatory chores, (8) mild corporal punishments (including spankings, punches, kicks, or ear and hair-pulling), (9) severe corporal punishments (including with a plank or a wet rope), (10) physical isolation (forcing the child to stand in a corner), (11) isolation from group (isolating the child from other children when they were playing), and (12) other punishments. The measurement of these 12 methods of punishment had a binary distribution (*no* versus *yes*). Those institutionalized children who answered *yes* to any of these items were coded as having been punished by staff. Those children who answered *no* to all items were coded as not having been punished by the staff. Based on these 12 responses, the composite variable was created summing up the responses (0 = *no*; 1 = *yes*). It is important to highlight that this composite variable does not show the number of times a child was punished but is a count of the different types of punishments they received (for more information about these variable, see Chap. 3). Additionally, child-level predictors also included the provenance of the child or the setting from where they came before entering the current institution (0 = *from their biological family*; 1 = *from another long-term residential center*), knowledge of projected duration of stay in institution (0 = *no, the child was not told how long he/she would stay in the center*; 1 = *yes, the child was told how long he/she would stay in the center*), presence of trusted adult(s) in institution (0 = *no*; 1 = *yes, one* or *more than one*), presence of trusted child in institution (0 = *no*; 1 = *yes*), presence of siblings in institution (0 = *no*; 1 = *yes*), being offered help with homework (0 = *no*; 1 = *yes*), presence of parental relationship (0 = *no*; 1 = *yes*), and child's level of education which was coded into four categories (0 = *primary*, 1 = *gymnasium* [grades 5 to 8; including special gymnasium schools], 2 = *vocational* [trade schools, grades 9 to 10; including special complementary apprentice and special vocational schools], and 3 = *lyceum* [high school; including special lyceums]).

4.3.2 Institution-Level Predictors

Here we included several variables deemed relevant for characterizing the institutional environment, and this information was included in SCARCIR. These were optimal ratio of children to caregivers during the night shift (for more information about these standards, see American Academy of Pediatrics, American Public Health Association, and National Resource Center for Health and Safety in Child Care and Early Education, 2011), number of children in dormitory room, institution location (*urban* vs. *rural*), institution size (*small* vs. *medium* vs. *large*), and type of institution (*traditional* vs. *family type* vs. *mixed type*). Additionally, we assessed the institution's openness to respect universal human rights such as the right to education and health (for more information about how these variables were computed and their definitions, see Chap. 2). The mean for how well the institution protected the right to education was 2.59 ($SD = 0.69$) which ranged from 0 to 3, and the mean for how well the institution protected the right to health was 3.01 ($SD = 1.45$) which ranged from 0 to 5, with higher scores the better.

4.4 Data Analysis Plan

All analyses, including accuracy of data coding and entry and the statistical assumptions of the tests, were conducted using SPSS version 19.0 (IBM SPSS, 2010) and the R program (R Development Core Team, 2016). As detailed below, for most of the variables no data were missing. For the dependent variables and variables regarding children's characteristics (i.e., education performance; gender; age at assessment and at first placement; time spent in institutions; presence of intellectual handicap; experience and/or awareness of punishments, exploitation by peers, and sexual abuse; provenance of the children; knowledge of duration of stay in institution; trusted adults and peers in institution; sibling in institutions; help with homework; parental relationship), the percentage of missing data ranged from 0.7% to 23%. In the case of institution-related variables (i.e., institution location, institution size, institution's openness to respect universal human rights such as the right to identity, personal history, free expression of opinion, information, periodic review of the protective measure, protective measure and legal status, have a family, personalized care, and quality care), the percentage of missing data was between 0.7% and 12%. Each analysis was conducted with all available data (pairwise deletion) and no imputation was conducted for the missing cases.

Because the data was hierarchical in nature with institutionalized children (N = 1479) nested within 53 institutions, and the measurement of self-reported educational performance had a binary distribution (poor/fair versus good/very good), multilevel (hierarchical) logistic regression models (Gelman & Hill, 2007) were used to examine the effects of individual level experience of punishments and institution-level variables on academic achievement and to account for the clustering of the children within institutions. Multilevel analysis was performed primarily using the *lme4* (Bates, Maechler, Bolker, & Walker, 2015) and *R2MLwiN* packages (Browne, 2012; Rasbash, Steele, Browne, & Goldstein, 2012; Zhang, Charlton, Parker, Leckie, & Browne, 2016) which are additional statistical software packages for the *R* program (R Development Core Team, 2016).

Institution, county, and region were tested both individually and combined. A statistical comparison of the empty models revealed that institution alone as the random intercept accounted for more variance. As a preliminary step, each predictor was tested in a separate logistic model with institution as the random intercept. Predictors that were significant at $p < 0.10$ were considered for inclusion in the subsequent models. Next, the predictors selected from the preliminary step were combined with each of the others in order to determine which variables to include in the final models.

Additionally, those variables considered conceptually important for the authors were included in the models even though they were not found significant within the preliminary step. The fit of each nested model was compared with the previous model using the likelihood ratio test (−2 log-likelihood), wherein each successive model was compared with previous models: the first model was compared with the empty (unconditional) model without explanatory variables, and the second model was compared with the first model. Using a chi-squared distribution, the differences between models were compared to determine significant changes between models.

The child-level predictors that were verified in the models but that were not found to be significantly predictive of self-reported academic performance included age at placement, time spent in institution, presence of intellectual disability, exploitation by peers, sexual abuse, and the awareness of peers being punished by staff, exploited by peers, or sexually abused. Institution-level predictors that that were verified in the models but that were not found to be significantly predictive of self-reported academic performance included institution location (urban vs. rural), institution size, institution openness to respect universal human rights such as the right to identity, personal history, free expression of opinion, information, periodic review of the protective measure, protective measure and legal status, have a family, personalized care, and quality care (for more information, see Chap. 2).

5 Results

5.1 Descriptive Analysis

As seen in Table 4.1, the majority of children reported good (45.0%) and fair (38.4%) academic performance. When the responses were combined, more than half of the children (53.5%) stated that they had a very good/good academic performance. Most of the children were enrolled in primary (40.9%) and gymnasium (44.8%) level of education.

The majority of the children (53.5%) had been placed in the institutions direct from their biological families, and 44.9% of them reported that they had been severely punished by a staff member. The majority of the children (66.7%) were not told how long they would stay in the institution, most of them (78.3%) declared that there were adults in the institution that they trusted, and the vast majority (93.6%) said that they received help with their homework.

For the purpose of the current study, these institutions were grouped as (a) small institutions with up to 100 children (18.9% of children), (b) medium institutions with 101–200 children (43.3% of children), and (c) large institutions with 201–400 children (37.9% of children). Out of 1479 institutionalized children, 58.6% were placed within institutions ($N = 33$) that had a traditional type of organization, 9.9% were placed within institutions ($N = 6$) that had a familial type of organization, and 31.5% were placed in institutions ($N = 14$) with a mixed-type model of organization. Mixed-type organizations were institutions in which the two previous models (traditional and familial) coexisted in varying proportions. Most of the children (81.5%) were placed in long-term residential centers that did not meet the optimal night child–staff ratio. Out of 53 institutions, 36 were located in urban areas, comprising 69.7% of the children in our sample.

Table 4.1 Frequencies and percentages of child and institution characteristics

			Type of institutional organization					
	Overall		Traditional		Familial		Mixed	
	N	%	*n*	%	*n*	%	*n*	%
Child level[a]								
Number of children	1479	100	866	58.6	147	9.9	466	31.5
Education performance								
Very good	125	8.5	72	8.3	14	9.5	39	8.4
Good	666	45.0	375	43.2	53	36.1	239	51.3
Fair	568	38.4	338	39.0	71	48.3	159	34.1
Poor	120	8.1	82	9.5	9	6.1	29	6.2
Type of education								
Primary	599	40.9	358	41.8	47	32.2	194	42.1
Vocational	128	8.7	65	7.6	17	11.6	46	10
Gymnasium	656	44.8	396	46.3	81	55.5	179	38.8
Lyceum/other	80	5.5	37	4.3	1	0.7	42	9.1
Gender								
Male	783	52.9	454	52.4	85	57.8	244	52.4
Female	696	47.1	412	47.6	62	42.2	222	47.6
Provenance								
From family	786	53.5	448	52.2	67	45.9	271	58.4
From a different center	682	46.5	410	47.8	79	54.1	193	41.6
Punishments from staff								
No	785	55.1	416	49.8	75	52.4	294	65.9
Yes	640	44.9	420	50.2	68	47.6	152	34.1
Knowledge of duration of stay								
No	987	66.7	563	65.0	88	59.9	363	72.1
Yes	492	33.3	303	35.0	59	40.1	130	27.9
Trusted adults in institution								
No	313	21.7	194	23.0	30	20.8	89	19.6
Yes	1128	78.3	649	77.0	114	79.2	365	80.4
Help with homework								
No	93	6.4	62	7.3	11	7.5	20	4.3
Yes	1361	93.6	785	92.7	135	92.5	441	95.7
Optional child–staff ratio met								
No	1205	81.5	761	87.9	107	72.8	337	72.3
Yes	274	18.5	105	12.1	40	27.2	129	27.7
Institution size								
Small (up to 100 children)	279	18.9	222	25.6	5	3.4	52	11.2
Medium (101–200 children)	640	43.3	332	38.3	84	57.1	224	48.1
Large (201–400 children)	560	37.9	312	36.0	58	39.5	190	40.8
Institution level[b]								
Number of residential centers	53	100	33	62.3	6	11.3	14	26.4
Institution location								
Rural	17	32.1	10	29.4	3	50	4	30.8
Urban	36	67.9	24	70.6	3	50	9	69.2

[a]Child level shows the number of children in each type of institution

[b]Institution level shows the number of long-term residential centers corresponding to the type of institutional organization

5.2 Multilevel Model of Academic Performance

In the final model (see Table 4.2), predicting self-reported educational performance, 1187 children with complete data (pairwise deletion) were clustered in a total of 53 institutions. The estimates, standard errors, confident intervals, odds ratios, and *p*-values for the model predictors are shown along with the Bayesian deviance information criterion values and variances. In this model (Table 4.2; Model 2), an increase of 1 year of age predicted a decrease in the odds of reporting very good/good academic performance by a factor of 0.89 ($p < 0.001$). Female children were 1.35 times more likely to report a very good/good academic performance compared with males ($p = 0.025$).

Children who had a history of institutionalization and were placed in the current institution from a different center were 0.64 times less likely to report a very good/good academic performance compared with children who came from their families ($p < 0.001$). Children reporting being punished by the institutional staff were 0.54 times less likely to report a very good/good academic performance compared to children who were not punished ($p < 0.001$). Children enrolled in gymnasium level of education were 0.43 ($p < 0.001$) less likely to report a very good/good academic performance compared with children enrolled in the primary level of education. Children who were told how long they would stay in the long-term residential center were 1.49 more likely to report a very good/good academic performance compared to children who were not given this information ($p = 0.009$). Children who had trusted adult(s) in their institution had greater odds of reporting a very good/good academic performance ($OR = 1.88$, $p < 0.001$) compared to children with no trusted adult(s). Children who had help with homework had lower odds of reporting a very good/good academic performance ($OR = 0.53$, $p = 0.016$) compared to children with no help. An increase of one point in the institution's openness to protect children's right to education predicted an increase in the odds of declaring very good/good academic performance by a factor of 1.32 ($p = 0.005$). An increase of one point in the institution's openness to protect children's right to health predicted a decrease in the odds of declaring very good/good academic performance by a factor of 0.88 ($p = 0.009$). Importantly in terms of results, the mean for how well the institution protected the right to education was 2.59 ($SD = 0.69$) which ranged from 0 to 3 and the mean for how well the institution protected the right for health was 3.01 ($SD = 1.45$) which ranged from 0 to 5, with higher scores the better. Additionally, institutions which had the optimal night child–staff ratio predicted increased odds of children reporting a very good/good academic performance by 1.77 times ($p = 0.005$). Finally, being in a familial type of institutional organization decreased the odds of children reporting a very good/good academic performance by 0.59 times compared to a traditional institution ($p = 0.033$).

Table 4.2 Multilevel model predicting child self-reported academic performance

	Estimate	*SE*	*Z*	*95% CI*[a]	*OR*[b]	*p*	
Model 1 (child-level variables)							
Age (years)	−0.12	0.03	−3.73	−0.19, −0.06	0.89	<0.001	***
Gender (male vs. female)	0.32	0.14	2.34	0.05, 0.57	1.36	0.019	*
Provenance (family vs. different institution)	−0.51	0.14	−3.71	−0.77, −0.23	0.60	<0.001	***
Punishments from staff (no vs. yes)	−0.60	0.14	−4.40	−0.87, −0.33	0.54	<0.001	***
Type of education (primary vs. vocational)	−0.63	0.33	−1.91	−1.28, 0.02	0.52	0.056	
Type of education (primary vs. gymnasium)	−0.77	0.17	−4.43	−1.14, −0.43	0.46	<0.001	***
Type of education (primary vs. lyceum/ other)	−0.12	0.35	−0.35	−0.79, 0.56	0.86	0.724	
Knowledge duration of stay (no vs. yes)	0.36	0.15	2.46	0.07, 0.66	1.42	0.014	*
Trusted adults in institution (no vs. yes)	0.59	0.16	3.75	0.29, .89	1.77	<0.001	***
Help with the homework (no vs. yes)	−0.61	0.25	−2.41	−1.12, −0.12	0.53	0.016	*
Model 2 (child and institution-level variables)							
Age	−0.13	0.04	−3.56	−0.20, −0.07	0.89	<0.001	***
Gender (male vs. female)	0.30	0.13	2.24	0.03, 0.56	1.35	0.025	*
Provenance (family vs. different institution)	−0.45	0.14	−3.30	−0.73, −0.20	0.64	<0.001	***
Punishments from staff (no vs. yes)	−0.62	0.13	−4.77	−0.89, −0.36	0.54	<0.001	***
Type of education (primary vs. vocational)	−0.64	0.37	−1.73	−1.32, 0.15	0.49	0.083	
Type of education (primary vs. gymnasium)	−0.79	0.19	−4.01	−1.15, −0.38	0.43	<0.001	***
Type of education (primary vs. lyceum/ other)	−0.18	0.38	−0.47	−0.90, 0.58	0.75	0.637	

(continued)

Table 4.2 (continued)

	Estimate	*SE*	*Z*	*95% CI*[a]	*OR*[b]	*p*	
Knowledge duration of stay (no vs. yes)	0.39	0.15	2.61	0.11, 0.69	1.49	0.009	**
Trusted adult(s) in institution (no vs. yes)	0.63	0.16	3.85	0.32, 0.97	1.88	<0.001	***
Help with the homework (no vs. yes)	−0.64	0.27	−2.42	−1.13, −0.10	0.53	0.016	*
Right to education	0.28	0.10	2.83	0.09, 0.46	1.32	0.005	**
Right to health	−0.13	0.05	−2.61	−0.22, −0.03	0.88	0.009	**
Optimal night child–staff ratio met (no vs. yes)	0.56	0.19	2.80	0.16, 0.95	1.77	0.005	**
Institutional organization (traditional vs. familial)	−0.54	0.26	−2.13	−1.05, −0.04	0.59	0.033	*
Institutional organization (traditional vs. mixed)	−0.05	0.19	−0.25	−0.42, 0.32	0.94	0.799	
Random effects	*DIC*[c]		*Variance*	*SE*	*95% CI*[a]		
Unconditional model	1584.172						
Institution			0.39	0.14	0.18, 0.73		
Level 1	1459.847						
Institution			0.21	0.09	0.06, 0.44		
Level 2	1457.703						
Institution			0.08	0.07	0.00, 0.24		

*$p < 0.05$; **$p < 0.01$; ***$p < 0.001$
[a]*CI* confidence intervals for estimate
[b]*OR* odd ratio
[c]*DIC* Bayesian deviance information criterion

6 Discussion

In a nationally representative sample of institutionalized children, 1479 children aged 7–19, placed in 53 long-term residential centers for school-aged children, and having three different types of institutional organization (i.e., traditional, family-type, and mixed), 53.5% of them declared that they had a very good/good academic performance.

6.1 Child-Level Explanatory Variables

Regarding child-level explanatory variables, the multilevel analysis revealed that an increase of 1 year in age predicted a decrease of the odds of reporting very good or good academic performance. Similarly, the results also showed that children who arrived in the current residential care facility from a different residential care facility performed more poorly in school. One interpretation of these results could be explained by the fact that children with longer institutionalization and more frequent moves from one residential center to another might have suffered more harmful physical, psychosocial, and intellectual consequences due to their prolonged institutional rearing as some studies have shown (Beckett et al., 2006; Kumsta et al., 2015; Loman et al., 2009; Pollak et al., 2010; Rutter et al., 1998; 2010; Zeanah et al., 2003) or that placement disruptions are harmful in themselves (Humphreys et al., 2015). Specifically, longer periods of time spent in institutions may be associated with increased impairment of executive functions (Bos et al., 2009; Loman et al., 2009; Pollak et al., 2010), thus likely affecting academic success. Interestingly, Attar-Schwartz (2009) showed an opposite result, namely, that children with a longer period of residence within institutions had lower levels of problems in school functioning.

Furthermore, being female predicted self-reports of a very good/good academic performance, and this finding is consistent with the result of another study of the normal population (Pomerantz, Saxon, & Altermatt, 2002) that found girls outperforming boys regarding grades during elementary school and into adolescence. A similar result was found by Attar-Schwartz (2009) studying more than 4000 children in 54 Israeli residential care facilities, suggesting that this finding could be also extended to the institutionalized children population.

Our results also showed that being told how long the child would stay in the long-term institution as well as having trusted adult(s) in their institution predicted higher odds of reporting very good/good academic performance. Knowing how long their stay in the institution may provide children with a sense of safety, predictability, and perceived control, which could help them adjust more readily to academic challenges. Additionally, the beneficial effects of the presence of trusted adult(s) on academic performance could be explained by the fact that having a sense of relatedness (connectedness or belonging) to caregivers may function as a motivational resource (Furrer & Skinner, 2003) and help children to better cope with difficulties in the school environment. Because these factors (i.e., child's knowledge of duration of stay and having a trusted adult in institution) have not been studied thoroughly within care facilities, further studies should be carried out to investigate these findings in more depth.

Institutionalized children were also less likely to report a very good/good academic performance if they reported having been punished by the institutional staff. This is not surprising given that exposure to victimization in the absence of institutionalization has been linked to poor functioning in a number of developmental domains. Specifically, it has also been shown that maltreatment (i.e., sexual abuse, physical abuse, physical neglect, and emotional maltreatment) is negatively linked to children's academic performance, and there were also found various deficits in academic engagement, social competencies, ego resiliency, and ego control (Shonk et al., 2001). Childhood maltreatment was similarly associated with low-grade point average and problems completing homework assignments, with maltreatment effects moderated by cognitive deficits related to attention problems (Slade & Wissow, 2007). A longitudinal study also showed that early physical maltreatment predicts adolescent school-related problems such as absenteeism and college attendance (Lansford et al., 2002).

In addition, children were less likely to report a very good/good academic performance if they were enrolled in gymnasium level of education compared with those enrolled in primary education. In Romania and other countries, children learn literacy and other basic academic skills in the primary grades that provide a foundation for the more challenging demands of the middle grades. As they transition to middle school, students are expected to master literacy and academic abilities that are unique to different disciplines and with increasing difficulty. For those who did not master basic skills in the primary grades, there is typically less support to recover these skills in later grades, and students can fall behind quickly due to their inability to keep up with more complex demands (see Biancarosa & Snow, 2006; Lee & Spratley, 2010). The effort to adequately address the educational needs of adolescents has been an ongoing challenge for many countries around the globe for decades, including the United States (Jacobs, 2008). Thus, the transition from the primary to secondary school grades is often the most challenging time for students in general, and given the higher levels of adversity experienced by institutionalized children, it is not surprising that our participants in the middle school grades self-reported less positive outcomes regarding their academic performance than those in the primary grades.

Furthermore, the present research revealed an outcome that may seem counterintuitive, namely, that children were less likely to report a very good/good academic performance if they had help with homework. However, it is likely that the students receiving help with homework were those who were struggling academically. Those who were able to complete homework without help were likely not having significant problems with academic work. In addition, the survey does not indicate whether the homework help was implemented by trained tutors or other academic professionals able to provide individualized, evidence-based instruction for each student's particular difficulty. Such instruction could target the root of the academic problem and help children become increasingly more capable of independent learning over time. On the other hand, if homework help was provided by regular institutional staff, this type of help may have been inadequate because many institutions were understaffed, provided inadequate training for employees, or simply lacked nonmedical specialists (psychologists, physical therapists, or social workers; see Stephenson et al., 1993; Rosenberg, Pajer, & Rancurello, 1992; Williams, 1990) due to the abolishment of social work in 1969, sociology, psychology, and pedagogy in

1977 as academic disciplines by the communist regime due to political and ideological reasons that lasted until 1989 (Universitatea Bucuresti, Facultatea de Sociologie si Asistenta Sociala, n.d.; Universitatea Babes-Bolyai, Facultatea de Psychologie si Stiinte ale Educatiei, n.d.). In addition, these staff may have perceived this duty as an extra burden to their already stressful jobs or they may have expressed frustration with children when they did not see improvement in children's abilities over time, further reinforcing children's lack of confidence in their academic abilities.

6.2 Institution-Level Explanatory Variables

With respect to institution-level explanatory variables (see Table 4.2), the multilevel analysis revealed that an increase of one point in the institution's openness to protect children's right to education predicted an increase of the odds of declaring very good/good academic performance. Regarding children's access to education in general, it is important to highlight that long-term residential centers for Romanian children complied with the obligation to enroll their children in preschool and school education. For the *cămine spital* (institutions for children with disabilities), this regulation was later introduced and selectively applied, depending mainly on the intellectual potential of the children in these institutions. Specifically, our results showed that the long-term residential settings in which children had free access to the library, personal space for doing homework or study, and provided an age appropriate form of education facilitated children's academic performance.

Additionally, an increase of one point in the institution's openness to protect children's right to health predicted a decrease of the odds of declaring very good/good academic performance. The right to health was measured by items measuring whether or not the child had treatment and rehabilitation needs recorded in his/her medical file, received general medical assistance, had records of general medical examinations, received the treatment written in medical file, and had anthropometric measures (i.e., height and weight) completed (for more information, see Chap. 2). This counterintuitive result should be considered in the context that many institutional settings may have emphasized children's medical needs more than their psychological needs. This approach could have been particularly marked the institutional settings where the management staff had a medical background. At the time, many long-term residential centers lacked nonmedical specialists (psychologists, physical therapists, or social workers) who could have helped children from institutions to obtain better school results. Future studies should further examine these hypotheses.

Moreover, institutions which had the optimal child–staff ratio during morning, daytime, and nighttime (for more information about this variable, see Chap. 2) predicted increased odds of children reporting a very good/good academic performance. This result suggests that, by having an adequate number of caregivers around, institutionalized children were most likely better protected, supervised, and motivated to succeed academically. Alternatively, as highlighted above, with more caregivers around children might have a more predictable environment and a sense of connectedness or belonging to caregivers that function as a motivational resource helping children to better cope with difficulties in the school environment and, consequently, succeed academically. Future studies should further examine these hypotheses.

Finally, being in a familial type of institutional organization decreased the odds of children reporting a very good/good academic performance. This was an unexpected outcome knowing that familial type institutions housed fewer children in small houses or apartments, and daily activities were organized to resemble a family model and to provide individualized care. It might be that these facilities cared for children with more behavioral, emotional, and educational challenges, and consequently, they had more academic problems. In a similar context, however, Attar-Schwartz (2009) found that children in small family-like settings showed fewer problems in school functioning. Such an inconsistency in the literature should be further explored.

7 Strengths and Limitations

The current study is the only comprehensive investigation we are aware of that measured the self-reported academic performance in a large sample of Romanian institutionalized children. By using a nationally representative sample of children in 53 long-term residential centers across all eight administrative regions of Romania in rural and urban areas, we were able to model using multilevel analyses a large number of child- and institution-level variables in order to study how they were associated with the dependent variable. Additionally, this investigation used the social–ecological model (Bronfenbrenner, 1977; Bronfenbrenner & Morris, 1998), a conceptual framework which guided us to assess institutionalized children's academic performance taking into account a multidimensional approach, in which both individual and contextual institutional characteristics were accounted for regarding children's performance.

Our results should be considered in view of several limitations. First, self-report data is subject to bias, and children generally may be more inclined to perceive themselves in a more positive manner, particularly with regard to school performance (Gramzow, Elliot, Asher, & McGregor, 2003), as this is likely to increase their self-esteem as well as perception of the adults around them. Whether institutionalized children would perceive themselves in a slightly more negative manner than their non-institutionalized counterparts is unknown at this point. Future studies should employ multiple informants in and outside of care institutions (i.e., children, caregivers, and teachers) in order to enhance our understanding of institutionalized children's academic functioning. Most of the measurements of academic performance in the studies that we reviewed in the beginning of this chapter were objective measures (e.g., report cards) and adult reports (e.g., academic performance items in adult questionnaires). Our search was able to identify only two studies (Tan, 2009; Tan et al., 2015) that also made use of self-reports in addition to the questionnaire items completed by the parents. Their analyses proved that the self-report scale had good internal consistency properties and results correlated well with the adult measure (Tan, 2009), which shows that child questionnaires of academic competence are reliable to use in previously institutionalized children. This is encouraging given the scarcity of studies that made use of self-report in measuring school performance.

Second, we collected concurrent data on the academic performance of institutionalized children and some of the potentially contributing factors at a single point in time, which only provided us with a snapshot into the lives of these children who grew up in institutions from a very young age and who had been most probably subjected to severe deprivation throughout many years. Our cross-sectional design does not allow us to infer causality between the variables that we studied. Investigations with institutionalized children should include collecting information longitudinally from early in life and from multiple domains to be able to interpret the data from a developmental perspective.

8 Implications for Improving Children's Care

The present study clearly shows that both individual and institutional characteristics function as risk and protective factors regarding children's academic performance. The results are useful because they highlight the relationship between the environmental context in which institutionalized children live and their academic outcomes. Consequently, in addressing institutionalized children's educational performance, child welfare policymakers and practitioners should take into account a multidimensional approach. Specifically, we recommend focusing on the institutional level characteristics (e.g., type of institution, child–staff ratio) to prevent the abuse and neglect that children so often experience within long-term residential centers. In addition, to improve children's academic performance, there is a need for a structural intervention designed to increase the readiness of institutional settings to respect most basic human rights and personalized interventions for children that target their individual intellectual characteristics and needs.

9 Summary

Most importantly, the multilevel analyses revealed that reporting a very good/good academic performance was predicted by (a) child's age, (b) being a female child, (c) being told how long they would stay in the long-term residential center, and (d) having trusted adult(s) in their institution. Moreover, children were less likely to report a very good/good academic performance if they (e) were placed in the current institution from a different center, (f) reported having been punished by the institutional staff, (g) were enrolled in gymnasium level of education, and (h) had help with homework.

With respect to institution-level explanatory variables, the analysis also revealed that reporting (h) an increase of one point in the institution's openness to protect children's right to education predicted an increase in the odds of declaring very good/good academic performance; and (i) an increase of one point in the institution's openness to protect children's right to health predicted a decrease in the odds of declaring very good/good academic performance. Additionally, (j) institutions which had the optimal child–staff ratio predicted increased odds of children reporting a very good/good academic performance; and (k) being in a familial type of institutional organization decreased the odds of children reporting a very good/good academic performance.

Questions for Discussion

1. Identify two important academic performance-related consequences of maltreatment (i.e., neglect and emotional, physical, or sexual abuse) of children, either with or without a history of institutionalization. Substantiate your responses using published research.
2. Based on your knowledge of living conditions in Romanian institutions, imagine the daily experiences of institutionalized children vs. children living with biological parents. In addition to variables described in this study, think of other types of experiences that were common among institutionalized children and describe how these experiences could impact their educational outcomes.
3. What kind of intervention could be employed with institutionalized children that would improve their educational outcomes? Describe why it could be helpful.

References

Alloway, T. P., & Alloway, R. G. (2010). Investigating the predictive roles of working memory and IQ in academic attainment. *Journal of Experimental Child Psychology, 106*, 20–29.

American Academy of Pediatrics (AAP), American Public Health Association (APHA), & National Resource Center for Health and Safety in Child Care and Early Education (NRCHSCCEE). (2011). *Caring for our children: National health and safety performance standards; guidelines for early care and education programs* (3rd ed.). Elk Grove Village, IL/Washington, DC: American Academy of Pediatrics/American Public Health Association.

Attar-Schwartz, S. (2009). School functioning of children in residential care: The contributions of multilevel correlates. *Child Abuse and Neglect, 33*(7), 429–440.

Attar-Schwartz, S. (2011). Maltreatment by staff in residential care facilities: The adolescents' perspectives. *Social Service Review, 85*(4), 635–664.

Attar-Schwartz, S. (2013). Runaway behavior among adolescents in residential care: The role of personal characteristics, victimization experiences while in care, social climate, and institutional factors. *Children & Youth Services Review, 35*(2), 258–267. doi:10.1016/j.childyouth.2012.11.005.

Attar-Schwartz, S. (2014). Experiences of sexual victimization by peers among adolescents in residential care settings. *Social Service Review, 88*(4), 594–629.

Attar-Schwartz, S., & Khoury-Kassabri, M. (2015). Indirect and verbal victimization by peers among at-risk youth in residential care. *Child Abuse & Neglect*, 4284–4298. doi:10.1016/j.chiabu.2014.12.007.

Barnett, W. S. (1998). Long-term cognitive and academic effects of early childhood education on children in poverty. *Preventive Medicine, 27*, 204–207.

Bates, D., Maechler, M., Bolker, B., & Walker, S. (2015). Fitting linear mixed-effects models using lme4. *Journal of Statistical Software, 67*(1), 1–48. doi:10.18637/jss.v067.i01.

Beckett, C., Maughan, B., Rutter, M., Castle, J., Colvert, E., Groothues, C., … Sonuga-Barke, E. J. S. (2006). Do the effects of early severe deprivation on cognition persist into early adolescence? Findings from the English and Romanian adoptees study. *Child Development, 77*, 696–711.

Beckett, C., Maughan, B., Rutter, M., Castle, J., Colvert, E., Groothues, C., … Sonuga-Barke, E. J. S. (2007). Scholastic attainment following severe early institutional deprivation: A study of 242 adoptees adopted from Romania. *Journal of Abnormal Child Psychology, 35*, 1063–1073.

Biancarosa, C., & Snow, C. E. (2006). *Reading next – A vision for action and research in middle and high school literacy: A report to Carnegie Corporation of New York* (2nd ed.). Washington, DC: Alliance for Excellent Education.

Bos, K. J., Fox, N., Zeanah, C. H., & Nelson, C. A. (2009). Effects of early psychosocial deprivation on the development of memory and executive function. *Frontiers in Behavioral Neuroscience, 316*. doi:10.3389/neuro.08.016.2009.

Braitstein, P., Ayaya, S., Nyandiko, W. M., Kamanda, A., Koech, J., Gisore, P., … Ayuku, D. O. (2013). Nutritional status of orphaned and separated children and adolescents living in community and institutional environments in Uasin Gishu county, Kenya. *PloS One, 8*(7), e70054. doi:10.1371/journal.pone.0070054.

Bronfenbrenner, U. (1977). Toward an experimental ecology of human development. *American Psychologist, 32*(7), 513–531.

Bronfenbrenner, U., & Morris, P. A. (1998). The ecology of developmental processes. In W. Damon & R. M. Lerner (Eds.), *Handbook of child psychology, Theoretical models of human development* (Vol. 1, 5th ed., pp. 993–1028). New York, NY: Wiley.

Browne, W. J. (2012). *MCMC estimation in MLwiN, v2.26*. Centre for Multilevel Modelling, University of Bristol.

Diamond, A. (2010). The evidence base for improving school outcomes by addressing the whole child and by addressing skills and attitudes, not just content. *Early Education and Development, 21*(5), 780–793.

Eckenrode, J., & Laird, M. (1993). School performance and disciplinary problems among abused and neglected children. *Developmental Psychology, 29*(1), 53–62. doi:10.1037/0012-1649.29.1.53.

Egeland, B., Sroufe, L. A., & Erickson, M. (1983). The developmental consequence of different patterns of maltreatment. *Child Abuse & Neglect, 7*(4), 459–469.

Escueta, M., Whetten, K., Ostermann, J., & O'Donnell, K. (2014). Adverse childhood experiences, psychosocial well-being and cognitive development among orphans and abandoned children in five low income countries. *BMC International Health & Human Rights, 14*(1), 1–13. doi:10.1186/1472-698X-14-6.

Euser, S., Alink, L. A., Tharner, A., van IJzendoorn, M. H., & Bakermans-Kranenburg, M. J. (2016). The prevalence of child sexual abuse in out-of-home care: Increased risk for children

with a mild intellectual disability. *Journal of Applied Research in Intellectual Disabilities, 29*, 83–92. doi:10.1111/jar.12160.
Euser, S., Alink, L. R., Tharner, A., van IJzendoorn, M. H., & Bakermans-Kranenburg, M. J. (2014). Out of home placement to promote safety? The prevalence of physical abuse in residential and foster care. *Children and Youth Services Review, 37*, 3764–3770.
Furrer, C., & Skinner, E. (2003). Sense of relatedness as a factor in children's academic engagement and performance. *Journal of Educational Psychology, 95*(1), 148.
Gelman, A., & Hill, J. (2007). *Data analysis using regression and multilevel/hierarchical models*. New York: Cambridge University Press.
Gramzow, R. H., Elliot, A. J., Asher, E., & McGregor, H. A. (2003). Self-evaluation bias and academic performance: Some ways and some reasons why. *Journal of Research in Personality, 37*(2), 41. doi:10.1016/S0092-6566(02)00535-4.
Gray, C. L., Pence, B. W., Ostermann, J., Whetten, R. A., O'Donnell, K., Thielman, N. M., & Whetten, K. (2015). Prevalence and incidence of traumatic experiences among orphans in institutional and family-based settings in 5 low- and middle-income countries: A longitudinal study. *Global Health, Science and Practice, 3*(3), 395–404. doi:10.9745/GHSP-D-15-00093.
Gresham, F. M., & Elliott, S. N. (1990). *Social skills rating system manual*. Circle Pines, MN: AGS.
Haarr, R. N. (2011). *Violence against children in state-run residential institutions in Kazakhstan: An assessment*. Astana, Kazakhstan: United Nations Children's Fund. Retrieved September 20, 2016, from http://www.ceecis.org/ccc/publications/Violence_against_children_in_state-run_residential_institutions_in_Kazakhstan_2011_ENG.pdf
Hermenau, K., Hecker, T., Elbert, T., & Ruf-Leuschner, M. (2014). Maltreatment and mental health in institutional care-comparing early and late institutionalized children in Tanzania. *Infant Mental Health Journal, 35*(2), 102–110. doi:10.1002/imhj.21440.
Hermenau, K., Hecker, T., Ruf, M., Schauer, E., Elbert, T., & Schauer, M. (2011). Childhood adversity, mental ill-health and aggressive behavior in an African orphanage: Changes in response to trauma-focused therapy and the implementation of a new instructional system. *Child & Adolescent Psychiatry & Mental Health, 5*(1), 29–37. doi:10.1186/1753-2000-5-29.
Hodges, J., & Tizard, B. (1989). IQ and behavioural adjustment of ex-institutional adolescents. *Journal of Child Psychology and Psychiatry and Allied Disciplines, 30*, 53–75.
Humphreys, K. L., Gleason, M. M., Drury, S. S., Miron, D., Nelson 3rd, C., Fox, N. A., & Zeanah, C. H. (2015). Effects of institutional rearing and foster care on psychopathology at age 12 years in Romania: Follow-up of an open, randomised controlled trial. *The Lancet Psychiatry, 2*(7), 625–634. doi:10.1016/S2215-0366(15)00095-4.
IBM Corp. (2010). *IBM SPSS statistics for Windows (Version 19.0)*. Armonk, NY: Author.
Jacobs, V. A. (2008). Adolescent literacy: Putting the crisis in context. *Harvard Educational Review, 78*(1), 7–39.
Kaplan, C., Schene, P., DePanfilis, D., & Gilmore, D. (2009). Introduction: Shining light on chronic neglect. *Protecting Children, 24*(1), 1–7.
Kendall-Tackett, K. A., & Eckenrode, J. (1996). The effects of neglect on academic achievement and disciplinary problems: A developmental perspective. *Child Abuse & Neglect, 20*(3), 161–169. doi:10.1016/S0145-2134(95)00139-5.
Kumsta, R., Kreppner, J., Kennedy, M., Knights, N., Rutter, M., & Sonuga-Barke, E. (2015). Psychological consequences of early global deprivation. *European Psychologist, 20*, 138–151.
Lansford, J. E., Dodge, K. A., Pettit, G. S., Bates, J. E., Crozier, J., & Kaplow, J. (2002). A 12-year prospective study of the long-term effects of early child physical maltreatment on psychological, behavioral, and academic problems in adolescence. *Archives of Pediatrics & Adolescent Medicine, 156*(8), 824–830.
Lee, C. D., & Spratley, A. (2010). *Reading in the disciplines: The challenges of adolescent literacy*. New York, NY: Carnegie Corporation of New York.
Loman, M. M., Wiik, K. L., Frenn, K. A., Pollak, S. D., & Gunnar, M. R. (2009). Post-institutionalized children's development: Cognitive, academic, and health outcomes. *Behavioral and Developmental Pediatrics, 30*(5), 1–9.

McDermott, J. M., Westerlund, A., Zeanah, C. H., Nelson, C. A., & Fox, N. A. (2012). Early adversity and neural correlates of executive function. Implications for academic adjustment. *Developmental Cognitive Neuroscience*, *2*(Suppl. 1), S59–S66.

Miyake, A., Friedman, N. P., Rettinger, D. A., Shah, P., & Hegarty, M. (2001). How are visuo-spatial working memory, executive functioning, and spatial abilities related? A latent variable analysis. *Journal of Experimental Psychology: General*, *130*, 621–640.

National Authority for the Protection of Child's Rights & Phare 2003 "Educational Campaign on Child's Rights". (2006). *Child welfare in Romania: The story of a reform process*. Bucharest, Romania. Retrieved December 3, 2016, from https://www.unicef.org/ceecis/Rom_RefHist.pdf

Nelson, C. A., Fox, N. A., & Zeanah, C. H. (2014). *Romania's abandoned children: Deprivation, brain development, and the struggle for recovery*. Cambridge, MA: Harvard University Press.

Nelson, C. A., Zeanah, C. H., Fox, N. A., Marshall, P. J., Smyke, A. T., & Guthrie, D. (2007). Cognitive recovery in socially deprived young children: The Bucharest Early Intervention Project. *Science*, *318*, 1937–1940.

Pollak, S. D., Nelson, C. A., Schlaak, M. F., Roeber, B. J., Wewerka, S. S., Wiik, K. L., ... Gunnar, M. R. (2010). Neurodevelopmental effects of early deprivation in postinstitutionalized children. *Child Development*, *81*, 224–236.

Pomerantz, E. M., Saxon, J. L., & Altermatt, E. R. (2002). Making the grade but feeling distressed: Gender differences in academic performance and internal distress. *Journal of Educational Psychology*, *94*(2), 396.

R Development Core Team. (2016). *R: A language and environment for statistical computing*. Vienna, Austria: R Foundation for Statistical Computing. ISBN:3-900051-07-0. Retrieved June 27, 2013, from https://www.r-project.org/

Rasbash, J., Steele, F., Browne, W. J. & Goldstein, H. (2012). *A user's guide to MLwiN, v2.26*. Centre for Multilevel Modelling, University of Bristol.

Rosenberg, D. R., Pajer, K., & Rancurello, M. (1992). Neuropsychiatric assessment of orphans in one Romanian orphanage for "unsalvageables". *JAMA*, *268*(24), 3489–3490.

Rowe, E., & Eckenrode, J. (1999). The timing of academic difficulties among maltreated and non-maltreated children. *Child Abuse & Neglect*, *23*(8), 813–832.

Rus, A. V., Parris, S., Cross, D., Purvis, K., & Drăghici, S. (2011). Reforming the Romanian child welfare system: 1990–2010. *Review of Research and Social Intervention*, *34*, 56–72.

Rus, A. V., Stativa, E., Pennings, J. S., Cross, D. R., Ekas, N., Purvis, K., & Parris, S. R. (2013). Severe punishment of children by staff in Romanian placement centers for school-aged children: Effects of child and institutional characteristics. *Child Abuse and Neglect*, *37*(12), 1152–1162. doi:10.1016/j.chiabu.2013.07.003.

Rutter, M., Kreppner, J. M., O'Connor, T. G., & The English Romanian Adoptees (ERA) Study Team. (2001). Specificity and heterogeneity in children's responses to profound institutional privation. *British Journal of Psychiatry*, *17*, 97–103.

Rutter, M., Sonuga-Barke, E., Beckett, C., Castle, J., Kreppner, J., Kumsta, R., ... Gunnar, M. (2010). Deprivation-specific psychological patterns: Effects of institutional deprivation. *Monographs of the Society for Research in Child Development*, *75*, 1–242.

Rutter, M., & the English and Romanian Adoptees (ERA) study team. (1998). Developmental catch-up and deficit following adoption after severe global early privation. *Journal of Child Psychology and Psychiatry*, *39*(4), 465–476.

Segura, A., Pereda, N., Abad, J., & Guilera, G. (2015). Victimization and polyvictimization among Spanish youth protected by the child welfare system. *Children and Youth Services Review*, *59*, 105–112.

Segura, A., Pereda, N., Guilera, G., & Abad, J. (2016). Poly-victimization and psychopathology among Spanish adolescents in residential care. *Child Abuse & Neglect*, 5540–5551. doi:10.1016/j.chiabu.2016.03.009.

Shonk, S. M., Cicchetti, D., Susan, M. S., & Dante, C. (2001). Maltreatment, competency deficits, and risk for academic and behavioral maladjustment. *Developmental Psychology*, *37*(1), 3.

Slade, E. P., & Wissow, L. S. (2007). The influence of childhood maltreatment on adolescents' academic performance. *Economics of Education Review, 26*(5), 604–614. doi:10.1016/j.econedurev.2006.10.003.

Stativa, E., Anghelescu, C., Palicari, G., Stanescu, A., & Nanu, R. (2002). *Child abuse in residential care institutions in Romania.* Bucharest, Romania: Extrem Group.

Stephenson, P., Anghelescu, C., Fumarel, S., Georgescu, A., Iorgulescu, D., McCreery, R., … Stanescu, A. (1993). Training needs of staff in Romanian institutions for young children. *Child: Care, Health and Development, 19*(3), 221–234.

Tan, T. X. (2009). School-age adopted Chinese girls' behavioral adjustment, academic performance, and social skills: Longitudinal results. *American Journal of Orthopsychiatry, 79*(2), 244–251.

Tan, T. X., Rice, J. L., & Mahoney, E. E. (2015). Developmental delays at arrival and postmenarcheal Chinese adolescents' adjustment. *American Journal of Orthopsychiatry, 85*(1), 93–100.

Tibu, F., Sheridan, M., McLaughlin, K. A., Fox, N. A., Zeanah, C. H., & Nelson, C. A. (2016). Disruptions of working memory and inhibition mediate the association between exposure to institutionalization and symptoms of attention-deficit/hyperactivity disorder. *Psychological Medicine, 46*, 529–541.

UN General Assembly. (1989, November 20). *Convention on the rights of the child* (United Nations, Treaty Series, Vol. 1577, p. 3).

Universitatea Babes-Bolyai, Facultatea de Psychologie si Stiinte ale Educatiei (n.d.). *Scurt istoric al facultatii de Psihologie si Stiinte ale Educatiei* [Brief history of the Faculty of Psychology and Educational Sciences]. Retrieved July 15, 2016, from http://psiedu.ubbcluj.ro/index.php?id=11-istoric-psihologie

Universitatea Bucuresti, Facultatea de Sociologie si Asistenta Sociala. (n.d.). *Trecut* [Past]. Retrieved July 15, 2016, from http://sas.unibuc.ro/trecut_ro

van IJzendoorn, M. H., Juffer, F., & Klein Poelhuis, C. W. (2005). Adoption and cognitive development: A metaanalytic comparison of adopted and nonadopted children's IQ and school performances. *Psychological Bulletin, 131*, 301–316.

Vorria, P., Ntouma, M., & Rutter, M. (2015). The cognitive development and school achievement of adopted adolescents: The Greek "Metera" study. *European Journal of Developmental Psychology., 12*(1), 1–14.

Whetten, K., Ostermann, J., Whetten, R., O'Donnell, K., & Thielman, N. (2011). More than the loss of a parent: Potentially traumatic events among orphaned and abandoned children. *Journal of Traumatic Stress, 24*(2), 174–182. doi:10.1002/jts.20625.

Whetten, K., Ostermann, J., Whetten, R. A., Pence, B. W., O'Donnell, K., Messer, L. C., & Thielman, N. M. (2009). A comparison of the wellbeing of orphans and abandoned children ages 6–12 in institutional and community-based care settings in 5 less wealthy nations. *PloS One, 4*(12), e8169. doi:10.1371/journal.pone.0008169.

Williams, C. J. (1990, December 10). The unwanted children: Casualties left by a tyrant. *Los Angeles Times.*

Zeanah, C. H., Nelson, C. A., Fox, N. A., Smyke, A. T., Marshall, P., Parker, S., & Koga, S. (2003). Designing research to study the effects of institutionalization on brain and behavioral development: The Bucharest Early Intervention Project. *Development and Psychopathology, 15*, 885–907.

Zhang, Z., Charlton, C., Parker, R., Leckie, G. & Browne, W. J. (2016). *R2MLwiN: Running MLwiN from within R. R package version 0.8-2.* Retrieved June 24, 2016, from http://CRAN.R--project.org/package=R2MLwiN

Chapter 5
The Prevalence of Stunting Among the Romanian Institutionalized Children Placed in Long-Term Institutional Settings in the 1990s

Ecaterina Stativa, Adrian V. Rus, Sheri R. Parris, Jacquelyn S. Pennings, Bogdan Simion, and Reggies Wenyika

Living within the context of an institution, many factors converge to limit the growth of the individual, across a spectrum of domains

Sheri R. Parris, personal communication, December 7, 2016

E. Stativa (✉)
Social Pediatrics and Obstetrics Research Department, The National Institute for Mother and Child Health "Alessandrescu-Rusescu",
B-dul Lacul Tei 120, cod 0209395 Bucharest, Romania
e-mail: kattyshu@yahoo.com; ecaterina.stativa@gmail.com

A.V. Rus
Department of Social and Behavioral Sciences, Southwestern Christian University, Bethany, OK, USA
e-mail: adrian.rus@swcu.edu

S.R. Parris
Texas Christian University, Fort Worth, TX, USA
e-mail: sheri.parris@gmail.com

J.S. Pennings
Elite Research, LLC, Irving, TX 75063, USA
e-mail: jacspen@gmail.com

B. Simion
Fundatia SERA, Bucharest, Romania
e-mail: bogdan.simion@sera.ro

R. Wenyika
Southwestern Christian University, Bethany, OK, USA
e-mail: reggies.wenyika@swcu.edu

A.V. Rus et al. (eds.), *Child Maltreatment in Residential Care*,
DOI 10.1007/978-3-319-57990-0_5

1 Introduction

Children's growth is the result of many factors, among which health and nutrition play a very important role, yet various environmental conditions can also disrupt normal development. Worldwide, there are millions of children whose growth is disrupted by undernutrition and malnutrition, as well as adverse environmental factors. Low height for age, an indicator of stunting, is most relevant to this disturbance. The World Health Organization (WHO) states that a child is stunted if their length/height-for-age z-scores are less than −2 standard deviations based on Child Growth Standards (de Onis, 2015; de Onis, Blössner, & Borghi, 2010; de Onis, Onyango, Borghi, Garza, & Yang, 2006).

Stunting of linear growth in children can result from antenatal, intrauterine, and/or postnatal undernutrition (Waterlow, 1994). Additionally, stunting can occur from environmental conditions (Espo et al., 2002; Martorell, Ramakrishnan, Schroeder, Melgar, & Neufeld, 1998), socioeconomic conditions, and education levels of parents (Semba et al., 2008; Van de Poel, Hosseinpoor, Speybroeck, Van Ourti, & Vega, 2008). Stunting in childhood can lead to long-term consequences in later years such as poor cognition and academic performance, low wages, lost productivity, and increased risk of nutrition-related chronic diseases if excessive weight gain occurs later in childhood (Victoria et al., 2008).

Within this chapter, we present (1) a very brief literature review of stunting within residential centers across the globe, (2) a history of the health status of Romanian institutionalized children, and (3) the results of the present study that highlighted significant difference in children's stunting across institutional settings.

1.1 Stunting of Institutionalized Children

Various studies have shown that children living within institutional care settings experience a substantial global growth suppression of their height, weight, and head circumference (for a review, see Johnson et al., 2010; Johnson & Gunnar, 2011; Rutter, 1998; Smyke et al., 2007; Van IJzendoorn, Bakermans-Kranenburg, & Juffer, 2007).

Regarding stunting, a retrospective chart review of 193 children (2–72 months) residing in orphanages in Russia (Miller et al., 2007) found that 25% had short stature (Z scores ≤ -2) at orphanage entry, and for 39% of those with stunting at entry, the height remained compromised throughout their orphanage residence. Additionally, Dobrova-Krol and colleagues (Dobrova-Krol, van IJzendoorn, Bakermans-Kranenburg, Cyr, & Juffer, 2008), studying 16 institution-reared children (3–6 years old) placed in four children's homes in Ukraine, found that at 3 months of age, the supine lengths of the stunted institution-reared children were significantly lower than the supine lengths of the native noninstitutionalized family-reared children. This trend persisted even at 24 months of age; however, the researchers noticed a relative improvement from 24 months through 48 months of age. In a different study of 146 children (0–72 months) residing in two Eastern Indian orphanages, Routray and colleagues (2015) found that 36.7% were stunted (no information regarding the prevalence of stunting at entry was offered).

1.2 The Historical Context of the Current Study

After 1989, the situation of institutionalized children in Romania was over-publicized through images sometimes purposely sought to shock the public opinion in Western European countries. The images were real, but every time only images were shown of institutions that housed children with severe chronic illnesses. However, the life experience of Romanian institutionalized children varied across all types of institutional settings, a reality that was not presented in detail to the public at the time. As shown by Correll and colleagues, the neighboring countries such as Ukraine, Bulgaria, and other countries in Eastern Europe (i.e., Belarus and Russia) had a similar situation (Correll, Correll, & Predescu, 2006), yet only Romania's situation was heavily publicized by the western mass media and shocked the world (Correll et al., 2006). The authors of the abovementioned report highlighted that residential institutions that provided social protection for unwanted children during the Ceausescu regime were among the most serious problems that faced the newly established Romanian democracy in the early 1990s (Correll et al., 2006).

Connecting the high number of institutionalized children to the pronatalist policies of Ceausescu's communist regime is legitimate when considering the growing numbers of unwanted and abandoned children between 1966 and 1989. After coming to power in 1965, Nicolae Ceausescu believed that numerical population growth was one of the main ways to improve the country's economic development. As shown previously (Muresan & Copil, 1974; Trebici, 1976), demographic indicators from 1966 and before, however, did not foreshadow a growing population. Specifically, between 1957 and 1966, there was a decreased trend in crude birthrate from 24.2‰ in 1957 to 14.3‰ in 1966 that coincided with the liberalization of abortion in Romania in 1957, following the Soviet Union model in this regard. Thus, by 1965, there were 408 abortions recorded per 100 live births, or about 80% of the total number of conceptions ended up in abortions (Muresan & Copil, 1974; Trebici, 1976). Given these circumstances, the communist Romanian government decided to reverse the declining birthrate trend and aimed to achieve an 18–19‰ birth rate, believing that this rate would improve the economic progress of the country. Accordingly, the population growth target was to reach 24–25 million people by 1990 and 30 million by 2000 (from 19 million in 1966) (Muresan & Copil, 1974; Trebici, 1976). To achieve these goals, the November 1966 Decree 770 was issued which banned the practice of abortion on demand (with some exceptions), given that this was the most important instrument of fertility control used by women in Romania at the time. The result was that in 1 year, the birthrate almost doubled from 14‰ to 27.4‰ (Muresan & Copil, 1974; Trebici, 1976). These demographic policies were extremely unpopular in Romania, and women resorted to every means to limit their fertility, risking their health or even their lives. In the 1980s, these demographic policies become even more unpopular given that Romania's population was experiencing a period of extremely restrictive living conditions following the communist government's decision to pay in full the country's foreign debt. These policies were imposed through the specific repressive means of the communist regime's political police. Party propaganda tried to justify the prohibition of abortion by highlighting its interest for women's health care. However, that argument was shaky because after a woman gave birth to four children (before 1985), and then five children (starting in 1985 and after), they were allowed to use legal abortion for the purpose of their fertility control.

Subsequent retrospective studies showed that these demographic policies deeply affected the health and lives of women and children. The medically unsupervised methods used for clandestine abortions during this time probably damaged the cervixes of many women, as well as causing chronic infections and severe anemia, which in turn increased the risk for postpartum hemorrhage and infections. Thus, many women who survived remained infertile or frequently gave birth to children who had low birth weight, or were premature or stillborn. The exact figures are not known about the prevalence of post-abortion morbidity during this period (Stephenson, Wagner, Badea, & Serbanescu, 1992). According to one retrospective study conducted in 2001 (Glavce, Dragomirescu, Valentin, & Apavaloae, 2001), in the beginning of 1967, the trend showed a 30% surge in children with low weight at birth (under 2500 grams), a 4% decrease in the number of children with an average weight, and a stagnation in the percentage of overweight children. For decades, the average birth weight of babies born in Romania did not exceed 3000 grams, which is 200 grams less than the European average (Stanescu, 2002). Infant and maternal mortality rates rose to very high levels in the years following establishment of pronatalist policies. While infant mortality decreased steadily, after increasing by 10% in one single year, the maternal mortality due to abortions continuously increased year by year. Between 1966 and 1989, about 10,000 women died due to complications of clandestine abortions (Stephenson et al., 1992). In the absence of social services to support vulnerable mothers who faced unwelcome pregnancies, they abandoned their unwanted newborn children (who usually also had health problems) in maternities and hospitals. After shorter or longer periods, these children were institutionalized in long-term residential institutions specific for their age.

But there was also another reason for children's institutionalization. Some children were born with low birth weight due to intrauterine growth retardation. To aid the growth and recovery for these children, they were housed in maternity wards until they reached the normal weight, but mothers were not allowed in these wards. Consequently, by separating the children from their mothers, the relationship between them ceased and sometimes mothers with low socioeconomic status chose to abandon their children. In these circumstances, the absence of the biological mother, of the breast milk, and of the nurturing interactions between mother and child negatively affected and delayed the child's growth retardation recovery (Ministry of Health, Institute for Mother and Child Care, & UNICEF, 1991). The abandonment of the children was also somehow "encouraged" by the medical personnel. When parents sought to take their children home after a "temporary abandonment" in maternities or hospitals, they were subject to some informal regulations; the most important one was the ability of the parents to take care of their children (i.e., presence of parenting skills and economic preparedness). These regulations were aimed at reducing infant mortality at home, which was considered an indicator of neglect by the health authorities and a sign of "undermining" the pronatalist policies of the communist regime. Importantly, during the communist regime, doctors from the primary healthcare dispensaries were investigated and could be punished if a child residing within their territory died outside a hospital; thus, there was a tendency on their part to unduly send children to hospitals or institutions for protection. A study conducted in the beginning of 1991 (Ministry of Health, Institute for Mother and Child Care, & UNICEF, 1991) in nurseries and dystrophic centers showed that 74% of children were institutionalized due to the recommendation of a pediatrician. These recommendations must be understood within the context of this time period, when vulnerable children had special nutritional needs (special food, formula, etc.) and their parents did not have the means to provide. In general, hospitals and nurseries had priority, and they were supplied with such products. Purchasing formula from pharmacies was costly for an average parent at that time. According to the same study (Ministry of Health, Institute for Mother and Child Care, & UNICEF, 1991), 80% of children in nurseries had medical problems of which the majority were nutritional or growth disorders, and, consequently, children showed a substantial global growth suppression of their height and weight.

The magnitude of child abandonment during the years of the pronatalist decree is not known exactly. In the early 1990s, the media promoted the notion that there were hundreds of thousands of abandoned or institutionalized children in Romania. However, these estimates were not confirmed by subsequent empirical research. Also, there was much confusion about how to define which children were considered abandoned or institutionalized under the law 3/1970. In the absence of a clear definition, children were considered abandoned if they had special needs and were living with their biological families, but were enrolled in special schools (designed for children with deficiencies). There were only a few of these special schools in Romania, and children who attended them had to have a decision from the Commission for Child Protection (Law 3/1970). The institutions that were included in this category were spread across all levels of education and included special kindergartens, primary, gymnasium, vocational, and lyceum institutions as well as rehabilitation centers. In addition, there were children who were placed in the care of their relatives or other people, and they were incorrectly considered abandoned (DPC & EU/PHARE, 1997).

After the wave of adoptions in the early 1990s (an estimated 3000 children were adopted), there were 8000 children living within nurseries and 1675 children placed in dystrophic centers (Stephenson, Anghelescu, Stativa, & Pasti, 1997). We highlight that, although dystrophic centers were medical institutions and not child protection entities, they housed both dystrophic children and abandoned children with health problems (growth and nutritional disorders). Many of these children had no birth certificates and therefore, according to the law, they could not be placed in nurseries. In the beginning of 1991, 30,325 children were in long-term residential institutions for children older than 3 years (Stephenson et al., 1997). There were no data from this period about children placed in long-term residential centers for the severely disabled. These were institutions which housed children over 3 years with chronic illnesses and disabilities, believed to be irrecoverable by the authorities.

The pronatalist decree was repealed in 1989, shortly after the fall of the communist regime and the installation of the new democratic regime. Contrary to expectations, the number of children abandoned in maternities and hospitals did not drop under the new democratic regime, although contraception and abortions were fully liberalized. One reason for this is that social and economic problems facing families increased after the fall of the communist regime, but social services were not created yet at the local community level to counteract these difficulties, including services to prevent child abandonment.

Before 1990 and until 1990–1992, most children in residential institutions were sent there from maternities and pediatric hospitals. But after 1992, children had begun to be placed in long-term institutions (especially those over 7 years) coming directly from their biological families without having a previous history of institutionalization. The cause of this phenomenon was the country's economic collapse when many factories were closed and numerous families were unable to provide the necessities for their children, especially for school-age children. In 1997, a census conducted in long-term residential centers in Romania showed there were 35,165 children in institutions for preschool- and school-aged children, 9309 children in nurseries, and 4473 were in residential centers for children with severe disabilities (DPC & EU/PHARE, 1997). The same census showed that 54% of the children in centers for school-aged children came directly from their biological families and did not have a prior history of institutionalization.

The number of children in the protection system in Romania was comparable to other Western European countries. The major difference was that in Romania the residential institutions were almost the only protective solution for these children, whereas in Western European countries children in difficulty benefited from a variety of local community services allowing them not to be removed from their biological families for economic reasons (Stephenson et al., 1997). Also, preventive services could have deterred the abandonment of children in maternity wards or placing young children in residential care institutions. In Romania, the first reform of the child protective system was started in 1997. But it took another 7 years to lay the foundation of local community level services to aid in the prevention of child abandonment and removal from families for economic reasons.

Romania is one of a few countries in the region that conducted several cross-sectional and longitudinal studies focusing on institutionalized and noninstitutionalized children after the fall of communism in the 1990s. A particular interest was to evaluate children's health through the nutritional status indicators. The unusually high infant and maternal mortality rate in Romania between 1967 and 1990s, compared to most countries in the region, was the main justification for this interest. In 1989, the maternal mortality ratio was 170 maternal deaths per 100,000 live births. In real terms, 627 mothers died, and 545 of these died through abortion. In 1991, after the abolition of the pronatalist decree, there was a spectacular drop to 114 maternal deaths through abortion. The infant mortality rate increased from 46.6‰ in 1966 to 59.5‰ (deaths per 1000 live births) in 1967. In 1989, the infant mortality rate was 27‰, dropping to 22‰ in 1991 (Ministry of Health, Institute for Mother and Child, UNICEF, & WHO, 1993). Because of these studies, we have information about the nutritional status of children (inclusive of growth retardation) in the 1990s.

The first benchmark study on nutritional status was conducted in 1991 and showed that the prevalence of stunting in noninstitutionalized Romanian children age 0–24 months was 7.3% (95% CI, 6.0–8.6) and was 8.5% for children ages 24–59 months (95% CI, 7.0–10.0) (Ministry of Health, 'Alfred Rusescu' Institute for Mother and Child Care, Center for Disease Control and Prevention, International Micronutrient Malnutrition Prevention and Control, & UNICEF, 1993). By 1999, the situation had improved, and the prevalence of stunting was 5–6% for noninstitutionalized children 0–24 months old (Stanescu et al., 2002). Regarding institutionalized children, the first study (Stanescu, 2002) that examined the status of children's growth in Romanian nurseries was conducted in 1995 on a sample of 2813 children (4–60 months of age) placed in 27 nurseries (out of 59 open that time). Results showed that 50% of children up to 6 months old had short stature for their age (less than −2 standard deviations), and for children ages 37–60 months, 70% had the same issue (Stanescu, 2002). In another study conducted in Romania in 1999, using a representative sample of 3164 institutionalized children (0–18 months), the prevalence of low height ranged from 36% among children under 2 years old (31.4% among infants and 41.4% among children between 1 and 2 years of age), 51.7% among children in the 2–5-year age group, and 34.4% among school-aged children (Stativa, Anghelescu, Palicari, Stanescu, & Nanu, 2002). The aforementioned studies showed that the prevalence of stunting among children in the 1990s in long-term residential institutions was very high. It should be noted that in the study conducted in 1995 (Stanescu, 2002), data were collected by measuring children's growth indicators, whereas the study conducted in 1999 (Stativa et al., 2002) was based on data collected from children's medical records regardless of the year in which the measures were made and recorded. For this reason, any comparison between these two studies should be made with caution.

1.3 Purpose of the Current Study

The major goals of the current study were twofold. First, using the WHO length/height-for-age (HAZ) z-scores (de Onis, 2015; de Onis et al., 2006, 2010), this study sought to investigate the prevalence of stunting among Romanian institutionalized children placed in long-term residential centers (i.e., nurseries, centers for preschool- and school-aged and disabled children). Second, the research aimed to compare the magnitude of children's stunting across these four types of centers.

2 Methods

This study is a secondary analysis of data from the Survey on Child Abuse in Residential Care Institutions in Romania (SCARCIR) (for detailed information about the SCARCIR; Stativa et al., 2002).

2.1 *Participants*

Two criteria were used to include data from the original study in the current analysis. First, children had to have information regarding their height recorded in their files at the time when original SCARCIR data were collected in October and November of 1999 (consequently, we selected only participants whose height data was recorded in 1999). Second, children's height-for-age *z*-scores had to be considered biologically plausible. Consequently, participants from the original SCARCIR data set who did not meet the two abovementioned criteria were excluded ($N = 205$), resulting in a final sample for the current study of 1178 (651 boys and 527 girls) children with ages between 0 and 19 years ($M = 6.61$; $SD = 5.17$; $Mdn = 5.0$) living in 57 long-term residential centers (i.e., nurseries, centers for pre-, school-aged, and disabled children; for detailed information about how the centers were selected in the original study, see Rus et al., 2013; Stativa et al., 2002).

2.2 *Measures*

2.2.1 Height

Information about height was obtained from children's medical records. Length/height-for-age *z*-scores were computed using the height and weight data from the SCARCIR (Stativa et al., 2002) and the relatively new WHO standards for assessing the growth and development of children from birth to 5 years of age (WHO Multicentre Growth Reference Study Group, 2006a, 2006b) employing the SPSS macro provided by WHO Anthro (2010). Similarly, the *z*-scores for children 5–19 years old were computed using the SPSS Macros and WHO AnthroPlus (2009).

2.2.2 Stunting

The nutritional status of each child (chronic malnutrition or stunting) was computed using HAZ *z*-scores which show a child's height in terms of the number of standard deviations above or below the median height of healthy children in the same age group or in a reference group (WHO Multicentre Growth Reference Study Group, 2006a). Thus, children with a HAZ z-score of less than −2 were classified as stunted (de Onis, 2015; de Onis et al., 2006, 2010). Accordingly, the dependent variable (i.e., stunting) was expressed as a binomial variable (0 = *not stunted* vs. 1 = *stunted*).

2.2.3 Institution Type

Children in four types of institutions were assessed, namely, (a) nurseries, and long-term residential centers for (b) preschool-aged, (c) school-aged, and (d) severely disabled children. Very young Romanian children and infants often began their institutional experience in cradles or nurseries ("leagăne"; long-term residential care for children ages 0 to 3). If they were not retrieved by their families by the age of three, they were likely placed in long-term residential centers for children ("case de copii"), including centers for preschool children ("case de copii preşcolari") and school-aged children ("case de copii şcolari"). Typically, those with severe physical or mental problems were placed in residential centers for children with severe disabilities ("cămine spital"). The quality of care or children's needs and basic rights were not homogenously respected across these institutions (for more information, see Chap. 2).

2.3 Data Analysis Plan

The analyses were conducted using SPSS version 19.0 (IBM SPSS, 2010). Frequencies of missing data were assessed. For most of the variables, there was no missing data. Additionally, HAZ scores that were lower than minus six or higher than six were assumed to be inaccurate or extreme (i.e., biologically implausible) and eliminated from the analysis. Statistical analysis included descriptive analysis in the form of frequencies and percentages and crosstabulations with chi square test of association.

3 Results

3.1 Descriptive Analysis

Out of 1178 institutionalized children measured in this study, 547 (46.4%) were stunted. The mean time children had spent in their current institution was 32.41 months ($SD = 31.43$; $Mdn = 22.0$) ranging from 0 to 179 months, and mean age at first placement was 31.79 months ($SD = 42.92$; $Mdn = 9.0$) ranging from 0 to 212 months. As shown in Table 5.1, only 23.2% of children had malnutrition and 11.7%

Table 5.1 Frequencies and percentages of child and institution characteristics

	Type of institutional organization									
	Overall		Nursery		Preschool-aged		School-aged		Disabled	
	N	%	*n*	%	*n*	%	*n*	%	*n*	%
Child level[a]										
Number of children	1178	100	554	47.0	179	15.2	373	31.7	72	6.1
Gender										
Male	651	55.3	291	52.5	106	59.2	217	58.2	37	51.4
Female	527	44.7	263	47.5	73	40.8	156	41.8	35	48.6
Malnutrition at entry in center										
No	880	76.8	344	62.2	159	88.8	316	92.4	61	84.7
Yes	266	23.2	209	37.8	20	11.2	26	7.6	11	15.3
Chronic disease at entry in center										
No	1015	88.3	462	83.5	174	97.2	322	93.3	57	79.2
Yes	134	11.7	91	16.5	5	2.8	23	6.7	15	20.8
Physical disability at assessment										
No	1015	88.3	467	84.3	172	96.1	337	98.0	39	54.2
Yes	134	11.7	87	15.7	7	3.9	7	2.0	33	45.8
Institution level[b]										
Number of residential centers	57	100	17	29.8	10	17.5	25	43.9	5	8.8

[a]Child level shows the number of children in each type of institution
[b]Institution level shows the number of long-term residential centers corresponding to the type of institutional organization

had a chronic disease (as documented in their files when they were placed in the current institution). Furthermore, 11.7% of children had a physical disability when the data were collected.

3.2 *Children's Stunting Across Institutional Settings*

The first two columns of Table 5.2 show the overall frequencies and percentages of children with and without stunting. The remaining columns show the results of a series of crosstabulations with chi square test of association to determine differences in children's stunting between children in nurseries, institutions for preschool-aged and school-aged children, and those placed in institutions for the disabled. Cramer's *V* statistics are reported as a measure of effect size.

Table 5.2 Children's stunting differences across type of institutional organization

	Type of institutional organization												
	Overall		Nursery		Preschool-aged		School-aged		Disabled				
	N	%	*n*	%	*n*	%	*n*	%	*n*	%	χ^2	*Cramer's V*	*p*
Stunting											**81.547**	**0.263**	**<0.001**
No	631	53.6	262	47.3[a]	95	53.1[a]	260	69.7[b]	14	19.4[c]			
Yes	547	46.4	292	52.7[a]	84	46.9[a]	113	30.3[b]	58	80.6[c]			

Note. Differences are tested within stunting items using z-test of proportions. Across rows, proportions with different superscripts within the same block are significantly different ($p < 0.05$). Differences are tested within item using z-test of proportions with Bonferroni corrections

These results show that stunting was found in 292 (52.7%) children in nurseries, 84 (46.9%) in centers for preschool-aged children, 113 (30.3%) in centers for school-aged children, and 58 (80.6%) in centers for disabled children. A significantly lower percentage of children in school-aged centers (30.3%) were stunted compared to those in nurseries (52.7%), preschool-aged centers (46.9%), and centers for disabled children (80.6%). In addition, a significantly higher percentage of children in centers for disabled children (80.6%) was stunted compared to those in nurseries (52.7%), preschool-aged (46.9%), and school-aged centers (30.3%).

4 Discussion

In this study, a relatively large sample of institutionalized children (0–19 years old) was used to measure the prevalence of stunting. The overall prevalence of stunting in 1999 among Romanian institutionalized children across all institutional settings was 46.4%. Regarding children in nurseries, the present study found that 52.7% were stunted, and this result shows that the magnitude of stunting in 1999 was lower compared to another previous study conducted in 1991 (57% were stunted) (Ministry of Health, Institute for Mother and Child Care, & UNICEF, 1991), and it was relatively similar compared to a study conducted in 1995 (Stanescu, 2002), as well as higher when compared to what was found by a study conducted in 1996 (41% were stunted) (Stephenson et al., 1997). The worldwide prevalence of low height-for-age has been found to vary from 5% to 65% (de Onis & Blossner, 1997). According to the same report published in 1997, the prevalence of low height-for-age rose at around 3 months of age, and then it slowed down at 3 years of age. Thus, according to the report's author, for children below the age of 2–3 years, low height-for-age probably reflects "*a continuing process of "failing to grow" or "stunting"; for older children, it reflects a state of "having failed to grow" or "being stunted"*" (de Onis, 1997, p. 47).

Summarizing the results, a significantly lower percentage of children in school-aged centers were stunted compared to those in preschool-aged centers or nurseries. Certainly, the highest percentage of children with stunting was at the centers for the disabled (see Table 5.2), but this percentage cannot be compared to the percentage of stunting in children in other centers (for preschool- and school-aged children) because only children over 3 years of age with serious health problems, chronic diseases, frequently associated with genetic diseases, malformations, or handicaps were placed in centers for the disabled. The decrease in the prevalence of stunting in centers that housed children older than 3 years (centers for preschool- and school-aged children) compared to nurseries unfortunately cannot be attributed to the recovery of growth disorders during institutionalization.

With the exception of institutions for children with serious chronic illnesses and handicaps, most children with stunting were found in nurseries. These results are explained by the health of children at the time of admission to these institutions. Of the children in nurseries, most had health problems, including those that affect growth and lead to malnutrition, such as chronic illness or disabilities. The vast majority (80%) of children in these nurseries were placed there directly from maternity wards, pediatric hospitals, and other nurseries (DPC & EU/PHARE, 1997). Thus, these children spent most of their early lives in institutions, which deprived them of having nurturing emotional interactions with caregivers. These early experiences often irreversibly affected children's growth development (Rutter, 1998). After age 3, children who did not leave the child protection system were placed in other long-term residential centers. Healthy children without severe chronic diseases and disabilities were next placed in institutions for preschool ages and those with chronic diseases and disabilities in centers for the disabled. This explains the low percentage of children with chronic diseases at entry into preschool-aged centers (see Table 5.1). However, this low severe chronic illness frequency is not reflected in a decreased prevalence of growth delays for those placed in centers for preschool-aged children (46.9%) as we would have expected. This confirms that the recovery of stunting in the context of institutional care is difficult, especially if the recovery does not begin before the child reaches 2 years of age and is not removed from residential institutional environment (Rutter, 1998).

The school-aged children placed in long-term residential centers had a significantly lower prevalence of stunting than those placed in a nursery or preschool-aged center. These results may be explained by the fact that 54% of children placed in school-aged centers came from their biological families and did not have a prior history of institutionalization (DPC & EU/PHARE, 1997; Stephenson et al., 1997). Parents placed them in institutions due to a variety of economic reasons, including a lack of boarding schools for children from rural communities. Boarding schools were common in Romania during that time period as a way to provide education to children. Most of these boarding schools were abolished after 1989 or became too expensive. Therefore, for many children living in rural areas, placement within the long-term residential centers became the only solution for continuation of their education.

Knowing that children living within institutional care settings are shown to experience a substantial global suppression of their growth, including their height (for a review, see Dobrova-Krol et al., 2008; Johnson et al., 2010; Johnson & Gunnar, 2011; Miller et al., 2007; Routray et al., 2015; Rutter, 1998; Smyke et al., 2007; Van IJzendoorn et al., 2007), we suspect that the overall experience of institutionalization (including social and emotional deprivation) may also have contributed to the stunting of the children in our sample.

Regarding malnutrition, the causes are complex and may include more factors than a lack of adequate nutrition (Stativa, 2002). For children placed in long-term residential centers where they may experience privation, malnutrition should also be considered an indicator of a dysfunctional child-caregiver affective relationship. Thus, any recovery program designed to prevent or alleviate stunting in institutionalized children should require the active participation of a nurturing caregiver. To improve outcomes, we need a comprehensive and multidisciplinary approach where many potential risk factors are taken into consideration and addressed, such as nutrition, hygiene, health condition, abuse, neglect, and not least the attachment between child and caregiver (Stativa, 2002).

5 Implications for Improving Children's Care

Institutionalized children in Romania experienced various forms of neglect during the communist era, which continued even after the collapse of the communist regime in 1989. However, as part of profound reforms of the child protection system, Romania ratified the United Nations Convention on the Rights of the Child (UNCRC) in 1990 (UN General Assembly, 1989) and adopted its own national plan of action for child protection based on the World Summit for Children in the mid-1990s (UNICEF, 1990). At the root of the problem of institutionalization of children was denial by the communist regime of the existence of various social problems that needed a solution. Residential institutions were the only solution for many children in difficulty. In the absence of psychosocial professionals, children typically had access to inadequate and inappropriate solutions for their problems. Without community support services, most of the children entered the child protection system at an early age, with virtually no personalized care. The first steps toward regulatory reform included the restructuring of long-term residential centers, development of alternatives to institutions (i.e., familial model), and implementation of measures to prevent child abandonment ("Protecția drepturilor copilului – experiența României," n.d.). Reforms of institutional care continued after data was collected in 1999, and the Romanian child protection system now includes more types of services provided to prevent the entry of children into residential centers (e.g., public and private day care centers, after-school programs, public and private maternal centers, shelters for women and children victims of domestic abuse, counseling centers for parents and children, day care centers for children with disabilities, and services for monitoring, assistance, and support of pregnant women predisposed to abandon their children, etc.). Additionally, there are minimum mandatory standards for care and safety in place for residential facilities (Bejenaru & Tucker, 2014). In 2006, a social inspection mechanism was created to unify monitoring and control activities regarding implementation of the minimum quality standards for all types of social services. The health of the child was the most important predictor of institutionalization and by default for stunting; thus, the Ministry of Health developed various screening programs for children designed for early detection and treatment of diseases such as hypothyroidism, phenylketonuria, cystic fibrosis, celiac disease, retinopathy of prematurity, hip dislocation, and deafness, and the development of disability rehabilitation services has decreased the magnitude of institutionalization in Romania during the last years. At present, there is a law in place requiring that each maternity ward or pediatric hospital hire a social worker to prevent child abandonment at birth. After 2004, children up to 3 years old could no longer be placed in residential institutions; instead, they are cared for by foster parents. Nowadays, there are about 19,000 children in the care of professional foster parents (assistant maternal profesionist), a full-time occupation with salary provided by the state or private organizations (ANPDC, 2016). Furthermore, presently, there are about 20,000 children over 3 years of age placed within public and private residential centers. Also, it is encouraged for abandoned children to be placed with their relatives (up to the fourth degree relatives), and about 19,000 are currently in the care of their extended families or other persons (ANPDC, 2016).

6 Limitations

There are some limitations to our study. First, this research did not precisely define the nature of children's malnutrition, chronic or physical problems at entry, or when data were collected, and researchers relied on the accuracy of children's medical records. Second, even though there is strong evidence supporting the assumption that the experience of institutionalization (which often includes deprivation and abuse) per se is associated with significant global growth suppression (for a review, see Johnson et al., 2010; Johnson & Gunnar, 2011; Rutter, 1998; Smyke et al., 2007; Van IJzendoorn et al., 2007), we know little about other potential risk factors that children in our sample might have experienced, such as prenatal exposure to alcohol, low birth weight, or nutritional insufficiencies. Thus, this study lacked a control for those variables related with participant's personal histories. Third, WHO standards (WHO Anthro, 2010; WHO Multicentre Growth Reference Study Group, 2006a, 2006b) were used to compute children's length/height-for-age z-scores using data that were collected prior to when these standards were published. Therefore, it may be possible that the estimation of stunting was influenced by this difference. Finally, the data only allowed us to examine the association between children's stunting across various types of institutions (i.e., nurseries, and centers for preschool, school-aged, and disabled children). Thus, the present cross-sectional design does not allow us to infer a causal relationship between these variables.

7 Summary

The present study provided a novel perspective regarding the stunting among Romanian institutionalized children placed in long-term residential centers, such as nurseries, centers for pre-, school-aged, and disabled children. The study included a historical perspective of the Romanian child protection system useful for understanding the determinants and magnitude of the phenomenon of stunting among children institutionalized in long-term residential centers. The present research revealed that, overall, 46.4% of children were stunted when they were measured in 1999.

Questions for Discussion

1. Some studies found that stunted children can experience a "catch-up" in growth in some circumstances. Define these circumstances and explain why these would contribute to a catch-up.

2. In the literature, there are frequent assertions highlighting that undernutrition and malnutrition are major causes for stunting. Meanwhile, research in recent years has shown that in residential institutions where food was adequate quantitatively and qualitatively, the growth of children was still disrupted, and with little hope for their normalization with advancing age. How do you explain this phenomenon?
3. What are the policies in your country to help prevent disturbances in nutritional status of children in the first years of life?

References

Autoritatea Nationala pentru Protectia Drepturilor Copiilor (ANPDC). (2016). *Statistici* [Statistics]. Retrieved from http://www.copii.ro/statistici/?lang=en

Bejenaru, A., & Tucker, S. (2014). Challenging dominant representations of residential childcare in Romania: An exploration of the views of children and young people living in the care system. *Journal of Youth Studies*, 1–14. doi:10.1080/13676261.2014.918250. (ahead-of-print).

Correll, L., Correll, T., & Predescu, M. (2006). *USAID and child welfare reform in Romania: Challenges, successes, and legacy*. Washington, DC: USAID/DGST/E&E, JBS International, Aguirre Division. Retrieved October 27, 2016, from http://pdf.usaid.gov/pdf_docs/Pdach405.pdf

de Onis, M. (2015). World Health Organization reference curves. In M. L. Frelut (Ed.), *The ECOG's eBook on child and adolescent obesity*. Retrieved June 16, 2016, from http://ebook.ecog-obesity.eu/

de Onis, M., & Blossner, M. (1997). *WHO global database on child growth and malnutrition*. Geneva, Switzerland: World Health Organization. Retrieved February 18, 2017, from http://www.who.int/nutgrowthdb/about/introduction/en/index2.html

de Onis, M., Blössner, M., & Borghi, E. (2010). Global prevalence and trends of overweight and obesity among preschool children. *The American Journal of Clinical Nutrition*, *92*(5), 1257–1264. doi:10.3945/ajcn.2010.29786.

de Onis, M., Onyango, A. W., Borghi, E., Garza, C., & Yang, H. (2006). Comparison of the World Health Organization (WHO) Child Growth Standards and the National Center for Health Statistics/WHO international growth reference: Implications for child health programmes. *Public Health Nutrition*, *9*(7), 942–947.

Department of Child Protection (DPC) & EU/PHARE. (1997). *Recensamantul copiilor/tinerilor plasati in institutiile de ocrotire din Romania* [Census of children/youth placed in child protection institutions in Romania] (Vol. 1–3). Bucharest, Romania: Childhood Protection Program Technical Assistance Unit.

Dobrova-Krol, N. A., van IJzendoorn, M. H., Bakermans-Kranenburg, M. J., Cyr, C., & Juffer, F. (2008). Physical growth delays and stress dysregulation in stunted and non-stunted Ukrainian institution-reared children. *Infant Behavior & Development*, *31*(3), 539–553. doi:10.1016/j.infbeh.2008.04.001.

Espo, M., Kulmala, T., Maleta, K., Cullinan, T., Salin, M. L., & Ashorn, P. (2002). Determinants of linear growth and predictors of severe stunting during infancy in rural Malawi. *Acta Paediatrica (Oslo, Norway: 1992)*, *91*(12), 1364–1370.

Glavce, C., Dragomirescu, L., Valentin, C., & Apavaloae, L. (2001). L'évolution du poids à la naissance en fonction des conditions socio-économiques différentes. *Revue de la Societe de Biometrie Humaine et Anthropologie*, *Tome 19*, 1–2.

IBM Corp. (2010). *IBM SPSS statistics for Windows (version 19.0)*. Armonk, NY: Author.

Johnson, D. E., & Gunnar, M. R. (2011). IV. Growth failure in institutionalized children. *Monographs of the Society for Research in Child Development*, *76*(4), 92–126.

Johnson, D. E., Guthrie, D., Smyke, A. T., Koga, S. F., Fox, N. A., Zeanah, C. H., & Nelson III, C. A. (2010). Growth and associations between auxology, caregiving environment, and cognition in socially deprived Romanian children randomized to foster vs ongoing institutional care. *Archives of Pediatrics & Adolescent Medicine, 164*(6), 507–516. doi:10.1001/archpediatrics.2010.56.

Martorell, R., Ramakrishnan, U., Schroeder, D. G., Melgar, P., & Neufeld, L. (1998). Intrauterine growth retardation, body size, body composition and physical performance in adolescence. *European Journal of Clinical Nutrition, 52*(Suppl. 1), S43–S52.

Miller, L. C., Chan, W., Litvinova, A., Rubin, A., Tirella, L., & Cermak, S. (2007). Medical diagnoses and growth of children residing in Russian orphanages. *Acta Paediatrica, 96*(12), 1765–1769.

Ministry of Health, 'Alfred Rusescu' Institute for Mother and Child Care, Center for Disease Control and Prevention, International Micronutrient Malnutrition Prevention and Control, & UNICEF. (1993). *Studiul national de nutritie a copilului sub varsta de 5 ani* [National nutrition survey of children under age 5]. Report.

Ministry of Health, Institute for Mother and Child Care, UNICEF. (1991). *Cauze ale institutionalizarii copiilor in leagane si sectii de distrofici in Romania* [Causes of children's institutionalization in "leagane" and dystrophic centers in Romania]. Retrieved http://iomc.ro/uploads/documents/Cauzele_institutionalizarii_1991.pdf

Ministry of Health, Institute for Mother and Child, UNICEF, & WHO. (1993). *Preventing maternal death in Romania: An analysis of maternity care and maternal mortality with recommendations for a safe motherhood programme*. Bucharest, Romania: Ministry of Health.

Muresan, P., & Copil, I. M. (1974). Romania. In B. R. Berelson (Ed.), *Population policy in developed countries* (pp. 367–368). New York, NY: McGraw-Hill.

Protecția drepturilor copilului – experiența României. (n.d.). Retrieved October 16, 2016, from http://www.drepturilecopiilor.ro/downloads/conference/Bogdan%20Adrian%20Panait%20-%20RO.pdf

Routray, S., Meher, B. K., Tripathy, R., Parida, S. N., Mahilary, N., & Pradhan, D. D. (2015). Growth and development among children living in orphanages of Odisha, an Eastern Indian state. *IOSR Journal of Dental and Medical Sciences, 14*(1), 38–41.

Rus, A. V., Stativa, E., Pennings, J. S., Cross, D. R., Ekas, N., Purvis, K., & Parris, S. R. (2013). Severe punishment of children by staff in Romanian placement centers for school-aged children: Effects of child and institutional characteristics. *Child Abuse and Neglect*. doi:10.1016/j.chiabu.2013.07.003.

Rutter, M. (1998). Developmental catch-up, and deficit, following adoption after severe global early privation. English and Romanian Adoptees (ERA) Study Team. *Journal of Child Psychology and Psychiatry, and Allied Disciplines, 39*(4), 465–476.

Semba, R. D., de Pee, S., Sun, K., Sari, M., Akhter, N., & Bloem, M. W. (2008). Effect of parental formal education on risk of child stunting in Indonesia and Bangladesh: Across-sectional study. *Lancet (London, England), 371*(9609), 322–328. doi:10.1016/S0140 6736(08)60169-5.

Smyke, A. T., Koga, S. F., Johnson, D. E., Fox, N. A., Marshall, P. J., Nelson, C. A., & Zeanah, C. H. (2007). The caregiving context in institution-reared and family-reared infants and toddlers in Romania. *Journal of Child Psychology and Psychiatry, and Allied Disciplines, 48*(2), 210–218.

Stanescu, A. (Ed.). (2002). *Programul național de supraveghere nutrițională 1993–2000: Evoluția situației nutritionale și a comportamentului alimentar de la naștere la 5 ani* [National nutritional surveillance program 1993–2000: Evolution of the nutritional status and of feeding practices from birth to the age of 5]. Bucharest, Romania: Mar Link.

Stativa, E., Anghelescu, C., Palicari, G., Stanescu, A., & Nanu, R. (2002). *Child abuse in residential care institutions in Romania*. Bucharest, Romania: Extrem Group.

Stephenson, P., Anghelescu, C., Stativa, E., & Pasti, S. (1997). *Cauzele institutionalizarii copiilor din Romania* [The causes of children from Romania]. Bucharest, Romania: UNICEF, Fundatia Internationala pentru Copil si Familie.

Stephenson, P., Wagner, M., Badea, M., & Serbanescu, F. (1992). Commentary: The public health consequences of restricted induced abortion – Lessons from Romania. *American Journal of Public Health, 82*(10), 1328–1331.

Trebici, V. (1976). *Romania's population and demographic trends*. Bucharest, Romania: Meridiane Publishing House.

UN General Assembly. (1989, November 20). *Convention on the rights of the child* (United Nations, Treaty Series, Vol. 1577, p. 3). Retrieved July 15, 2016, from http://www.ohchr.org/Documents/ProfessionalInterest/crc.pdf

UNICEF. (1990). World declaration on the survival, protection and development of children. Retrieved July 20, 2016, from http://www.unicef.org/wsc/declare.htm

Van de Poel, E., Hosseinpoor, A. R., Speybroeck, N., Van Ourti, T., & Vega, J. (2008). Socioeconomic inequality in malnutrition in developing countries. *Bulletin of the World Health Organization, 86*(4), 282–291.

Van IJzendoorn, M. H., Bakermans-Kranenburg, M. J., & Juffer, F. (2007). Plasticity of growth in height, weight, and head circumference: Meta-analytic evidence of massive catch-up after international adoption. *Journal of Developmental and Behavioral Pediatrics: JDBP, 28*(4), 334–343.

Victoria, C. G., Adair, L., Fall, C., Hallal, P. C., Martorell, R., Richter, L., & Sachdev, H. S. (2008). Maternal and child undernutrition: Consequences for adult health and human capital. *Lancet, 371*(9609), 340–357.

Waterlow, J. C. (1994). Introduction. Causes and mechanisms of linear growth retardation (stunting). *European Journal of Clinical Nutrition, 48*(Suppl. 1), S1–S4.

WHO Anthro. (2010). *WHO Anthro for personal computers, version 3.2.2: Software for assessing growth and development of the world's children*. Geneva, Switzerland: WHO. Retrieved June 16, 2016, from http://www.who.int/childgrowth/software/en/

WHO AnthroPlus. (2009). *WHO AnthroPlus for personal computers manual: Software for assessing growth of the world's children and adolescents*. Geneva, Switzerland: WHO. Retrieved June 16, 2016, from http://www.who.int/growthref/tools/en/

WHO Multicentre Growth Reference Study Group. (2006a). *WHO child growth standards: Length/height-for-age, weight-for-age, weight-for-length, weight-for-height and body mass index-for-age: Methods and development*. Geneva, Switzerland: World Health Organization.

WHO Multicentre Growth Reference Study Group. (2006b). WHO child growth standards based on length/height, weight and age. *Acta Paediatrica, 450*, 76–85.

Chapter 6
Psychopathology Following Severe Deprivation: History, Research, and Implications of the Bucharest Early Intervention Project

Kathryn L. Humphreys, Nathan A. Fox, Charles A. Nelson, and Charles H. Zeanah

> *Policy makers may need a strong method of proof to be willing to accept a given intervention, especially when it conflicts with their biases. Even if some experts claim to know, based on observational evidence or experience, that a particular intervention is effective in producing a given outcome, or is better than an alternative intervention, positive results from a well-designed randomized trial may be necessary to persuade policy makers to change standard practice.*
>
> Franklin G. Miller (2009)

1 Introduction

The Bucharest Early Intervention Project (BEIP) is the first-ever randomized controlled trial (RCT) of foster care for children who experienced institutional care due to abandonment at or soon after birth (Zeanah et al., 2003). Although experiences of

K.L. Humphreys (✉)
Department of Psychology, Stanford University, Stanford, CA 94305, USA
e-mail: k.humphreys@stanford.edu; humphrkl@gmail.com

N.A. Fox
Human Development and Quantitative Methodology (HDQM), University of Maryland, College Park, MD, USA
e-mail: fox@umd.edu

C.A. Nelson
Boston Children's Hospital/Harvard Medical School, Harvard Graduate School of Education, Boston, MA, USA
e-mail: Charles.Nelson@childrens.harvard.edu

C.H. Zeanah
Department of Psychiatry and Behavioral Sciences, Tulane University School of Medicine, New Orleans, LA, USA
e-mail: czeanah@tulane.edu

A.V. Rus et al. (eds.), *Child Maltreatment in Residential Care*,
DOI 10.1007/978-3-319-57990-0_6

psychosocial deprivation associated with institutional care were considered harmful for child development for a century (Chapin, 1915), the extent of recovery from such circumstances was not well established. In fact, prior to the BEIP, adoption studies had documented improvement in children who had experienced early institutional rearing, although it was difficult to determine how potential sample bias (i.e., who was and was not adopted) contributed to outcome. Only a RCT is capable of determining if foster care is a better intervention than institutional care.

In this chapter, we provide the theoretical and scientific foundations of this study, including the historical context and the study design. Furthermore, we discuss the key psychopathology findings from the BEIP, focusing on associations with institutional care history, the effects of a high-quality foster care intervention, and mediators and moderators of psychopathology following early adversity:

1. We discuss the unique value of conducting a randomized controlled trial of family-based care for abandoned children.
2. We provide evidence of significant intervention effects in a number of psychopathology domains.
3. We also highlight policy implications from our work, including that children should be placed into high-quality and child-centered family-based care, that this placement should occur as early in life as is possible, and that these placements should be stable across the child's life.

2 What's Out There Today: Established Research and Practice

The quality of care provided to abandoned or orphaned children varies widely, from none at all (e.g., "street children" who receive no societal intervention) to ideal (e.g., adoption into a family providing child-centered care). Nevertheless, the vast majority of these children receive caregiving that is between these extremes, and yet there is little consensus regarding best practices for abandoned children. Historically, many countries created institutions specifically to provide for the basic needs of these children (e.g., food, clothing, and shelter). And though the quality of care received in institutions can vary widely, some features are noted repeatedly: a regimented daily schedule, rotating caregivers, low levels of stimulation, and nonindividualized care, resulting in little psychological investment in each particular child (Zeanah, Smyke, & Settles, 2006). Given the low levels of individual attention and diminished opportunities to interact contingently with a caregiver, it is not surprising that the psychosocial deprivation experienced in institutions is linked to poorer outcomes in children. A century of research has linked institutional rearing for young children to negative outcomes in multiple domains, including physical growth, motor development, cognition, language, social functioning, attachment, and psychopathology (Zeanah et al., 2006). In this chapter, we focus on psychopathology. However, in most of the research conducted, one cannot explicitly link outcomes to the type of care the child received. And for obvious ethical reasons, children cannot be randomly assigned to institutional care, further constraining putative demonstrations of causal links between institutional care and outcomes.

Still, adoption from orphanages has provided a "natural experiment" in which the degree of recovery from deprivation can be examined. Several research groups, particularly in the Europe and North America, have studied the development and outcomes of adopted children who were formerly in orphanage care in other countries. These studies have often compared adopted children to those reared in their biological families and found that, as a group, children with a history of prior institutional care had poorer outcomes in a number of domains, including increased rates of psychiatric disorders and elevated levels of psychopathology (Gunnar, Bruce, & Grotevant, 2000). In fact, a framework developed by Rutter and colleagues in their studies of institutionalized children identified behavioral patterns that appeared uniquely clustered in children who had experienced psychosocial deprivation (Rutter, Sonuga-Barke, Beckett et al., 2010). Specifically, work from the English and Romanian Adoption Study (ERAS; Rutter, Sonuga-Barke, & Castle, 2010) led the researchers to identify four deprivation specific patterns, of which three are forms of psychopathology: quasi-autism, disinhibited attachment, and inattention/overactivity (the fourth was cognitive impairment). Furthermore, their group provided evidence of the benefit of earlier placement into families (which were largely British and middle-class). The ERAS found that children adopted before age 6 months fared significantly better than children adopted after 6 months across all developmental domains assessed and specifically in these psychopathological deprivation-specific patterns. In fact, though developmentally all children appeared behind typical at the age of adoption, children adopted by age 6 months achieved almost complete developmental catch-up by age 4 years. These gains were sustained for years after adoption into these highly supportive families. Those adopted after 6 months showed some recovery as well but to a lower extent compared to those placed in families very early in life.

Although adoption designs provide important information about the impact of psychosocial deprivation as well as when and how recovery from this form of early adversity may be possible, one important limitation is that children who are adopted (compared to those who remain in institutions) are not randomly assigned to this "intervention." Here, we reemphasize that children are not randomly assigned to institutional care, as it is unclear what factors are associated with decisions to place children (even selected children from within the same family) to institutional care and how children placed versus not placed in orphanages may differ. Thus, while children who were adopted have better outcomes across numerous domains compared to their non-adopted counterparts who remained in institutional care, it is clearly plausible that the children who were higher functioning in the first place were the ones selected by families for adoption. Other biases, including children's racial features, have been documented as a factor related to selection for adoption (e.g., Tizard & Tizard, 1967). This raises questions about the generalizability of findings from these results. RCTs do not guarantee that groups randomly selected for each group are identical, but the nature of random selection minimizes selection bias to interventions. The BEIP sought to use the RCT design to determine what effect, if any, family placement had for children in orphanage care without the limitation of potential selection biases into the intervention (Zeanah et al., 2003).

The context for BEIP and implementing an RCT in Romania early in the twenty-first century is that the country at that time was a fledgling democracy attempting to cope with a child protection crisis of unprecedented scope. Nicolae Ceauşescu rose to power in Romania in the 1960s and served as the General Secretary of the Communist Party in Romania from 1965 to 1989. His regime was characterized by brutality, oppression, and policies designed to increase Romania's population and industrial productivity. Specifically, his policies banned contraception, criminalized abortion, and required women, through incentives and punishments, to have at least five children by the time they were 45 years of age. His policies led to significant increases in the Romanian population but also increased child abandonment substantially. Because many women carried unwanted pregnancies and delivered children they could not afford, increasing numbers of infants were abandoned to the large, impersonal institutions that were characteristic within the Soviet bloc.

After Ceauşescu's fall from power, Western media discovered the magnitude of the problem and broadcast images of horribly neglected children living in overcrowded state-sponsored institutions in Romania. An estimated 170,000 children lived in these institutions in 1990 after Ceausescu was overthrown (Rosapepe, 2001).

A decade later, there was still a debate within Romania about how best to care for abandoned children. Some believed that institutional care was not only a reasonable alternative to family-based care but that it may have actually been superior in meeting children's needs. Others were interested in reforms (see Nelson, Fox, & Zeanah, 2014, for a fuller discussion).

In this context, the BEIP team was invited to design a study to provide data to inform the debate. The investigators proposed a true experimental design contrasting care as usual (i.e., continued institutional care) and placement in child-centered, high-quality foster care. Several important ethical considerations were made in designing and implementing the study, including (1) conducting research with implications for the population being studied, (2) procedures involving no more than minimal risk, (3) intense oversight to protect vulnerable participants, and (4) a policy of noninterference when it came to the placements of children in the study. In other words, the study team pledged not to interfere with placement of any child as these decisions were to be left entirely to the local Child Protection Commission in Bucharest. Therefore, if the Commission directed, children in either the care as usual group (CAUG) or foster care group (FCG) could return to their families or be adopted. This noninterference policy meant that several children in the CAUG eventually were returned to their biological families, were adopted domestically, or were placed into government-sponsored foster care that did not exist when the study began. In addition, some children randomly assigned to the foster care intervention were also reunited with their biological families, adopted domestically, and eventually as they approached adolescence, some who were determined to be unsafe in families were returned to an institution. The ethical issues have been discussed at length elsewhere by us and others (Miller, 2009; Millum & Emanuel, 2007; Nelson et al., 2014; Rid, 2012; Zeanah, Fox, & Nelson, 2012).

Following careful deliberation within the MacArthur Foundation Research Network on Early Experience and Brain Development, as well as with permission from the Romanian Ministry of Health, the local Child Protection Commission in Bucharest, and the Institution for Maternal and Child Health, the BEIP was launched. All children residing in six institutional settings in Bucharest, Romania, who were less than age 31 months (n = 187) were assessed for participation in the study. Exclusion criteria for the study included medical conditions (e.g., genetic syndromes, signs of fetal alcohol syndrome, and microcephaly) and resulted in the exclusion of 51 children. This resulted in a final sample of 136 children between 6 and 31 months of age (mean 22 months) who had been abandoned at or shortly after birth and placed in institutions.

After extensive baseline assessments (Zeanah, Smyke, Koga, & Carlson, 2005), the 136 institutionalized children were randomized into either CAUG (n = 68) or FCG (n = 68). Randomization was accomplished by assigning a number to each of the 136 study children and then writing these numbers on slips of paper and drawing them from a hat at random. The first number drawn was assigned to the CAUG, and the second number was assigned to the FCG, and this pattern was repeated until all 136 numbers had been drawn. In the cases of siblings, both siblings were listed on the same slip of paper so they were subsequently placed together. Families who fostered children as part of this study were demographically distinct from adoptive parents in the ERAS. BEIP foster families, though Romanian, were working class, had fewer resources, and had less access to health and social safety net programs available to middle-class adoptive families in the UK.

In addition to the foster care and care as usual groups that comprised the RCT, a third group of children was assessed at baseline to provide a comparison group of children from within Romania. These comparison children were required to have never experienced institutionalization (never institutionalized group [NIG], n = 72) and were recruited from public pediatric clinics in Bucharest. In addition to a baseline assessment, the original RCT included assessments at 30, 42, and 54 months of age. At age 54 months, the trial concluded, and per prior arrangement, the BEIP foster care network was turned over to local government authorities who began to support and oversee the foster families' care. Follow-up assessments of children were conducted when children were 8 and 12 years old, and at present a follow-up at age 16 years is underway. In addition, over the course of the study, to keep the number of NIG participants sizable enough to provide statistical power for analyses, additional NIG children were recruited to serve as comparison children. Generally, these children were recruited from schools attended by the BEIP participants.

3 New Research/Developments in This Area

The BEIP has resulted in numerous publications. The study is ongoing, and results are continuing to be reported, so only a selective presentation of findings is possible. Therefore, we summarize and discuss results from the BEIP that have focused on

Table 6.1 Measures used to assess psychopathology outcomes from the Bucharest Early Intervention Project by assessment wave and psychopathology domain

Assessment age	Internalizing	Externalizing	ADHD	RAD	DSED
Baseline	–	–	–	DAI	DAI
30 months	–	–	–	DAI	DAI
42 months	–	–	–	DAI	DAI
54 months	PAPA	PAPA	PAPA	DAI	DAI
8 years	HBQ	HBQ	HBQ	DAI	DAI
12 years	DISC	DISC; ICU	DISC	DAI	DAI

ADHD attention-deficit/hyperactivity disorder, *RAD* reactive attachment disorder, *DSED* disinhibited social engagement disorder, *PAPA* preschool age psychiatric assessment, *HBQ* MacArthur Health and Behavior Questionnaire, *DISC* diagnostic interview schedule for children, *ICU* Inventory of Callous-Unemotional Traits

Table 6.2 Comparison of intent-to-treat analyses following the formal end to the intervention at age 54 months

Assessmentage	Internalizing	Externalizing	ADHD	RAD	DSED
54 months	CAUG > FCG[a]	CAUG ≈ FCG	CAUG ≈ FCG	CAUG > FCG	CAUG > FCG
8 years	CAUG ≈ FCG	–	CAUG ≈ FCG	CAUG > FCG	CAUG > FCG
12 years	CAUG≈,>FCG[a]	CAUG > FCG[b]	CAUG ≈ FCG	CAUG > FCG	CAUG > FCG

ADHD attention-deficit/hyperactivity disorder, *RAD* reactive attachment disorder, *DSED* disinhibited social engagement disorder, *CAUG* care as usual group, *FCG* foster care group

≈ no statistically significant difference

[a]Girls only

[b]Boys only

psychopathology. Though parts of this review will be similar to a previously published paper from our group (Bos et al., 2011), much has been learned since that review appeared. Rather than organize the findings by the children's age during the assessment wave, as many of the prior empirical articles have done, this review will examine broad domains of psychopathology (internalizing, externalizing, attention-deficit/hyperactivity disorder [ADHD], reactive attachment disorder [RAD], and disinhibited social engagement disorder [DSED]) and outline key findings from throughout the follow-up period, starting from baseline (age 22 months) until the most current completed assessment (age 12 years) (see Table 6.1 for an overview of the measures used to assess psychopathology in the BEIP).

In addition to discussing whether group differences based on history of institutional care (e.g., ever institutionalized group [EIG] vs. NIG) and based on intent-to-treat analyses (e.g., CAUG vs. FCG; Table 6.2) were found, we provide findings, when possible, of mediators and moderators of psychopathology (e.g., attachment, genetics, foster care placement age, etc.). This lens allows a potential window into the mechanisms by which early experiences predict psychopathology risk as well as groups (e.g., boys or girls) that may be more or less vulnerable to psychopathology as a function of psychosocial deprivation and/or intervention.

3.1 *Internalizing Psychopathology*

3.1.1 54 Months: RCT Completion

Internalizing psychopathology, which consists of depression and anxiety symptoms and disorders, has been examined in follow-up assessments at ages 54 months, 8 years, and 12 years (see Table 6.1 for measures used). At 54 months, interviews were conducted with each child's parent, foster parent, or closest caregiver in institutional care, depending on the child's current living situation. Preschool-aged children from the EIG had higher rates of internalizing disorders than those from the NIG (32 vs. 14%; Zeanah et al., 2009). In addition, this study examined whether children randomly assigned to the FCG differed in internalizing psychopathology compared to those assigned to the CAUG. While an intent-to-treat intervention effect for FCG vs. CAUG was found (44 vs. 22%), this was explained by differences in girls. Girls assigned to the FCG had significantly lower rates of internalizing disorders than their CAUG counterparts, whereas there was no significant effect of the intervention on boys' internalizing psychopathology.

We also examined predictors of internalizing psychopathology at 54 months. Two different studies within the BEIP identified that observed attachment security with a caregiver at age 42 months predicted lower rates of internalizing disorders in both sexes. In fact, among girls, level of attachment security fully mediated the effects of the high-quality foster care intervention effects on internalizing disorders (McLaughlin, Nelson, Fox, & Zeanah, 2012). Further, attachment security at 42 months mediated association between caregiving quality at age 30 months and internalizing symptoms at age 54 months (McGoron et al., 2012). Taken together, these findings suggest that the manner in which the intervention reduced internalizing symptoms was through improvements in caregiving quality, which in turn positively affected children's attachment security.

Two published papers examined brain electrical activity (EEG) in relation to internalizing symptoms at age 54 months. McLaughlin, Fox, Zeanah, and Nelson (2011) examined frontal EEG asymmetry at age 42 months, which indexes the degree to which the right hemisphere has greater activation than the left hemisphere. This asymmetry was significantly associated with internalizing symptoms at 54 months after controlling for asymmetry at the baseline assessment (McLaughlin et al., 2011). The second analysis examined event-related potentials (ERPs), which assess brain response resulting from a specific stimulus. Slopen, McLaughlin, Fox, Zeanah, and Nelson (2012) examined various components of the ERP response that correspond to the time following stimulus presentation and found that reduced P100 and P700 amplitudes in response to facial stimuli were associated with higher levels of anxiety symptoms. These papers point to neural differences potentially resulting from institutional care history that may help to explain mechanisms by which internalizing symptoms were manifested at higher levels.

In addition to main effects of the intervention, Tibu, Humphreys, Fox, Nelson, and Zeanah (2014) designed, after the start of the BEIP, a post hoc analysis to examine outcomes of children who experienced child-centered and high-quality

MacArthur foster care (Smyke, Zeanah, Fox, & Nelson, 2009) and those who experienced government-sponsored foster care. Children in government-sponsored foster care had significantly higher levels of internalizing symptoms at age 54 months, which was qualified by a sex by group interaction. Similar to the main intent-to-treat findings (Zeanah et al., 2009), girls appeared to demonstrate the greatest recovery from institutional care through the placement into high-quality foster care. Furthermore, these findings highlight that placement into any foster care may not be sufficient for fostering healthy outcomes, as foster care placements characterized by being child centered and having high levels of caregiver support appeared to better placements for children in terms of internalizing psychopathology outcomes.

3.1.2 Follow-Up at 8 Years of Age

Internalizing symptoms in a follow-up at age 8 years were assessed via teacher report using the MacArthur Health and Behavior Questionnaire (HBQ; Essex et al., 2002), which does not yield clinical diagnoses but provides a dimensional assessment of symptoms. History of institutional care was associated with higher levels of depression and anxiety symptoms (Bick, Fox, Zeanah, & Nelson, 2015). Importantly, however, the intervention effect found at 54 months was no longer present at age 8, as children in the CAUG and FCG did not significantly differ from one another.

3.1.3 Follow-Up at 12 Years of Age

Similar to the findings at age 8 years, using the total number of symptoms, the EIG adolescents had significantly higher levels of internalizing symptoms than their NIG counterparts (Humphreys, Gleason et al., 2015). Yet, when boys and girls were examined separately, this group difference was found only among girls, such that girls with a history of institutional care had higher levels of internalizing than those girls who were never institutionalized. In addition, and similar to the findings from the follow-up assessment at age 8 years, there was no intent-to-treat effect, indicating that the role of the intervention on girls' internalizing psychopathology was not evident past the preschool age assessment.

However, importantly, in order to understand the impact of placement changes among individuals originally placed in the FCG, in this study we also conducted analyses that set aside the original intent-to-treat groupings. Thus, in addition to the CAUG and NIG designations, adolescents in the FCG were divided into two groups, approximately half of whom were still living in their original MacArthur foster care placements, whereas the other half had been disrupted from that placement (e.g., reunited with their biological family; foster caregiver became too ill to provide care). Within the FCG children, those who were in a stable foster care placement had lower levels of internalizing symptoms, and this was particularly true for girls.

It should be noted that those children who did and did not disrupt from their MacArthur placements were compared on a number of variables at age 54 months, when formal support for the intervention ended. Those children who later disrupted did not differ from those who remained stable on measures of IQ, psychopathology symptoms, and time spent in institutional care at 54 months, suggesting that disruptions were unlikely to be the result of child-specific challenging behaviors.

Teacher reports provided slightly different results. While those in the EIG had greater depression symptoms than those in the NIG, girls in the CAUG showed significantly higher levels of depression symptoms when compared with both the FCG and NIG participants (Bick et al., 2015), indicating a sex-specific intervention effect that had reemerged. For anxiety symptoms, there were no group differences based on institutional care history or intervention group for boys. However, for girls, the CAUG had significantly higher anxiety symptoms compared to both FCG and NIG.

Discrepancies among informants is a common issue in child psychopathology research (De Los Reyes & Kazdin, 2005), and to date it is not clear how best to make use of multiple informants, particularly when they disagree. Traditionally, differences in informant reports would be evidence of measurement bias, but it is also possible that each informant provides uniquely useful information about the child's functioning. Within the BEIP, these challenges are also complicated by rater consistency and the degree of familiarity with the child over time. Specifically, never institutionalized children often have the same parent provide reports on their child's behavior at all assessments. On the other end of the spectrum, children who remained in institutional care may have a different caregiver providing information at each assessment. The consistency in measurement, as well as the probability that a new caregiver will know less about a child compared to those caregivers who have long-term relationships with a biological or fostered child, is worth noting as a limitation and challenge to this work.

In terms of predictors of internalizing symptoms at age 12 years, two studies identified links to this form of psychopathology. First, using diffusion tensor imaging (DTI) to examine white matter tracts, Bick et al. (2015) found that alterations in the external capsule and body of the corpus callosum partially mediated the association between institutional care history and anxiety and depression symptoms. Most recently, Troller-Renfree et al. (2016) found that, using a dot-probe task, a positive attention bias, a measure of increased attention to happy (vs. neutral) faces, may be protective in children who experienced early psychosocial deprivation. Positive bias was associated with lower levels of teacher-reported internalizing problems.

3.2 *Externalizing Psychopathology*

3.2.1 54 Months: RCT Completion

Externalizing psychopathology, which consists of aggressive and oppositional behaviors, has been examined in assessments at ages 54 months and 8 and 12 years. The EIG participants (27%) had significantly higher rates of externalizing disorders than those in the NIG (7%) at age 54 months. There was no significant difference, however, based on the intervention group overall (i.e., CAUG [29%] vs. FCG [25%]; Zeanah et al., 2009). Attachment security at 42 months mediated association between caregiving quality at age 30 months and externalizing symptoms at age 54 months (McGoron et al., 2012).

The effect of the serotonin transporter genotype significantly moderated these effects (Brett et al., 2015). Specifically, individuals with the more "susceptible" *s/s* genotype had significantly lower levels of externalizing symptoms at age 54 months than their counterparts with at least one *l* allele. Conversely, among the CAUG, those with the *s/s* genotype had significantly higher levels of internalizing than those with an *l* allele. These findings suggest that individuals with a "susceptible" genotype may be more responsive to the environment, such that in good caregiving conditions, individuals thrive, whereas in harsher conditions they fare worse. Follow-up data from this study supports this conclusion, as externalizing symptoms at age 54 months were lowest among those with an organized attachment at 42 months and the *s/s* genotype, and those with this same genotype but with an atypical attachment at 42 months had the highest externalizing symptoms at the next assessment wave (Humphreys, Zeanah, Nelson, Fox, & Drury, 2015). Individuals with an *l* allele did not differ in externalizing symptoms regardless of intent-to-treat group or attachment status at 42 months.

In addition to potential differences based on genotype, other work examined type of foster care in relation to externalizing symptoms at age 54 months. Children placed in MacArthur foster care did not differ in externalizing symptoms compared to those children in the government-sponsored foster care (Tibu et al., 2014). One analysis examined whether attachment security at age 42 months explained the association between caregiving quality at 30 months and externalizing symptoms at 54 months and found evidence for a significant indirect effect (McGoron et al., 2012), indicating that the intervention's effort to improve caregiving quality for children may have had important downstream consequences on externalizing symptoms through creating secure attachments.

3.2.2 Follow-Up at 12 Years of Age

At age 12 years, ADHD symptoms were assessed independent of externalizing psychopathology. Among both boys and girls, those in the EIG had significantly higher levels of externalizing symptoms than those in the NIG (Humphreys, Gleason et al., 2015). In adolescence, for the first time, a significant intent-to-treat effect for externalizing psychopathology was found, such that children in the CAUG had higher levels of symptoms than those in the FCG. Yet, this specific intent-to-treat effect was accounted for by boys, indicating that the placement into foster care significantly reduced externalizing psychopathology only in boys at age 12 years. Among girls, there was no intent-to-treat effect.

Setting aside group designations based on random assignment, and, instead, looking at stability of the foster care placement for the FCG, indicated that those who remained in their MacArthur foster families had significantly reduced externalizing compared to those girls originally placed in the FCG but who had disrupted from their placement. As a reminder, evidence of differing levels of psychopathology found at 12 years were likely to result from placement disruptions rather than preexisting child behavior problems as the groups did not differ from each other at age 54 months on measures of externalizing symptoms. It is unclear if observed differences based on foster care placement stability were due to being disrupted from a placement, from the quality of the placement following disruption from the foster care intervention, from the number of disruptions experienced overall, or some other factors.

Callous-unemotional (CU) traits, often seen as a precursor to psychopathy, and a correlate of conduct disorder, are an important variety/type of externalizing psychopathology. Using caregiver reports of CU traits at age 12 years, we found higher rates of CU traits among children who experienced institutional rearing as young children compared to the NIG participants (Humphreys, McGoron et al., 2015). Intent-to-treat analysis indicated that, among boys, CU traits were significantly lower among those in the FCG compared to CAUG. These findings provide the first-ever evidence that CU traits can be prevented and also provided insight into the possible mechanism by which the intervention was able to prevent high levels of CU traits among boys with a history of psychosocial deprivation.

We also examined whether specific caregiving behaviors may have explained the lower levels of CU traits found among those children placed in the FCG. In particular, both caregiver warmth and caregiver responsiveness to their child when he or she was distressed were examined. Ratings of each were obtained via caregiver-child interactions at the 42-month assessment. We found that caregiver responsiveness to distress, but not caregiver warmth, mediated the intervention effect on CU traits in boys. These findings suggest that the promotion of empathic responding to children's distress may be an important target for parenting interventions that aim to prevent or reduce CU traits in children.

3.3 ADHD Psychopathology

It is important to point out that there is debate regarding whether ADHD should be considered as a form of externalizing psychopathology and that some measures include symptoms of inattention, hyperactivity, and impulsivity in dimensional assessments of externalizing behavior, whereas others do not. Though ADHD symptoms often correlate with the symptoms of oppositional defiant disorder and conduct disorder, their differential responses to intervention provide support that these represent separable constructs. In addition, as noted above, symptoms of inattention and overactivity are highly prevalent following early deprivation, seeming to represent a deprivation-specific pattern of behavior (Kreppner, O'Connor, & Rutter, 2001).

3.3.1 54 Months: RCT Completion

At age 54 months, the EIG (21%) had significantly higher rates of externalizing disorders than the NIG (3%). In addition, there was no significant difference based on the intervention group (i.e., CAUG [23%] vs. FCG [19%]; Zeanah et al., 2009). Analyses by Tibu et al. (2014) found that, after controlling for duration of time spent in foster care, there was a main effect of the type of foster care placement on level of ADHD symptoms. Specifically, children placed in the MacArthur foster care had significantly lower levels of ADHD symptoms than those in government-sponsored foster care.

Two analyses examined whether neural markers were associated with ADHD at age 54 months. Using EEG, both reductions in alpha relative power and increases in theta relative power, both thought to reflect a delay in cortical maturation, among EIG children predicted ADHD symptoms at age 54 months (McLaughlin et al., 2010). Furthermore, these EEG activations significantly mediated the association between institutionalization history and ADHD symptoms, which may indicate that atypical brain development related to psychosocial deprivation may be the cause of increased ADHD symptomatology among this population. A second study, using ERP to examine neural responses to facial stimuli, found that peak amplitude of the P700 significantly mediated the association between institutional rearing and ADHD symptoms at 54 months (Slopen et al., 2012). These findings point to another biologically embedded neural response associated with institutional care that helps to explain the increased prevalence of ADHD.

3.3.2 Follow-Up at 8 Years of Age

Teacher report was used to assess inattention and hyperactivity at age 8 years, and EIG children had higher inattention and impulsivity than the NIG children (Tibu et al., 2016). As with the 54-month assessment, there was no intervention effect of foster care on symptoms of inattention or impulsivity. Poorer performance on working memory and response inhibition tasks were found to partially mediate the association between early institutionalization and ADHD symptoms (Tibu et al., 2016). These findings suggest that interventions targeting these specific deficits (e.g., working memory training) may be beneficial for reducing ADHD symptoms among children who experienced severe psychosocial deprivation.

3.3.3 Follow-Up at 12 Years of Age

At age 12 years, we again found that the EIG had significantly higher rates of ADHD and higher levels of ADHD symptoms than the NIG (Humphreys, Gleason, et al., 2015). Unlike findings obtained from community samples, our results indicated that ADHD was elevated equally in boys and girls, suggesting that perhaps there is an etiological route to ADHD following deprivation that is unique to neglect and/or that the ADHD presented following psychosocial deprivation may represent a unique variant of ADHD. Although heritability estimates of ADHD are high, a growing body of evidence indicates that early adverse experiences likely play a role in elevated inattention, hyperactivity, and impulsivity (Humphreys & Zeanah, 2015). In addition, given that the psychopathology data from the DISC at age 12 years did not show differences based on intent-to-treat groupings or the stability of the foster care placement, this provides further support that the sensitive period for recovery from negative effects that may contribute to the development of ADHD symptoms is very early – earlier than the average age of 22 months in which the BEIP placements occurred.

3.4 Reactive Attachment Disorder

Reactive attachment disorder (RAD), also described as inhibited social behavior, has been carefully assessed at all assessment periods in the study, as attachment problems were hypothesized to be a major domain in which the foster care intervention would have positive effects.

3.4.1 Baseline to Age 54 Months

Signs of RAD were higher among the EIG than the NIG at the baseline assessment, and the CAUG and FCG did not differ, supporting the randomization procedure (Smyke et al., 2012). Across the intervention, the rates of RAD in the NIG remained stable and low, whereas rates in the CAUG remained stable and higher. Importantly, as early as the 30-month assessment, there was a significant intent-to-treat effect on signs of RAD, such that those children assigned to the FCG had significantly lower rates of RAD than the CAUG and were similar to the NIG from age 30 months through 54 months. Attachment security at 42 months mediated association between caregiving quality at age 30 months and RAD symptoms at age 54 months (McGoron et al., 2012).

3.4.2 Follow-Up at 8 Years of Age

Follow-up at age 8 years showed a similar trend, such that signs of RAD were three times as high among the CAUG than the FCG (Smyke et al., 2012). However, at this age group, both the CAUG and FCG had higher RAD signs than the NIG. Predictors of RAD signs at 8 years included a bias away from happy facial expressions (Troller-Renfree et al., 2015), indicating that social biases toward happy faces may help to protect children with a history of severe psychosocial deprivation from RAD.

3.4.3 Follow-Up at 12 Years of Age

At age 12 years, the EIG had more signs of RAD than the NIG, although males who had spent time in institutions had higher levels of inhibited social behavior than all other groups (Humphreys, Nelson, Fox, & Zeanah, 2016). In addition to a significant intent-to-treat effect at age 12 years, such that the FCG continued to have lower RAD signs than the CAUG, a timing of placement was also found. Those children in the FCG who were placed after age 24 months had marginally higher scores than those placed prior to age 24 months. In addition, a greater number of placement disruptions and a greater proportion of the child's life spent in institutional care were each associated with higher levels of RAD. These findings indicate that events both earlier and later in childhood may be important in adolescent presentations of RAD.

3.5 *Disinhibited Social Engagement Disorder*

Disinhibited social engagement disorder (DSED), also described as disinhibited social behavior (or "indiscriminate sociability" or "indiscriminate friendliness") also has been examined throughout the study and follow-up assessment.

3.5.1 Baseline Through Age 54 Months

Signs of DSED at baseline did not significantly differ by institutional care history (i.e., EIG vs. NIG) (Smyke et al., 2012) or by randomization into groups among children in institutions. Following this baseline assessment, the NIG had lower signs of DSED than both the CAUG and FCG at ages 30, 42, and 54 months. In addition, a significant intent-to-treat effect was found, emerging at the age 42-month assessment and continued to be present at age 54 months, such that children randomized to the FCG had lower signs of DSED than the CAUG. An age of placement effect for children placed in foster care was found, such that children placed after age 24 months had more signs of DSED at ages 30 and 54 months than those placed in foster care younger than 24 months. These findings support earlier placements for abandoned children. Further, attachment security at 42 months mediated association between caregiving quality at age 30 months and DSED symptoms at age 54 months (McGoron et al., 2012).

DSED, by definition, requires the presence of insufficient caregiving (American Psychiatric Association, 2013), yet individual differences following deprivation point to a possible genetic contribution. Indeed, children with either the *l* allele of the serotonin transporter or *val/val* genotype of BDNF gene were relatively stable in signs of DSED over time (Drury et al., 2012). However, children with the *s/s* genotype and *met* allele had the most signs of indiscriminate behavior at 54 months if they were randomized to the CAUG but the fewest signs if randomized to the FCG.

These findings indicate that there may be differential susceptibility to both positive and negative environmental experiences based on genotype that can be reflected in signs of DSED.

3.5.2 Follow-Up at 8 Years of Age

At age 8 years, there continued to be an effect of institutional care history (EIG had greater signs than the NIG) (Smyke et al., 2012). In addition, signs of DSED from the DAI were over twice as high among the CAUG than the FCG (Smyke et al., 2012).

3.5.3 Follow-Up at 12 Years of Age

Most recently, signs of DSED were examined from the follow-up at age 12 years, and again the EIG had higher levels than the NIG (Humphreys et al., 2016). An intent-to-treat effect was found to be statistically significant, indicating that those in the FCG had reduced signs of DSED than the CAUG, which indicates that differences from the randomization on this domain were detectable over 10 years since the formal end of the intervention. There was a significant association between proportions of a child's life spent in institutional care predicting higher levels of indiscriminate social behavior, even after controlling for time in institutions before 54 months. These findings indicate that even later childhood experiences may be important in adolescent presentations of his attachment problem.

4 How This Knowledge Can Improve Children's Care

The findings from the BEIP have significant practical applications for improving the well-being of children experiencing early neglect, the most common form of child maltreatment (U.S. Department of Health and Human Services & Services, 2015). Although the study did not explicitly test outcomes as a function of varying qualities of institutional care, it can be said that there is "no such thing as a good institution" (Nelson, 2003). The results from the BEIP show clear and dramatic effects of family placement for children who experienced institutional care. In addition, unlike studies such as the ERAS that provided a significant socioeconomic and cultural intervention in addition to family-based care, the fact our families were Romanian and, on average, had lower economic, educational, and health resources than families from the UK or USA makes it more remarkable that such robust intervention effects were found. Though the present chapter focused on psychiatric outcomes, it is important to point out that in nearly every domain studied, children who were randomly selected to be placed in high-quality foster care had better outcomes than their counterparts who were randomized to care as usual (Nelson et al., 2014). Additionally, these findings are likely underestimate of the true power of the foster care intervention for several reasons. First, a conservative intent-to-treat approach was used to test the intervention's effect. Second, the study's noninterference policy meant that only half of children in the FCG were no longer in their original placements by age 12 years (Humphreys, Gleason, et al., 2015). Third, very few of the children randomized to the CAUG were still residing in institutional care at this age. Thus, the primary policy implication of this study is that children should be placed in families rather than continue in an environment that is characterized by psychosocial deprivation.

A second policy implication from the BEIP derives from the findings considering the age of placement into foster care. Not all outcomes demonstrated evidence of a recovery (e.g., attention problems), perhaps because the period of development in which intervention would have had the strongest impact was outside of the range in which children were placed (i.e., before age 6 months). For example, in the ERAS, children adopted prior to 6 months of age were very unlikely to develop signs of inattention/overactivity compared to children adopted after 6 months of age. For many outcomes, there were clear advantages found in those children who were placed into families at younger ages, particularly in relation to attachment (Smyke, Zeanah, Fox, Nelson, & Guthrie, 2010) and cognitive domains (Nelson et al., 2007). The brain is plastic, but this plasticity decreases over time.

Our work, along with many other researchers studying the effects of early experiences of adversity, provides a clear incentive to prioritize intervention to enhance caregiving environments for children who have been abandoned as early as possible. In fact, the Romanian government passed a law in 2005 that banned the placement of children younger than 24 months in institutions. Although no doubt many factors contributed to this legislation, several of the major findings from this study identified 24 months as an important age in which children placed prior to this age typically fared better than those placed after age 24 months (Nelson et al., 2014). More recently, in 2014, the Romanian government extended the ban on institutional care for children younger than 36 months.

The third policy implication is that the foster care placement must be of high quality and child centered. While family placement is considered to be a better alternative for abandoned children than institutional care, not all family placements are equal (Zeanah, Shauffer, & Dozier, 2011). Children who have been abused or neglected may pose special difficulties for caregivers, and foster parents must be adequately prepared to be sensitive caregivers and required to receive regular support for specially trained mental health providers. The foster care program designed by the BEIP team was informed by the most recent research on child development and infant mental health and was equipped with local social workers who met regularly with foster parents (Smyke et al., 2009). In turn, these social workers received regular consultation from psychologists and psychiatrists in the USA. This approach requires significant time, effort, and training. The benefits can be found both anecdotally, with the reported support received by the study sponsored foster care parents compared to those parents working with the Romanian government-sponsored foster care system, as well as with child outcomes. At the level of psychopathology in early childhood, as noted above, we found that there were lower levels of psychopathology among children in the high-quality government-sponsored foster care compared to the government-sponsored foster care (Tibu et al., 2014). As a related point, the BEIP has also provided evidence into the quality of caregiving as an important mediator of the effects of the intervention. Caregivers in the foster care intervention were found to be more sensitive to the child's needs, which in turn resulted in greater empathy in the children (Humphreys, McGoron, et al., 2015) as well as reduced internalizing, externalizing, RAD, and DSED psychopathology (McGoron et al., 2012). Fostering sensitive caregiving within programs that train new and existing foster care providers is an additional important practical implication from the work of the BEIP.

Based on these results, we have advocated for placement into family-based care for abandoned children. We believe that the placement should occur as early in the child's life as is feasible and that the placement should be one of high quality, in which foster care providers are adequately prepared for their task and engage in sensitive caregiving.

The fourth policy implication from the BEIP is about the stability of such placements. It is not enough to merely experience a "dose" of foster care. Our research indicates that the stability of ones' foster placement is of great importance. In fact, those children who received high-quality foster care but then were disrupted from that placement fared nearly as poorly as those children who never received the foster care intervention (Humphreys, Gleason, et al., 2015; Troller-Renfree et al., 2016). An unfortunate consequence of prioritizing placements only for young children may mean that older children in stable placements become displaced from those families. Thus, finding foster care placements that are long term, with a substantial commitment to the child, are all essential ingredients for maintaining the positive outcomes that result from living with a family.

5 Summary

The BEIP was the first RCT of foster care for abandoned children placed in institutional care. Findings from this study spanned multiple domains, and this chapter focused on psychopathology, finding that across most outcomes placement into foster care resulted in better outcomes. Furthermore, being placed earlier in life tended to be associated with larger gains for attachment disorders, and experiencing placement disruptions could undermine recovery from early psychosocial deprivation. In terms of psychopathology, ADHD symptoms appear to be the most resistant to intervention, while attachment problems appear to be the most responsive. Individuals' sex and genetic predispositions were important within person moderators of effects, while the type of early experience, intervention received, and timing of the intervention were important extrinsic moderators of the association between institutional care history and psychopathology.

Questions for Discussion

1. Why was a randomized controlled trial required to evaluate the effectiveness of the high-quality foster care intervention? In other words, what could an RCT provide that was not previously known?
2. What is the benefit of studying child outcomes related to the age of placement into foster care? How might knowledge of sensitive periods guide policy and practice?
3. What are the potential advantages and disadvantages of improving the quality of existing institutions versus creating a government-sponsored network of foster placements?

Acknowledgments Funding was provided by the National Institute of Mental Health (MH091363 and MH107129), the John D. and Catherine T. MacArthur Foundation, and the Brain & Behavior Research Foundation (formerly NARSAD) Young Investigator Award 23819. The authors thank the Bucharest Early Intervention Project staff in Romania and the children and caregivers who participated in this study.

References

American Psychiatric Association. (2013). *Diagnostic and statistical manual of mental disorders (DSM-5)*. Arlington, VA: Author.

Bick, J., Fox, N., Zeanah, C., & Nelson, C. A. (2015). Early deprivation, atypical brain development, and internalizing symptoms in late childhood. *Neuroscience*. doi:10.1016/j.neuroscience.2015.09.026.

Bos, K., Zeanah, C. H., Fox, N. A., Drury, S. S., Mclaughlin, K. A., & Nelson, C. A. (2011). Psychiatric outcomes in young children with a history of institutionalization. *Harvard Review of Psychiatry, 19*(1), 15–24. doi:10.3109/10673229.2011.549773.

Brett, Z. H., Humphreys, K. L., Smyke, A. T., Gleason, M. M., Nelson, C. A., Zeanah, C. H., … Drury, S. S. (2015). Serotonin transporter linked polymorphic region (5-HTTLPR) genotype moderates the longitudinal impact of early caregiving on externalizing behavior. *Development and Psychopathology, 27*(1), 7–18. doi:10.1017/S0954579414001266.

Chapin, H. (1915). Are institutions for infants really necessary? *Journal of the American Medical Association, LXIV*, 1–3.

De Los Reyes, A., & Kazdin, A. E. (2005). Informant discrepancies in the assessment of childhood psychopathology: A critical review, theoretical framework, and recommendations for further study. *Psychological Bulletin, 131*, 483–509. doi:10.1037/0033-2909.131.4.483.

Drury, S. S., Gleason, M. M., Theall, K. P., Smyke, A. T., Nelson, C. A., Fox, N. A., & Zeanah, C. H. (2012). Genetic sensitivity to the caregiving context: The influence of 5httlpr and BDNF val66met on indiscriminate social behavior. *Physiology and Behavior, 106*, 728–735. doi:10.1016/j.physbeh.2011.11.014.

Essex, M. J., Boyce, W. T., Goldstein, L. H., Armstrong, J. M., Kraemer, H. C., Kupfer, D. J., & MacArthur Assessment Battery Working Group. (2002). The confluence of mental, physical, social, and academic difficulties in middle childhood. II: Developing the Macarthur Health and Behavior Questionnaire. *Journal of the American Academy of Child and Adolescent Psychiatry, 41*(5), 588–603. doi:10.1097/00004583-200205000-00017.

Gunnar, M. R., Bruce, J., & Grotevant, H. D. (2000). International adoption of institutionally reared children: Research and policy. *Development and Psychopathology, 12*, 677–693. doi:10.1017/S0954579400004077.

Humphreys, K. L., Gleason, M. M., Drury, S. S., Miron, D., Nelson, C. A., Fox, N. A., & Zeanah, C. H. (2015). Effects of institutional rearing and foster care on psychopathology at age 12 years in Romania: Follow-up of an open, randomised controlled trial. *The Lancet Psychiatry, 2*(7), 625–634. doi:10.1016/S2215-0366(15)00095-4.

Humphreys, K. L., McGoron, L., Sheridan, M. A., Mclaughlin, K. A., Fox, N. A., Nelson, C. A., & Zeanah, C. H. (2015). High-quality foster care mitigates callous-unemotional traits following early deprivation in boys: A randomized controlled trial. *Journal of the American Academy of Child & Adolescent Psychiatry, 54*, 977–983. doi:10.1016/j.jaac.2015.09.010.

Humphreys, K. L., Nelson, C. A., Fox, N. A., & Zeanah, C. H. (2016). Signs of reactive attachment disorder and disinhibited social engagement disorder at age 12 years: Effects of institutional care history and high-quality foster care. *Development and Psychopathology, 29*(2), 675–684.

Humphreys, K. L., & Zeanah, C. H. (2015). Deviations from the expectable environment in early childhood and emerging psychopathology. *Neuropsychopharmacology, 40*(1), 154–170. doi:10.1038/npp.2014.165.

Humphreys, K. L., Zeanah, C. H., Nelson, C. A., Fox, N. A., & Drury, S. S. (2015). Serotonin transporter genotype (5HTTLPR) moderates the longitudinal impact of atypical attachment on externalizing behavior. *Journal of Developmental & Behavioral Pediatrics, 1*. doi:10.1097/DBP.0000000000000171.

Kreppner, J. M., O'Connor, T. G., & Rutter, M. (2001). Can inattention/overactivity be an institutional deprivation syndrome? *Journal of Abnormal Child Psychology, 29*(6), 513–528.

McGoron, L., Gleason, M. M., Smyke, A. T., Drury, S. S., Nelson, C. A., Gregas, M. C., … Zeanah, C. H. (2012). Recovering from early deprivation: Attachment mediates effects of caregiving on psychopathology. *Journal of the American Academy of Child and Adolescent Psychiatry, 51*, 683–693. doi:10.1016/j.jaac.2012.05.004.

McLaughlin, K. A., Fox, N. A., Zeanah, C. H., & Nelson, C. A. (2011). Adverse rearing environments and neural development in children: The development of frontal electroencephalogram asymmetry. *Biological Psychiatry, 70*, 1008–1015. doi:10.1016/j.biopsych.2011.08.006.

McLaughlin, K. A., Fox, N. A., Zeanah, C. H., Sheridan, M. A., Marshall, P., & Nelson, C. A. (2010). Delayed maturation in brain electrical activity partially explains the association between early environmental deprivation and symptoms of attention-deficit/hyperactivity disorder. *Biological Psychiatry, 68*, 329–336. doi:10.1016/j.biopsych.2010.04.005.

McLaughlin, K. A., Nelson, C. A., Fox, N. A., & Zeanah, C. H. (2012). Attachment security as a mechanism linking foster care placement with improved mental health outcomes in previously institutionalized children. *Journal of Child Psychology and Psychiatry, 53*, 46–55.

Miller, F. G. (2009). The randomized controlled trial as a demonstration project: An ethical perspective. *American Journal of Psychiatry, 166*, 743–745. doi:10.1176/appi.ajp.2009.09040538.

Millum, J., & Emanuel, E. J. (2007). The ethics of international research with abandoned children. *Science, 318*, 1874–1875. doi:10.1126/science.1153822.

Nelson, C. A. (2003). Developmental effects of deprived caregiving. In *American Association for the Advancement of Sciences Annual Meeting*, Denver.

Nelson, C. A., Fox, N. A., & Zeanah, C. H. (2014). *Romania's abandoned children: Deprivation, brain development, and the struggle for recovery*. Cambridge, MA: Harvard University Press.

Nelson, C. A., Zeanah, C. H., Fox, N. A., Marshall, P. J., Smyke, A. T., & Guthrie, D. (2007). Cognitive recovery in socially deprived young children: The Bucharest Early Intervention Project. *Science, 318*, 1937–1940. doi:10.1126/science.1143921.

Rid, A. (2012). When is research socially valuable? Lessons from the Bucharest Early Intervention Project: Commentary on a case study in the ethics of mental health research. *The Journal of Nervous and Mental Disease, 200*(3), 248–249.

Rosapepe, J. C. (2001). Half way home: Romania's abandoned children ten years after the revolution. *Report of the US Ambassador to Romania, 12*(05).

Rutter, M., Sonuga-Barke, E. J., Beckett, C., Bell, C. A., Kreppner, J., Kumsta, R., … Stevens, S. (2010). Deprivation-specific psychological patterns: Effects of institutional deprivation by the English and Romanian Adoptee Study Team. *Monographs of the Society for Research in Child Development, 75*(1), 1–252.

Rutter, M., Sonuga-Barke, E. J., & Castle, J. (2010). I. Investigating the impact of early institutional deprivation on development: Background and research strategy of the English and Romanian Adoptees (ERA) study. *Monographs of the Society for Research in Child Development, 75*(1), 1–20. doi:10.1111/j.1540-5834.2010.00548.x.

Slopen, N., McLaughlin, K. A., Fox, N. A., Zeanah, C. H., & Nelson, C. A. (2012). Alterations in neural processing and psychopathology in children raised in institutions. *Archives of General Psychiatry, 69*(10), 1022–1030. doi:10.1001/archgenpsychiatry.2012.444.

Smyke, A. T., Zeanah, C. H., Fox, N. A., & Nelson, C. A. (2009). A new model of foster care for young children: The Bucharest early intervention project. *Child and Adolescent Psychiatric Clinics of North America, 18*, 721–734. doi:10.1016/j.chc.2009.03.003.

Smyke, A. T., Zeanah, C. H., Fox, N. A., Nelson, C. A., & Guthrie, D. (2010). Placement in foster care enhances quality of attachment among young institutionalized children. *Child Development, 81*(1), 212–223. doi:10.1111/j.1467-8624.2009.01390.x.

Smyke, A. T., Zeanah, C. H., Gleason, M. M., Drury, S. S., Fox, N. A., Nelson, C. A., & Guthrie, D. (2012). A randomized controlled trial comparing foster care and institutional care for children with signs of reactive attachment disorder. *American Journal of Psychiatry, 169*, 508–514. doi:10.1176/appi.ajp.2011.11050748.

Tibu, F., Humphreys, K. L., Fox, N. A., Nelson, C. A., & Zeanah, C. H. (2014). Psychopathology in young children in two types of foster care following institutional rearing. *Infant Mental Health Journal, 35*(2), 123–131. doi:10.1002/imhj.21428.

Tibu, F., Sheridan, M. A., McLaughlin, K. A., Nelson, C. A., Fox, N. A., & Zeanah, C. H. (2016). Disruptions of working memory and inhibition mediate the association between exposure to institutionalization and symptoms of attention deficit hyperactivity disorder. *Psychological Medicine, 46*(3), 529–541. doi:10.1017/S0033291715002020.

Tizard, J., & Tizard, B. (1967). *The social development of two year old children in residential nurseries.*

Troller-Renfree, S., McDermott, J. M., Nelson, C. A., Zeanah, C. H., Fox, N. A., Troller-Renfree, S., … Fox, N. A. (2015). The effects of early foster care intervention on attention biases in previously institutionalized children in Romania. *Developmental Science, 18*(5), 713–722. doi:10.1111/desc.12261.

Troller-Renfree, S., McLaughlin, K. A., Sheridan, M. A., Nelson, C. A., Zeanah, C. H., & Fox, N. A. (2016). The beneficial effects of a positive attention bias amongst children with a history of psychosocial deprivation. *Biological Psychology, 122*, 110–120.

U.S. Department of Health and Human Services (2015). *Child maltreatment 2013*. Washington, DC: Administration for Children and Families, Administration on Children, Youth and Families, Children's Bureau. doi:10.1016/j.mppsy.2008.05.001.

Zeanah, C. H., Egger, H. L., Smyke, A. T., Nelson, C. A., Fox, N. A., Marshall, P. J., & Guthrie, D. (2009). Institutional rearing and psychiatric disorders in Romanian preschool children. *The American Journal of Psychiatry, 166*(7), 777–785. doi:10.1176/appi.ajp.2009.08091438.

Zeanah, C. H., Fox, N. A., & Nelson, C. A. (2012). The Bucharest Early Intervention Project: Case study in the ethics of mental health research. *The Journal of Nervous and Mental Disease, 200*, 243–247. doi:10.1097/NMD.0b013e318247d275.

Zeanah, C. H., Nelson, C. A., Fox, N. A., Smyke, A. T., Marshall, P., Parker, S. W., & Koga, S. (2003). Designing research to study the effects of institutionalization on brain and behavioral development: The Bucharest Early Intervention Project. *Development and Psychopathology, 15*, 885–907. doi:10.1017/S0954579403000452.

Zeanah, C. H., Shauffer, M. C., & Dozier, M. (2011). Foster care for young children: Why it must be developmentally informed. *Journal of the American Academy of Child and Adolescent Psychiatry, 50*(12), 1199–1201. doi:10.1016/j.jaac.2011.08.001.

Zeanah, C. H., Smyke, A. T., Koga, S. F., & Carlson, E. (2005). Attachment in institutionalized and community children in Romania. *Child Development, 76*(5), 1015–1028. doi:10.1111/j.1467-8624.2005.00894.x.

Zeanah, C. H., Smyke, A. T., & Settles, L. D. (2006). Orphanages as a developmental context for early childhood. In *Blackwell handbook of early childhood development* (pp. 424–454). Malden, MA: Blackwell.

Chapter 7
Poly-victimization and Mental Health Problems Among Adolescents in Residential Facilities in Spain

Anna Segura, Noemí Pereda, Georgina Guilera, and Soledad Álvarez-Lister

Don't turn your face away.
Once you've seen, you can no longer act like you don't know.
Open your eyes to the truth. It's all around you.
Don't deny what the eyes to your soul have revealed to you.
Now that you know, you cannot feign ignorance.
Now that you're aware of the problem, you cannot pretend you don't care.
To be concerned is to be human.
To act is to care.

Vashti Quiroz-Vega (2013)

This research was supported by research grants from RECERCAIXA 2013, the Directorate General for Children and Adolescents [Direcció General d'Atenció a la Infància i l'Adolescència] of the Generalitat de Catalunya and the Agustí Pedro i Pons Foundation.

A. Segura (✉) • N. Pereda • S. Álvarez-Lister
Research Group on Child and Adolescent Victimization (GReVIA), University of Barcelona, Barcelona, Spain

Department of Clinical Psychology and Psychobiology, Faculty of Psychology, University of Barcelona, Passeig Vall d'Hebron, 171, 08035 Barcelona, Spain
e-mail: annasegura89@gmail.com; npereda@ub.edu; sole.alvarez@gmail.com

G. Guilera
Research Group on Child and Adolescent Victimization (GReVIA), University of Barcelona, Barcelona, Spain

Department of Social Psychology and Quantitative Psychology, Faculty of Psychology, University of Barcelona, Barcelona, Spain
e-mail: gguilera@ub.edu

A.V. Rus et al. (eds.), *Child Maltreatment in Residential Care*,
DOI 10.1007/978-3-319-57990-0_7

1 Introduction

Interpersonal violence constitutes a serious health and social problem for all children and adolescents (World Health Organization, 2013). Studies in European countries show that a large number of children and adolescents in the general population suffer victimization, especially in the form of violence committed by family members (see, for example, Ellonen & Salmi, 2011 in Finland; Pereda, Guilera, & Abad, 2014 in Spain; or Radford, Corral, Bradley, & Fisher, 2013 in the UK). In addition, children and youth removed from violent homes are at a higher risk of suffering multiple forms of victimization (e.g., Cyr et al., 2012; Segura, Pereda, Abad, & Guilera, 2015) or what has been defined as poly-victimization (Finkelhor, Ormrod, Turner, & Hamby, 2005). The issue is an important one, since a significant number of children and youths are being cared for by child welfare systems in European countries. Research on poly-victimization is a recent phenomenon, and some studies have already highlighted its significance for predicting mental health problems (Finkelhor, Ormrod, & Turner, 2009).

This chapter explores the phenomenon of poly-victimization in an at-risk sample of children and adolescents in residential care in Spain. Its overall aim is to establish whether they are receiving effective protection from the child welfare system. Its specific objectives are the following: (1) to analyze the current state of research into child abuse and neglect in Spain; (2) to describe the evolution of the child welfare system in Spain, specifically in the region of Catalonia; (3) to review studies of victimization experiences among children and adolescents cared for by the child welfare system in Spain; (4) to provide empirical data on the prevalence of victimization and poly-victimization among adolescents in residential care in Catalonia; and (5) to analyze the relationship between poly-victimization and mental health problems among adolescents in residential care.

2 Social and Academic Attention to Children's Victimization in Spain

2.1 The Study of Child Abuse and Neglect in Spain

Ever since Henry Kempe and colleagues defined the battered child syndrome in the 1960s (Kempe, Silverman, Steele, Droegemueller, & Silver, 1962), child abuse and neglect have attracted growing attention among scholars all over the world. In Spain, however, research into this serious problem has been quite slow to develop. It should be kept in mind that the country was immersed in a civil war from 1936 to1939, and under the Franco dictatorship which lasted until 1975, the prevalent attitude toward attention to children and youth placed the emphasis on moral and ideological control (Amich Elías, 2009). Additionally, three social and academic problems have held back the study of child victimization in Spain and have made it difficult to establish its true incidence.

Firstly, cultural factors related to the vision of family, violence, and childhood act against the notification of child abuse and neglect (De Paúl & Arruabarrena, 2001) and generally discourage professionals from reporting cases to the public services (Inglés, 2000; Saldaña, Jiménez, & Oliva, 1995; Sanmartín, 2002). Nationwide studies of child abuse reports by official social and medical services suggest that the prevalence of child victimization within the family is exceptionally low. However, Lachica (2010) stated that reports of child maltreatment represent only 10% of the actual cases, which suggests that official reports show only the tip of the iceberg (Morales & Costa, 1997). A recent study of a community sample of 1105 adolescents in Catalonia (Pereda, Abad, & Guilera, 2016) found that only 9.3% of those who suffered sexual victimization reported the event to the police or the courts. There seems no doubt that studies using reports from the health and social services to establish prevalence rates are underestimating the reality of child abuse in Spain.

Secondly, although some Spanish studies have observed that some victimization experiences tend to co-occur (e.g., Arruabarrena & De Paúl, 1999; Saldaña et al., 1995), most have explored only specific types of victimization (e.g., bullying), a focus that has contributed to the fragmentation of the field of developmental victimology (Finkelhor, 2007). As in many other countries, researchers have studied the type of victimization they were interested in rather than analyzing the wide range of victimizations experienced by children and adolescents and the consequences for their mental health (Finkelhor, 2011). Therefore, not all types of victimization have been paid equal attention. Arruabarrena and De Paúl (1999) state that in Spain, research on child victimization initially focused on physical abuse. Other types of violence against children have also been studied, mostly related to caregiver victimization, such as neglect and emotional abuse (e.g., De Paúl & Arruabarrena, 1995), and generally based on the analysis of social service files. More recently, the prevalence of sexual victimization (Pereda et al., 2016), dating violence (González Méndez & Santana Hernández, 2001), or electronic victimization (Montiel, Carbonell, & Pereda, 2015) has also been analyzed on the basis of interviews with children and youths and self-reports.

Thirdly, few studies on childhood victimization in Spain have been conducted at a national level. The studies that have applied a nationwide approach (e.g., Saldaña et al., 1995; Sanmartín, 2002) used data from social service reports and restricted their study to experiences of victimization within the family. The only studies that have analyzed multiple forms of victimization were conducted at a regional level with youth from community samples (e.g., Lila, Herrero, & Garcia, 2008; Pereda et al., 2014) or high-risk samples (e.g., child welfare, see Segura et al., 2015; immigrants, see Cedeño, Martínez-Arias, & Bueno, 2015; juvenile justice, see Pereda, Abad, & Guilera, 2015). It is difficult to extrapolate the results to the whole country; therefore, a nationwide study analyzing the prevalence of multiple forms of victimization among Spanish children and adolescents is still clearly needed.

In the last decade, the study of child victimization has taken a turn in many countries, and Spain is no exception. In the United States (USA), Finkelhor and his group have proved that children and adolescents constitute one of the most victimized groups in society and that these individuals often experience more than one type of victimization (Turner, Finkelhor, & Ormrod, 2006). Finkelhor and co-workers defined the term "poly-victimization" to refer to the experience of multiple forms of victimization in childhood (Finkelhor, Ormrod et al., 2005). These studies have had a significant influence in Spain, and several research teams have studied the extent of this phenomenon in different regions (e.g., Játiva & Cerezo, 2014), including Catalonia (Pereda et al., 2014; Soler, Paretilla, Kirchner, & Forns, 2012). Two studies with community samples in Catalonia found that 71.6% of adolescents had experienced two victimizations during the previous year (Soler et al., 2012), while the mean number of victimizations during the past year was between three and four (2.86 according to Pereda et al., 2014; 3.94 according to Soler et al., 2012).

In addition, Spanish studies with community samples have corroborated the results of international research in observing that poly-victimization is a potential predictor of clinical symptoms: for example, internalizing symptomatology such as depression and anxiety (Guerra, Pereda, Guilera, & Abad, 2016; Soler, Forns, Kirchner, & Segura, 2014), externalizing symptoms (Soler et al., 2014), suicidal phenomena (Soler, Segura, Kirchner, & Forns, 2013), and post-traumatic stress symptoms (Soler et al., 2012). Pereda and Gallardo-Pujol (2014) also found that children who experienced poly-victimization were more likely to be re-victimized in adulthood.

2.2 *The Development of the Child Welfare System*

In instances of interpersonal victimization, institutions such as the police, the courts, and the social services tend to intervene in a way that is often not considered necessary after other stresses and traumas, such as accidents or serious illness (see Finkelhor, 2007). The special nature of interpersonal victimization may require the intervention of the child welfare system, and so the estimated lifetime cost of child maltreatment may be high (for the USA, see Fang, Brown, Florence, & Mercy, 2012).

The protection of children is a value that is shared worldwide today (Schene, 2006). Until the twentieth century, however, it was not a priority. The Convention on the Rights of the Child (CRC), the first international, mandatory law on children's rights (United Nations General Assembly, 1989), constituted a turning point. The CRC emphasized that children must be considered not only as vulnerable subjects to be protected but also as people with rights. It also stated that all actions involving children should be based on the best interests of the child.

In Spain, before the twentieth century, abandoned children and offenders received scarce attention from the state, and children were assisted almost exclusively in private hospices (Sánchez Vázquez & Guijarro Granados, 2002). The Organization and Attributions of Courts for Children Act was passed in 1918; with regard to the creation of special courts for children, its implementation throughout the country was slow and irregular (González, 1999; Sánchez et al., 2002). In the following years, the juvenile courts were directed to reeducate and take charge of children and youths (under the age of 16) who had committed offenses or had experienced severe forms of interpersonal violence (e.g., sexual exploitation or abandonment), to whom measures such as reprimands, juvenile probation, or confinement in reformatory institutions were applied (Amich Elías, 2009). The juvenile courts remained in place under the Franco dictatorship, but their judgments were now underpinned by the doctrine of the fascist state (Amich Elías, 2009). The system was used to keep families and children of different ideologies under the control of the regime (Valiente, 1996). As a result, legislation on child protection was slower to emerge than in other European countries (del Valle, Canali, Bravo, & Vecchiato, 2013).

After the return of democracy in 1975, several child protection laws were introduced. In 1987, new state legislation on child protection (Law *21/1987*, Reform of the Civil Code and the Civil Procedure in Relation to Adoption and Other Forms of Child Protection) represented a profound modification of the Spanish child protection system (Casas & Montserrat, 2002) because the protection of children now became the responsibility of specific public agencies. This legislation aimed to improve the care of children and youths in a variety of ways, for instance, by enhancing child welfare workers' ability to detect cases of both severe and non-severe abuse, by promoting measures other than institutionalization (e.g., being cared for by family relatives), by working with each family and child on an individual basis, and by including psychologists in the child welfare teams (De Paúl, 2009). The 1996 Legal Protection of Children and Young People Act defined the basic rights of the child. This legislation embraced the CRC and stipulated that children's rights should be taken into account in all actions involving minors, especially in public agencies (Vidal Casero, 2002).

In addition, in 1987 responsibility for the social services was transferred to each specific Spanish region (De Paúl, 2009), and each regional government introduced its own legislation in order to protect vulnerable children and adolescents. As a result, Spain today does not have a nationwide child welfare system, and until now each regional child welfare system has evolved in its own way. Catalonia, in the northeast of the country, is unique in having developed a body of legislation on child protection (De Paúl & Arruabarrena, 2001). The decentralization of the social services has hindered the development of research and statistical studies of the child welfare system at nationwide level, although Domínguez Alonso and Mohedano Menéndez (2014) reported that in 2011, 8405 children and adolescents were placed in residential facilities, and 3055 were fostered by relatives. These results reflect that placement in residential care is a frequent protective policy in Spain. Nevertheless, there have been changes since the 1980s and 1990s, thanks to the decrease in the numbers of children attended at each center, the professionalization of child welfare workers, and the integration of protected children into normalized daily life routines, among other factors (De Paúl & Arruabarrena, 2001).

In Catalonia, the protection of vulnerable minors (mainly orphans and abandoned children) was traditionally organized by the church or by charities (Pinilla, 2011). When the Spanish government transferred responsibilities for child protection to the regional authorities, the Catalan government set up a network of social services and resources that covered the entire region (Casas, 2012). Some of these powers were assigned to the Department of Health and others to the Department of Justice. This situation of fragmentation lasted until 1988, when the Directorate General for Children was created.

Currently, the Catalan child welfare system, known as the Directorate General for Children and Adolescents (DGAIA)[1] is part of the Catalan Ministry for Social Welfare and the Family. Its priority is to assist and protect children and adolescents at social risk or victims of family abuse or neglect. In this system, several multidisciplinary and specialized professional teams assess and review situations of risk and propose protective measures for each case – for example, care within the child's own family; fostering within the extended family (kinship care), non-relative family care, or pre-adoptive care; residential care (short and long term, and other institutions such as open centers or residential treatment centers); and adoption.

The residential care system looks after children from 0 to 18 years old who have had to be removed from unsafe homes. Residential care is the last measure that should be implemented, when all other possibilities have been exhausted; it is applied when the separation of the child from the family is expected to be temporary or when foster care is not recommended. Residential care facilities are defined as either short term or long term. Short-term centers provide limited and temporary shelter (for a few months) for children who need to be immediately removed from their families. During the institutionalization, the situation of children and their families is examined and diagnosed, and an appropriate proposal for the child's future care is put forward. Long-term centers provide permanent shelter and offer care and education for children who live in violent families or whose parents have serious difficulties in meeting their child's basic needs, due to mental health problems, substance abuse, and so on.

According to the official data, 7104 children and adolescents were attended by the DGAIA in 2013. The largest group was in residential facilities (n = 2719, 38.3%). Others were fostered in kinship care (n = 2494, 35.1%), non-relative family care (n = 964, 13.6%), or other measures (n = 927, 13.0%) (Síndic de Greuges, 2014). Although in the 1970s and 1980s the Catalan government started to deinstitutionalize the child welfare system (Bravo & Fernández del Valle, 2009), residential care is still the most used protective measure (Síndic de Greuges, 2014); against this background, Casas (2012) proposed that future studies should assess the impact of the protective measures taken by the welfare system on children's and adolescents' lives.

[1] More information is available at http://sac.gencat.cat/sacgencat/AppJava/organisme_fitxa.jsp?codi=5157 and http://treballiaferssocials.gencat.cat/ca/el_departament/funcions_i_estructura/organismes/secretaria_dinfancia_i_adolescencia/.

3 Poly-victimization and Mental Health Problems Among Adolescents in Residential Facilities

Some studies have reported that even when children and adolescents are cared for in residential facilities, they continue to experience victimization (Ellonen & Pöso, 2011; Segura et al., 2015) in the form of emotional, sexual, and physical abuse (Euser, Alink, Tharner, van Ijzendoorn, & Bakermans-Kranenburg, 2013; Gavrilovici & Groza, 2007; Green & Masson, 2002; Rus et al., 2013). Rates of interpersonal violence may reach alarming levels, both prior to entry (Carrasco-Ortiz, Rodríguez-Testal, & Hesse, 2001; Gearing, MacKenzie, Schwalbe, Brewer, & Ibrahim, 2013; Hobbs, Hobbs, & Wyne, 1999) and while in the care of the child welfare system (Cyr et al., 2012; Ellonen & Pösö, 2011; Euser et al., 2013; Gavrilovici & Groza, 2007).

In spite of these worrying findings, poly-victimization among children and adolescents cared for by the child welfare system has not been examined in depth. Exceptions are the studies conducted in Canada by Collin-Vézina, Coleman, Milne, Sell, and Daigneault (2011) and Cyr et al. (2012); in Norway by Greger, Myhre, Lydersen, and Jozefiak (2015); in the United States by Kolko et al. (2010) and Salazar, Keller, Gowen, and Courtney (2013); and in Spain by Segura et al. (2015). In the latter study, 129 adolescents from 18 residential facilities in Spain reported a mean number of 4.57 victimizations over the past year. Using a similar methodology with a sample of 220 children and youths in the child welfare system in Canada that included those living in reception centers (i.e., short-term residential centers), Cyr et al. (2012) found that 93% of those who suffered one episode of victimization had suffered at least one other type of victimization during the past year. Both studies found that around half of children and adolescents cared for by the child welfare system were considered as poly-victims who had suffered four or more victimizations, according to the criteria established by Finkelhor, Ormrod et al. (2005).

Moreover, studies in both Spain and abroad have found that the experience of lifetime poly-victimization or multiple types of victimization in youths in the child welfare system (including those in foster care, in residential facilities, or living with their primary/biological parents) was relevant to the development of psychological problems, both internalizing and externalizing (e.g., Collin-Vézina et al., 2011; Greeson et al., 2011; Greger et al., 2015; Segura, Pereda, Guilera, & Abad, 2016). However, no research has analyzed the impact of poly-victimization on mental health problems among adolescents under care at residential facilities and its influence on the effectiveness of the protection measures.

3.1 Objectives and Hypothesis

To our knowledge, the relationship between poly-victimization and mental health problems among youth under care in residential facilities in Spain has not been analyzed to date. Taking these adolescents as the target sample, we designed our study with the following objectives and hypotheses in mind: (a) to determine the prevalence of past-year victimization and poly-victimization (although previous studies have focused on many types of victimization in child welfare samples (see Segura et al., 2015), none have analyzed victimization while in care) and (b) to examine the relationship between past-year poly-victimization and the risk of mental health problems.

3.2 *Method*

3.2.1 Participants

The initial sample included 129 adolescents in care at residential facilities. Those who had been at the facility for less than a year were excluded. The final sample thus comprised 95 adolescents (51.6% males and 48.4% females), aged 12–17 years old ($M = 14.49$, $SD = 1.64$) recruited from 16 residential care facilities (92.6% from long-term and 7.4% from short-term centers) in Catalonia, Spain. Based on an adaptation of the Hollingshead Four-Factor Index (Hollingshead, 1975), subjects' families corresponded to the following socioeconomic categories: low (40.0%), medium-low (18.9%), medium (7.4%), medium-high (2.1%), and high level (3.2%). This information was not available for approximately one third (28.4%) of the sample. Most adolescents (73.7%) were born in Spain, while 14.7% were born in Central or South America, 7.4% in Africa, 3.2% in other European countries, and 1.1% in Asia.

In most cases (90.9%), the reason for implementing child protection measures was related to victimization experiences (such as neglect, physical or sexual abuse, witnessing domestic violence, among others), whereas in the rest (16.8%), an undefined risk situation was determined or this information was unavailable (the sum is more than 100% because more than one reason could be given). The mean length of stay in residential care facilities was 4.51 years ($SD = 3.19$, $range = 1–13.67$, $Mdn = 3.25$, $IQR = 12.67$). Most parents (88.4%) still had visitation rights with their children.

3.2.2 Procedure

To conduct this study, a convenience sampling method was used, including 13.67% of the residential facilities run by the Directorate General for Children and Adolescents (DGAIA) of the Catalan Ministry for Social Welfare and the Family. Two inclusion criteria were applied: age between 12 and 17 years old and sufficient cognitive and language ability to understand the interview questions. Of the adolescents who met the inclusion criteria and were invited to participate, 69.2% were eventually recruited. This figure represented 6.7% of all adolescents (aged 12–17) in residential care facilities in 2013 in Catalonia according to data provided by the DGAIA (personal communication, March 4, 2014). Adolescents were interviewed individually by researchers who were trained in collecting data on violence against children (United Nations Children's Fund, 2012). The study was conducted in accordance with the basic ethical principles of the Declaration of Helsinki in Seoul (World Medical Association, 2008) and was approved by the Institutional Review Board of the University of Barcelona. Youths did not receive economic compensation for their participation.

3.2.3 Measures

Sociodemographic Data Information including age, gender, country of birth (Spanish born vs. foreign), educational level, and parents' occupation was obtained from the participants.

Child Welfare Data Information including type of residential center, reason for being taken into care, time in care, and contact with parents was obtained from child welfare system files.

Victimization Experiences The Juvenile Victimization Questionnaire (JVQ; Finkelhor, Hamby, Ormrod, & Turner, 2005) is a self-report instrument developed to assess 36 different types of victimization against children and youths, for both lifetime and past-year time frames. To analyze the victimization experiences suffered by adolescents while in care at residential facilities, we used the past-year time frame. In this study the interview version was used, which had previously been translated into Catalan and Spanish with the authors' permission. The 36 victimizations are grouped into six modules including conventional crime (e.g., robbery, assault with weapon), caregiver victimization (e.g., neglect, psychological/emotional abuse), victimization by peers and siblings (e.g., dating violence, peer or sibling assault), sexual victimization (e.g., sexual assault/assault by known adult, flashing/sexual exposure), witnessing and indirect victimization (e.g., witness to domestic violence, witness to murder), and electronic victimization (e.g., online harassment, online sexual solicitations). The presence or absence of each victimization experience was scored as 1 or 0, respectively. The total number of victimizations (out of 36 items) was computed for each participant (Finkelhor, Ormrod et al., 2005). Good psychometric properties were shown in the original version of the instrument (Finkelhor, Hamby et al., 2005), and evidence of the validity of its Spanish/Catalan adaptation has been reported (Pereda, Gallardo-Pujol, & Guilera, 2016).

Psychopathology The Youth Self-Report/11-18 (YSR; Achenbach & Rescorla, 2001) was designed to assess adolescents' emotional and behavioral problems over the last 6 months. The instrument comprises 119 items that are scored on a three-point Likert scale ranging from 0 (not at all) to 2 (very often). Items are grouped into two broadband dimensions and internalizing and externalizing symptoms. T scores ≥64 can be interpreted as indicating clinical severity. The self-report version of YSR was used, which was translated into Spanish and Catalan by the Epidemiology and Diagnosis in Developmental Psychopathology Unit of the Autonomous

University of Barcelona. Good reliability (Cronbach's alpha, $\alpha = .90$) was reported for both internalizing and externalizing symptom dimensions (Achenbach & Rescorla, 2001). The Spanish version of the YSR has shown adequate psychometric properties (Zubeidat, Fernández-Parra, Ortega, Vallejo, & Sierra, 2009).

3.2.4 Data Analysis

SPSS v.21 was used for all the data analysis, with the level of statistical significance being set at $p < .05$. Poly-victimization was studied using Finkelhor, Ormrod et al.'s (2005) criteria, which identify youth who experience at least one victimization more than the mean number among the victim group as a whole as past-year poly-victims (e.g., the threshold was set at four or more types of victimization). The relationship between non-poly-victim and poly-victim groups and each specific JVQ victimization experience was analyzed using either the chi-square test (χ^2) or Fisher's exact test, as appropriate. When statistically significant associations were found, odds ratios (*OR*) and 95% confidence interval (CI) were calculated. Finally, the extent to which poly-victimization might predict the clinical severity of symptoms was examined by means of logistic regression. After controlling for sociodemographic variables (i.e., gender, males vs. females; age, 15–17 vs. 12–14; and country of birth, Spain vs. foreign origin [Step 1]), the poly-victimization variable was entered (the non-poly-victim group vs. the poly-victim group [Step 2]). The Hosmer-Lemeshow test indicated a good fit to each regression model.

3.3 *Results*

3.3.1 Victimization Rates by Modules

Most adolescents ($n = 80$, 84.2%) reported at least one type of victimization during the past year (77.6% of males and 91.3% of females, χ^2 ($df = 1$) = 2.329, $p = .127$).[2] Victims had experienced a mean of 4.09 victimizations ($SD = 2.45$). The most common types of victimization were conventional crime (68.4%, $n = 65$), witnessing and indirect victimization (52.6%, $n = 50$), and peer and sibling victimization (47.4%, $n = 45$). A quarter of the sample reported caregiver (26.3%, $n = 25$) and electronic (24.2%, $n = 23$) victimization, and 8.4% ($n = 8$) reported sexual victimization.

3.3.2 Poly-victimization

The 44.2% of protected adolescents in residential facilities were past-year poly-victims. Table 7.1 shows rates for the JVQ modules for both the non-poly-victim group (comprising non-victims and victims who suffered fewer than four types of

[2] Since female participants were older, age was controlled using the Mantel-Haenszel procedure.

Table 7.1 Descriptive statistics (%, *n*) for JVQ victimization modules were shown for non-poly-victim and poly-victim groups

	Non-poly-victim group (*n* = 53)		Poly-victim group (*n* = 42)		Statistic	
Victimization modules	%	*n*	%	*N*	χ^2 (*df* = 2)	*OR*
Any victimization	71.7	38	100	42	11.533**	**16.58**
Conventional crime	45.3	24	97.6	41	29.704**	**49.54**
Caregiver victimization	13.2	7	42.9	18	10.623**	**4.93**
Peer and sibling victimization	26.4	14	73.8	31	21.112**	**7.85**
Sexual victimization	3.8	2	14.3	6	3.358[a,b]	4.25
Witnessing and indirect victimization	30.2	16	81.0	34	24.220**	**9.83**
Electronic victimization	9.4	5	42.9	18	14.165**	**7.20**

In bold, odds ratio (*OR*) whose confidence intervals did not include the value of 1
Significance is shown by multiple asterisks *$p < .01$ and **$p < .001$
[a]Given that 20% of the expected frequencies were less than 5, the *p*-value was obtained by *Fisher's exact test*
[b]Adjusted by adding 1 to each cell of the 2 × 2 table

victimization in the past year) and the poly-victim group (comprising those who suffered at least four types of victimizations in the past year). Significant differences were found between groups regarding all victimization modules, with the exception of sexual victimization. Poly-victims were more likely to report any type of victimization during the past year (*OR* = 16.58, 95% CI [2.09, 131.55]) and also conventional crimes (*OR* = 49.54, 95% CI [6.34, 387.20]), witnessing and indirect victimization (*OR* = 9.83, 95% CI [3.73, 25.87]), peer and sibling victimization (*OR* = 7.85, 95% CI [3.13, 19.70]), electronic victimization (*OR* = 7.20, 95% CI [2.38, 21.75]), and caregiver victimization (*OR* = 4.93, 95% CI [1.81, 13.44]) than non-poly-victims.

3.3.3 Poly-victimization and Psychopathology Among Adolescents in Care

In the regression analysis of the internalizing symptoms (Table 7.2, left), poly-victimization was a significant predictor, increasing the variance explained by the model by 15%. Thus, poly-victims were more likely to present a clinical level of internalizing symptoms than non-poly-victims (*OR* = 5.21, 95% CI [1.88, 14.41]). Age was also statistically significant for this broadband dimension, with younger adolescents being more likely to present internalizing symptoms within clinical ranges (*OR* = 3.63, 95% CI [1.88, 10.21]).

As for the regression analysis of the externalizing symptoms (Table 7.2, right), poly-victimization was a significant predictor for this broadband dimension overall,

Table 7.2 Past-year victimization experiences (percentages) in a sample of adolescents in residential care

	Internalizing symptoms		Externalizing symptoms	
Step 1	Model χ^2 (3) = 4.478 Nagelkerke's R^2 = .065		Model χ^2 (3) = 1.080 Nagelkerke's R^2 = .015	
Step 2	Model χ^2 (4) = 15.773* $\Delta\chi^2$ (1) = 11.295** Nagelkerke's R^2 = .215		Model χ^2 (4) = 8.723 $\Delta\chi^2$ (1) = 7.643* Nagelkerke's R^2 = .119	
	Wald F	*OR*	*Wald F*	*OR*
Female gender	1.568	1.89	0.199	1.23
Younger youths	5.964*	**3.63**	0.045	0.91
Foreign origin	1.425	0.50	1.891	0.48
Poly-victims	10.084**	**5.21**	2.266*	**3.43**

Note. Step 1 – demographics. Step 2 – demographics and poly-victimization compared to non-poly-victims
In bold, odds ratio (*OR*) whose confidence interval did not include the value of 1
Significance is shown by multiple asterisks *$p < .01$ and **$p < .001$

increasing the variance explained by the model by 10%. Poly-victimized youths were three times (*OR* = 3.43, 95% CI [1.40, 8.44]) more likely to present a clinical level of externalizing symptoms than non-poly-victims.

4 Discussion

The current study examined the poly-victimization experienced by adolescents while in residential care and its relation to the risk of mental health problems. We stress that it is an exploratory study, and our findings should not be extrapolated to all adolescents being cared for by the child welfare system in Spain.

With regard to prevalence, we observed that adolescents in care at residential facilities reported a high prevalence of all past-year victimization experiences. These results are in agreement with those of previous studies with child welfare samples (e.g., Euser et al., 2013; Euser, Alink, Tharner, van IJzendoorn, & Bakermans-Kranenburg, 2014; Gavrilovici & Groza, 2007), which found that adolescents continued to experience victimization even when in care at residential facilities.

Moreover, we found that adolescents in care experienced high levels of poly-victimization. Our results are closer to those recorded in the study of a Canadian child welfare sample (Cyr et al., 2012) that used the same methodology to identify poly-victims. In addition, the results of the poly-victim and the non-poly-victim groups differed for all kinds of victimization, with the exception of sexual victimization. In general, these results are in line with previous studies (Ford, Wasser, & Connor, 2011; Turner, Finkelhor, & Ormrod, 2010) with community samples, which have found that poly-victims experience higher rates of all forms of victimization than non-poly-victims. Nevertheless, the finding that poly-victims did not experience higher rates of sexual victimization was at odds with the results of previous studies in adolescents involved in different public service systems (e.g., child welfare, juvenile justice, alcohol/drug services, see Hazen, Connelly, Roesch, Hough, & Landsverk, 2009) and community samples (Ford et al., 2011). Our results suggest that at residential facilities, sexual victimization is prevented better than other types of victimization, although of course it is a very serious form of violence that continues to occur inside the centers.

Regarding the association between poly-victimization and mental health problems, we found that past-year poly-victimization was a significant predictor of symptom severity: poly-victims were more likely to report internalizing and externalizing symptoms within the clinical range. Previous studies found similar results with adolescents in residential care (Collin-Vézina et al., 2011; Greger et al., 2015; Segura et al., 2016) and community samples (e.g., Cyr, Clément, & Chamberland, 2013). These results emphasize that the persistence of victimization during residential care has a notable impact on the development of clinically severe symptoms. In studies with community samples, individual variables such as self-esteem and mastery have been found to be mediators and/or moderators between poly-victimization and psychological distress (Soler, Kirchner, Paretilla, & Forns, 2013; Turner, Shattuck, Finkelhor, & Hamby, 2015). Thus, the accumulation of multiple victimization experiences in vulnerable children and adolescents who are removed from their families and continue to experience victimization once they are placed out of home may seriously impact their individual resources for facing adversity and may increase the risk of mental health problems. Moreover, younger youths may be more likely to show internalizing symptoms due to their earlier entry to residential care; indeed, the United Nations General Assembly (2010) repeatedly recommended that new children and adolescents should not be placed in long out-of-home placements, especially younger ones.

5 Strengths and Limitations

To our knowledge, this is the first attempt to analyze the relationship between the most recent victimization experiences and internalizing and externalizing symptom severity among adolescents in residential care in Spain. However, the study has several limitations that should be highlighted. First, because of its cross-sectional design, no causal relationship can be inferred between poly-victimization and psychopathology. Second, the relatively small sample obtained using convenience sampling does not allow for generalization. Third, as the confidence intervals of some *OR* were very wide, caution is required when interpreting their values. For all these reasons, future studies should aim to replicate these results with more representative and larger samples.

6 Implications for Children's Care

The current findings have several implications for those who work with adolescents in residential care. Firstly, the child welfare system and its staff should focus their efforts toward ensuring that residential care facilities are free from violence and provide a safe environment. The United Nations General Assembly (2006) recommended reducing the numbers of children in residential care facilities by promoting alternative measures such as foster care. Moreover, since children and adolescents in residential care are exposed to the risk of violence from other children, the United Nations (Pinheiro, 2006) suggested that child welfare workers should bear in mind the importance of differences in age and developmental stage and vulnerability as risk factors. Therefore, in addition to designing strategies for preventing violence in residential facilities, periodic monitoring is required to determine whether the measures taken truly protect children and adolescents from suffering new forms of victimization. Future studies should also try to determine what kinds of victimization adolescents in care at residential facilities are most likely to suffer and to identify risk situations and the most likely perpetrators.

Secondly, multidisciplinary teams in the child welfare system should assess the risk level of future re-victimization on a case-to-case basis, paying particular attention to scientifically established risk factors such as the experience of previous poly-victimization (Pereda & Gallardo-Pujol, 2014) and the presence of psychopathology (Cuevas, Finkelhor, Ormrod, & Turner, 2009). In addition, child welfare staff should receive specialized training in developmental victimology before conducting the victimization and re-victimization assessments in order to prevent secondary victimization.

Thirdly, both clinicians and child welfare staff should be aware that poly-victimization increases the risk of developing mental health problems. Practitioners should identify adolescent poly-victims and bear this risk in mind in their treatment and refer those who already present psychopathology to the mental health services. Additionally, as Pereda et al. (2014) suggested, researchers and clinicians should develop and apply intervention programs designed to treat a wide range of victimizations, rather than focusing on a single type.

7 Conclusions

This chapter, which includes a literature review and an original report, raises several important questions. Although studies of victimization focus on one of the most vulnerable samples of the child and adolescent population (e.g., foster care, juvenile detention, residential treatment facilities, among other settings, see Euser et al., 2014; Salazar et al., 2013), little research has been conducted on individuals in residential care. In Catalonia, Casas (2012) suggested that the impact of child protection laws on this vulnerable population and the effects of specific protection measures (e.g., residential care facilities and foster care) should be regularly assessed. We propose that the Catalan government and the child welfare system should conduct periodic studies to evaluate the effectiveness of the protection measures in place and to identify ways of improving preventive policies for each type of abuse. The communication between law- and policy-makers and professionals working directly with these children should be reinforced. The conclusions of governmental reports and studies need to reach child welfare workers, and at the same time, practitioners must inform the authorities of children's and adolescents' victimization experiences.

Further, according to Casas (2012), the proportion of children and adolescents with foster families in relation to the total number of young people in care provides a benchmark indicator for the child welfare system. A study based on data from 2008 showed that our child welfare system had the lowest rate of children in foster care (Jackson & Cameron, 2011) in a sample of European countries. According to Casas (2012), approximately half of protected children are still in residential care; the other half are in foster care, mainly in kinship care (see Sect. 2.2). Thus, although child welfare policies both in Catalonia and abroad state that residential care should be the last resort (Síndic de Greuges, 2009; United Nations General Assembly, 2010), in practice very few children in our country are fostered by non-relative families. Therefore, in view of the advantages of foster care over residential care, and also of the increased social spending that residential care entails, there is an imperative need to develop policies to promote foster care especially with trained families (i.e., non-relatives) (Síndic de Greuges, 2014).

Finally, our findings showed that children and adolescents in residential care experience multiple types of victimization in spite of the fact that they are under the tutelage of the child welfare system. The strategies implemented to protect these children and youths have proved insufficient, given that adolescents in residential care experienced more poly-victimization during the past year than a community sample in the same cultural context (see Pereda et al., 2014). Furthermore, the accumulation of multiple types of victimization increases the risk of internalizing and externalizing symptoms within the clinical range. As poly-victimization has a poor prognosis in terms of psychological adjustment, child and adolescent welfare staff should be particularly alert to its development. Issues related to residential care facilities such as overcrowding and the lack of coordination with mental health services, and also the likelihood that on leaving the centers youths will return to the violent contexts from which they came, call for an urgent reflection on the suitability of the measures provided by the child welfare system (Síndic de Greuges, 2009, 2014).

Questions for Discussion

1. Can you think of different ways (both before and after the intervention of the child welfare system) of preventing the experience of victimization during the time children and adolescents are in residential facilities?
2. In terms of costs and benefits, for children and young people, for society, and for the country's social spending, what resources should be promoted in order to offer better protection for those children and adolescents in residential facilities?

3. Which factors do you think might explain the similarities and differences between countries in terms of the prevalence of victimization while children are in residential facilities?

References

Achenbach, T. M., & Rescorla, L. A. (2001). *Manual for the ASEBA school-age forms & profiles*. Burlington, VT: University of Vermont, Research Center for Children, Youth, & Families.

Amich Elías, C. (2009). Normativa jurídico-penal sobre infancia y juventud delincuente en la dictadura franquista [Juvenile criminal Law under the Francoist dictatorship]. *Cuadernos de Historia del Derecho, 16*, 75–109.

Arruabarrena, M. I., & De Paúl, J. (1999). *Maltrato a los niños en la familia: Evaluación y tratamiento* [Child abuse within the family: Evaluation and treatment]. Madrid, Spain: Ediciones Pirámide.

Bravo, A., & Fernández del Valle, J. (2009). Crisis y revisión del acogimiento residencial. Su papel en la protección infantil [Crisis and review of residential care. Its role in child protection]. *Papeles del Psicólogo, 30*(1), 42–52.

Carrasco-Ortiz, M. A., Rodríguez-Testal, J. F., & Hesse, B. M. (2001). Problemas de conducta de una muestra de menores institucionalizados con antecedentes de maltrato [Behavioral problems of a sample of institutionalized children with a history of abuse]. *Child Abuse & Neglect, 25*(6), 819–838.

Casas, F. (2012). *La protecció dels infants i adolescents en situació de risc social i desemparament a Catalunya* [The protection of children and adolescents at risk and social distress in Catalonia]. Barcelona, Spain: UNICEF Comitè Catalunya.

Casas, F., & Montserrat, C. (2002). Interdisciplinary teams and decision making in child protection systems: The experience of Catalonia. *International Journal of Child and Family Welfare, 5*(4), 146–158.

Cedeño, L. F., Martínez-Arias, R., & Bueno, J. A. (2015). Retrospective assessment of multiple victimization among immigrants in Spain. *International Journal of Psychological Studies, 7*(4), 78–85.

Collin-Vézina, D., Coleman, K., Milne, L., Sell, J., & Daigeault, I. (2011). Trauma experiences, maltreatment-related impairments, and resilience among child welfare youth in residential care. *International Journal of Mental Health and Addiction, 9*(5), 577–589.

Cuevas, C. A., Finkelhor, D., Ormrod, R., & Turner, H. (2009). Psychiatric diagnosis as a risk marker for victimization in a national sample of children. *Journal of Interpersonal Violence, 24*(4), 636–652.

Cyr, K., Chamberland, C., Lessard, G., Clément, M.-È., Wemmers, J.-A., Collin-Vézina, D., … Damant, D. (2012). Polyvictimization in a child welfare sample of children and youths. *Psychology of Violence, 2*(4), 385–400.

Cyr, K., Clément, M.-E., & Chamberland, C. (2013). Lifetime prevalence of multiple victimizations and its impact on children's mental health. *Journal of Interpersonal Violence, 29*(4), 616–634.

De Paúl, J. (2009). La intervención psicosocial en protección infantil en España: Evolución y perspectivas [Psychosocial intervention in child protection in Spain: Trends and Prospects]. *Papeles del Psicólogo, 30*(1), 4–12.

De Paúl, J., & Arruabarrena, M. I. (1995). Behavior problems in school-aged physically abused and neglected children in Spain. *Child Abuse & Neglect, 19*(4), 409–418.

De Paúl, J., & Arruabarrena M. I. (2001). *Manual de protección infantil* [Manual of child protection] (2nd ed.). Barcelona, Spain: Masson.

Del Valle, J. F., Canali, C., Bravo, A., & Vecchiato, T. (2013). Child protection in Italy and Spain: Influence of the family supported society. *Psychosocial Intervention, 22*, 227–237.

Domínguez Alonso, J., & Mohedano Menéndez, R. (2014). El acogimiento de menores en el actual sistema de protección a la infancia: La importancia del contexto [The placement of minors in the current system of child protection: The importance of context]. *Revista Internacional de Trabajo Social y Bienestar, 3*, 149–155.
Ellonen, N., & Pösö, T. (2011). Violence experiences in care: Some methodological remarks based on the finnish child victim survey. *Child Abuse Review, 20*(3), 197–212.
Ellonen, N., & Salmi, V. (2011). Poly-victimization as a life condition: Correlates of poly-victimization among Finnish children. *Journal of Scandinavian Studies in Criminology and Crime Prevention, 12*, 20–44.
Euser, S., Alink, L. R. A., Tharner, A., Van IJzendoorn, M. H., & Bakermans-Kranenburg, M. J. (2013). The prevalence of child sexual abuse in out-of-home care: A comparison between abuse in residential and in foster care. *Child Maltreatment, 18*(4), 221–231.
Euser, S., Alink, L. R. A., Tharner, A., Van IJzendoorn, M. H., & Bakermans-Kranenburg, M. J. (2014). Out of home placement to promote safety? The prevalence of physical abuse in residential and foster care. *Child and Youth Services Review, 37*, 64–70.
Fang, X., Brown, D. S., Florence, C. S., & Mercy, J. A. (2012). The economic burden of child maltreatment in the United States and implications for prevention. *Child Abuse & Neglect, 36*(2), 156–165.
Finkelhor, D. (2007). Developmental victimology. The comprehensive study of childhood victimizations. In R. C. Davis, A. J. Luirigio, & S. Herman (Eds.), *Victims of crime* (3rd ed.pp. 9–34). Thousand Oaks, CA: Sage.
Finkelhor, D. (2011). Prevalence of child victimization, abuse, crime, and violence exposure. In J. W. White, M. P. Koss, & A. E. Kazdin (Eds.), *Violence against women and children: Mapping the terrain* (pp. 9–29). Washington, DC: American Psychological Association.
Finkelhor, D., Hamby, S. L., Ormrod, R., & Turner, H. (2005). The Juvenile Victimization Questionnaire: Reliability, validity, and national norms. *Child Abuse & Neglect, 29*, 383–412.
Finkelhor, D., Ormrod, R. K., & Turner, H. A. (2009). Lifetime assessment of poly-victimization in a national sample of children and youth. *Child Abuse & Neglect, 33*, 403–411.
Finkelhor, D., Ormrod, R., Turner, H., & Hamby, S. L. (2005). Measuring poly-victimization using the Juvenile Victimization Questionnaire. *Child Abuse & Neglect, 29*(11), 1297–1312.
Ford, J. D., Wasser, T., & Connor, D. F. (2011). Identifying and determining the symptom severity associated with polyvictimization among psychiatrically impaired children in the outpatient setting. *Child Maltreatment, 16*(3), 216–226.
Gavrilovici, O., & Groza, V. K. (2007). Incidence, prevalence and trauma associated with exposure to violence in Romanian institutionalized children. *International Journal of Child & Family Welfare, 10*(3–4), 125–138.
Gearing, R. E., MacKenzie, M. J., Schwalbe, C. S., Brewer, K. B., & Ibrahim, R. W. (2013). Prevalence of mental health and behavioral problems among adolescents in institutional care in Jordan. *Psychiatric Services, 64*(2), 196–200.
González, M. (1999). Los tribunales para niños. Creación y desarrollo [Juvenile Courts. Creation and development]. *Historia de la Educación, 18*, 111–125.
González Méndez, R., & Santana Hernández, J. D. (2001). La violencia en parejas jóvenes [Violence in young couples]. *Psicothema, 13*, 127–131.
Green, L., & Masson, H. (2002). Adolescents who sexually abuse and residential accommodation: Issues of risk and vulnerability. *British Journal of Social Work, 32*, 149–168.
Greeson, J. K. P., Briggs, E. C., Kisiel, C. L., Layne, C. M., Ake, G. S., Ko, S. J., … Fairbank, J. A. (2011). Complex trauma and mental health in children and adolescents placed in foster care: Findings from the national child traumatic stress network. *Child Welfare, 90*(6), 91–108.
Greger, H. K., Myhre, A. K., Lydersen, S., & Jozefiak, T. (2015). Previous maltreatment and present mental health in a high-risk adolescent population. *Child Abuse & Neglect, 45*, 122–134.
Guerra, C., Pereda, N., Guilera, G., & Abad, J. (2016). Internalizing symptoms and polyvictimization in a clinical sample of adolescents: The roles of social support and non-productive coping strategies. *Child Abuse & Neglect, 54*, 57–65.

Hazen, A. L., Connelly, C. D., Roesch, S. C., Hough, R. L., & Landsverk, J. A. (2009). Child maltreatment profiles and adjustment problems in high-risk adolescents. *Journal of Interpersonal Violence, 24*(2), 361–378.

Hobbs, G. F., Hobbs, C. J., & Wynne, J. M. (1999). Abuse of children in foster and residential care. *Child Abuse & Neglect, 23*(12), 1239–1252.

Hollingshead, A. B. (1975). *Four factor index of social status. Working paper.* New Haven, CT: Yale University.

Inglés, A. (2000). *El maltractament d'infants a Catalunya. Quants, com, i perquè* [Child abuse in Catalonia. How many, how, and why]. Barcelona, Spain: Centre d'Estudis Jurídics i Formació Especialitzada, Departament de Justícia, Generalitat de Catalunya.

Jackson, S., & Cameron, C. (2011). *Final report of the YiPPEE project (WP12). Young people from a public care background: Pathways to further and higher education in five European countries.* London, UK: Thomas Coram Research Unit, University of London.

Játiva, R., & Cerezo, M. A. (2014). The mediating role of self-compassion in the relationship between victimization and psychological maladjustment in a sample of adolescents. *Child Abuse & Neglect, 38*(7), 1180–1190.

Kempe, C. H., Silverman, F. N., Steele, B. F., Droegemueller, W., & Silver, H. K. (1962). The battered-child syndrome. *Journal of the American Medical Association, 181*(17), 17–24.

Kolko, D. J., Hurlburt, M. S., Zhang, J., Barth, R. P., Leslie, L. K., & Burns, B. J. (2010). Posttraumatic stress symptoms in children and adolescents referred for child welfare investigation: A national sample of in-home and out-of-home care. *Child Maltreatment, 15*(1), 48–63.

Lachica, E. (2010). Síndrome del niño maltratado: Aspectos médico-legales [Battered child syndrome: Forensic aspects]. *Cuadernos de Medicina Forense, 16*(1–2), 53–63.

Lila, M., Herrero, J., & Garcia, E. (2008). Multiple victimization of Spanish adolescents: A multilevel analysis. *Adolescence, 43*(170), 333–350.

Montiel, I., Carbonell, E., & Pereda, N. (2015). Multiple online victimization of Spanish adolescents: Results from a community sample. *Child Abuse & Neglect, 52*, 123–134.

Morales, J. M., & Costa, M. (1997). Tendencias actuales en la investigación del maltrato infantil [Current trends in research of child abuse]. In J. Casado, J. A. Díaz, & C. Martínez (Eds.), *Niños maltratados* [Abused children] (pp. 309–324). Madrid, Spain: Díaz de Santos.

Pereda, N., Abad, J., & Guilera, G. (2015). Victimization and polyvictimization of Spanish youth involved in juvenile justice. *Journal of Interpersonal Violence, 30*, 1–29.

Pereda, N., Abad, J., & Guilera, G. (2016). Lifetime prevalence and characteristics of child sexual victimization in a community sample of Spanish adolescents. *Journal of Child Sexual Abuse, 25*(2), 142–158.

Pereda, N., & Gallardo-Pujol, D. (2014). One hit makes the difference: The role of polyvictimization in childhood in lifetime revictimization on a southern European sample. *Violence and Victims, 29*(2), 217–231.

Pereda, N., Gallardo-Pujol, D., & Guilera, G. (2016). Good practices in the assessment of victimization: The Spanish adaptation of the Juvenile Victimization Questionnaire from a causal indicators approach. *Psychology of Violence.* doi:10.1037/vio0000075

Pereda, N., Guilera, G., & Abad, J. (2014). Victimization and polyvictimization of Spanish children and youth: Results from a community sample. *Child Abuse & Neglect, 38*(4), 640–649.

Pinilla, J. (2011). *La infància, una història fosca. Les condicions de vida dels nens a Catalunya a través dels segles* [Childhood, a dark history. The living conditions of children in Catalonia through the centuries]. Lleida, Spain: Pagès Editors.

Pinheiro, P. S. (2006). *World report on violence against children.* New York, NY: United Nations.

Quiroz-Vega, V. (2013). *The basement: Robbie's rite of passage.* Liverpool: Tate Publishing and Enterprises.

Radford, L., Corral, S., Bradley, C., & Fisher, H. L. (2013). The prevalence and impact of child maltreatment and other types of victimization in the UK: Findings from a population survey of caregivers, children and young people and young adults. *Child Abuse & Neglect, 37*(10), 801–813.

Rus, A. V., Stativa, E., Pennings, J. S., Cross, D. R., Ekas, N., Purvis, K. B., & Parris, S. R. (2013). Severe punishment of children by staff in Romanian placement centers for school-aged children: Effects of child and institutional characters. *Child Abuse & Neglect, 37*(12), 1152–1162.
Salazar, A. M., Keller, T. E., Gowen, L. K., & Courtney, M. E. (2013). Trauma exposure and PTSD among older adolescents in foster care. *Social Psychiatry and Psychiatric Epidemiology, 48*(4), 545–551.
Saldaña, D., Jimenez, J., & Oliva, A. (1995). El maltrato infantil en España: Un estudio a través de los expedientes de menores [Child abuse in Spain: A research on child care files]. *Infancia y Aprendizaje, 71*, 59–68.
Sánchez Vázquez, V., & Guijarro Granados, T. (2002). Apuntes para una historia de las instituciones de menores en España [Notes for a history of juvenile institutions in Spain]. *Revista de la Asociación Española de Neuropsiquiatría, 22*(84), 121–138.
Sanmartín, J. (Dir.). (2002). *Maltrato infantil en la familia en España* [Child maltreatment in the family in Spain (1997/1998)]. Valencia, Spain: Centro Reina Sofía para el Estudio de la Violencia.
Schene, P. (2006). Forming and sustaining partnerships in child and family welfare: The American experience. In N. Freymond & G. Cameron (Eds.), *Towards positive systems of child and family welfare: International comparisons of child protection, family service, and community caring systems* (pp. 84–117). Toronto, Canada: University of Toronto Press.
Segura, A., Pereda, N., Abad, J., & Guilera, G. (2015). Victimization and polyvictimization among Spanish youth protected by the child welfare system. *Children and Youth Services Review, 59*, 105–112.
Segura, A., Pereda, N., Guilera, G., & Abad, J. (2016). Poly-victimization and psychopathology among Spanish adolescents in residential care. *Child Abuse & Neglect, 55*, 40–55.
Síndic de Greuges de Catalunya. (2009). *The protection of children at high social risk in Catalonia*. Barcelona, Spain: Síndic de Greuges de Catalunya.
Síndic de Greuges de Catalunya. (2014). *Informe sobre el seguiment dels infants acollits en família* [Report on the monitoring of children in foster family]. Barcelona, Spain: Síndic de Greuges de Catalunya.
Soler, L., Forns, M., Kirchner, T., & Segura, A. (2014). Relationship between particular areas of victimization and mental health in the context of multiple victimizations in Spanish adolescents. *European Child & Adolescent Psychiatry, 24*(4), 417–425.
Soler, L., Kirchner, T., Paretilla, C., & Forns, M. (2013). Impact of poly-victimization on mental health: The mediator and/or moderator role of self-esteem. *Journal of Interpersonal Violence, 28*, 2695–2712.
Soler, L., Paretilla, C., Kirchner, T., & Forns, M. (2012). Effects of poly-victimization on self-esteem and post-traumatic stress symptoms in Spanish adolescents. *European Child & Adolescent Psychiatry, 21*, 645–653.
Soler, L., Segura, A., Kirchner, T., & Forns, M. (2013). Polyvictimization and risk for suicidal phenomena in a community sample of Spanish adolescents. *Violence and Victims, 28*(5), 899–912.
Turner, H. A., Finkelhor, D., & Ormrod, R. (2006). The effect of lifetime victimization on the mental health of children and adolescents. *Social Science and Medicine, 62*(1), 13–27.
Turner, H. A., Finkelhor, D., & Ormrod, R. (2010). Poly-victimization in a national sample of children and youth. *American Journal of Preventive Medicine, 38*(3), 323–330.
Turner, H. A., Shattuck, A., Finkelhor, D., & Hamby, S. (2015). Effects of poly-victimization on adolescent social support, self-concept, and psychological distress. *Journal of Interpersonal Violence*, 1–26.
United Nations Children Fund (UNICEF). (2012). *Ethical principles, dilemmas and risks in collecting data on violence against children: A review of available literature*. New York, NY: UNICEF, Statistics and Monitoring Section, Division of Policy and Strategy.
United Nations General Assembly. (1989). *Convention on the rights of the child*, United Nations, Treaty Series, Vol. 1577, p. 3, A/RES/44/25.

United Nations General Assembly. (2006). *Report of the independent expert for the United Nations study on violence against children*, A/61/299.
United Nations General Assembly. (2010). *Guidelines for the alternative care of children: Resolution adopted by the General Assembly,* A/RES/64/142.
Valiente, C. (1996). The rejection of authoritarian policy legacies: Family policy in Spain (1975–1995). *South European Society and Politics*, *1*, 95–114.
Vidal Casero, M. C. (2002). La evolución legislativa de la protección del menor, la defensa de sus derechos y la atención a su salud [Legislative developments of child protection, the defense of their rights and their health care]. *DS: Derecho y salud*, *10*(2), 219–230.
World Health Organization (WHO). (2013). *European report on preventing child maltreatment*. Geneva, Switzerland: WHO.
World Medical Association (WMA). (2008). *Ethical principles for medical research involving human subjects*. Adopted by the 59th WMA General Assembly, Seoul, Korea.
Zubeidat, I., Fernández-Parra, A., Ortega, J., Vallejo, M. A., & Sierra, J. C. (2009). Características psicosociales y psicopatológicas en una muestra de adolescentes españoles a partir del Youth Self-Report/11-18 [Psychosocial and psychopathological characteristics of Spanish adolescents simple throw Youth Self-Report/11-18]. *Anales de Psicología*, *25*(1), 60–69. doi:10.6018/analesps.25.1.71501.

Chapter 8
Child Sexual Abuse in Religiously Affiliated and Secular Institutions in Germany

Miriam Rassenhofer, Nina Spröber-Kolb, Paul L. Plener, Michael Kölch, and Jörg M. Fegert

In Germany, only very few institutions have a prevention concept. Unfortunately, the willingness to develop such concepts usually only occurs when a case becomes known. There is often a great deal of insecurity concerning prevention concepts.

Johannes W. Rörig (2016) (German Independent Commissioner for Child Sexual Abuse Issues)

1 Introduction

In the last few years, research about child sexual abuse has increased considerably producing a fair amount of results and literature internationally. However, the specific aspect of sexual abuse in institutions where children and adolescents live or where care is taken of them, like (boarding) schools, orphanages or residential child welfare institutions, is still being rather neglected in research (see also Chap. 9). Not much is known about its frequency, dynamics and consequences.

As the state and the churches are the most important organizations funding and running institutions working with children and adolescents in Germany, we

M. Rassenhofer (✉) • N. Spröber-Kolb • P.L. Plener • J.M. Fegert
University Hospital Ulm, Child and Adolescent Psychiatry/Psychotherapy, Steinhövelstr. 5, 89075 Ulm, GERMANY
e-mail: miriam.rassenhofer@uniklinik-ulm.de; nina.sproeber@gmail.com; nina.sproeber@uniklinik-ulm.de; paul.plener@uniklinik-ulm.de; joerg.fegert@uniklinik-ulm.de

M. Kölch
Vivantes Hospital, Berlin, Germany
e-mail: m.koelch@ruppiner-kliniken.de

A.V. Rus et al. (eds.), *Child Maltreatment in Residential Care*,
DOI 10.1007/978-3-319-57990-0_8

dedicated some of our research to examining child sexual abuse within state- and church-run institutions.

In this chapter, we want to cover the following objectives:

1. Description of an approach that invites victims to participate in the political reappraisal process of child sexual abuse in Germany
2. Presentation of two studies, resulting from this approach, concerning child sexual abuse in institutions: The comparison of victim's testimonials about abuse in the context of Catholic, Protestant, or secular institutions and the comparison of information about abuse in the context of the Catholic Church
3. Description of political and societal changes as well as developments concerning prevention and intervention following the abuse affair and the reappraisal process in Germany

2 What's Out There Today

Child sexual abuse has been a taboo in the German society for quite a long time. Several attempts to raise the public consciousness about this topic, for example, the newspaper articles "Der Lack ist ab" (The glamour is gone) by Jörg Schindler (Frankfurter Rundschau, November 1999) or "Unbarmherzige Schwestern" (Merciless nuns) by Peter Wensierski (Der Spiegel, May 2003) triggered very little public reaction. A few years later, in 2006, some former residents of orphanages and residential child welfare institutions submitted petitions concerning maltreatment in these institutions to the German Parliament. The response was the establishment of a round table aimed to reappraise maltreatment in residential care in the 1950s and 1960s. Approximately one third of the former residents reported having experienced sexual abuse in institutions in that era (Runder Tisch Heimerziehung, 2010), but the German Government decided to investigate this topic separately. For some years, nothing happened as child sexual abuse seemed to elicit little interest and remained a taboo. Then, at the beginning of the year 2010, some former students of an elite school of the Jesuit Order in Germany disclosed having been victims of sexual abuse in their school (Anker & Behrendt, 2010). A growing surge of disclosures of cases in further elite schools and more institutions followed and triggered a public debate about the topic (see also Chap. 9). It seemed as if the revelation of child sexual abuse being a problem also present in elite institutions, higher education and high social classes changed people's minds and raised public consciousness about sexual abuse. The following reappraisal process is described in more detail in Chap. 9. The main focus of the current chapter is the participatory approach that used the expertise of victims (citizen science) as the basis for a political and societal reappraisal process and its results concerning abuse in institutions.

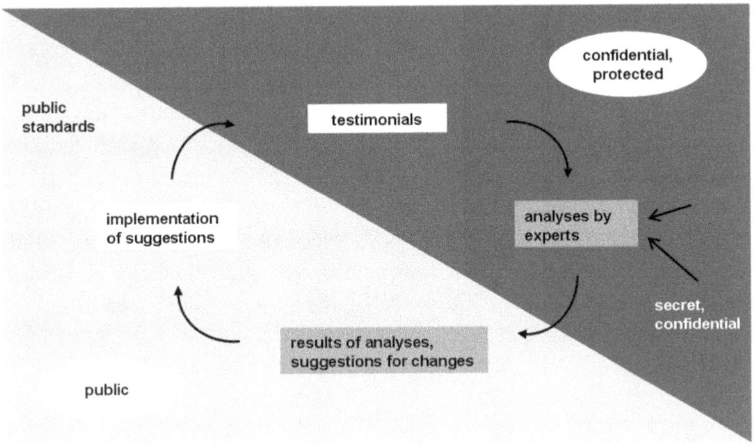

Fig. 8.1 Functionality of a critical incident reporting system (Fegert, Ziegenhain, & Fangerau, 2010)

3 New Research/Developments in This Area

3.1 Participatory Approach of a Political and Societal Reappraisal Process

Critical incident reporting systems (CIRSs) were first used in aviation (Flanagan, 1954) and have since become common instruments for risk management and patient safety in the medical system (e.g. Graaf et al., 2015; Kusano et al., 2015). A basic principle of a CIRS is guaranteed anonymity. Critical incidents are reported anonymously and then analysed by experts. The results of these analyses are published with the objective to learn from former errors and prevent similar incidents in the future. Judicial proceedings are explicitly not the purpose of a CIRS. Figure 8.1 schematically shows the functionality of a CIRS.

To our knowledge, it was for the first time in 2010 that a CIRS was used in a political and societal process. The Independent Commissioner who was appointed by the German Government as a contact person for victims of sexual abuse, their relatives and people interested in the issue established a contact point staffed with professionals that could be reached by phone or e-mail. Individuals of the target group were thus provided with the possibility to address themselves anonymously to the contact point in order to share their experiences or comment on political topics concerning child sexual abuse. Information was documented in a web-based template. There were predefined categories to choose as well as free text fields to capture information literally. Participants were not systematically interrogated but information was gathered in a free and non-directive conversation. Hence, we avoided suggestion and gave participants the opportunity to mention aspects that were relevant for them personally.

The accompanying research process included analyses of the information gathered at the contact point (quantitatively for categorical data and qualitatively for free text data) and their periodic publication on the website of the Independent Commissioner and in the media. Commenting on the results and the development of the process was possible at the contact point. A CIRS with an included feedback loop was hence realized. For a more detailed description of the participatory approach and the accompanying research process, see Rassenhofer et al. (2013).

The Independent Commissioner used the testimonials, experiences and messages of victims as a base for her recommendations (see Unabhängige Beauftragte, 2011) that were integrated in the work of the Round Table (see Runder Tisch Sexueller Missbrauch, 2011).

3.2 *Results of the CIRS Data*

Between May 2010 and October 2011, over 20,000 calls and more than 3,000 letters or e-mails reached the contact point of the Independent Commissioner. Six thousand five hundred forty-seven data sets were statistically analysable, among them 4,750 data sets of victims. Victims were on average 46 years old and predominantly female (66.7%). They mostly reported on abuse in the past that took place repeatedly within the family or institutions. We found a shift towards severe forms of abuse. For more detailed descriptions of the data, analyses and results, see Rassenhofer et al. (2013) or Fegert et al. (2013).

3.2.1 Sexual Abuse in Religiously Affiliated and Secular Institutions

The fact that the data set of the CIRS included over 1,000 victims of sexual abuse in institutions enabled us to compare testimonials about cases in religiously affiliated and secular institutions on differences in the nature of the sexual abuse, its effect on victims and their adjustment to adult life (Spröber et al., 2014). Religiously affiliated institutions were divided into a Protestant or a Roman Catholic context, so that we had three groups for the comparison: (1) Roman Catholic context ($N = 404$), (2) Protestant context ($N = 130$) and (3) non-religiously affiliated context ($N = 516$). Due to heterogeneous group sizes and different populations for each aspect or variable, statistic comparisons were carried out by non-parametric tests (Kruskal-Wallis- and Mann-Whitney-U-Test). Victims that reported having been abused in an institution were predominantly male (60%) and on average 52 years old, with victims from a religiously affiliated context being significantly older than those from a secular context and more men in the Catholic group than in the other two groups. Gender of offender as well as patterns of abuse (time, frequency, type and extent) did not differ statistically between the three groups. The percentages of victims who reported psychiatric diagnoses as a consequence of the abuse were similar in all three groups, whereas the Protestant group reported more psychosocial problems than the other two groups. Patterns of abuse seemed very similar in all three settings: repeated, ongoing assaults committed by male offenders predominated in all three groups. Offenders used situations when they were alone with the victims or even purposely created such situations and tried to gain the victim's trust. A strategy of offenders in all three settings was to disguise abuse as something educational. Disclosure often resulted in punishment or ignorance. We concluded from the testimonials of victims and their above-described similarities that sexual abuse is not attributable to specific religious or confessional attitudes towards sexuality but rather to the nature of structures typical for institutions like hierarchical power structures, dependence or group cohesion as well as to assumptions in society concerning the rights of children and attitudes towards authorities and towards sexuality.

This first exploratory study about patterns and consequences of child sexual abuse in religious and non-religiously affiliated institutions that was based on a large amount of data and a great sample helped to increase knowledge about this issue and may serve as a starting point for hypotheses and the development of effective prevention strategies.

3.2.2 Sexual Abuse in the Roman Catholic Church: Data from Two Independent CIRSs

In 2010, at the same time the government set up a reappraisal process with the Round Table, Independent Commissioner and contact point, the Roman Catholic Church in Germany – that stood in the focus of many disclosures during the abuse affair – responded by also building up a telephonic contact point for victims in terms of a CIRS. People in charge of this Catholic hotline and those in charge of the governmental contact point cooperated very early so some design matchings were possible. This enabled us later on to compare information that were collected at these two different and independent CIRSs in order to see if there are differences in the use depending on who has sponsored a CIRS (Rassenhofer et al., 2015).

We created a merged data set including information from victims that reported having experienced child sexual abuse in the context of the Roman Catholic Church in Germany. As the process at the two contact points and the structure of the data were quite similar, merging was quite straightforward. We examined the two data sets for overlap in the type of information. Variables including demographic information as well as characteristics and consequences of the abuse were comparable. After converting them to the same format we merged the two subsets into one single data set that contained information on 927 victims. Data were obtained through the church CIRS on 571 individuals and through the government CIRS on 356 individuals.

Statistical comparisons were carried out by non-parametric tests (Mann-Whitney-U-Test for independent samples). Overall, victims were on average 55 years old and predominantly male (65%) with no age difference between the two groups but with a higher percentage of men in the government data set than in the church data set. We found an underlying similarity in the data of mainly past cases of sexual abuse with a peak of occurrence in the 1960s but also further differences between the two groups concerning the setting within the Catholic Church, in which the abuse took place, the percentage of priests as offenders, type and extent of abuse, psychosocial consequences and claims for compensation. The government data set contained more male victims, more repeated acts, more acts in children's homes and (boarding) schools, more acts with physical contact, more psychosocial problems as consequences of the abuse and more claims for compensation. On the other hand, the church data set reported more acts within congregational activities and more priests as offenders.

Because of the nature of the data without systematic interrogation, different populations for each aspect and without correction for multiple testing, these statistical differences should be interpreted cautiously. But alone the fact that there are existing differences between the data gathered at different CIRSs leads to the conclusion that there are different underlying motives and expectations in individuals that address themselves to different contact points. Furthermore, we concluded that in order to reach as many people as possible, it is helpful or rather necessary to set up different programmes and several CIRSs that are sponsored by different entities. The results and the usage of these two contact points confirm the feasibility and value of a participatory CIRS approach.

4 How This Knowledge Can Improve Children's Care

The results of the two described studies confirm that institutions bear the risk of child sexual abuse. Furthermore, it is important to mention that this is not a specific problem of the Roman Catholic Church or religiously affiliated institutions but of all kinds of institutions due to the nature of institutional structures as well as the perception of the rights of children. Regarding prevalence and severity of the consequences, we conclude that effective prevention and intervention strategies in institutions are needed.

One essential aspect is education of professionals working with children and adolescents in institutions. They need a special training about specific risks, warning signals, handling of suspected cases of abuse, intervention strategies and consequences of sexual abuse, for example, in an e-learning programme (Liebhardt et al., 2015). Our experience in Germany of an e-learning programme for the prevention of child sexual abuse has been excellent (Hoffmann et al., 2013; König et al., 2015), and an extensive e-learning curriculum in the area of child protection for further qualification in trauma-focused pedagogy and therapy as well as prevention concepts and risk analyses in institutions is being developed at the moment (ECQAT, 2016).

Prevention concepts including a complaint management system need to be implemented by default in institutions. In the testimonials of victims, we often heard that residents of institutions had not been able to find anyone to tell about the abuse. Institutions were/are often closed systems, which made it difficult or even impossible for victims to find a trustful person within or outside the institution to disclose their experiences to. We conclude that there is the need for a complaint management system like a CIRS where incidents can be reported anonymously as well as an independent contact person for the children and adolescents that does not belong to the staff of the institution. Furthermore, participation of children and adolescents in their institutions has to be promoted to strengthen their position and to enable them to be actively involved in the development of rules and structures in their institutions. Beyond the institutions themselves, we identified the necessity of raising consciousness about sexual abuse in policy and society. We have seen some progress in this area since 2010 (c.f. Rassenhofer et al., 2013), but there is still a way to go.

5 Summary

The German reappraisal process of child sexual abuse included the participation of victims who were provided an opportunity to share their experiences anonymously at an independent contact point sponsored by the government. This contact point led to a unique database of information about sexual abuse. The database included testimonials of 4,570 victims, among them over 1,000 that reported experiencing child sexual abuse in institutions. We compared information about abuse in religiously affiliated institutions (Roman Catholic or Protestant context) and in secular institutions. We did not find fundamental differences and concluded that the dynamics of child sexual abuse and its consequences is rather influenced by nature of structures typical for institutions and to assumptions in society concerning the rights of children than to religion- or confession-related aspects. Another comparison study compared data about abuse in the context of the Roman Catholic Church stemming from the mentioned database and data assessed at the victim hotline of the Catholic Church. We found some differences between these groups, indicating that individuals address themselves with different expectations and different motives to specific contact points. In order to reach as many individuals as possible, it is necessary to set up more than one contact point.

The participation of victims through a complaint management system working as a critical incident reporting system (CIRS) has been proven feasible and valuable and furthermore led to a unique collection of testimonials about child sexual abuse. We confirmed that children and adolescents in institutions are at risk to experience sexual abuse. Prevention concepts, complaint management systems and participation in institutions are needed to reduce this risk.

Questions for Discussion

1. What are the advantages of a critical incident reporting system (CIRS), and what has to be considered when implementing a CIRS as a complaint management system in an institution?
2. The comparison of religiously affiliated and secular institutions indicated that child sexual abuse is attributable to the nature of institutional structures. Please describe the nature of such structures and point out potential risk factors.

3. What would you expect to be included in an e-learning programme about prevention of child sexual abuse for the staff in institutions working with children and adolescents?

References

Anker, J., & Behrendt, M. (2010, January 28). Das Schweigen muss gebrochen warden. *Berliner Morgenpost*. Retrieved from http://www.morgenpost.de/berlin-aktuell/article104884741/Das-Schweigen-muss-gebrochen-werden.html. 10 Jan 2017.

ECQAT. (2016, December 20). *E-Learning Kinderschutz*. Retrieved from https://ecqat.elearning-kinderschutz.de/

Fegert, J. M., Rassenhofer, M., Schneider, T., Spröber, N., & Seitz, A. (2013). *Sexueller Kindesmissbrauch – Zeugnisse, Botschaften, Konsequenzen: Ergebnisse der Begleitforschung für die Anlaufstelle der Unabhängigen Beauftragten der Bundesregierung zur Aufarbeitung des sexuellen Kindesmissbrauchs, Frau Dr. Christine Bergmann*. Weinheim, Germany: Beltz Juventa.

Fegert, J. M., Ziegenhain, U., & Fangerau, H. (2010). *Problematische Kinderschutzverläufe – Mediale Skandalisierung, fachliche Fehleranalyse und Strategien zur Verbesserung des Kinderschutzes*. Weinheim, Germany: Juventa.

Flanagan, J. C. (1954). The critical incident technique. *Psychological Bulletin*, *51*(4), 327.

Graaff, J. C., Sarfo, M. C., Wolfswinkel, L., Werff, D., & Schouten, A. N. (2015). Anesthesia related critical incidents in the perioperative period in children; a proposal for an anesthesia-related reporting system for critical incidents in children. *Pediatric Anesthesia*, *25*(6), 621–629.

Hoffmann, U., König, E., Niehues, J., Seitz, A., Fegert, J. M., & Liebhardt, H. (2013). Onlinekurs “Prävention von sexuellem Kindesmissbrauch”. Erste Erfahrungen und Forschungsergebnisse. *Nervenheilkunde*, *32*, 856–865.

König, E., Hoffmann, U., Liebhardt, H., Michi, E., Niehues, J., & Fegert, J. M. (2015). Ergebnisse der Evaluation des Online-Kurses „Prävention von sexuellem Kindesmissbrauch“. In J. M. Fegert, U. Hoffmann, E. König, J. Niehues, & H. Liebhardt (Eds.), *Sexueller Missbrauch von Kindern und Jugendlichen. Ein Handbuch zur Prävention und Intervention für Fachkräfte im medizinischen, psychotherapeutischen und pädagogischen Bereich* (pp. 15–24). Berlin, Germany/Heidelberg, Germany: Springer.

Kusano, A. S., Nyflot, M. J., Zeng, J., Sponseller, P. A., Ermoian, R., Jordan, L., … Ford, E. C. (2015). Measurable improvement in patient safety culture: A departmental experience with incident learning. *Practical Radiation Oncology*, *5*(3), e229–e237.

Liebhardt, H., Hoffmann, U., König, E., Niehues, J., & Fegert, J. M. (2015). Didaktisches und inhaltliches Konzept des Online-Kurses „Prävention von sexuellem Kindesmissbrauch“. In J. M. Fegert, U. Hoffmann, E. König, J. Niehues, & H. Liebhardt (Eds.), *Sexueller Missbrauch von Kindern und Jugendlichen. Ein Handbuch zur Prävention und Intervention für Fachkräfte im medizinischen, psychotherapeutischen und pädagogischen Bereich* (pp. 9–14). Berlin, Germany/Heidelberg, Germany: Springer.

Rassenhofer, M., Spröber, N., Schneider, T., & Fegert, J. M. (2013). Listening to victims: Use of a critical incident reporting system to enable adult victims of childhood sexual abuse to participate in a political reappraisal process in Germany. *Child Abuse & Neglect*, *37*, 653–663.

Rassenhofer, M., Zimmer, A., Spröber, N., & Fegert, J. M. (2015). Child sexual abuse in the Roman Catholic Church in Germany: Comparison of victim-impact data collected through church-sponsored and government-sponsored programs. *Child Abuse & Neglect*, *40*, 60–67.

Rörig, J. W. (2016, June 14). Welcoming Speech at the Pontifical Gregorian University, on the occasion of The Discharge of the first diploma course “Safeguarding of Minors”, Rome, Italy. Retrieved from https://beauftragter-missbrauch.de/fileadmin/Content/pdf/Presse_Service/Reden/Rede_Rom.pdf. Accessed 20 Dec 2016.

Runder Tisch Heimerziehung. (2010). Runder Tisch Heimerziehung in den 50er und 60er Jahren. Abschlussbericht. Arbeitsgemeinschaft für Kinder- und Jugendhilfe, Berlin, Germany. Retrieved from http://www.rundertisch-heimerziehung.de/documents/RTH_Abschlussbericht_000.pdf. 10 Jan 2017.

Runder Tisch Sexueller Missbrauch. (2011). Sexueller Kindesmissbrauch in Abhängigkeits- und Machtverhältnissen in privaten und öffentlichen Einrichtungen und im familiären Bereich. Abschlussbericht, Berlin, Germany. http://www.bmjv.de/SharedDocs/Downloads/DE/Fachinformationen/Abschlussbericht_RTKM.html. 8 Dec 2016.

Spröber, N., Schneider, T., Rassenhofer, M., Seitz, A., Liebhardt, H., Konig, L., & Fegert, J. M. (2014). Child sexual abuse in religiously affiliated and secular institutions: A retrospective descriptive analysis of data provided by victims in a government-sponsored reappraisal program in Germany. *BMC Public Health*, *14*, 282.

Unabhängige Beauftragte. (2011). Abschlussbericht der Unabhängigen Beauftragten zur Aufarbeitung des sexuellen Kindesmissbrauchs, Dr. Christine Bergmann, Berlin, Germany. Retrieved from https://beauftragter-missbrauch.de/fileadmin/Content/pdf/Presse_Service/Publikationen/Abschlussbericht-der-Unabhaengigen-Beauftragten-zur-Aufarbeitung-des-sexuellen-Kindesmissbrauchs.pdf. 8 Dec 2016.

Chapter 9
Research on Child Sexual Abuse in Institutions in German-Speaking Countries: A Summary

Nina Spröber-Kolb, Miriam Rassenhofer, Marc Allroggen, Paul L. Plener, Michael Kölch, and Jörg M. Fegert

The protection of children from abuse and violence is one of our most important issues. Children can't defend themselves against abuse and violence and very often suffer from consequences of child sexual abuse and maltreatment for all their life.

Dr. Christine Bergmann, (German Independent Commissioner for Child Sexual Abuse Issues, 2010).

1 Introduction

In this chapter, we describe the changes in society and the development of the research about child sexual abuse in institutions in German-speaking countries (Austria, Germany, and Switzerland), which has been neglected for a long time.

In 2010, the so-called abuse scandal in Germany ignited a political debate in all three German-speaking countries over the extent of abuse committed by professional educators. Although there had already been an increasing amount of research in this field, development of trauma therapy, and changes in the educational system since the late 1980s, this "abuse scandal" acted as a catalyst for politics, changes in society, and reinforced research in this field. We will illustrate the different reap-

N. Spröber-Kolb (✉) • M. Rassenhofer • M. Allroggen • P.L. Plener • J.M. Fegert
Klinik für Kinder- und Jugendpsychiatrie /-psychotherapie, Universitätsklinikum Ulm, Steinhövelstraße 5, 89075 Ulm, Germany
e-mail: nina.sproeber@uniklinik-ulm.de; nina.sproeber@gmail.com; miriam.rassenhofer@uniklinik-ulm.de; marc.allroggen@uniklinik-ulm.de; paul.plener@uniklinik-ulm.de; joerg.fegert@uniklinik-ulm.de

M. Kölch
Clinics of Ruppin, Clinic of the Medical University of Brandenburg, Neuruppin, Germany
e-mail: M.Koelch@ruppiner-kliniken.de

A.V. Rus et al. (eds.), *Child Maltreatment in Residential Care*, DOI 10.1007/978-3-319-57990-0_9

praisal processes in the three countries using different methodological approaches to assess the prevalence of child sexual abuse in institutions, dynamics and structures of the institutions that facilitated the maltreatment, and consequences for the victims and the offenders. In addition, we will report on the current research on child sexual abuse in institutions. At the end of the chapter, we will conclude with future research and ideas for prevention and intervention of child sexual abuse in practice.

In this chapter, we will cover the following objectives:

- Description of the changes in society in the three German-speaking countries Austria, Germany, and Switzerland in the twentieth century as a background for the development of research on child sexual abuse in institutions
- Research on child sexual abuse in institutions in the past and reappraisal processes
- Summary of the current research on child sexual abuse in institutions in the three German-speaking countries

2 What's Out There Today: Established Research and Practice

Education of children in institutions has been discussed in society from time to time in the past, even in the early 1950s (e.g., closing of reformatory Sonnenberg, Switzerland, 1944/1945; see Akermann, Furrer, & Jenzer, 2012; Bühler, 2009; Loosli, 2006). Although society has been shocked by the media reports of severe physical, emotional, and sexual abuse, public attention has each time decreased after a short while. Without starting to think about changing the system for the long term, consequences have been restricted to the affected institutions such as closing a residential home, transferring offenders to other institutions, or – rarely – dismissing the reports (Isely & Isely, 1990; Lengwiler, 2013). It became obvious in the last decade that children who would have needed special protection were exposed to a toxic environment in many institutions in the last century and so have been at high risk of maltreatment (Commission of Investigation into Catholic Archdiocese of Dublin, 2009; Scicluna, 2010). Survivors of child sexual abuse in institutions have shown high rates of mental health and psychosocial problems in later life, even more than survivors of child physical or emotional abuse (Fitzpatrick et al., 2010).

The environment of children who are raised in institutions, and the situation of children in general, has been undergoing a continuing process of improvement in all three European German-speaking countries – Austria, Germany, and Switzerland. While children had previously been taught to be an obedient part of society, in the late 1960s/1970s, education started to focus more on encouraging the individual personality of children, promoting their talents and abilities and comfort with independence, critical thinking, and sense of responsibility for society.

At this particular time, there has already been a systematic appraisal process of the child welfare system in Austria, provoked by the documentary "Bambule" by Ulrike Meinhof (Iben, 1972). Effects of being reared in an institution on personality were examined (Mader & Sluga, 1969). In 1975, first reforms (e.g., implementing of a control system, better education of staff, participation of children and adolescents) of the child welfare system have been drafted and implemented (Berger, 2015). Similar developments could be seen in Germany and Switzerland in the 1970s. Child protection has been intensified, and first helplines for child sexual abuse have been founded in these days. Since their introduction, child protection in all three countries has been strengthened in a continuing process.

Child maltreatment and sexual abuse has gained more and more attention in public and in research (both internationally and in the German-speaking countries) and has been assessed in surveys, first mainly in families (Finkelhor, 1984; Kavemann & Lohstöter, 1984; Raupp & Eggers, 1993). In Germany, the first representative study (N = 3,241 adolescents and adults between 16 and 60 years) has been conducted. Experiences of participants in childhood have been assessed retrospectively (Wetzels, 1997). Results show prevalence rates of child sexual abuse of 7.3% for males and 18.1% for females (3.4% for males and 10.1% for females if protection age limit of 14 years has been considered). Besides assessing the prevalence rates and starting to look at the dynamics of child sexual abuse, researchers focused on establishing behavior checklists and psychiatric symptoms following sexual abuse and determining characteristics for credibility (Steller & Köhnken, 1989).

The UN convention on the rights of children in 1989 has been a milestone in the implementation of children's rights. The governments of all three countries have ratified the convention (Austria in 1989, Germany in 1992, and Switzerland in 1997). The conditions of the convention have been implemented in national law since then. In 1992, the Swiss Department of the Interior (Arbeitsgruppe Kindesmisshandlung, 1992) authorized a multidisciplinary expert team to do research on child maltreatment as a basis for changes in the Swiss system.

Another important milestone in the legal framework has been the right to nonviolent education which was granted by the law in Austria in 1998 and in Germany in 2000 (note: still no such regulations in Switzerland). Linked to this development, research studies started to examine more detailed consequences of child sexual abuse. Findings of neuroimaging studies in the USA and development of new approaches in trauma therapy pointed to the need for early protection of children and a close collaboration between the youth welfare system and health care. Studies in German-speaking countries showed that children and adolescents in the youth welfare system very often have experienced multiple traumata (Fegert & Besier, 2009). Few of them have received tailored trauma therapy and pedagogics as those approaches have not been evaluated in German-speaking countries and there has been a lack of trained professionals to distribute this skill set (Fegert, Ziegenhain, & Goldbeck, 2013). Government-sponsored research projects also started to prevent sexual abuse of minors in institutions (Fegert & Wolff, 2002, 2006).

Triggered by victims in other countries, child sexual abuse in institutional settings (e.g., Commission to Inquire into Child Sexual Abuse, 2009; John Jay College, 2004) has been investigated more and more. In line with that, until 2008 there was a broad reappraisal process in Germany that considered how children were treated in institutional care in the 1950s and 1960s. A commission in Germany (Round Table) revealed a huge amount of coercion and unethical pedagogic interventions in institutional care during this time, which was followed by numerous impairments of the children in later life, such as psychiatric disorders, social problems, and the inability to cope with their life (Arbeitsgemeinschaft für Kinder- und Jugendhilfe, 2010). One recommendation from the work of this commission was that the prevalence of child sexual abuse in institutions was to be assessed in-depth during a special examination.

All in all, improving the prevention of child sexual abuse in families as well as in institutions has been an ongoing process since the late 1960s in all three German-speaking countries that can be seen in the legal system – another milestone has been the ratification of the Council of Europe Convention for the Protection of Children against Sexual Exploitation (Austria 2011, Germany 2015, Switzerland 2014) – as well as in research.

Though none of these developments reached as much attention in the public and society as the occasions in 2010. On the 29th of January 2010, Pater Mertens, the headmaster of the "Canisius-Kolleg" (ruled by the Jesuit fraternity) in Berlin published a letter in a newspaper that was addressed to former students of the school. Pater Mertens wrote this letter after having talked to three former students that told him about child sexual abuse in the Canisius-Kolleg in the years 1970–1980, committed by two priests. Mertens himself said that this occasion has provoked a "Knall" (Mertens, 2015, p. 495). More and more people have started to disclose about their history of sexual, physical, and emotional abuse in institutions in the past. At first, the main focus was on institutions run by the Roman Catholic Church, disclosures by victims who were abused in Protestant-affiliated and secular institutions followed. A current case of sexual abuse of a handicapped person in an institution by a male nurse has been an additional catalyst for reactions and changes in society in Switzerland (Tschan, 2015).

In this chapter, we use the term "institution" to mean facilities or services that take definitive duties of society (e.g., education in schools, taking care of children in a residential home). In the context of child sexual abuse, the term "institution" is used in four different ways (according to Kindler & Fegert, 2015, pp. 167–168):

- Institutions can be locations where something can happen; these locations hold special territorial characteristics which influence behavior and safety.
- Institutions serve also as a connection for people of different groups (e.g., in residential homes, a nexus for children who live there and educators who work there); depending on the job and on the personality of a person, the experiences can be quite different (e.g., differing levels of adults' sensitivity to children, differing levels of children's ability to confide in adults). Research of child sexual abuse in institutions focuses on sexual exploitation when the meeting of victim and offender has been initiated in an institution, whereas actual sexual assaults can then happen in the home of an adult or while being on a trip in a car.
- Institutions are also social actors that structure their formal and informal sequences to the inside, that form characteristics (e.g., climate) and that act to the outside; institutions are seen as actors that regulate distance, sexuality, trust, power, and aggression which is the basis for an "offender-victim-institution-dynamic."
- Institutions are a system within a system, with superior influences that are the organization, the law, the administration, and society.

The Roman Catholic Church and the Protestant Church have strong traditional roots in Austria, Germany, and Switzerland. According to the national census (2013 and 2014), between 60% and 70% of Austrian, German, and Swiss people are Roman Catholic or Protestant. The Roman Catholic Church and the Protestant Church are influential institutions as care providers for children and adolescents in kindergartens, private schools, residential homes, and extracurricular activities.

The Roman Catholic Church and the governments of Germany and Austria have started a broad reappraisal process of past child sexual abuse in institutions which is interlocked with the political recognition of the suffering experienced and compensation considerations. Switzerland followed a bit later in doing so (starting in 2013).

In the following part of this chapter we will illustrate research on child sexual abuse and reappraisal processes for each country.

3 New Research/Developments in This Area

3.1 Germany

In 2010, the German government established a Round Table committee, titled "Child Sexual Abuse in Relationships of Dependence, and Imbalance of Power in Private and Public Institutions and Families," which was chaired by the federal ministries responsible for family matters, justice, and education. Their task was to develop recommendations and strategies concerning support for victims, prevention of future abuse, education of professionals, and judicial questions. Concurrently, the Roman Catholic Church apologized for the suffering of the victims and promised to examine the accusations. Responsible commissioners were appointed by the government ("Independent Commissioner for the Reappraisal of Child Sexual Abuse") and the Roman Catholic Church ("Commissioner of the German Conference of the Bishops to Inquire about Child Sexual Abuse of Minors in Church Affiliated Institutions").

Commissioners' tasks were to gather information about past cases of child sexual abuse and to develop a set of recommendations for the Parliament and the German Conference of Bishops Round Table, respectively, regarding the provision of services for victims. The Roman Catholic Church and the Round Table set up independent anonymous reporting systems that could be accessed through various contact points: hotline telephone numbers, mailing, and e-mail addresses.

Callers to the hotlines were allowed to control the conversation with experienced therapists and counselors and to choose what to talk about. Although standardized interviews would have been preferable with respect to statistical methodology, it was felt to be more important that victims are able to speak about whatever they themselves felt to be relevant. Another consideration was the fact that even 20 years after the fall of the Berlin Wall, many Germans are highly suspicious of revealing their private affairs to state establishments. The guarantee of anonymity and the assurance of no initiation of any criminal investigation were regarded as necessary measures to instill trust. If the callers agreed, the hotline staff documented their experiences and messages using a web-based template. Independent research teams analyzed the data. Both entities set up websites to keep victims informed about the results and outcomes based on a Critical Incident System (Fegert, Ziegenhain, & Fangerau, 2010). Of note, the government did not restrict the reappraisal process to child sexual abuse that has happened in institutions, but also assessed child sexual abuse in families. Although the two telephonic contact points/hotlines were developed and worked independently, they cooperated by supporting each other via delegates in the advisory board.

The establishment of the reporting system, data collection, and comparison of results are described in more detail elsewhere (Fegert, Rassenhofer, Schneider, Seitz, & Spröber, 2013; Rassenhofer, Spröber, Schneider, & Fegert, 2013; Rassenhofer, Zimmer, Spröber, & Fegert, 2015, Chap. 8 in this book).

Between May 2010 and October 2011, the telephonic contact point of the Independent Commissioner of the Round Table handled over 20,000 telephone calls and over 3,000 letters or e-mails. About 10,000 of the calls included conversations, but not all of them agreed to take part in the research part of the project and thus refused documentation. After excluding these calls as well as test calls, prank calls, and repeat calls, 6,754 analyzable data sets were left, of which 4,570 were from victims of sexual abuse. The average age of victims was 46.2 years (range: 8–89). The majority of contacts were from victims (66.3%), but some were received from confidants or acquaintances of victims (16.2%), from offenders (0.6%), from contact persons of offenders (0.4%), and from people who were reporting physical abuse or neglect or who just wanted to transmit a message to politicians (16.5%). Approximately two-thirds of the victims were female. Most cases of abuse were reported to have taken place in the past (95%), to have happened several times or recurrently (91%), and to have been committed by men (87%). More than half of the victims experienced different forms of maltreatment. All but 4% of the cases had involved touching or other physical contact by the offender; in 34% of the cases, the victim was penetrated. The two most common contexts were family members (58%) and institutions (31%), followed by persons from the social environment (8%) and strangers (5%) (Rassenhofer et al., 2013). Many victims ($n = 1,132$) reported suffering from psychiatric disorders such as depression, PTSD, and anxiety disorders, and $n = 2,081$ victims stated severe long-term psychosocial consequences among other physical complaints, relationship problems, and reduction of performance (Fegert et al., 2013).

The victim hotline of the Roman Catholic Church in Germany finished its work at the end of 2012. 8,465 contacts were documented (telephone calls, emails, letters), and 1,596 analyzable data sets have been gained (Zimmer et al., 2014). The findings of both hotlines showed that many victims suffered from severe maltreatment in institutions in the past; increased psychosocial limitations and high rates of psychiatric symptoms are correlated to these toxic environments (Rassenhofer et al., 2015). Victims that contacted the Catholic victim hotline illustrated most cases of child sexual abuse in the institution as relationship crimes in which religious employees took advantage of the trust of wards. For a more detailed comparison between religiously affiliated and secular institutions, see Chap. 8 in this book.

The telephonic contact point of the government is still at work. However, the first phase, in which data collection and analysis was accompanied by a research group, was terminated in 2011, right before the Round Table finished its work with publishing concluding recommendations. The results of the work of the first Independent Commissioner (data of telephonic contact point, results of research projects) were integrated in these recommendations (Bergmann, 2011):

- Development of guidelines for handling suspicious cases
- Involving external experts in cases of suspicion
- Implementation of child-focused measures to guarantee quality of development of personnel
- Development and implementation of an internal and external complaint management system
- Topic-specific qualifying of professionals by external experts
- Establishing risk-analysis of institutions
- Implementation of participation for children and youth
- Development of institutional-specific prevention concepts
- Documentation of suspicious cases

The Roman Catholic Church in Germany has improved prevention of child sexual abuse since then (e.g., establishing a clearing center to check requests for compensation in 2011, developing an E-learning course for child protection, update of the guidelines for exposure to child sexual abuse and to abuse of dependent adults in Roman Catholic institutions in 2013, supporting prevention projects in practice, appointing a contact person for children/ parents in each diocese).

For the government as well as for the Roman Catholic Church, the appointees to inquire on child sexual abuse are still on duty, collecting information, developing prevention strategies, and monitoring the implementation of planned changes.

Both entities (government and Roman Catholic Church) instructed research teams to assess more information about the prevalence of child sexual abuse in institutions: The Roman Catholic Church commissioned different surveys (Raue, 2010, 2011; Zinsmeister, 2011) to estimate the number of victims and offenders and kind of offenses. Independent surveys (Hegenberg-Miliu, 2014; Obermeyer & Stadler, 2011) assessed the views of victims and institutional dynamics. Besides that, the Roman Catholic Church ordered two research projects: The first project was an analysis of psychiatric-psychological surveys of priests that have abused children (Leygraf, König, Kröber, & Pfäfflin, 2012) and an examination of the characteristics of offenders. In 2013, there was a qualitative analysis of the psychosocial consequences for victims as well as of the institutional dynamics of a boarding school in a convent (Klosterinternat Ettal) where children have been sexually abused (Keupp, Straus, Mosser, Gmür, & Hackenschmied, 2013).

Another research project tried to assess the extent of child sexual abuse in institutions of the Roman Catholic Church. As the research team and the bishops conference were not able to come to an agreement about publishing, the research team interviewed 100 victims of child sexual abuse by Catholic priests (Hellmann, Fernau, Baier, & Pfeiffer, 2015). The investigators reported that children in boarding schools and residential homes have been at high risk for maltreatment and sexual abuse. Offenders exploited their power to abuse their wards. People in the social environment often knew or at least suspected that children had been abused. And, again, they found severe psychosocial consequences for the victims.

An interdisciplinary research project conducts quantitative analysis of personnel files and dynamics between offenders, victims, and institutions and conducts a secondary analysis of national and international empirical results (Dölling et al., 2016). Preliminary results of this secondary analysis (based on 40 international studies) show that 78.6% of offenders in the Roman Catholic Church have been male (45.1% in other institutions), mostly priests or teachers, 52.2% of offenses have been planned, and 82.9% of 14,488 analyzed acts have been hands-on acts.

There has been strong cooperation between the government and the Roman Catholic Church in this reappraisal process. In 2012, the Center for Child Protection (CCP) was founded with cooperation between the Archdiocese of Freising (Munich), the Department of Child and Adolescent Psychiatry and Psychotherapy at the University of Ulm, and the Pontifical University Gregoriana in Rome. Staff of the Roman Catholic Church were empowered to prevent child sexual abuse and support victims and their parents in an effective way by developing and implementing an E-learning curriculum "prevention of child sexual abuse for pastorale occupations." Good feasibility and high motivation was shown during a pilot phase including N = 716 learners (German, English, Spanish, Italian speakers), even in areas where the Internet was hard to use reliably (Fegert, Böhm, Rassenhofer, & Witt, 2015).

The Protestant Churches have agreed with the implementation of the recommendations of the Round Table like many sports clubs and social institutions up to 2012, but they have rarely investigated maltreatment in a structured way in Protestant-affiliated institutions in the past (Ladenburger, Lörsch, Enders, & Bange, 2014).

All the efforts that have been undertaken show initial success. The Independent Commissioner has published a monitoring interim report about the implementation of the recommendations of the Round Table (UBSKM, 2013): 70% of the N = 585 congregations have appointed a contact person for children and parents if there are acts of sexual violence, in almost 60% of congregations at least one prevention strategy has been implemented in Germany (UBSKM, 2013).

Beyond studies about specific subsamples in institutions, a survey about lifetime prevalence of sexual abuse in institutional settings examined a sample (N = 2,513) representative for the German general population (Witt et al., in preparation). Participants (n = 2,437 adults and n = 76 adolescents) answered a questionnaire about whether they had ever experienced abuse in an institution and were asked to specify type of institution (e.g., child welfare residential home, school, club), relationship of offender to victim (e.g., peer, staff member), as well as nature of abuse (hands-on, hands-off, forced sexual intercourse). Results showed that 3.1% of adult participants and 6.6% of adolescents had experienced some type of sexual abuse in an institution. Among the adults, women reported higher rates of all types of abuse than men (hands-on, 3.9% vs. 0.8%; hands-off, 1.2% vs. 0.3%; with penetration, 1.7% vs. 0.2%). Adolescents merely reported incidents of hands-on abuse (9.4% girls, 4.5% boys). The authors conclude that sexual abuse in institutions is a substantial problem within the general population in Germany. They emphasize the need for developing and enhancing protective strategies (Witt et al., in preparation).

A recent study funded by the Federal Ministry of Education and Research (BMBF) for the first time examined the prevalence of sexual victimization of adolescents in institutional care in Germany. In this study, 322 adolescents (mean age 16.69 years, 43% female) from 20 residential care facilities and 12 boarding schools were included. The mean time of living in the institution was 3.08 years. Lifetime prevalence for severe sexual victimization like (attempted) oral, vaginal, or anal penetration (in and outside of the institution) was 46.7% for girls and 8.0% for boys. Any type of sexual victimization including sexual harassment was reported by 37% of the boys and 82% of the girls. It is remarkable that a high proportion of the severe sexual victimization (boys 14% of the incidents, girls 22% of the incidents) took place after admission to the current institution. Examination of the circumstances of the offenses shows that adolescents of about the same age were mostly named as offenders, while staff members played a minor role as perpetrators (Allroggen, Ohlert, Rau, & Fegert, submitted-a). When asking the adolescents from this sample about their own sexually aggressive behavior, 31% of the boys and 13% of the girls reported to have exhibited sexually aggressive behavior in some form or other in their lives, 7% of the boys and 1% of the girls reported to have committed sexual assault with (attempted) penetration (Allroggen, Ohler, Rau, & Fegert, submitted-b). The authors conclude that the high rate of sexual victimization among adolescents in institutional care should be considered during decision-making processes concerning out-of-home placement and during a stay in residential care.

However, despite the high prevalence of sexual victimization of adolescents in institutional care, another study from Germany shows that adolescents seem to feel quite safe during their stay in institutional care. This study uses a combination of quantitative (online questionnaire) and qualitative (group discussions) research approaches and discusses that the feeling of security is probably a consequence of underestimation of threats in institutions (Allroggen et al., 2016).

3.2 Austria

Although there was very early improvement of the child welfare system in Austria, disclosure of victims of child sexual abuse in 2010 initiated a broad process in Austria as well as in Germany. Just like in Germany, the reappraisal process has been twofold: one part from the state and the other from the Roman Catholic Church. In 2010, the state of Tyrol was the first that implemented a "commission for victim protection." This commission prepared suggestions for reappraisal and compensation (Schreiber, 2013). The suggested implementation of a country-wide commission was refused by the government. So, there is no overview of child sexual abuse in institutions in Austria. Thus, investigations have generally been executed in individual institutions (Bauer, Hoffmann, & Kubek, 2013; Helige, John, Schmucker, & Wörgötter, 2013; Schreiber, 2013) with most of these initiated by state or city governments. In addition, information has also been collected by interdisciplinary research teams that have looked at recorded files and conducted interviews with survivors of institutional abuse. Findings have been analyzed quantitatively and qualitatively, and high rates of maltreatment have been found in all studies.

We have chosen one of the studies that is based on a broad empirical data set and considers long-term consequences to illustrate the procedure of the investigations in Austria: The "Wiener Heimkinderstudie" (Berger & Katschning, 2013) is based on information from survivors of child sexual abuse in institutions in the broader area of Vienna between 1945 and 1990. Between March 2011 and March 2012, interviews were conducted with N = 130 survivors of maltreatment in residential homes. Those participants were recruited from N = 1,500 persons (average age: 53.6 years, range: 23.5–79.4) who contacted the Independent Commission for Victim Protection. Forty-six percent of those 130 participants were in a residential home for 5–10 years, 34% were there for more than 10 years. Almost all persons reported having experienced psychological (98.5%) and physical violence (96.2%), and almost half of them (48.5%) reported having experienced child sexual abuse. Many survivors have experienced psychosocial problems in their later life (e.g., unstable relationships, unstable careers, problematic social contacts, delinquency) and high rates of psychiatric problems (around 60% of the sample). These findings were independent from time period (they have compared 1945–1975 to 1976–1990) or familiar risk factors (such as unstable families, violence). Child sexual abuse also seems to have a closer correlation with later psychopathology, problems in having relationships, and in social contacts than other forms of maltreatment. However, there is a significant reduction in the amount of physical violence experienced between the two-time periods.

In addition to these studies, a research team (Dietrich-Daum & Hoffmann, 2013) investigated the environment and conditions of the child and adolescent psychiatry institutional unit in Innsbruck from 1954 to 1987 under the management of the head of the department Maria Nowak-Vogl based on personal files, records, literature, and interviews with former patients. They concluded that patients were at high risk for maltreatment and abuse in the past. Thus, under the management of Nowak-Vogl, a medication (Epiphysan to treat hypersexuality) was tested on abusing inpatients. There is no permission to use this medication for children since 1983.

In 2010, the Roman Catholic Church in Austria established a country-wide commission ("Klasnic-Kommission"), supported by the Bishops' conference. The commission that operated until 2015 had the following tasks:

- Acting as a contact point for survivors of child sexual abuse in the Roman Catholic Church
- Legal and psychological counseling
- Suggestions for individual interventions (e.g., therapy, financial aid, mediation)
- Giving general recommendations
- Documentary
- Public relations
- Coordination of centers of society, the Church, and government

Up to 2015, 1,355 persons had contacted the commission, and 1,051 victims had received financial compensation. Meanwhile, the Roman Catholic Church appointed an experienced advocate in all dioceses that investigate cases of child sexual abuse and recommend consequences for the offender.

The commission also initiated a research project that started 2011. Several findings have been published so far based on this sample (e.g., Lueger-Schuster et al., 2014, 2015). Participants have experienced institutional abuse and disclosed these experiences to the independent victims' protection commission. This commission carried out a clearing process that included analyses of documents confirming whether a person was actually registered in an institution and interviews with clinical psychologists assigned by the commission to assess abuse-related symptoms. The reports were judged for their credibility by the commission to readdress survivors of abuse and to determine the extent of the financial compensation and psychotherapeutic treatment. Both the data from the clearing documents and the questionnaire data, which was collected in a study after survivors had reported to the commission, were examined in a study (Lueger-Schuster et al., 2014, 2015). A clinical psychologist handed out the first information about the study after the compensation had been approved. Of N = 795 readdressed survivors, more than half (n = 448, 56.4%) agreed to an analysis of their documents. Almost half of those (n = 185, 76.4% male) filled out a set of questionnaires (e.g., questionnaires regarding PTSD symptoms, resilience, coping strategies, factors of disclosure, psychiatric symptoms). Participants were 56.28 years on average (range 26–80 years). Results revealed that the majority of the participants had experienced emotional abuse (83.3%), while sexual and physical abuse had been experienced by around 69% of the participants. Overall, the survivors reported a great diversity of exposure to physical, sexual, and emotional abuse during their childhood. Although survivors with PTSD reported significantly more family risk factors, familial characteristics were not found to influence the development of PTSD in later life. However, maltreatment in institutions was associated with long-term sequelae on mental health. Furthermore, reacting less emotionally during disclosure, task-oriented coping, as well as optimism, were correlated with better mental health outcomes of the participants (Lueger-Schuster et al., 2014, 2015).

3.3 Switzerland

The reappraisal process in Switzerland differs from Austria and Germany as there has not been a country-wide procedure either by the government or by the Roman Catholic Church for a very long time. As recently as 2013, the government apologized for the suffering of all the children that had been reared in institutions before. Besides being reared in institutions, children have often been taken to families by authorities and lived there either as foster children or "Verding-Kinder" (which is special for Switzerland and means that children had to work for families). In 2016, the national convention agreed to a suggestion for paying compensation to the survivors of maltreatment in institutions.

In general, there have been numerous special research studies about individual institutions and organizations in Switzerland – even very early ones – but no summary that compares in a systematic way institutions and the youth welfare system considering regional differences in the federalistic country (Lengwiler, 2013, p. 22). The website of the "Independent Expert Commission for Administrative Provision" gives an overview about all single research projects. In 2004, the ministry for education and research ordered a report about research on children that have been reared in institutions. Most Swiss studies to assess experiences of children reared in institutions in the past are drafted as "historical studies," conducted by an interdisciplinary research team. As an example, we illustrated the study of Akermann and colleagues (2012).

An interdisciplinary research team in Luzern investigated economic, societal, legal, and pedagogical conditions of the era between 1930 and 1970. The historical study (see Akermann et al., 2012) is based on oral history and analysis of discourse through the examination of files and analysis of survivors' testimonials. The aim was to understand the influence of society on the living conditions of children in institutions. In addition to the file analysis, 54 survivors were interviewed (in-depths interviews). Survivors were able to contact the contact point for incidents that have occurred in residential homes in Luzern. For the first part of the interviews, participants were able to talk in an unstructured way; in a second step, researchers asked manual-based questions for topics that had not been mentioned by the survivors. Of these, 42 interviews were transcribed, and categories were determined to find "typical profiles." In addition, written sources (files from institutions such as house rules, annual reports, files about residents, files of authorities such as court files, records, writings about education in institutions) have been analyzed.

Findings demonstrate several problems of the youth welfare system during this time period (Akermann et al., 2012, p. II):

- Discrimination of abnormal and socially disadvantaged families.
- A strong religious moral in the education of educators.
- Arbitrariness of the consequences handed by authorities.
- Financial problems of the residential homes.
- Deficient control by authorities of the management of institutions.
- No participation for children and adolescents in institutions in making decisions that affect them.
- Stigmatization of residents.
- Children had to work; education was neglected.
- Repressive punishments.
- Sexual violence.
- Consensus in society that children who were brought up in an institution have behavior problems.

Results show severe forms of physical, emotional, and sexual abuse that survivors have experienced. 27 of the 42 transcribed interviews contain information about child sexual abuse. Usually, offenders were members of the religious staff, but survivors also reported about child sexual abuse in their families. Risk factors for sexual abuse have been deduced from the analyzed data: isolation of the institution ("total institution"), suppression of offenses by offenders and colleagues, no information/education for children about sexuality, and a focus on sexual incidents between peers (Akermann et al., 2012, p. III). Examinations indicated frequent and long-lasting forms of severe neglect, physical violence, and emotional and sexual child abuse in residential homes and boarding schools. The results of the historical analyses of the dynamics of society, institutions, and the incidences of child maltreatment and child sexual abuse were very interesting (Akerman et al., 2012, p. 120 ff.). The aim of the residential homes was to "norm" the children, but also to give them a home (especially for orphanages). Many problems for children in residential homes stemmed from societal beliefs and norms during this period. For instance, a bio-political way of thinking, and specifically an eugenic way of thinking (which was very strong during the Nazi reign in Germany and Austria, but also had an impact in Switzerland up to the 1980s), meant that children in residential care were considered as genetically weak and in need of improvement. Religious thinking considered these children as sinful. Also, children who were reared in institutions were considered as non-credible and children had no independent contact point; though, disclosure has been difficult, because they were not believed.

Although, physical punishment was limited by rules in residential homes, the rules were not enforced. There are several reasons for that (Akermann et al., 2012, p. 120 ff.):

- First of all, it was a common way of thinking for educators that children needed to be punished.
- Educators were poorly educated.
- Sometimes circumstances in the residential homes (particularly before the 1960s) were very hard/poor.
- Corporal punishment was still allowed by law.

But there is still the question of why some educators used excessive forms of physical or emotional violence. Akermann et al. (2012) concluded that residents were punished so harshly and cruelly because they were viewed as sinful, that there was a lack of external control of institutions, and that most institutions had too many rules (which meant that children were not able to fulfill one rule without being against the other rule). In addition, some educators just enjoyed using force. The interaction of these factors kept the cycle of violence and abuse going.

Currently, the prevalence of child sexual abuse is being assessed in Swiss studies by asking adolescents about their experience of such (Averdijk, Müller-Johnson & Eisner, 2012; Mohler-Kuo et al., 2014). Mohler-Kuo and colleagues (2014) assessed child sexual abuse in an epidemiological survey using self-report computer-assisted questionnaires. A nationally representative sample of 6,787 students in the ninth grade, who were M = 15.5 years old (SD = 0.66), were questioned. The results revealed that 40.2% of the girls and less than half as many boys (17.2%) had experienced at least one type of sexual abuse. Lifetime prevalence rates for sexual abuse without physical contact was 35.1% for girls and 14.9% for boys, while reported rates of sexual abuse including physical contact but no penetration were lower

(14.9% for girls and 4.8% for boys). Penetrative sexual abuse was reported by 2.5% of the girls and 0.6% of the boys. Sexual harassment was the most frequently experienced type of sexual abuse. In more than half of the cases of sexual abuse on girls and over 70% of the cases of sexual abuse on boys, the perpetrators were adolescents. Moreover, the results of the study revealed that only about half of the female victims and even fewer male victims (44.4–58.4% and 5.8–38%, respectively, depending on the event) disclosed their experience to someone, mainly to peers. Overall, the prevalence rates of child sexual abuse, the high numbers of sexual harassment via the Internet, as well as the frequent sexual abuse by adolescent perpetrators in the study by Mohler-Kuo and colleagues (2014) align with current prevalence trends and information on child sexual abuse found in research. Especially when considering the low disclosure rates, in particular toward family members and officials, interventions and recommendations for actions have to be made.

4 How This Knowledge Can Improve Children's Care

The research that has been conducted within the framework of the reappraisal processes of institutional care of children in the three European German-speaking countries has found a high prevalence of child sexual, physical, and emotional abuse in institutions in the past. Even when familial risk factors are controlled for, child sexual abuse, in particular, has a deep impact on the development of psychiatric problems and psychosocial deficits. The reappraisal processes show that it is very important for all the survivors that they are heard and that their suffering is recognized. Survivors should know who they can talk to, and the procedures of compensation should be transparent. Research on the efficacy of trauma therapy has been improved within the last decades, but there is still a need for a better education of medical and psychological specialists to know more about PTSD and to offer trauma therapy. To support access to a better education on child sexual abuse, E-learning programs are a promising approach. Also, well-grounded practical training in trauma therapy should be an important part of the education of all pedagogical, medical, and psychological experts.

Moreover, the results of the research have shown that the understanding of education, rights of children, and protection of children have been undergoing a continuing change toward more freedom, as well as strengthening the abilities and the personality of children. To eliminate child sexual abuse in institutions, it is important that the staff of institutions are well selected (e.g., education, certificate of good conduct) and that all staff members have knowledge about child sexual abuse, know the procedures of the institution to handle suspicious cases, and are encouraged to show moral courage (e.g., by offering supervision, being able to talk about a suspicious case anonymously). Children and parents/relatives should also know the procedures. There should be a transparent complaint management system for children and their relatives. Analysis of the life pathways of child sexual abuse survivors has illustrated that listening to children, taking them and their problems seriously, and offering effective help can prevent the development of severe psychiatric problems.

Actual prevalence studies have clarified that there is still a high risk for children in institutions to become victims of child sexual abuse, but children underestimate the risk; education on child sexual abuse – also peer-to-peer – victimization – should be improved.

Although there has been quite a good amount of research on the prevalence of child sexual abuse in institutions in the three German–speaking countries in recent years, there is still a need for representative studies of child and adolescent sexual abuse in institutions. To achieve this, cooperation between institutions, organizations, and political experts must be intensified, and the definition of child sexual abuse must be standardized. Data collection should be easy for institutions to implement. Future research studies should be conducted as stratified random samples and population studies that ask adolescents for their actual experiences.

5 Summary

In this chapter, we first illustrated the development of research on child sexual abuse in institutions against the background of changes in society, especially implementation of rights of children and promoting personality, capabilities, and talents of children. Although there have been reports and documentaries on child sexual abuse in institutions – even very early ones in the 1940s/1950s – the situation of children in institutions has only undergone improvement as a continuing process as recently as the late 1970s. Research on child sexual abuse in institutions and families has been expanded since the 1990s. The first representative studies (retrospective studies) on the prevalence of child sexual abuse have been conducted, the first helplines for children have been implemented, and prevention and intervention strategies for institutions have been published.

Societal and political awareness of this problem in Austria, Germany, and Switzerland since 2010 has brought outrage, initially triggered by the disclosure of child sexual abuse in institutions run by the Roman Catholic Church, followed by secular institutions and protestant-affiliated institutions.

In all three European German-speaking countries, reappraisal processes were mainly initiated by state or city governments and then started by the Roman Catholic Church. Survivors of child sexual abuse were able to give reports to telephonic contact points or contacts points. Survivors were listened to and their reports have been documented in order to provide compensation/financial help for medical services and so on. Collected data has also been evaluated for research. Studies in different countries have been drafted in different ways (unstructured data collection, interviews with survivors, historical studies). All studies show a high prevalence of child sexual abuse in institutions in the past, with physical and emotional abuse also reported as frequent occurrences. Swiss historical studies try to explain the reason for this through analysis of education, the situation of institutions, and way children in institutions have been perceived. Long-lasting psychosocial consequences of the abuse were increased when children were not listened to or believed if they tried to get help. Current representative studies to assess prevalence of child sexual abuse in institutions still show there is a high risk of abuse for children in institutions, particularly the problem of peer-to-peer victimization.

Since 2010, many recommendations based on the results of research and reappraisal processes have been transferred to practice. However, it is important that the effectiveness of the implementation of prevention and intervention strategies is monitored.

Questions for Discussion

1. Why did reports on child sexual abuse and maltreatment in institutions not reach broad interest in society before 2010?
2. What are the advantages and disadvantages of the data on child sexual abuse in institutions that was collected by the hotlines sponsored and managed by the government or the Roman Catholic Church?
3. Why do residents feel quite safe in institutions today, even though there is still a high risk of being sexually abused?

References

Akermann, M., Furrer, M., & Jenzer, S. (2012). *Kinderheime im Kanton Luzern im Zeitraum von 1930–1970*, Luzern. http://www.disg.lu.ch/schlussbericht_aufarbeitung_kinderheime_120731.pdf. 29 Jan 2017.

Allroggen, M., Domann, S., Strahl, B., Schloz, C., Fegert, J. M., & Kampert, M. (2016). How much insecurity does security need? – The discrepancy in assessing the sense of security of children, adolescents and caregivers in institutions. *Child and Youth Services*, *37*(4), 381–397. doi:10.1080/0145935X.2016.1210447.

Allroggen, M., Ohlert, J., Rau, T., & Fegert, J. M. (Submitted-a). Lifetime prevalence and incidence of sexual victimization of adolescents in institutional care.

Allroggen, M., Ohlert, J., Rau, T., & Fegert, J. M. (Submitted-b). Sexual violence by juveniles in institutions – A descriptive study on prevalence and circumstances.

Arbeitsgemeinschaft für Kinder- und Jugendhilfe. (2010). Abschlussbericht des Runden Tisches „Heimerziehung in den 50ern und 60er Jahren", Berlin. http://www.rundertisch-heimerziehung.de/documents/RTH_Abschlussbericht.pdf. 29 Jan 2017.

Arbeitsgruppe Kindesmisshandlungen. (1992). *Kindesmisshandlungen in der Schweiz. Schlussbericht zuhanden des Vorstehers des Eidgenössischen Departments des Inneren*. Bern, Switzerland: Department des Inneren.

Averdijk, M., Müller-Johnson, K., & Eisner, M. (2012). Sexuelle Viktimisierung von Kindern und Jugendlichen in der Schweiz. Schlussbericht für die UBS Optimus Foundation, Zürich. www.optimusstudy.org/fileadmin/user_upload/documents/Full_Report_Schweiz/Optimus_Studie_WissenschaftlicherSchlussbericht_2012_d.pdf. 29 Jan 2017.

Bauer, I., Hoffmann, R., & Kubek, C. (2013). Abgestempelt und ausgeliefert. Fürsorgeerziehung und Fremdunterbringung in Salzburg nach 1945, Salzburg. http://service.salzburg.gv.at/lkorrj/XBeilage?cmd=dateiAusliefern&klasse=beilagen.ABeilagen&beilagenid=239&nachrid=50885. 29 Jan 2017.

Berger, E. (2015). Gewalt in pädagogischen Institutionen in Österreich. In Fegert, J. M., & Wolff, M. (Eds.), *Kompendium „Sexueller Missbrauch in Institutionen" – Entstehungsbedigungen, Prävention und Intervention* (pp. 697–706). Weinheim, Germany: Beltz Juventa.

Berger, E., & Katschning, T. (2013). Gewalt in Wiener Heimen zwischen 1945 und 1990 – eine restrospektive Studie aus psychotraumatologischer Perspektive. *Neuropsychiatrie, 27*, 188–195.

Bergmann, C. (2011). *Abschlussbericht der Unabhängigen Beauftragten zur Aufarbeitung des sexuellen Kindermissbrauchs, Dr. Christine Bergmann*. Berlin, Germany: Geschäftsstelle der Unabhängigen Beauftragten zur Aufarbeitung des sexuellen Kindesmissbrauchs.

Bühler, L. (2009). *Der Skandal um die Erziehungsanstalt Sonnenberg 1944: Das Medienereignis von den Wertekonflikten im Anstaltswesen bis zur Anstaltskrise*. Bachelor thesis, Universität Luzern, Lucerne, Schweiz.

Commission of Investigation into Catholic Archdiocese of Dublin. (2009). *Report by Commission of Investigation into Catholic Archdiocese of Dublin*. Part 1: http://www.justice.ie/en/JELR/DACOI%20Part%201.pdf/Files/DACOI%20Part%201.pdf, Part 2: http://www.justice.ie/en/JELR/DACOI%20Part%202.pdf/Files/DACOI%20Part%202.pdf. 6 Feb 2017.

Commission to Inquire into Child Abuse. (2009). *Final report of the commission to inquire into child abuse dated 20th May 2000: Executive summary*. http://www.childabusecommission.ie/rpt/pdfs/CICA-Executive%20Summary.pdf. 29 Jan 2017.

Dietrich-Daum, E., & Hoffmann, B. (2013). Die Innsbrucker *Kinderbeobachtungsstation von Maria Nowak-Vogl*. Bericht der Medizin-Historischen ExpertInnenkommission. https://www.i-med.ac.at/pr/presse/2013/Bericht-Medizin-Historische-ExpertInnenkommission_2013.pdf. 29 Jan 2017.

Dölling, D., Hermann, D., Horten, B., Bannenberg, B., Dreßing, H., Kruse, A., ... Schmitt, E. (2016). Metaanalyse zum sexuellen Missbrauch an Minderjährigen im Rahmen der katholischen Kirche. *Forensische Psychiatrie, Psychologie und Kriminologie, 10*, 103–115.

Fegert, J. M., & Besier, T. (2009). *Psychisch belastete Kinder und Jugendliche an der Schnittstelle zwischen Kinder- und Jugendhilfe und Gesundheitssystem. Expertise zum 13. Kinder- und Jugendbericht der Bundesregierung*. München, Germany: DJI-Deutsches Jugendinstitut e.V.

Fegert, J. M., Böhm, B., Rassenhofer, M., & Witte, S. (2015). Reaktionen auf die Missbrauchsfälle in der katholischen Kirche in Deutschland. *Nervenheilkunde, 34*(7), 501–513.

Fegert, J. M., Rassenhofer, M., Schneider, T., Seitz, A., & Spröber, N. (2013). *Sexueller Kindesmissbrauch – Zeugnisse, Botschaften, Konsequenzen: Ergebnisse der Begleitforschung für die Anlaufstelle der Unabhängigen Beauftragten der Bundesregierung zur Aufarbeitung des sexuellen Kindesmissbrauchs, Frau Dr. Christine Bergmann*. Weinheim, Germany: Beltz Juventa.

Fegert, J. M., & Wolff, M. (Hrsg.). (2002). Sexueller Missbrauch durch Professionelle in Institutionen. Münster, Germany: Votum.

Fegert, J. M., & Wolff, M. (Hrsg.). (2006). Sexueller Missbrauch durch Professionelle in Institutionen – Prävention und Intervention – ein Werkbuch. Weinheim, Germany: Juventa.

Fegert, J. M., Ziegenhain, U., & Fangerau, H. (2010). *Problematische Kinderschutzverläufe – Mediale Skandalisierung, fachliche Fehleranalyse und Strategien zur Verbesserung des Kinderschutzes*. Weinheim, Germany: Juventa.

Fegert, J. M., Ziegenhain, U., & Goldbeck, L. (Hrsg.). (2013). *Traumatisierte Kinder und Jugendliche in Deutschland: Analysen und Empfehlungen zu Versorgung und Betreuung*. Weinheim, Germany: Beltz.

Finkelhor, D. (1984). *Child sexual abuse: New theory and research*. New York, NY: Free Press.

Fitzpatrick, M., Carr, A., Dooley, B., Flanagan-Howard, R., Flanagan, E., Shevlin, K., ... Egan J. (2010). Profiles of adult survivors of severe sexual, physical and emotional institutional abuse in Ireland. *Child Abuse Review, 19*, 387–404.

Hagenberg-Miliu, E. (Hrsg.). (2014). Unheiliger Berg. Das Bonner Aloisiuskolleg der Jesuiten und die Aufarbeitung des Missbrauchsskandals. Stuttgart, Germany: Kohlhammer.

Helige, B., John, M., Schmucker, H., & Wörgötter, G. (2013). Endbericht der Kommission Wilhelminenberg. http://www.kommission-wilhelminenberg.at/presse/jun2013/Bericht-Wilhelminenberg-web_code.pdf. 29 Jan 2017.

Hellmann, D. F., Fernau, S., Baier, D., & Pfeiffer, C. (2015). Sexueller Missbrauch durch katholische Geistliche in Deutschland. *Nervenheilkunde, 34*(7), 525–530.

Iben, G. (1972). Selbst- und Mitbestimmung in sozialpädagogischen Institutionen. In A. Leber & H. Reiser (Eds.), *Sozialpädagogik, Psychoanalyse und Sozialkritik* (pp. 123–144). Neuwied, Germany: Luchterhand.

Isely, P. J., & Isely, P. (1990). The sexual abuse of male children by church personnel: Intervention and prevention. *Pastoral Psychology*, *39*(2), 85–99.

John Jay College. (2004). The nature and scope of sexual abuse of minors by Catholic priests and deacons in the United States 1950–2002. http://www.usccb.org/issues-and-action/child-and-youth-protection/upload/The-Nature-and-Scope-of-Sexual-Abuse-of-Minors-by-Catholic--Priests-and-Deacons-in-the-United-States-1950-2002.pdf. 29 Jan 2017.

Kavemann, B., & Lohstöter, I. (1984). *Väter als Täter*. Reinbek, Germany: Rowohlt.

Keupp, H., Straus, F., Mosser, P., Gmür, W., & Hackenschmied, G. (2013). *Sexueller Missbrauch, psychische und körperliche Gewalt im Internat der Benediktinerabtei Ettal. Individuelle Folgen und organisatorisch-strukturelle Hintergründe*. München: Institut für Praxisforschung und Projektberatung. www.ipp-muenchen.de/texte/ap_10.pdf. 27 Jan 2017.

Kindler, H., & Fegert, J.M. (2015). Missbrauch in Institutionen. Empirische Befunde zur grundlegenden Orientierung. In J. M. Fegert, & M. Wolff (Eds.), *Kompendium „Sexueller Missbrauch in Institutionen". Entstehungsbedingungen, Prävention und Intervention* (pp. 167–185). Weinheim, Germany: Beltz Juventa.

Ladenburger, P., Lörsch, M., Enders, U., & Bange, D. (2014). *Schlussbericht der unabhängigen Kommission zur Aufarbeitung von Missbrauchsfällen im Gebiet der ehemaligen Nordelbischen evangelisch-lutherischen Kirche, heute evangelisch-lutherische Kirche in Norddeutschland.* https://www.kirchegegensexualisiertegewalt.de/fileadmin/user_upload/baukaesten/Baukasten_Kirche_gegen_sexualisierte_Gewalt/Dokumente/Untersuchungsbericht.pdf. 29 Jan 2017.

Lengwiler, M. (2013). *Bestandsaufnahme der bestehenden Forschungsprojekte in Sachen Verding- und Heimkinder. Basel: Bundesamt für Justiz.* www.fuersorgerischezwangsmassnahmen.ch/pdf/Bericht_Lengwiler_de.pdf. 28 Jan 2017.

Leygraf, N., König, A., Kröber, H.L., & Pfäfflin, L. (2012). *Sexuelle Übergriffe durch Geistliche in der katholischen Kirche Deutschlands*. Eine Analyse forensischer Gutachten 2000–2010. http://www.dbk.de/fileadmin/redaktion/diverse_downloads/Dossiers_2012/2012_Sex-Uebergriffe-durch-katholische-Geistliche_Leygraf-Studie.pdf. 28 Jan 2017.

Loosli, C. A. (2006). *Anstaltsleben*. Zürich, Switzerland: Rotpunktverlag.

Lueger-Schuster, B., Butollo, A., Moy, Y., Jagsch, R., Glück, T., Kantor, V., … Weindl, D. (2015). Aspects of social support and disclosure in the context of institutional abuse – Long-term impact on mental health. *BMC Psychology*, *3*(1), 1–9. doi:10.1186/s40359-015-0077-0.

Lueger-Schuster, B., Kantor, V., Weindl, D., Knefel, M., Butollo, A., Moy, Y., … Glück, T. (2014). Institutional abuse in the Catholic Church in Austria: Types of abuse and impact on adult survivors' mental health. *Child Abuse & Neglect*, *8*(1), 52–64.

Mader, R., & Sluga, W. (1969). Persönlichkeitsänderung durch langen Heimaufenthalt. *Acta Paedopsychiatrica*, *36*, 36–45.

Mertens, P. K. (2015). Kirche und Missbrauch – ein Rückblick. *Nervenheilkunde*, *34*(7), 495–500.

Mohler-Kuo, M., Landolt, M. A., Maier, T., Meidert, U., Schönbucher, V., & Schnyder, U. (2014). Child sexual abuse revisited: A population-based cross-sectional study among Swiss adolescents. *Journal of Adolescent Health*, *54*, 304–311.

Obermeyer, B., & Stadler, R. (2011). *Bruder, was hast du getan? – Kloster Ettal. Die Täter, die Opfer, das System*. Köln, Germany: Kiepenheuer & Witsch.

Rassenhofer, M., Spröber, N., Schneider, T., & Fegert, J. M. (2013). Listening to victims: Use of a critical incident reporting system to enable adult victims of childhood sexual abuse to participate in a political reappraisal process in Germany. *Child Abuse & Neglect*, *37*(9), 653–663.

Rassenhofer, M., Zimmer, A., Spröber, N., & Fegert, J. M. (2015). Child sexual abuse in the Roman Catholic Church in Germany: Comparison of victim-impact data collected through church-sponsored and government-sponsored programs. *Child Abuse & Neglect*, *40*, 60–67.

Raue, U. (2010). *Bericht über Fälle sexuellen Missbrauchs an Schulen und anderen Einrichtungen des Jesuitenordens, Deutsche Provinz der Jesuiten*. Online: www.jesuiten.org/fileadmin/Redaktion/Downloads/Bericht_27_05_2010_aktuell.pdf. 27 Jan 2017.

Raue, U. (2011). *Bericht über Grenzverletzungen gegenüber Kindern und Jugendlichen im Jesuiten-Kolleg St. Blasien, Deutsche Provinz der Jesuiten*. Online: www.jesuiten.org/fileadmin/Redaktion/Downloads/Bericht_Raue_St._Blasien_-_15.02.11.pdf. 27 Jan 2017.

Raupp, U., & Eggers, C. (1993). Sexueller Missbrauch von Kindern: Eine regionale Studie über Prävalenz und Charakteristik. *Monatsschrift Kinderheilkunde, 141*, 316–322.

Schreiber, H. (2013). *Im Namen der Ordnung. Heimerziehung in Tirol*. Innsbruck, Austria: Studien-Verlag.

Scicluna, C. J. (2010). *Sexueller Missbrauch Vatikan: Topinterview mit Kirchenanwalt Scicluna*. Online: http://www.internetpfarre.de/blog/archives/240-SEXUELLER-MISSBRAUCH-VATIKAN-TOPINTERVIEW-MIT-KIRCHENANWALT-SCICLUNA.html

Steller, M., & Köhnken, G. (1989). Criteria-based statement analysis. In D. C. Raskin (Ed.), *Psychological methods for investigation and evidence* (pp. 217–245). New York, NY: Springer.

Tschan, W. (2015). Übergriffe in Institutionen in der Schweiz. In J. M. Fegert, & M. Wolff (Eds.), *Kompendium „Sexueller Missbrauch in Institutionen". Entstehungsbedingungen, Prävention und Intervention* (S. 707–719). Weinheim, Germany: Beltz Juventa.

Unabhängiger Beauftragter für Fragen des sexuellen Kindesmissbrauchs (UBSKM). (2013). *Bilanzbericht 2013*. Berlin. Online: https://www.fonds-missbrauch.de/fileadmin/content/UBSKM_Bilanzbericht_barrierefrei.pdf. 29 Jan 2017.

Witt, A., Rassenhofer, M., Allroggen, M., Brähler, E., Plener, P., & Fegert, J. M. (in preparation). The Prevalence of Sexual Abuse in Institutions: Results from a Representative Population-Based Sample in Germany.

Wetzels, P. (1997). *Zur Epidemiologie physischer und sexueller Gewalterfahrungen in der Kindheit: Ergebnisse einer repräsentativen retrospektiven Prävalenzstudie für die BRD*. Hannover, Germany: Kriminologisches Forschungsinstitut Niedersachsen e.V.

Zimmer, A., Lappehsen-Legner, D., Weber, M., & Götzinger, K. (2014). *Sexueller Kindesmissbrauch in kirchlichen Institutionen – Zeugnisse, Hinweise, Prävention. Ergebnisse der Auswertung der Hotline der Deutschen Bischofskonferenz für Opfer sexueller Gewalt*. Weinheim, Germany/Basel, Switzerland: Beltz Juventa Verlag.

Zinsmeister, J. (2011). *Abschlussbericht der Untersuchung schwerer Grenzverletzungen zum Nachteil von Kindern und Jugendlichen am Aloisiuskolleg Bonn – Bad Godesberg (1950–2010)*, Deutsche Provinz der Jesuiten. www.jesuiten.org/fileadmin/Redaktion/Downloads/Abschlussbericht_AKO_Zinsmeister.pdf. 27 Jan 2017.

Chapter 10
Family Environment in Institutions for Young Children in Russia: Mental Health and Development Versus Medical Care

Maria Solodunova, Oleg Palmov, and Rifkat J. Muhamedrahimov

...we become ourselves through others...

Lev Vygotsky (1966, p. 43)

1 Introduction

The history of orphanages in the Russian Federation has deep roots. According to the Tsar Peter the First Decree, foster homes were opened in all provinces at the beginning of the eighteenth century. Continuing to exist through charitable funds, during the reign of Catherine the Second (1762–1796), the foster homes were converted to governmental organizations. The high level of morbidity and mortality in foster homes led to the creation of a childcare placement system in peasant families and small shelters at almshouses. However, despite efforts toward the development of a family care and foster care system, at the beginning of twentieth century, thousands of children without parental care lived in large urban orphanages. After the 1917 revolution, large orphanages, as well as the family care system, were abolished. For orphaned young children and babies, so-called baby homes (BH) were created inside the healthcare system. In 1946, according to "the Regulations on BH", baby homes were a place for the public care of orphaned children, children of single mothers, and children who had lost touch with their parents or whose parents had been deprived of their parental rights. The number of children had to be from 30 up to 100 (Muhamedrahimov et al., 2003). The dominancy of "good health" is fixed in the system of children's distribution to institutions. All children from birth to 4 years of age, left without parental care, placed under control in the BHs, belonged to the Ministry of Health. Thus, the BHs are hospitals in fact.

M. Solodunova (✉) • O. Palmov • R.J. Muhamedrahimov
Division of Child and Parent Mental Health and Early Intervention, St. Petersburg State University, University Embankment, 7/9, 199034 St. Petersburg, RF, Russia
e-mail: m.solodunova@spbu.ru; oleg_palmov@mail.ru; rjm@list.ru

A.V. Rus et al. (eds.), *Child Maltreatment in Residential Care*,
DOI 10.1007/978-3-319-57990-0_10

The transition from a purely healthcare to medical-pedagogical childcare model is associated with the addition of assistant teachers to the staff of baby homes in 1986. In contrast to the ward nurses providing hygienic care and medical procedures, assistant teachers were responsible for child development and conducted individual and group sessions for children by age level. It should be noted that no assistant teachers were assigned to the wards for children with developmental disabilities. Medical nurses remained the only staff in these wards since it was believed that the basic needs of children with special needs were healthcare and treatment, and their future was to reside in specialized children's homes for children with disabilities from ages 4–18.

In the mid-1990s and early 2000s, the current medical-pedagogical model was supplemented by defectological and rehabilitative practices. Speech therapists, special teachers (defectologists), and instructors of therapeutic physical training were included in the staffing of baby homes. Among rehabilitation techniques, the presence of Sensory Rooms in baby homes was highly appreciated by the professional community, as well as Montessori rooms. Equipment and training of professionals demanded huge costs and efforts. However, multidisciplinary rehabilitation and adult-directed early education were not coordinated and were carried out outside the context of the social-emotional experience of the child and his/her relationships with caregivers.

For many years, the majority of institutions for orphans and children without parental care did not value the mental health of the children, despite the fact that the majority of children entering institutions had special needs and behavioral problems. Traditionally, it was thought that the main "problem" of children in the orphanage system was innate and acquired in the early postnatal period due to dysfunctional parents (drug or alcohol addiction, social risks) rather than considered as mental health problems. Therefore, the "care" of children was increasingly understood in terms of the "correction" of violations of physical health and behavior.

In 1992 the first Russian Federation early childhood intervention program was founded and implemented in St. Petersburg (Kozhevnikova, Muhamedrahimov, & Chistovich, 1995). The team members of the program were willing to address their work to the orphanages, and BH #13 has become a platform for educational activities, joint early intervention practice, and research. Thus, BH professionals started using assessments of children's development to guide educational activities and to stimulate children with severe disabilities who had previously been considered untrainable. New understanding about early interventions for institutionalized children required moving on from the idea of medical and educational treatment to the concept of child mental health and development and to interdisciplinary early intervention, aimed at the children and their social environment.

Cooperation between the BH and the early intervention team produced workshops on early social-emotional development and intervention programs, as well as studies of the characteristics of the social environment of children in the BHs (Muhamedrahimov, 1999a; Muhamedrahimov, Palmov, & Nikiforova, 1996). The study of institutional environment showed that the children's living arrangements in traditional institutions were very different from the family. First of all, the stability and responsiveness of the immediate social environment are different. For instance, children reside among 12–14 others in the same age group, with regular transfers from one group to another to a certain age. This means that if a child spends his/her early childhood in a BH, he/she changes the "family" about four times. At the same time, children from these groups, as well as caregivers, whom the child has already managed to remember and established "rules" of interaction, are not transferred together. Employees' schedules at BH are also a source of instability for the child: adults have interchangeable schedules. Some of them may have two working days and then 2 days off, while others work for 1 day with a break of 3 days (Muhamedrahimov, 1999b; The St. Petersburg-USA Orphanage Research Team, 2008). Thus, a child's caregiver will change every 2 or 3 days, also during which he will have to interact with other collaborators who have different personality characteristics, attitudes, values, and experience of working with children. In such circumstances a child finds him-/herself in a situation where the integration of experience with one primary caregiver who can provide continuous and systematic interaction is impossible. Moreover, working with a group of 12–14 children of the same age, a BH employee is unable to give personal, individual attention to each child. Studies have shown that the duration of the individual contact with each child is not more than 17 min per day (Muhamedrahimov, 1999b), which is clearly not enough to establish relations and create an attachment between child and adult. As a result, children who are brought up in BHs have early experiences that do not allow them to maintain relationships with adults and peers. This creates future obstacles to the establishment of families and educating their own children. Thus, the consequence of staying in institutions in infancy and early childhood is the development of numerous problems that accompany a person throughout later life (Nelson, Fox, & Zeanah, 2014; Rutter & Sonuga-Barke, 2010; The Leiden Conference, 2012; The St. Petersburg-USA Orphanage Research Team, 2008).

This collaboration fostered ideas for possible ways to provide a better social-emotional environment, a more family-like environment, and more consistent caregiving in the orphanages (Muhamedrahimov, 1999a; Muhamedrahimov, Palmov, & Nikiforova, 1996). More than 30 workshops and 20 conference presentations for baby homes all over the Russian Federation were conducted over 5 years after 1995 and changed the attitudes of many individual professionals. The Saint Petersburg BH #13 was characterized by its new professional attitudes and openness to collaboration in the interests of children. After 2000, due to collaboration with the joint research team from St. Petersburg State University Division of Child and Parent Mental Health and Early Intervention (RF) and University of Pittsburg Office of Child Development (USA), this institution became the T + SC (training + structural changes) intervention BH in "The Effects of Improving Caregiving on Early Mental Health" study (2000–2005)[1] (The St. Petersburg-USA Orphanage Research Team, 2008) and in the follow-up study, aimed to maintain provided social-emotional

[1] This research was funded by Grant R01 HD39017-01from the National Institute of Child Health and Human Development of the US Public Health Service (to Robert B. McCall).

intervention (2007–2012)[2] (McCall et al., 2013; McCall, Groark et al., 2016; McCall, Muhamedrahimov et al., 2016a, 2016b; Muhamedrahimov et al., 2014). Below presented the short description of these projects, the dissemination of the projects' results to BHs in different regions of RF, and the influence of results on the RF national policy for orphan children and children left without parental care.

2 "The Effects of Improving Caregiving on Early Mental Health" Project

The study "The Effects of Improving Caregiving on Early Mental Health" was aimed at demonstrating the role of early caregiver-child social-emotional interactive and relationship experiences on orphanage children's development in a more direct and comprehensive manner than before, by experimentally improving the social-emotional relationship experience of orphanage children (The St. Petersburg-USA Orphanage Research Team, 2008). It is one of the largest institutional intervention studies, involving three orphanages and a maximum of 530 caregivers and 954 children (The St. Petersburg-USA Orphanage Research Team et al., 2005).

The study represents a quasi-experimental test of the role of early social-emotional experience and adult-child relationships in the development of typically developing children and those with disabilities from birth to 4 years of age living in orphanages in St. Petersburg, Russian Federation.

The main hypothesis was an improved social-emotional early environment and the opportunity to develop caregiver-child relationships in the first year or two of the lives of institutionalized children will produce better development and more mature social-emotional behaviors that reflect more positive relationships with caregivers. Three BHs participated in the study. There were few criteria to select the BHs: willing to cooperate, high institutional standards for medical, pedagogical services, rehabilitation, nutrition and sanitation, equipment and toys. In the same time, all three baby homes had the similar characteristics as many other orphanages in the literature: deficiency in social-emotional caregiver-child interactions and lack of relationship experiences provided to children, frequently changing adults, minimum social interaction with children. In addition, children had 9–12 caregivers per week, as many as 60–100 different caregivers over the first 2 years of life, and no caregiver today was the same as yesterday or tomorrow caregivers (The St. Petersburg-USA Orphanage Research Team et al., 2005).

There are two main components of the intervention: (1) training of caregivers to promote responsive caregiving and (2) changing of orphanage structure and employment patterns with the aim to increase staff stability and consistency. The purpose of the interventions was to promote the development of warm, caring, and socially

[2] This research was funded by Grants HD 050212 and 39,017 from the National Institute of Child Health and Human Development of the US Public Health Service (to Robert B. McCall & Cristina J. Groark).

responsive interactions and attachment relationships between children and caregivers. The methodology used required that both the training and structural changes interventions be provided to one orphanage, only the training to a second, and neither to a third (Groark et al., 2005; Muhamedrahimov et al., 2004; The St. Petersburg-USA Orphanage Research Team, 2008).

The *training intervention* was conducted using "train-the-trainer" approach for the professionals and the caregivers with the aim to develop new skills of reading children's cues and emotions, child-directed play, and responsive interactions, following the child's lead. Infant mental health issues were a special part of the training program with the emphasis on caregiver-infant interaction, attachment, emotional availability of caregivers, and coping with grief and loss in young children. Also, the modules on working with children with special needs were provided. Few additional modules for the team of professional were conducted: adult learning styles, team building, and supervision. The team members (special teachers) were trained to observe and evaluate caregivers' behaviors and give a feedback supporting positive behaviors according to the topics of training modules and discussing what could be improved. The observation criteria and guidelines for feedback and discussion were developed (Groark et al., 2005; Muhamedrahimov et al., 2004; The St. Petersburg-USA Orphanage Research Team, 2008).

A set of *structural changes* was aimed at improving the stability and consistency of caregivers and providing a family environment for each child that would support relationship building. This set of structural changes consisted of the following: (a) the group was decreased from 12 or 13 to 6 or 7, (b) two primary and four secondary caregivers assigned to each subgroup in which one of the primary caregivers was present for most of the children's waking hours 7 days a week, (c) a reduction from approximately nine to six caregivers assigned to a ward but minimum change in total caregiver hours, (d) integrating the children by age and disability status within a group, (e) periodic graduations of children to new wards were stopped, (f) the regular assignment of specific caregivers to be substitutes for a particular ward when needed, (g) the creation of an in-house monitoring and supervisory system, and (h) family hour in both the morning and afternoon in which visitors to the wards were not allowed and children were to be with their caregivers (Muhamdrahimov et al., 2004; The St. Petersburg-USA Orphanage Research Team, 2008). The caregivers in one BH received training + structural changes (T + SC). A second BH received training only (TO), and a third BH conducted business as usual and had no intervention (NoI).

Four categories of assessments and measures on the caregivers and children were included in to this study: those that assess (1) the implementation of the interventions, (2) outcomes in the caregivers, (3) outcomes in the children, and (4) outcomes of caregiver-child interactions (The St. Petersburg-USA Orphanage Research Team, 2008). In this chapter we will focus on characteristics of caregiver interactions with children in the natural environment of their ward and children's general behavioral development.

To measure caregiver social interaction with children, the HOME Inventory (24-mo. version; Caldwell & Bradley, 1984; see Bradley & Caldwell, 1995) was administered by independent observers at the baseline before any intervention, after implementation was complete, and annually thereafter for all primary (assistant teachers) and most secondary (medical nurses) caregivers. The results show that a combination of two interventions, training and structural changes (T + SC), produced a significant and sustained increase in HOME total and subscale scores. This increase was greater for training + structural changes than for training only, which showed some but smaller and less consistently significant increases (The St. Petersburg-USA Orphanage Research Team, 2008). During the first year after the T + SC intervention was completely implemented, improvements in total score and subscales occurred to nearly their maximum extent. Few improvements were found in TO. Achieving a high level within the first year, the score for T + SC group remained high over all post-intervention time points, even nearly 4 years after T + SC had been completely implemented.

General behavioral development was assessed with the Battelle Developmental Inventory (LINC, 1988), which produces a total score and the six subscales of personal-social, fine motor, gross motor, adaptive, communication, and cognition. Children were classified as typically developing or with disabilities, and within these groups there was a cross-sectional and a longitudinal sample.

The results for typically developing children had shown that the double intervention (T + SC) produced increases in developmental scores compared to both the training only (TO) and the no intervention (NoI) control groups for Battelle total score and the six subscales and were consistent for cross-sectional and longitudinal samples. For T + SC the intervention effects were more significant after 9+ months than after only 4–9 months of exposure for total score and most subscales especially in terms of effect size. This dose-response effect suggests that the T + SC intervention provided continuing and developmentally appropriate support to children as they increased in age and skills.

Children with disabilities showed improvements as a function of the interventions similar to those of typically developing children. For longitudinal children with disabilities, T + SC increased from an average of 23 to 41 or an average increase of 18 DQ points vs. −5 for NoI (The St. Petersburg-USA Orphanage Research Team, 2008).

The results show that the double intervention (T + SC) produced substantially more developmental improvement in children in essentially every domain than the single intervention (TO). Thus, the training of the new caregiving skills in social-emotional relationships within the context of structural changes led to children's developmental advancements in all major domains.

3 Maintaining a Social-Emotional Intervention in Baby Homes and Follow-Up of Children Transitioned to St. Petersburg (RF) Families

Once the intervention project ended, all additional financial support stopped, and the interventions had to be maintained on the BHs' government-provided budget. There were several components to promote maintenance in the original intervention.

After funds terminated, the number of caregivers and caregiver hours available in the T + SC BH did not change much. A train-the-trainer strategy was adopted. A brief training course was given during and after the intervention period by those specialists originally trained as "trainers". So, the staff training course was continually available to prepare new caregivers. An in-house monitoring and supervision system was established in which specialists (e.g., staff professionals in children with disabilities, early education) were responsible for monitoring the caregivers and encouraging them to implement the training on the wards on a continuing basis. Additional coaching and technical assistance were provided by outside professionals to both T + SC and TO, which consisted of weekly or bimonthly visitations, supervision, and assistance in periodic refresher training (McCall et al., 2013).

In the TO institution, separate funds were obtained after the intervention period to assist this BH to implement structural changes, especially reduced group size. This was only partly successful, because not all groups were reduced in size; integration by age and disability status was only partly accomplished, and family hour was not implemented. However, the in-house monitoring and supervisory system encouraging appropriate caregiver-child interactions that had been implemented in the T + SC were not fully created in TO.

It was hypothesized that these maintenance activities would preserve the intervention in two ways, first by maintaining the improved caregiver behavior and BH environment as reflected on the HOME Inventory and, second, as a result, maintaining the benefits to children's behavioral development as measured by the Battelle Developmental Inventory (McCall et al., 2013).

Up to approximately 50 caregivers in in each BH were individually assessed periodically with the HOME Inventory (24-month group version; Caldwell & Bradley, 1984; see Bradley & Caldwell, 1995). The results demonstrated increase in scores in T + SC, but not TO and NoI, after intervention compared to pre-intervention levels to approximately the last 1–2 years of the intervention project. The differences between three intervention conditions (BHs) remained significant across four assessments during 8 years and did not interact with time.

The Battelle Developmental Inventory's personal-social and communication subscales demonstrated similar trend as in HOME scores. Specifically, the multivariate differences in children's behavioral development scores produced by intervention conditions were maintained during the last years of the intervention project and for 6 years thereafter with no multivariate interaction with time. The results showed the increase of Battelle scores over post-intervention time period for TO and NoI but not for T + SC, and during the follow-up period TO's scores approached or exceeded those of T + SC after intervention project (McCall et al., 2013).

The maintenance of intervention effects on caregivers, the environment, and children's development might be connected with following factors: (a) intervention involved all baby home caregivers and professionals and designed to develop and support child-directed, responsive, and sensitive behaviors of the caregivers, who may use new skills and adjust to individual child within stable "family-like" environment of the ward; (b) the train-the-trainer strategy allows to keep educational activities for new caregivers and repeat training modules and develop new ones; (c) commitment and motivation of the director; and (d) certain activities during the follow-up period, for example, the monitoring and supervision system that was established in T + SC as part of the intervention and continued thereafter was designed to continuously encourage caregivers to implement on the wards the training they had received (McCall et al., 2013).

The core question of the follow-up project was to understand how staying during infancy and early childhood in the institution with a family-like socio-emotional environment affects the child's development after departing from the institution to a family (to adoptive, foster, and biological families and kin in the St. Petersburg region) (McCall et al., 2013; McCall, Groark et al., 2016; McCall, Muhamedrahimov et al., 2016a, 2016b; Muhamedrahimov et al., 2014). A literature review showed that there was quite a lot of research that follows up on children in foster care after living in institutions (Chisholm, 1998; Marcovitch et al., 1997; Nelson et al., 2007; O'Connor et al., 2003; Rutter et al., 2007; van IJzendoorn & Juffer, 2006). Many studies have shown that the lack of sensitive and responsive relationship between the child and adults in typical orphanage led to the development of chronic stress, which is subsequently followed by developmental delays and behavior disorders (Gunnar, 2001; Johnson & Gunnar, 2011; McCall, 2011, 2013). In contrast, high-quality interaction and relationship between the child and adult can smooth such adverse outcomes (e.g., Gunnar & Quevedo, 2007, 2008). However, in the literature there were no works (1) where the previously institutionalized children were observed after the placement to the families within the same country; (2) where the implementations had been made within the orphanage, and children were observed after staying in that institution and while living in different types of families; and (3) where the impact of staff training only and staff training plus structural changes intervention program consequences on the development and behavior of children were separately studied. The follow-up study intended to find out whether the children, brought up in institutions with warm emotional relationships between children and adults, were more successful after being placed into families in their country of birth and whether their parents described those children as developing better and having less problems in behavior than children from traditional institutions.

Participants in the current study were all children in the intervention study and during follow-up study who entered the three BHs (T + SC, TO, and NoI) – and remained in residence for at least 3 months before having their departure assessment and transitioning to domestic adoptive, biological (or kin), and foster families – and family-reared children who had never been placed to a BH (McCall, Groark et al., 2016; Muhamedrahimov et al., 2014). The parents rated their children's development on the set of forms after they had lived with them for an average of 33.5 months and were between 1.5 and 10.8 years of age (McCall, Groark et al., 2016).

The comparison between previously institutionalized (PI) and never institutionalized (NI) children showed that PI children were rated similarly to NI children on most behavioral measures, consistent with substantial catch-up growth typically displayed by children after transitioning to families. However, PI children were rated more poorly than NI children on certain competencies in early childhood and some attentional skills. In particular, children aged 18–59 months were rated as less competent on the Infant-Toddler Social and Emotional Assessment (ITSEA, Carter, Briggs-Gowan, Jones, & Little, 2003), especially in prosocial peer relationships, imitation and play, and attention. Given the relative lack of social and emotional interactions between caregiver and child in an institution, especially in the NoI BH, it is not surprising that PI children will have significantly reduced early social and emotional competencies (McCall, Muhamedrahimov et al., 2016b).

It was found that children in the combined sample of the three institutions were relatedly poorer on some indicators, if they had been transferred to the family at older ages. Those results suggested that children, transferred to the family at younger ages, adjusted well to the family, but improved conditions of social and emotional environment within the institution may lead to positive consequences in years after the transition to the family (McCall, Muhamedrahimov et al., 2016b).

The results showed that despite very substantial differences in the level of children's developmental level at the departure from three BHs, the significant differences between children from three BHs in the family placement were fewer than expected. Nevertheless, consistent with expectations, parents reported T + SC children displayed less indiscriminate friendliness than NoI children (McCall, Muhamedrahimov et al., 2016a).

Contrary to the expectations, T + SC children were more impulsive on the Child Behavior Questionnaire (CBQ/30–72, CBQ; Rothbart, Ahadi, Hersey, & Fisher, 2001) than NoI children. Note that T + SC children were more proactive, were involved in more different activities, and were more independent and creative. Perhaps this is why parents rated them as "impulsive," compared to the NoI children, in whose previous experience such behavior had been not supported. T + SC children showed lower scores in aggressive/defiant behavior and less externalizing behaviors assessed by the Child Behavior Checklist (CBCL/6–18; Achenbach & Rescorla, 2001) than NoI children the longer they were in the BH. It may connect with the longer period of time in improved conditions that gave more opportunities to learn appropriate behaviors with peers and adults at somewhat older ages (McCall, Muhamedrahimov et al., 2016a; Muhamedrahimov et al., 2014).

These results indicate that the improvement of the social and emotional experience of the child in an institution leads to the obvious positive effects over the years. The fact that produced differences between children are not so great does not mean that institutionalization is relatively harmless to the child and its effects can be decreased by the transition to the family. Furthermore, some authors (e.g., Fraley, Roisman, & Haltigan, 2013) suggest that small differences do not indicate that the intervention was useless; it may mean that the most noticeable effect of the intervention will come in a longer period of time and at older ages (McCall, Muhamedrahimov et al., 2016a).

4 Dissemination of the St. Petersburg Baby Home Social-Emotional Intervention Project to Other Baby Homes of Russian Federation

The results of the St. Petersburg Baby Home project were widely disseminated at specialized conferences in Russia, resulting in the formation of the professional community and NGOs' new effective approaches of helping institutionalized children.

In 2007 the National Foundation for the Prevention of Cruelty to Children (NFPCC), Russian nonprofit organization, invited the Saint Petersburg research group to implement training + structural changes (T + SC) model at the Krasnoyarsk Territory specialized orphanages #3 (Krasnoyarsk) and #5 (Sosnovoborsk) as part of the early intervention project "Reducing the level of abandonment and disability of children in BHs" (Muhamedrahimov et al., 2009). The project was a component of a program to improve health and enhance the quality of social and health services within the framework of the partnership program of the Krasnoyarsk Territory and the US Agency for International Development, "Promoting an integrated socioeconomic development of the region."

The project in Krasnoyarsk baby home #3 contained research-based intervention components developed in St. Petersburg Baby Home project: staff training and structural changes (The St. Petersburg-USA Orphanage Research Team, 2008). The *training* program was close to the program developed in St. Petersburg project and was aimed to increase baby home staff caregiving sensitivity and responsiveness as well as to develop a professional technology in work with young children, including children with special needs. The trainers from St. Petersburg conducted seminars, trainings, work on creation of the BH's new policies, training modules, etc. In addition to the baby home training program, two baby home groups (12–13 children in each) participated in the *structural changes* intervention. Each group was divided into two groups (of six and seven children) with allocation of separate facilities for each of the groups. The staff schedule was changed: assistant teachers who became potential primary caregivers for children had a schedule of five consistent working days and 2 day offs (before that they had had the changeable schedule with two working days and 2 day offs). Children were integrated by age and disability status. The "family hour" was implemented to work of each group to reduce the number of adults attending children. The "family hour" is one-hour time twice a day when nobody, except the group staff, can move into the group and take the children out; this is a time for "inter-family" plans, activities, recreation, and joy between "professional mothers" (the group's assistant teacher and medical nurse) and the children. In addition, a new rule according to which children were staying in the same group from the beginning until the departure from BH was introduced. All these changes were aimed at improving the stability and consistency of the social environment of children (Groark et al., 2005; Muhamedrahimov et al., 2003; The St. Petersburg-USA Orphanage Research Team, 2008).

Twenty-four children 4–48 months of age from two integrated by age and disability intervention groups were assessed at three points: at baseline (BL) before any intervention, 2.5 and 8 months after staff training, and structural changes. "The list of changes in children's behavior" (Muhamedrahimov & Shevchuk, 2009) was developed and used to assess the manifestation of disruptive behaviors, as well as indiscriminate friendliness in children. The expert records for 3 morning hours (from 9.00 to 12.00 am) included the number of manifestations of self-stimulation, body rocking, autoaggression (head banging, hitting him-/herself, etc.), unusual postures, aggression toward objects, aggression toward children, and gnawing items. In addition, the number of children displaying the indiscriminate friendliness

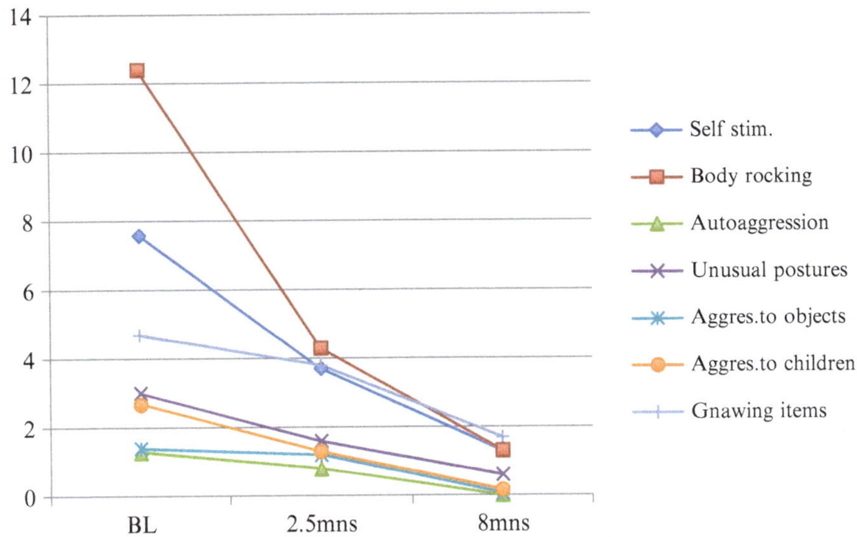

Fig. 10.1 The dynamics of disruptive behaviors manifestations in children (baseline to 2.5–8 months of the intervention project)

toward the stranger woman entering the ward was registered, and the BH doctor's regular records on the children's physical health were checked (Muhamedrahimov et al., 2009).

The results revealed a decrease for each type of the selected behavior manifestations from the baseline (before changes) to 2.5 and 8 months after the intervention program (see Fig. 10.1).

The results showed that a few months after implementation of the intervention program, children expressed less manifestation of indiscriminate friendliness (89% of observed children at BL vs. 33–50% of children at 2.5 and 8 months after intervention). In addition, the BH doctor's regular records on the children's physical health demonstrated a reduction in morbidity (respiratory catarrh, bronchitis, conjunctivitis, dermatitis) – 110 cases before vs. 57 cases after the project. According to informal group staff observations, children showed more manifestation of anxiety when meeting a stranger and less manifestation of the desire to rush outside the ward, returned to the primary caregiver after contact with stranger, and demonstrated the desire to be closer to the primary caregiver during walks outside. It was also observed that children demonstrated the preference of interaction with primary caregiver and lack of independent research activity in the early stages after the T + SC program implementation. Children with special needs, staying in a permanent environment and communicating with children of all ages and developmental levels, demonstrated their ability to imitate and initiate social interaction. The older children became more initiative in games; they developed imagination and played games that reflected the life of a family. For example, they asked to cover the slide with a blanket and made a "house" in which they "live." The relationships between children improved: they tended to agree with each other, shared toys, and organized cooperative games themselves. The children created dialogs with other children and caregivers, expressed their desires, and shared experiences and feelings with each other. When dressing, the children themselves chose the clothes they wore, and the girls decided which bow to tie. After dressing, the kids loved to look at themselves in the mirror. Children began to pay attention not only to how they looked themselves but also to how the caregivers looked: they noticed the changes and gave their opinion (Muhamedrahimov et al., 2009).

The Krasnoyarsk project results led us to the general conclusion that the attempt to implement the T + SC program to another BH after its approval in the BH #13 in St. Petersburg was successful, that the spread was effective, and that those experiences can be shared. To increase the conversion efficiency and further improve the development and behavior of children require a combination of increasing the stability and consistency of the social environment (through structural changes) with the strengthening of staff sensitivity and responsiveness (through training and supervision).

After 2009–2010 several nongovernmental child charity funds shifted from the purchase of equipment, toys, and providing leisure activities for the children in baby homes to "clever charity," organizing training and supporting structural changes in the baby homes. Thus, Children Charity Foundation "The Sun City" (Novosibirsk) initiated a collaboration with Division of Child and Parent Mental Health and Early Intervention at Department of Psychology, St. Petersburg State University, and has organized seminars, trainings, and conferences spreading the model of reforming the orphanages in Siberian region, and supported "T + SC" implementation in more than five baby homes.

In the baby home #2 in Novosibirsk the structural changes started in one pilot group and then were gradually implemented in all the wards during 2011–2012. The "Train the Trainers" model was used to educate professionals and caregivers (The St. Petersburg-USA Orphanage Research Team, 2008). Training modules included an initial set of topics developed for the main project (The St. Petersburg-USA Orphanage Research Team, 2008) and three additional modules: "care with respect" which focused on predictability of all events and adult behavior, value of child's independent play and physical activity, and cooperation with children in all aspects of daily care procedures (Pikler, 2007; Tardosh, 2007a, 2007b). Staff supervision after training and orientation training for newly hired caregivers have become the daily work of the senior assistant teacher, special teachers, and pediatricians. The interdisciplinary team has developed and implemented a number of new policies for caregivers and specialists. A comfortable home environment has been created in the wards; the playpens were taken out. The caregivers eventually learned to divide the ward space into areas according to the interests and needs of children of different ages and levels of development. Observations of the children and caregivers have demonstrated improvements in the quality of social interaction in dyads and a significant improvement in the development of children. It is important to note that all children with special needs from the pilot group were adopted or retuned to biological families.

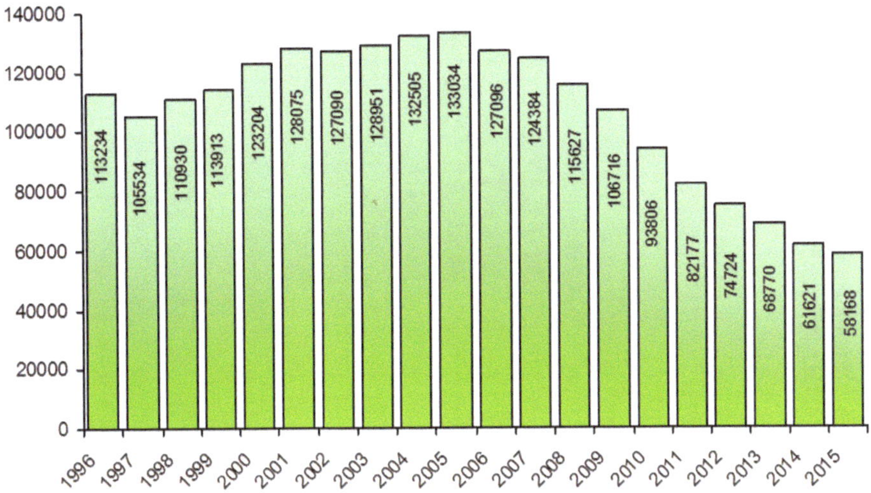

Fig. 10.2 The number of children left without parental care in 1996–2015 (Retrieved from http://www.usynovite.ru)

5 Russian Federation State Policies and University-Community Collaboration on Improvements of Caregiving Environment for Young Children Left Without Parental Care

Until 2006, the number of children in institutions remained consistently high. For example, in 2005 a record number of 133,034 children left without parental were reported (see Fig. 10.2). In recent years, however, the number of children left without parental care and brought up in institutions has been markedly reduced. According to the Ministry of Education and Science of the Russian Federation data, the number of children left without parental care in 2014 was 61,621, and at the end of 2015 it was 58,168 (see http://www.usynovite.ru).

With regard to children from birth to 4 years of age who are brought up in BHs, according to the Federal State Statistic Service of the Russian Federation, on January 1, 2014, the Russian Federation operated 194 BHs including 18,427 beds, with 13,977 children, including 9333 orphans and children left without parental care (on January 1, 2013, they operated 207 BHs including 19,819 beds with 15,993 children, including 11,145 orphans and children left without parental care) (see Fig. 10.3, see http://www.gks.ru).

The decreasing number of orphaned children is connected with the state policy of the RF, which is determined by the president and the government, and aimed at reducing social orphanhood. First of all, these solutions involve work with the biological families and support the development of the institute of foster families.

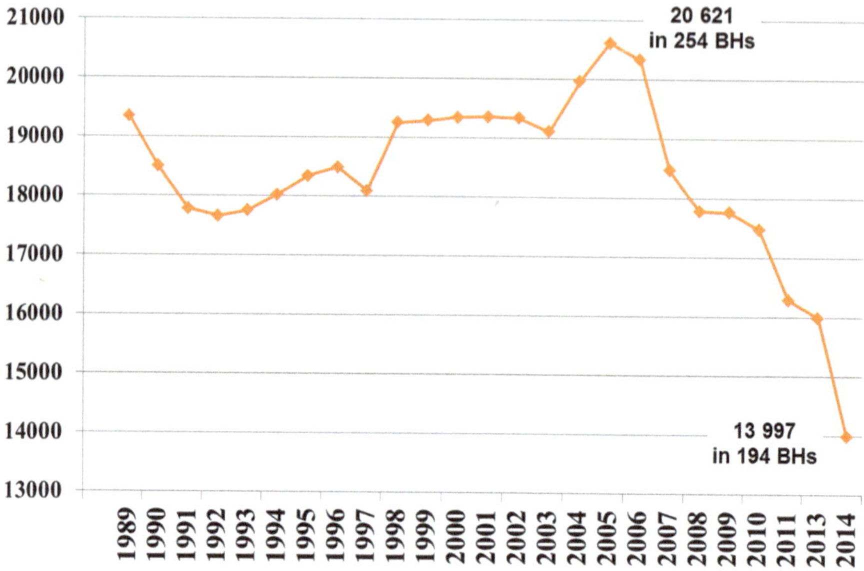

Fig. 10.3 Number of BH in the Russian Federation in 1989–2014 (Retrieved from http://www.gks.ru)

Among the regulations that contribute to this goal is the Presidential Decree of June 1, 2012, No761 (The Presidential Decree of June 1, 2012 No761 "On the National Strategy of Actions for Children" for 2012–2017, 2012). According to this document, the key principle is the fundamental right of every child to live and grow up in a family.

The care system for children left without parental care in the RF has always put as a priority to seek opportunities to return the child to the biological family or place him/her in substitute care of different types – adoption, foster, or relative/nonrelative kinship. However, for many years it was obvious that it takes a long time and considerable effort to develop the institute of foster families, as well as to establish a professional support system for foster families. In particular, regarding foster families, it was clear that Russian citizens were not ready to accept children with special needs, focusing only on healthy children. Also, the level of understanding for rearing nonbiological children remained quite low in the foster families. The situation was also aggravated by the "secret of adoption" in the legislation, whereby adoptive parents had the right to decide whether to report a child's true story to him/her or bring him/her up as a biological child. In addition, the system of professional support for foster families was also nonexistent; all the work in this direction was carried out only by nongovernmental organizations which were often a community of adoptive parents, who themselves had faced difficulties raising up children from institutions.

According to the reasons listed, for a long time orphans and children left without parental care were transferred for adoption to the United States and Western

Table 10.1 The number of orphaned children transferred to domestic and international families (2011–2015)

	2011		2012		2013		2014		2015	
Departure destinations	Under 1 year	1–3 years	Under 1 year	1–3 years	Under 1 year	1–3 years	Under 1 year	1–3 years	Under 1 year	1–3 years
Russia	7427	9476	6787	8358	7051	9050	6930	8910	5832	8023
Abroad	175	1931	112	1356	23	719	0	456	0	271

European countries. The situation changed dramatically in 2013 with the adoption of the so-called The Law of Dima Yakovlev (named after a Russian child who died while in the care of a US adoptive family). According to Article 4 of this Law, it is prohibited to transfer children of Russian citizenship to US adoptive families (The Federal Law No272, 2012). Later, a number of laws were adopted, involving a ban on the adoption of Russian children. For example, in 2014 the moratorium touched the citizens of countries where same-sex marriages were legalized (The Resolution No93, 2014).

The introduction of these laws had an effect in the form of decreasing the number of children transferred abroad to international families (see Table 10.1 and http://www.usynovite.ru), as well as an unwanted effect such as an increase in the number of siblings and children with disabilities in institutions and increase the number of secondary returns of children from substitute families to institutions from 176 in 2013 to 270 in 2015 (see Annual Report of the Ombudsman for Children's Rights in St. Petersburg, 2015).

In recent years, the state policy of the RF on caring for children without parental care has been largely directed at keeping children in birth families, placing children in different types of substitute families, and improving the quality of care in institutions for children who reside there. "The reform of institutions for orphans and children left without parental care, by downsizing, creating in these institutions conditions, close to family; creating new, modern apartment type children's homes and the formation of a children's village in accordance with international standards; and using modern methods of child development, education, and rehabilitation, with the active participation of volunteers and non-governmental organizations"; these are statements from the Presidential Decree of June 1, 2012 No761 "On the National Strategy of Actions for Children for 2012–2017" (The Presidential Decree No761, 2012). Difficulties in implementing the National Strategy in the closed, rigid institutional care system led to a broad discussion of the further steps of its reforming at the level of professional, nongovernmental, and government agencies. New regulations on improving institutions (The Resolution of the Government of the RF No481, 2014) signed in May 24, 2014, have been influenced by results of the intervention project in St. Petersburg BHs. Ultimately, the new policies require that living conditions in institutions should be similar to several aspects of the family environment, as implemented in the intervention. Specifically, group size should not exceed to six for children up to 4 years and eight for children over 4 years, groups should consist of children of different ages and disability status, the number of caregivers per group should be limited, and children should not be routinely transferred to new groups.

Professional observations and public control over the implementation of the Resolution No481 in BHs have found a lack of understanding the value of early social-emotional experience and child mental health concept as a basis of modernization. In 2015, new educational programs for graduates were established by Russian members of St. Petersburg-USA Orphanage Research Team at the Faculty of Psychology, St. Petersburg State University: "Child mental health and development. Creating family environment for children in of orphanages" and "Improving the quality of the social environment of children in baby homes: staff training." These two training courses provide the professionals from baby homes with basic knowledge needed to implement the Resolution of the Government of the RF No. 481 and give practical trainer skills to conduct five staff training modules at their work places. With financial support from the funds and NGOs, more than 300 professionals representing approximately 90 institutions all over the Russian Federation were trained, and in 25 of them the training and structural changes intervention model with the expert supervision was subsequently implemented.

In August 2016, the "Concept of Early Intervention Development in the Russian Federation for the period till 2020" was approved (The Resolution of the Government of the RF No1839-r, 2016). This resolution became a significant event for more than 20 years history of the development of services for vulnerable children and their parents in RF. The concept is based on the principles adopted in international early intervention practice and suggests to develop in the organizations of public health, education, and social protection of various kinds of services for families and their children at risk with age 0–3 and children with disabilities with the possibility to extend the service to 7–8 years of child's age. For the BHs, recent legislative initiatives of the government have provided the conditions for evolutionary changes. Thus, due to the introduction of the "National Strategy of Actions for Children for 2012–2017" and "The Law of Dima Yakovlev," the number of children in BH has decreased significantly; creating family-type social environment for 6 rather than 12 children in the group (The Resolution No481, 2014) became a possible task for the majority of BHs. Development of the early intervention system in RF brings opportunities to establish new family-centered services in baby homes: rehabilitation facility, unoccupied room, and available professional resources of BH could be used as interdisciplinary services for the children at risk and with disabilities growing up in biological or foster families. Elements of the social-pedagogical early intervention programs could be used by interdisciplinary BH teams without additional training. But, since the fields of physical and occupational therapy, behavioral approach, and augmentative and alternative communication were not included in to the traditional education of the majority of BH specialists, development and conducting of new training programs are one of the nearest perspectives of educational support of the baby homes. At the same time St. Petersburg BH #13 and other institutions – the pioneers of advanced experiences – are ready to deliver the following services for children being raised in families and their parents: interdisciplinary assessment and counseling, individual or group play and educational sessions for young children integrated by age and developmental level and their mothers, day care group for children with disabilities, respite care, department for the prevention of social orphanhood for daily, day and night, and 5-day stay of the mothers and their children including children with disabilities.

6 Summary

We believe that all children should live in families. Although the number of institutions in the Russian Federation decreased during last several years, and the foster care system is developing intensively, institutionalization of children left without parental care is still common, especially for those with special needs, those who have siblings, or for children at older ages. While institutionalization does exist, the social-emotional environment for children in institutions should be improved to meet their needs to grow and develop in close relationships with emotionally available sensitive and responsive primary caregiver. The St. Petersburg Baby Home intervention project aimed at providing the close to family caregiving environment for young orphan children demonstrated the effective influence of the staff training and structural changes on children's development and mental health. This research-based model of reorganization of caregiving environment for institutionalized children might be effectively used in order to change the life and early experience of orphan children and children left without parental care, including those with special needs. Development of childcare system in the Russian Federation could lead to reorganization of baby homes, and they might be developed to Centers for Children and Families aimed to provide interdisciplinary family-centered early intervention services both for children left without parental care and for family-reared children, including those with developmental disabilities and who experienced early deprivation and adversity.

Questions for Discussion

1. Identify the main components of the intervention program in the St. Petersburg Baby Home project. Compare and contrast this program a program used in your own country.
2. How did the intervention program influence the baby home social-emotional environment and children's development?
3. Describe the dissemination of the St. Petersburg Baby Home intervention program in other institutions of the Russian Federation. How did the project results influence the legislation of the Russian Federation concerning the life of orphan children and children left without parental care?

References

Achenbach, T. M., & Rescorla, L. A. (2001). *Manual for the ASEBA school-age forms & profiles*. Burlington, Canada: University of Vermont, Re- search Center for Children, Youth, and Families.

Annual Report of the Ombudsman for Children's Rights in St. Petersburg. (2015). (Ежегодный доклад за 2015 год Уполномоченного по правам ребенка в Санкт-Петербурге.) Retrieved from http://spbdeti.org

Bradley, R. H., & Caldwell, B. M. (1995). Caregiving and the regulation of child growth and development: Describing proximal aspects of caregiving systems. *Developmental Review, 15*, 38–85.

Carter, A. S., Briggs-Gowan, M. J., Jones, S. M., & Little, T. D. (2003). The infant-toddler social and emotional assessment (ITSEA): Factor structure, reliability, and validity. *Journal of Abnormal Child Psychology*, *31*, 495–514.

Chisholm, K. (1998). A three-year follow-up of attachment and indiscriminate friendliness in children adopted from Romanian orphanages. *Child Development, 69*, 1092–1106. http://www.jstor.org/stable/1132364

Fraley, R. C., Roisman, G. I., & Haltigan, J. D. (2013). The legacy of early experiences in development: Formalizing alternative models of how early experiences are carried forward over time. *Developmental Psychology*, *49*, 109–126. doi:10.1037/a0027852.

Groark, C. J., Muhamedrahimov, R. J., Palmov, O. I., Nikiforova, N. V., & McCall, R. B. (2005). Improvements in early care in Russian orphanages and their relationship to observed behaviors. *Infant Mental Health Journal*, *26*(2), 96–109.

Gunnar, M. (2001). Effects of early deprivation: Findings from orphanage-reared infants and children. In C. A. Nelson & M. Luciana (Eds.), *Handbook of developmental cognitive neuroscience* (pp. 617–629). Cambridge, MA: MIT Press.

Gunnar, M. R., & Quevedo, K. (2007). The neurobiology of stress and development. *Annual Review of Psychology*, *58*, 145–173.

Gunnar, M. R., & Quevedo, K. (2008). Early care experiences and HPA axis regulation in children: A mechanism for later vulnerability. *Progress in Brain Research*, *167*, 137–149.

Johnson, D. E., & Gunnar, M. R. (2011). Growth failure in institutionalized children. In M. C. RB, M. H. van IJzendoorn, F. Juffer, C. J. Groark, & V. K. Groza (Eds.), *Children without permanent parents: Research, practice, and policy. 4, Monographs of the society for research in child development. Serial no. 301* (vol. 76, pp. 92–126).

Kozhevnikova, E. V., Muhamedrahimov, R. J., Chistovich, L. A. (1995). (Кожевникова Е.В., Мухамедрахимов Р. Ж., Чистович Л.А. Санкт-Петербургская программа "Абилитация младенцев" – первая в России программа раннего вмешательства Педиатрия. 1995. №4. С. 112–113.)

LINC Associates. (1988). *The Battelle Developmental Inventory scoring booklet*. Itasca, IL: Riverside.

Marcovitch, S., Goldberg, S., Gold, A., Washington, J., Wasson, C., Krekewich, K., et al. (1997). Determinants of behavioural problems in Romanian children adopted in Ontario. *International Journal of Behavioral Development*, *20*, 17–31. doi:10.1080/016502597385414.

McCall, R. B. (2011). Research, practice, and policy perspectives on issues of children without permanent parental care. *Monographs of the Society for Research in Child Development*, *76*(4, Serial no. 301), 223–272. doi:10.1111/j.1540-5834.2011.00634.x

McCall, R. B. (2013). The consequences of early institutionalization: Can institutions be improved? Should they? *Child and Adolescent Mental Health*, *18*, 193–201. doi:10.1111/camh.12025.

McCall, R. B., Groark, C. J., Fish, L., Muhamedrahimov, R. J., Palmov, O. I., & Nikiforova, N. V. (2013). Maintaining a social-emotional intervention and its benefits for institutionalized children. *Child Development*, *84*(5), 1734–1749. doi:10.1111/cdev.12098.

McCall, R. B., Groark, C. J., Fish, L., Muhamedrahimov, R. J., Palmov, O. I., & Nikiforova, N. V. (2016). Characteristics of children transitioned to intercountry adoption, domestic adoption, foster care, and biological families from institutions in St. Petersburg, Russian Federation. *International Social Work*, *59*(6), 778–790.

McCall, R. B., Muhamedrahimov, R. J., Groark, C. J., Palmov, O. I., Nikiforova, N. V., Salaway, J. L., & Julian, M. M. (2016a). The development of children placed into different types of Russian families following an institutional intervention. *International Perspectives in Psychology: Research, Practice, Consultation*, *5*(4), 255–270. doi:10.1037/ipp0000060.

McCall, R. B., Muhamedrahimov, R. J., Groark, C. J., Palmov, O. I., Nikiforova, N. V., Salaway, J. L., & Julian, M. M. (2016b). The development of post-institutionalized vs. parent-reared Russian children as a function of age at placement and family type. *Development and Psychopathology*, *28*(1), 251–264.

Muhamedrahimov, R. J. (1999a). New attitude: Infant care facilities in Saint-Petersburg (Russia). In J. D. Osofsky & H. E. Fitzgerald (Eds.), *WAIMH Handbook of infant mental health. Vol. One: Perspectives on infant mental health* (pp. 245–294). New York, NY: Wiley.

Muhamedrahimov, R. J. (1999b). (Мухамедрахимов Р. Ж. Мать и младенец: психологическое взаимодействие. СПб.: Изд-во Санкт-Петерб. ун-та. 287с.)

Muhamedrahimov, R. J., Agarkova, V. V., Vershinia, E. A., Palmov, O. I., Nikiforova, N. V., & McCall, R. B. (2014). Behavior problems in children transferred from a social–emotionally depriving institution to families in St. Petersburg, Russian Federation. *Infant Mental Health Journal*, *35*, 87–93. doi:10.1002/imhj.21435.

Muhamedrahimov, R. J., Palmov, O. I., Konkova (Solodunova), M. Y., Yarusova, O. A., Kudina, O. E., Tutynina, L. V., … & Istomina, L. A. (2009). (Мухамедрахимов Р. Ж., Пальмов О. И., Конькова (Солодунова) М. Ю., Ярусова О. А., Кудина О. Е., Тутынина Л. В., …, Истомина Л. А. Опыт изменения социального окружения детей в домах ребенка. Внедрение технологии раннего вмешательства в домах ребенка Красноярского края. Красноярск: Национальный фонд защиты детей от жестокого обращения, издательство «Полис», 64с.)

Muhamedrahimov, R. J., Palmov, O. I., & Nikiforova, N. V. (1996). Infant-infant interaction in the orphanage. In A. Guedeney et al. (Eds.), *World Association for infant mental health conference abstracts*., 25–28 Jul 1996 (p. 152). Tampere, Finland: Vammalan Kirjapaino Oy.

Muhamedrahimov, R. J., Palmov, O. I., Nikforova, N. V., Groark, C. J., & McCall, R. B. (2004). Institution-based early intervention program. *The Infant Mental Health Journal*, *25*(N5), 488–501.

Muhamedrahimov, R. J., Palmov, O. I., Nikiforofa, N. V., Groark, C. J., & McCall, R. B. (2003). (Мухамедрахимов Р. Ж., Пальмов О. И., Никифорова Н. В., Гроарк К. Я., МакКолл Р. Б. Изменение социального окружения в домах ребенка: программа раннего вмешательства. Дефектология. № 4. С. 44–53.)

Muhamedrahimov, R. J., & Shevchuk, E. A. (2009). (Мухамедрахимов Р.Ж., Шевчук, Е.А. "Лист регистрации поведения".) Unpublished manuscript.

Nelson, C. A., Fox, N. A., & Zeanah, C. H. (2014). *Romania's abandoned children*. Cambridge, MA: Garvard University Press.

Nelson, C. A., Zeanah, C. H., Fox, N. A., Marshall, P. J., Smyke, A. T., & Guthrie, D. (2007). Cognitive recovery in socially deprived young children: The Bucharest Early Intervention Project. *Science*, *318*, 1937–1940. doi:10.1126/science.1143921.

O'Connor, T. G., Marvin, R. S., Rutter, M., Olrick, J. J., Britner, P. A., & The English and Romania Adoptees Study Team. (2003). Child–parent attachment following early institutional deprivation. *Development and Psychopathology*, *15*, 19–38. doi:10.1017/S0954579403000026.

Pikler, E. (2007). Give me time: Gross motor development under the conditions at Loczy. In A. Tardos (Ed.), *Bringing up and providing care for infants and toddlers in an institution* (pp. 127–135). Budapest, Hungary: Association Pikler – Loczy, Paros Print Bt.

Rothbart, M. K., Ahadi, S. A., Hershey, K. L., & Fisher, P. (2001). Investigations of temperament at three to seven years: The Children's Behavior Questionnaire. *Child Development*, *72*, 1394–1408. doi:10.1111/1467-8624.00355.

Rutter, M., Beckett, C., Castle, J., Colvert, E., Kreppner, J., Mehta, M., et al. (2007). Effects of profound early institutional deprivation: An overview of findings from a UK longitudinal study of Romanian adoptees. *European Journal of Developmental Psychology*, *4*, 332–350. doi:10.1080/17405620701401846.

Rutter, M., & Sonuga-Barke, E. J. (2010). X. Conclusions: Overview of findings from the era study, inferences, and research implications. *Monographs of the Society for Research in Child Development.*, *75*(1), 212–229. doi:10.1111/j.1540-5834.2010.00557.x.

Tardos, A. (2007a). From the hands of the caretaker. In A. Tardos (Ed.), *Bringing up and providing care for infants and toddlers in an institution* (pp. 39–55). Budapest, Hungary: Association Pikler – Loczy, Paros Print Bt.

Tardos, A. (2007b). The child as an active participant in his own development. In A. Tardos (Ed.), *Bringing up and providing care for infants and toddlers in an institution* (pp. 105–127). Budapest, Hungary: Association Pikler – Loczy, Paros Print Bt.

The Federal Law No272 (Федеральный закон от 28 декабря 2012 г. N 272-ФЗ "О мерах воздействия на лиц, причастных к нарушениям основополагающих прав и свобод человека, прав и свобод граждан Российской Федерации".) Retrieved from http://base.garant.ru/70291034/

The Federal State Statistic Service of the Russian Federation. Retrieved from http://www.gks.ru

The Leiden Conference. (2012). The development and care of institutionally reared children. *Child Development Prospectives*, *6*(2), 174–180. doi:10.1111/j.1750-8606.2011.00231.x.

The Ministry of Education and Science of the Russian Federation. Retrieved from http://www.usynovite.ru

The Presidential Decree No761 "On the National Strategy of Actions for Children for 2012–2017". (2012). (Указ Президента РФ от 1 июня 2012 г. N 761 "О национальной стратегии действий в интересах детей на 2012–2017.) Retrieved from http://base.garant.ru/70183566/

The Resolution No93. (2014). (Постановление от 10 февраля 2014 года №93 "О мерах по совершенствованию порядка передачи детей-сирот и детей, оставшихся без попечения родителей, на воспитание в семьи".) Retrieved from http://government.ru/dep_news/10470/

The Resolution of the Government of the Russian Federation No1839-r "Concept of Early Intervention Development in the Russian Federation for the period till 2020". (2016). (Распоряжение Правительства РФ №1839-р "О концепции развития ранней помощи в Российской Федерации на период до 2020 года».) Retrieved from http://government.ru/media/files/7NZ6EKa6SOcLcCCQbyMRXHsdcTmR9lki.pdf

The Resolution of the Government of the Russian Federation No481. (2014). (Постановление Правительства РФ от 24 мая 2014 г. N 481 "О деятельности организаций для детей-сирот и детей, оставшихся без попечения родителей, и об устройстве в них детей, оставшихся без попечения родителей". Retrieved from http://www.garant.ru/hotlaw/federal/544284/

The St. Petersburg-USA Orphanage Research Team. (2008). The effects of early social- emotional and relationship experience on the development of young orphanage children. *Monographs of the Society for Research in Child Development*, *73*(3), vii–viii, 1–262, 294–295. doi:10.1111/j.1540–5834.2008.00483.x.

The St. Petersburg-USA Orphanage Research Team, Muhamedrahimov, R. J., Palmov, O. I., Nikiforova, N. V., Groark, C. J., & McCall, R. B. (2005). Characteristics of children, caregivers, and orphanages for young children in St. Petersburg, Russian Federation. *Journal of Applied Developmental Psychology*, *26*, 477–506.

van IJzendoorn, M. H., & Juffer, F. (2006). The Emmanuel Miller memorial lecture 2006: Adoption as an intervention. Meta-analytic evidence for massive catch-up and plasticity in physical, socio-emotional, and cognitive development. *Journal of Child Psychology and Psychiatry*, *47*, 1228–1245. doi:10.1111/j.1469-7610.2006.01675.x.

Vygotsky, L. S. (1966). Development of the higher mental functions. In A. N. Leontyev, A. R. Luria, & A. Smirnov (Eds.), *Pyschological research in the USSR* (vol. 1, pp. 11–46). Moscow, Russia: Progress Publishers.

Chapter 11
Institutional Care in Ukraine: Historical Underpinnings and Developmental Consequences

Nataliya A. Dobrova-Krol and Marinus H. van IJzendoorn

> *Group care for children and adolescents is widely used as a rearing environment and sometimes used as a setting in which intensive services can be provided. This consensus statement on group care affirms that children and adolescents have the need and right to grow up in a family with at least one committed, stable, and loving adult caregiver. In principle, group care should never be favored over family care. Group care should be used only when it is the least detrimental alternative, when necessary therapeutic mental health services cannot be delivered in a less restrictive setting.*
>
> Dozier et al. (2014, p. 219)

N.A. Dobrova-Krol (✉)
Intercultural Psychiatry for Child, Youth and Family, ipsy de Jutters,
The Hague, The Netherlands

Centre for Child and Family Studies, Institute of Education and Child Studies, Graduate School of Social and Behavioural Sciences, Leiden University,
Wassenaarseweg 52, 2333, AK, Leiden, The Netherlands
e-mail: n.dobrova@i-psy.nl; natashad-k@live.nl

M.H. van IJzendoorn
Centre for Child and Family Studies, Institute of Education and Child Studies, Graduate School of Social and Behavioural Sciences, Leiden University,
Wassenaarseweg 52, 2333, AK, Leiden, The Netherlands
e-mail: vanijzen@fsw.leidenuniv.nl

A.V. Rus et al. (eds.), *Child Maltreatment in Residential Care*,
DOI 10.1007/978-3-319-57990-0_11

1 Introduction

After the downfall of the Soviet Union and the gaining of its independence as a sovereign state in 1991, Ukraine has gradually embarked on the path of reform and abolishment of institutional care as a child-rearing practice breaching the right of the child for family care and healthy development (Bilson & Carter, 2008; The Presidential Commissioner for Children's Rights, 2013, 2016). However, Ukraine still relies mainly on institutional rather than family-based care for children deprived of parental care. As a consequence, out of the 52 countries in the WHO European region, Ukraine has taken the third place as to the absolute number and the sixth place as to the relative number of institution-reared children under 3 years of age (Browne, Hamilton-Giachritsis, Johnson, & Ostergren, 2006; UNICEF, 2012). In order to understand the slow implementation of reforms of institutional care and the failure to break the vicious circle of approaches and attitudes feeding the phenomenon of the institutional placement of children, as well as the high number of children deprived of parental care, it is important to understand the broader context of historical, cultural, and social circumstances that have affected the entire Ukrainian population.

In this chapter, we will examine various aspects of institutional care in Ukraine. Before doing so, we will briefly describe the historical background of the present situation, as to underlying beliefs and circumstances. The present structure and functioning of institutional care in Ukraine and its impact on the development of children will be examined. A special focus will be on children with HIV infection, as Ukraine has the second largest HIV epidemic among the Eastern European and Central Asian countries, which also affects children and increases the risk of their institutionalization (UNAIDS, 2015). We will discuss the prospects of children graduating from institutional care and make some recommendations that follow from our analysis.

2 Institutional Care in Ukraine: A Brief Historical Overview

In modern history, the territory that now makes up Ukraine has been part of several countries; parts of the present Ukraine fell under Poland, Turkey, Austria, and Russia. During the eighteenth century, the major part of the Ukrainian territory was taken over by the Russian Empire. The main historical influence on the care for orphaned children in Ukraine and its current system of institutions stems therefore from the Russian tradition.

Beginning from the eighteenth century, the development of institutional care for children in the Russian Empire coincided in many aspects with the history of foundling care in Western Europe (Gorshkova, 1995; Gouroff, 1829; Pullan, 1989; Ransel, 1988). However, the Russian project, inspired by the ideas of the Enlightenment, was more far-reaching: the foundling homes were envisioned as incubators of an entirely new type of individual and as the breeding ground for people who would be especially useful to their nation. Children were to be made completely different from their parents, filled with enlightened morality, work ethic, civicmindedness, patriotism, and respect for constituted authority (Gorshkova, 1995; Ransel, 1988). Consequently, even legitimate children whose parents were alive were welcomed into the growing net of the institutions.

However, mortality rates in the children's homes went up to 98% (Langmeier & Matejeek, 1984), and, according to contemporary observers, children who survived early institutional upbringing looked reticent and disobedient and became involved in crime at later ages (Ransel, 1988). Despite these poor results, the conviction that in a carefully controlled institutional environment, by applying progressive pedagogical techniques, the outcasts of society could be transformed into loyal and conscious citizens was broadly accepted by the educated elite. This became a basis for the educational politics well into the twentieth century.

By the end of the nineteenth century and the beginning of the twentieth century, there was a short-lived shift in the policy of the government, aiming to support families in their parenting role (Ransel, 1988). Subsequent historical changes, the Bolshevik Revolution, and the emergence of the new Soviet state once more strongly revived the utopian ideals of institutional rearing. After the October Revolution in 1917, when the Bolsheviks came to power, all children were declared to be state children, and their rearing was to be unified (Oslon & Holmogorova, 2001). Adoption was outlawed, and it was not until 1926 that it was made legitimate again (Stolee, 1988). The new Soviet policy makers "expressed a wish that all families would be destroyed as soon as possible, so that there would be as many abandoned children as possible and the state would raise them in much greater numbers" (Lunacharsky, 1927/1991, p. 10). Children's homes for orphans and homeless children were viewed as a "wonderful rearing laboratory."

These new concepts of child-rearing in the institutions found their theoretical basis in Makarenko's theory of personality development "in the collective, by the collective and for the collective" (Bronfenbrenner, 1970, p. 51), formulated in the 1930s and a cornerstone of Soviet education ever since. The strength and continuity of this ideological conviction is shown by the project envisaged in 1956 by the Communist Party leader N. Khrushchev, who stated the necessity to establish new boarding schools for all children, in order to bring up "the constructors of the new society, people with a good heart and lofty ideals of utter devotional service to their nation" (Khrushchev, 1956, p. 2). Plans were made to increase the number of the institutionalized children up to at least 2.5 million by the year 1965 (Khrushchev, 1956).

The new institutions, often referred to as "schools of the future," were expected to raise model citizens, trained for specific occupations, to perform a welfare function by providing educational opportunities for children from underprivileged families or groups, to replace community-based services for vulnerable families and children, and to enhance the social and economic freedom for women. The voluntary cession of children by their parents was again encouraged (Dunstan, 1980). To fulfill the party's ambitions to institutionalize the highest possible number of children, schools and children's homes were to be reorganized into boarding schools (*internats*), and new facilities were built. *Internats* were to house about 400 children each, usually from 6 to 16–18 years of age, and often were equipped with small factories or farms where children could work and develop their skills (Bronfenbrenner, 1970; Dunstan, 1980).

It soon became clear, once more, that the Soviet state was unable to cope with the challenges of institutional child-rearing. The state had to reconsider the role and the responsibility of the family in child upbringing, returning that responsibility to the families. By the 1970s, the development of residential education slowed down and practically stopped, the standards in the institutions deteriorated, and boarding schools were turned into schools for "difficult" children, children deprived of parental care or lacking the conditions for family upbringing (Dunstan, 1980). The public care system for orphans and children deprived of parental care established in the 1960s all over the Soviet Union is still prevalent in Ukraine. As a direct consequence of its ideological origins, this system is structured in such a way as to keep children deprived of parental care from birth to young adulthood.

Ideologically driven developments in the care for orphaned children were not unique to Russia, Ukraine, and the former Soviet Bloc countries. The parallels can be found at different times in different parts of the world as well. For instance, in America in the nineteenth century, some Protestants and state-managed orphan asylums also "wanted to break children away from the culture, and often the religion, of their impoverished parents," and Catholic or Jewish asylums "intended to protect children's religious and/or cultural heritage from a world that asylum managers saw as hostile to it" (Hacsi, 1998, p. 54).

There are also more recent examples of the attempts to create an alternative collective form of child-rearing and to nourish a "new type" of citizen loyal to the state. Israeli Kibbutz movements strived to create collective rearing alternatives to family care in order to discourage individualism, to liberate women from childcare in order to involve them more in the socioeconomic life of the community, and to prepare children better for communal life (Aviezer, Van IJzendoorn, Sagi, & Schuengel, 1994). Also in China, after the 1948 revolution, most of the functions that traditionally belonged to the family, including child-rearing, were transferred to the people's communes. By the end of 1958, millions of nurseries and kindergartens had been established in the rural communes. Families were encouraged to send their children to the institutions for similar reasons as in the Soviet Union and Israeli Kibbutz movements, i.e., to free adults and especially women from the child-rearing responsibilities and facilitate their greater involvement in the production and to ensure the proper "socialist" upbringing of the children (e.g., Dixon, 1982; Shao Chuan, 1989).

Even though the role of the ideological principles in the advancement of institutional upbringing may not be unique and limited only to Ukraine, Russia, and the region, its persistence and scale of the influence on child welfare has gone far beyond similar developments in other parts of the world and was exacerbated by several traumatic events affecting the whole population of the country.

3 The Impact of Traumatic Events

For Ukraine, the twentieth century was marked by a number of traumatic events. The first was the devastation of the Civil War that followed the Bolshevik Revolution of 1917. Then the Stalinist mass repressions, especially targeting the Ukrainian political and intellectual elite (Conquest, 1986), culminating in the Holodomor of 1932–1933, a famine artificially created by the communist regime through the confiscation of harvests and all food products. Officially denied by the Soviet Union as long as it existed, after many decades the Holodomor has received general recognition as specifically targeting the Ukrainian population and therefore amounting to genocide (Conquest, 1986; Verkhovna Rada, 2006).

From 1941 to 1945, the Second World War raged on the territory of Ukraine. Two years after the war, Stalin's policy of confiscating grain from peasants caused the Famine of 1946–1947. Conservative estimates state the number of direct victims of the Holodomor at five million and of the Second World War again at five million Ukrainians (Magocsi, 2010). The Famine of 1946–1947, according to the data of various researchers, killed from 100,000 to 2.8 million people (Ellman, 2000). Added to that, indirect losses in the first part of the twentieth century are calculated to be many millions of lives: together more than the entire population of a country like Greece or Portugal.

Especially hard-hit were the children of Ukraine. As a consequence of World War I, civil war, famine, and spread of poverty and diseases, the estimates of the first wave of orphans, dating from 1914 through 1927, were ranging from two to seven and a half million orphaned and homeless children (Ball, 1994; Stolee, 1988). One-third of the Holodomor victims of 1932–1933 were children, and during this period, large numbers of them became orphaned and homeless. In late spring 1933, for example, over 300,000 homeless children were recorded in Kyiv region alone (Conquest, 1986).

The next wave of orphans appeared as a result of the Nazi invasion of Ukraine in 1941 and of the destruction of life and property caused by the war and four-year occupation. During the war, the number of homeless children grew rapidly, and by its end, the Soviet Union counted over one million orphaned children. The Famine of 1946–1947 also provoked massive orphanhood: saving their children, especially severely malnourished infants, from hunger, desperate parents were bringing them to cities and leaving them in the hope that they would be taken to an orphanage or children's homes (Ganson, 2006).

It is argued here that Ukraine's twentieth-century experience amounts to historical trauma that is conceptualized as a collective complex trauma inflicted on a group of people sharing a specific group identity. This can be seen as a legacy of traumatic events over the life-span and across generations. Historical trauma encompasses the psychological and social responses to cumulative wounding and affects not only survivors but also their descendants at the levels of the individual, family, community, culture, and society. Historical trauma, being collective, cumulative, and intergenerational in nature, can result in social malaise and weakened social structures, poverty, substance abuse, health problems, family dysfunction, and child maltreatment (Brave Heart, 2003; Evans-Campbell, 2008; Haskell & Randall, 2009; Maercker, & Hecker, 2016).

Not all studies show long-term intergenerational impact of collective trauma; for example, meta-analytic research on the aftermath of the Holocaust shows massive traumatization in the child survivor generation but surprisingly little impact on the second and the third generation. However, the same studies point out that the presence of supportive interpersonal relationships and successful social productivity help to shield against negative consequences of trauma, whereas repeated exposure to traumatic experiences and genetic predisposition may increase the vulnerability (Barel, Van IJzendoorn, Sagi-Schwartz, & Bakermans-Kranenburg, 2010; Sagi-Schwartz, Van IJzendoorn, & Bakermans-Kranenburg, 2008; Van IJzendoorn, Bakermans-Kranenburg, & Sagi-Schwartz, 2003). Besides, Shamai (2016) points out that the assessment of the impact of trauma should not only focus on the individual but also address systemic impact on families, culture, and society and take into consideration pre-trauma conditions, the functioning of the social system, as well as the possibility to process the trauma individually and collectively afterward.

Recent studies demonstrate that the Holodomor genocide, as a collective trauma that occurred in an already weakened society, followed by other massive traumatic events, continues to exert its intergenerational impact on Ukrainian families and is manifested in trauma-based behaviors, such as disrupted relationships and family roles, indifference toward others, increased social hostility, and risky health behaviors, including alcohol and drug abuse, and increased spread of HIV/AIDS (Bezeo & Maggi, 2015a, 2015b; Gornostay, 2014). Indeed, one-third of Ukrainians die before the age of 65 years, a rate that is much higher than in European countries; in 2004 mortality from alcohol abuse (including alcohol psychosis) in Ukraine was second highest across the entire WHO European Region; currently, Ukraine has the second biggest HIV epidemic among the Eastern European and Central Asian countries (Bailey et al., 2010; UNAIDS, 2007, 2015; World Bank, 2009).

Apart from historical trauma, modern Ukrainian families and communities have to deal with turbulent political and economic transformations of the more recent decades, which brought substantial financial insecurity and poverty. New atrocities and the current war cause loss of life, family disruption, and a growing number of internally displaced persons. So along with the ideological convictions, inherited from Russia and the Soviet Union, that presented institutions as beneficial for the rearing of the children and substituting family care, Ukraine had and still has to cope with extremely unfavorable circumstances that generate a high number of orphans. Historical trauma and persistently unfavorable economic and social situations disrupt the functioning of families and communities, undermine parenting practices, and cause health problems on a large scale. Institutional care, either by ideology or necessity, remains a prominent reality of child-rearing in Ukraine to this day. In fact, it can be said that a major feature of the Ukrainian situation at this moment is the phenomenon of social orphanhood.

4 The Phenomenon of Social Orphanhood

Ukraine has to deal with numerous cases of evasion of parental responsibilities and family dysfunction that, as a result, lead to social orphanhood. Every year about 600 newborns in maternity hospitals alone enlarge the social orphan population during the first hours of their life. According to different sources, in Ukraine 95–98% of children deprived of parental care are social orphans (e.g., Lopatchenko, 2014; UNICEF, 2010). Social orphanhood is defined as a distortion of parental behavior and a form of child maltreatment when parents, for various reasons, withdraw from fulfilling their parental duties, such as rearing and preparing children for socially meaningful activities, supporting minors and protecting young people's rights and interests (UNICEF, 2010).

The distortion of parental behavior can be caused by different factors that are in most cases interrelated (Lopatchenko, 2014; Ukrainian Institute of Social Studies, 2001):

- Socioeconomic: unemployment of the parents, financial difficulties, jobs that require parents' frequent and lasting absences from home or labor migration, lack of permanent housing, etc.
- Family dysfunction and/or deprivation of parental rights: early or nonmarital motherhood, parental illness, parental substance abuse, incarceration, lack of parenting skills as a consequence of institutional upbringing, family crises, domestic violence, and diverse kinds of child abuse.
- Child health condition: abandonment as a result of congenital conditions, developmental disorders or disabilities, or diseases; in such cases, the decision to have the child institutionalized is provoked by lack of objective information as to the family's future prospects or even recommendations of the medical doctors. 95% of children admitted to institutional care suffer from delays in physical and mental development (Kukuruza et al., 2015).
- Lack of community-based family-centered services, absence of an effective early childhood intervention system, and poor cross-sectoral cooperation (Dobrova-Krol, 2014).

The extensive presence of the phenomenon of social orphanhood suggests that Ukraine's children and families, on one hand, may suffer from the effects of historical trauma and ongoing hardships. On the other hand, they have to bear the consequences of the imposed ideological convictions that promoted institutional care over family care and for decades substituted community-based services. These effects seem to be transmitted through the generations, thus creating a vicious circle of adversity.

5 Institutional Care in Ukraine: Organizational Structure, Abuse, and Structural Neglect

The latest study of institutional care of children in Ukraine[1] conducted by The Presidential Commissioner for Children's Rights (2016) reports a total of 774 residential institutions that house 104,000 child residents or 1.4% of the child population of Ukraine. Although the number of orphans and children deprived of parental care decreased by 12 percent between 2008 and 2013 (UNICEF, 2015), in 2016 it increased again by at least 0.2% of the total number of children as compared to the data from 2008.

The majority of the childcare institutions in Ukraine are state-run, with a standardized structure and functioning across the country, inherited from the Soviet system of care. Institutions are organized in such a way as to maintain children who are deprived of parental care from birth to young adulthood. They are differentiated according to children's age (for the age groups from 0 to 3 years, 3 to 7 years, and 7 to 16–18 years); they are also specialized depending on children's physical condition (there are special boarding schools for children with various developmental and physical impairments). Usually, at age 4, depending on health condition and the level of functioning, each child is given a classification from 0 to 4 and placed in an institution under the Ministry of Education or Social Policy (Kukuruza et al., 2015; Mathews, Rosenthal, Ahern, & Kurylo, 2015):

- 0 – no disability (boarding school of the Ministry of Education)
- 1 and 2 – mild intellectual disability (specialized boarding school of the Ministry of Education)
- 3 and 4 – moderate to severe intellectual disability (children are considered to be "uneducable" and placed in the institutions of the Ministry of Social Policy)

While, in institutional care, children are frequently transferred within and between institutions until their graduation, children with moderate to severe disabilities rarely leave institutional care and remain institutionalized through the rest of their lives (Mathews et al., 2015; Ukrainian Institute of Social Studies, 2001).

Childcare institutions for young children in Ukraine may house up to 200 young residents and are usually characterized by high child-to-caregiver ratios, multiple shifts, and frequent change of caregivers, which, as research reveals, are common to institutional care across different countries (Dobrova-Krol, Van IJzendoorn, Bakermans-Kranenburg, & Juffer, 2008). By the age of three, children may have been exposed to as many as 50 different caregivers.

The conditions of rearing in the institutions may vary substantially: some provide fairly clean environments, medical care, and adequate nutrition, with usually limited cognitive and social stimulation, especially during the first year of life, whereas others fail to ensure appropriate nutrition, hygiene, medical care, and stimulation. The daily schedule across Ukrainian institutions is usually strictly

[1] Occupied territories of Donetsk and Crimea were not included in this study.

regimented. Apart from routines around sleeping, meals, and hygiene, it often includes group learning activities adjusted to age, and indoor and outdoor play activities. All children are expected to participate in the daily routine and may be exempt from it only if they are ill or as a form of punishment. The rearing conditions are especially poor in institutions for children with severe disabilities (level 3–4 institutions), where immobile children are often undernourished, do not receive proper medical care, and usually seen languishing in inactivity in rows of cribs (Mathews et al., 2015).

A recent report by experts from Disability Rights International (DRI) on a 3-year investigation of 33 Ukrainian institutions reveals extensive evidence of abuse in many of Ukraine's institutions for children and adults with and without disabilities who are subject to severe emotional and physical pain, restraint, seclusion, forced abortions and sterilization, sexual abuse and trafficking (especially in the war affected territories), and dangerous or neglectful medical care that constitute ill-treatment under international law. In some cases, abuse that DRI observed may even rise to the level of torture (Mathews et al., 2015). Other studies also report about maltreatment and abuse of children in Ukrainian institutions by personnel or other, usually older children (e.g., Balakireva et al., 2010).

In a survey that involved 110 care-leavers aged 15–26 years old, 438 children aged 13–19 years old still living in institutional care, and 55 experts, 18 out of 110 care-leavers reported that they were treated harshly by personnel in the institutions and 19 out of 110 care-leavers witnessed harsh treatment of other children (e.g., cases of harsh physical punishment, torture, and humiliation). These reports were supported by the data obtained from the representatives of NGOs and state-run institutions working with children in institutional care (Balakireva et al., 2010).

Even if a child does not become a victim of physical or emotional abuse while in institutional care, he or she suffers from the impact of this rearing environment. A body of empirical and theoretical studies has been consistent in demonstrating that the rearing failures of institutional care are associated with its radical departure from the conditions of the average expectable environment (Cicchetti & Valentino, 2006; Hartmann, 1958; Rutter, Kumsta, Schlotz, & Sonuga-Barke, 2012; Rutter, O'Connor, & The English and Romanian Adoptees (ERA) Study Team, 2004). Depending on the child's age, the average expectable environment encompasses consistent protective and sensitive caregiving, a supportive family, as well as socialization and open opportunities for exploration and mastery of the world. The presence of the average expectable environment is an essential prerequisite for the normal development of the child (Bowlby, 1997; Nelson et al., 2007).

Obviously, the environment in Ukrainian institutions falls outside the scope of the expected range of the average environment due to the risk of structural neglect that is embedded in the organization and functioning of childcare institutions (Dobrova-Krol et al., 2008; Van IJzendoorn, 2008): its regimented nature, high child-to-caregiver ratio, multiple shifts, and frequent change of caregivers almost inevitably deprive children of continuous and reciprocal interactions with stable caregivers, necessary to respond to their developmental needs.

6 Prospects of Graduates of Institutional Care in Ukraine

The regimented nature of the institutions provides little to no opportunities for socialization and mastery of the outside world, or development of self-efficacy and supportive networks. The lack of experience of family interaction and adequate positive social role models intensify the feeling of social alienation. The lack of skills for arranging their everyday life (e.g., where to get one's meals or clothes, what to do in case of financial or legal problems or in case of sickness, etc.) and lack of programs and services supporting the care-leavers after their graduation make their transition to adult life very abrupt and insecure. Young graduates often do not have a place to live, no financial means, and scarce opportunities for acquiring education or profession. Half of the graduates have no housing after they leave the residential institution (Ukrainian Institute of Social Studies, 2001).

A survey of 312 care-leavers aged 16–18 years old, aimed at the identification of possible social and psychological factors that can hinder the adaptation of care-leavers in society, shows that the care-leavers view financial problems and housing as the major problems after leaving the institutional care. Comparison with family-reared children demonstrates that the care-leavers have smaller if any supportive networks; they are more worried about their future, less motivated to choose a profession according to their interests, and tend to seek a pragmatic or convenient solution that will give more security (Sidorenko, 2013).

According to the survey of Balakirieva et al. (2010), the care-leavers report experiencing social exclusion and stigma and have difficulty establishing new friendships. One-third of the respondents reported concealing the fact that they grew up in institutional care to avoid biased attitudes when they apply for a job or meet new friends. The experts that participated in this study confirm that the young care-leavers show poor outcomes across a number of life domains, including accommodation, employment, education, and health. They are often discriminated against and end up in poverty, get involved in criminal activities, or become homeless. To support themselves financially, young people end up doing exhausting low-paid work or end up in criminal circles or prostitution (Balakirieva et al., 2010).

In neighboring Russia, according to survey data, 1 in 3 children who leave residential care becomes homeless, 1 in 5 ends up with a criminal record, and as many as 1 in 10 commits suicide. Also, 1 in 10 young offenders in Russia was raised in institutional care (Harwin, 1996; Tobis, 2000). In addition, the experience of residential care can impact family systems and roles and lead to family dysfunction. For instance, in Canada, where by 1960 over half of the First Nations and Métis children were placed in residential care, it is now generally acknowledged that this experience was not only traumatizing to these children but also led to secondary trauma in their offspring as a result of having parents reared in residential care who lacked parenting role models (Ball, 2010).

Thus, the life path of an institutionalized child is often full of perinatal adversities, starting with the trauma of separation from their own biological family and continued in an environment characterized by structural institutional neglect with a high risk of abuse. This experience often leads to significant developmental difficulties. After graduation from the institution, they are frequently exacerbated by the lack of support and security and do not adapt well to society, consolidating the cycle of the transmission of trauma. Institutional care, both for its graduates and their offspring, may very well prove to be a vicious circle of self-perpetuating need for state support.

7 Extreme Rearing Circumstances: Institutional Care Versus Multiple Problem Families

In the Western world, institutional care as a form of child-rearing never received the degree of idealization that it received in Russian and Soviet culture. Still its drawbacks and benefits have been the subject of debate, especially after John Bowlby gave the debate a historical impetus in his report to the World Health Organization on the mental health of homeless children in postwar Europe and the effect of institutional care on children's development (Bowlby, 1951).

There are modern researchers who maintain that institutions of good quality can provide a sense of permanence, security, structure, and camaraderie, absent in dysfunctional and abusive families, and that institutional care may be the best option for some children who are left homeless by such plagues of modern times as parental drug and alcohol abuse and AIDS (e.g., Carp, 2006; McKenzie, 1996; Seelye, 1997). Miller and colleagues (2007) suggest that, in case of extreme rearing circumstances, institutions can provide beneficial and for some children even life-saving interventions. Ferris and colleagues (2007) found a trend for survival advantage for Romanian HIV-infected children in institutional care as compared to children who resided with their biological families. McCall (2013) maintains that it is the quality and characteristics of the care within an environment, rather than the type of environment itself, that most likely impact the development of the child. Several studies show that institutional environments may sometimes be more favorable for children in need than their extended families and other family-based configurations of care (e.g., Braitstein, 2015; Whetten et al., 2009). However, Bakermans-Kranenburg and Van IJzendoorn (2009) in their comments to the study by Whetten et al. (2009) that describes better developmental outcomes for institution-reared children argue that such conclusions are limited to a specific age range, a specific set of countries and institutions, and a restricted set of measures on certain developmental domains and therefore are not generalizable.

As discussed earlier in this chapter, institutional rearing falls outside the scope of the expected range of the average environment due to the risk of structural neglect that is embedded in the organization and functioning of childcare institutions (Van IJzendoorn, 2008). It appears that the greater the deviation from the conditions of the average expectable environment is, the greater is the impact on the development of children and vice versa. Thus, the better the developmental outcomes institutional care provides, the closer it appears in its structure and functioning to the more regular family environment (e.g., Gunnar, 2001; McCall, 2013).

Of course, the notion of the average expectable environment is also applicable to families. Families may deviate from the average expectable norm for various reasons (e.g., family instability, economic hardships, child abuse, and neglect). This raises the question as to what may be more beneficial for the development of the child – a well-functioning institution or his or her own dysfunctional family.

However, after several decades of studies that compared the development of children in institutions with their family-reared counterparts from a socially disadvantaged environment, it can be said that John Bowlby's (1951, pp. 68–69) conclusion that "children thrive better in bad homes than in good institutions" seems to hold true remarkably well, even when keeping in mind his warning that much depends on how bad the home is and how good the institution.

Whether the rule applies also in Ukraine, with a distinct heritage of institutional care and its strong ideological underpinnings, with many families living under the poverty threshold, suffering from health problems and substance abuse, has been explored in several studies as discussed below.

8 Impact of Institutional Care and HIV on the Development of Preschoolers

In a series of studies (Bakermans-Kranenburg, Dobrova-Krol, & Van IJzendoorn, 2012; Dobrova-Krol, 2009; Dobrova-Krol, Van IJzendoorn, Bakermans-Kranenburg, Cyr, & Juffer, 2008; Dobrova-Krol, Van IJzendoorn, Bakermans-Kranenburg, & Juffer, 2010a, 2010b), the impact of the type of rearing environment (family vs. institution) and HIV infection status on different developmental domains (physical growth, regulation of stress, cognitive performance, theory of mind (ToM), attachment, indiscriminate friendliness) of 64 Ukrainian preschoolers reared in institutions or in their own disadvantaged biological families was examined.

Four ethnically homogeneous groups were compared: children with and without perinatal HIV infection reared in their biological families and childcare institutions. We assessed children who were put into care at 1 month after birth on average. These children permanently resided in institutions with similar organization and quality of care. Institutions involved in our study provided adequate nutrition and health care, but lacked stimulation and stability in child-caregiver relationships. Family-reared children, both uninfected and HIV-infected children, were raised in families with low to middle income. HIV-impacted families had lower monthly income and were more likely to experience multiple adversities, such as single parenting, substance abuse, unemployment, and criminal records, than families without HIV. HIV-infected children in families and institutions had about the same level of immune control over HIV as reflected by their CD4 T-lymphocyte count.

Institutional care was associated with less favorable outcomes in all examined developmental domains (see Table 11.1). Presence of HIV infection led to less favorable developmental outcomes; however, the negative impact of institutional care was greater than presence of HIV in several domains as discussed below.

HIV-Infected Children in Families and Institutions In three out of six developmental outcomes that we examined, HIV-infected children reared in disadvantaged families demonstrated better results than HIV-infected children reared in institutions. Thus, physical growth delays of HIV-infected children reared in families were less substantial (see Fig. 11.1).

They showed better cognitive performance than HIV-infected institution-reared children, who lagged behind by more than 15 IQ points. Ninety-six percent of the HIV-infected children reared in families managed to develop clearly discernable attachment relationships as opposed to only 46% of the HIV-infected children in institutional care. HIV-infected family-reared children were more often secure and less often disorganized than HIV-infected children in institutions (see Fig. 11.2).

Comparison of the quality of the rearing environment of HIV-infected children in families and institutions with the help of the HOME inventory (Bradley et al., 1993) did not reveal any significant differences on the HOME Total Score between these groups. Examination of the individual HOME scales demonstrated that institutional care was offering better physical environment, whereas families provided better child-caregiver interactions. In addition, families provided a more consistent rearing environment with a limited number of stable caregivers, which was not possible in institutions because of their structure and functioning, described earlier. We may conclude that due to the consistency, stability, and better quality of child-caregiver relationships, even compromised family care promoted more optimal development of HIV-infected children compared to institutions that provided better physical environments. Moreover, HIV-infected children reared in families tended to show more favorable developmental outcomes even in comparison to uninfected and relatively healthy children reared in institutions.

Compared to the institutions, HIV-impacted families facilitated better outcomes in several domains. However, HIV-impacted families failed to facilitate early Theory of Mind development. Also, the elevated levels of disorganized attachment and indiscriminate friendliness in comparison to uninfected family-reared children indicate that the rearing environment in HIV-impacted families was not optimal for the normal development of children. Still, on the basis of the findings of this study, we may conclude that the institutional rearing environment appeared to be more damaging for children's physical growth, cognitive development, and attachment formation than the presence of HIV in multiple-problem families.

Risk and Protective Factors Although, on average, institutional care was associated with less favorable outcomes in all developmental domains that we studied, there was individual variation in the responses of institution-reared children to apparently similar adverse experiences. In some cases, the outcomes in different domains were even close to normal. For instance, in almost 30% of children, height-for-age scores were within one standard deviation from population norms at the time of the

Table 11.1 Descriptive statistics for family-reared vs. institution-reared children

	Family-reared children						Institution-reared children					
	HIV−			HIV+			HIV−			HIV+		
	n^{*}	*M*	*(SD)*	n^{*}	*M*	*(SD)*	n^{*}	*M*	*(SD)*	n^{*}	*M*	*(SD)*
Age of mother (yrs)	17	32.12	(5.93)	14	32.47	(5.68)	11	30.18	(8.73)	8	30.38	(5.21)
Family income	12	234.75^{a}	(112.29)	13	149.54^{b}	(43.10)						
Age of child (mos)	19	51.44	(9.77)	16	52.01	(14.78)	16	48.14	(9.72)	13	52.28	(12.99)
Weight-for-age at birth	16	-0.32^{a}	(0.99)	15	$-1.15^{a,b}$	(1.21)	15	$-0.81^{a,b}$	(0.61)	13	-1.36^{b}	(0.56)
Height-for-age at assessment	19	0.20^{a}	(0.98)	16	$-0.54^{a,b}$	(1.06)	16	$-1.58^{b,c}$	(1.29)	13	-1.86^{c}	(1.30)
Cognitive performance	19	97.63^{a}	(19.40)	16	78.00^{b}	(16.87)	16	67.31^{b}	(18.97)	13	64.00^{b}	(14.32)
Attachment security	19	5.97^{a}	(1.74)	16	$4.63^{a,b}$	(1.31)	16	3.75^{b}	(1.94)	13	4.27^{b}	(1.87)
Indiscriminate friendliness	19	0.63^{a}	(0.90)	16	1.13^{a}	(1.20)	16	2.44^{b}	(1.31)	13	$1.69^{a,b}$	(1.70)
Positive caregiving	19	1.39^{a}	(1.43)	16	-0.19^{b}	(1.34)	16	-0.96^{b}	(1.62)	13	-0.62^{b}	(1.41)
		n	*(%)*		*n*	*(%)*		*n*	*(%)*		*n*	*(%)*
CD4 T-lymphocyte count				14	913.21	(459.91)				13	1147.69	(375.01)
Perinatal complications	19			16			16	5	(37.5)	13		
Antiretroviral therapy				16	6^{a}	(37.5)				13	12^{b}	(92.3)
Theory of mind	18		(61)	16		(25)	11		(18)	13		(23)

Note: Means in the same row that do not share superscripts differ at $p < .05$
*Number of cases with available data

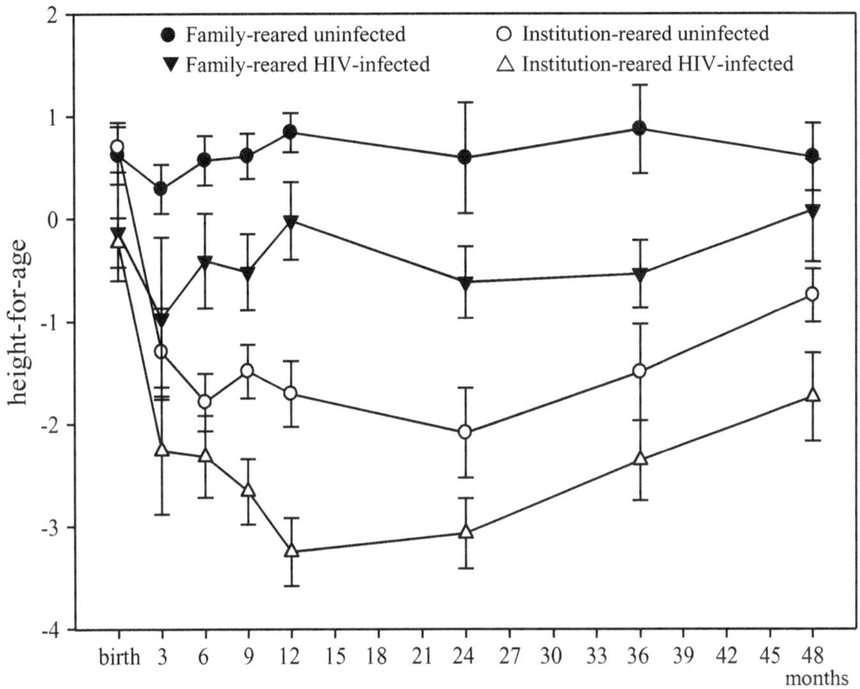

Fig. 11.1 Height-for-age (Z-scores, mean, SE) of uninfected and HIV-infected family- and institution-reared children. *Note*: at 36 months $N = 47$ (family-reared uninfected, 8; family-reared infected, 16; institution-reared uninfected, 10; institution-reared infected, 13) at 48 months $N = 35$ (family-reared uninfected, 8; family-reared infected, 11; institution-reared uninfected, 7; institution-reared infected, 9) (*Source*: Dobrova-Krol et al., 2010b, p. 243)

assessment; 7% of children demonstrated cognitive performance within the normal range; 21% of children succeeded in the Theory of Mind task. Finally, 28% of children managed to form secure, clearly developed attachment relationships with their favorite caregiver, and about 37% of children exhibited no or little signs of indiscriminate friendliness. These findings suggest the presence of certain factors which may buffer or exacerbate the influence of institutional care on the development of the child.

We found a moderating role of 5HTTLPR genotype for the association between adverse rearing environment and attachment disorganization. Carriers of one or two short alleles appeared to suffer most from the adverse institutional environment, whereas carriers of two long alleles seemed protected, suggesting that genetic layout may indeed play a role in this apparent resilience (Bakermans-Kranenburg, Dobrova-Krol, & Van IJzendoorn, 2011).

Perinatal adversities and less optimal physical and health condition of the child at birth were significantly associated with less favorable physical development in institutionalized children. An important but indirect finding was related to a sub-

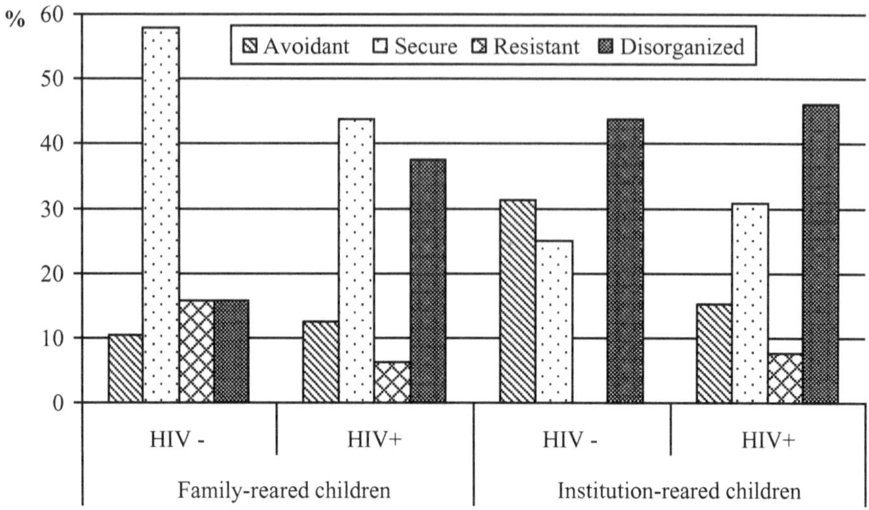

Fig. 11.2 Distribution of attachment patterns (*Source*: Dobrova-Krol et al., 2010a, p. 1372)

group of children with the so-called perinatal hypoxic conditions (see Miller, 2005). Children who were diagnosed with these conditions demonstrated persistent severe growth delays. Despite some improvement in the course of their development, at the time of the assessment, these children remained severely delayed. Their cortisol production also clearly deviated from other uninfected institution-reared children. Obviously, children with perinatal complications may be at increased risk for developmental delays in institutional care and require special attention.

Better quality of the rearing environment and especially better quality of caregiving was associated with better physical growth and with better cognitive performance in HIV-infected institution-reared children. The overall quality of the rearing environment within institutions that were involved in this study was fairly adequate. Moreover, with respect to physical characteristics, e.g., safety, quantity and variety of toys, and even structured learning activities in institutions appeared to be better than HIV-impacted families. Nevertheless, adequate physical aspects of the rearing environment of the childcare institutions appeared to be insufficient to facilitate normative physical and cognitive development of HIV-infected children and compensate for the conditions of structural institutional neglect.

This study emphasizes the harmful effect of structural institutional neglect especially during the first years of life. During these years, children in institutional care were most severely delayed in their physical growth. Findings on indiscriminate friendliness among institution-reared children also illustrate how the lack of consistent and sensitive caregiving during the first year of life may impede the formation of stranger anxiety and the development of preference for familiar caregivers. The findings of the study are supported by another empirical study that examined the impact of the quality of caregiving on the development of 100 4- to 8-year-old

Ukrainian children raised in institutions and their biological families (39 institution reared and 61 family reared) showing that institutionalized children's attachment and cognitive development were significantly compromised as compared to the family-reared children (Barone, Dellagiulia, & Lionetti, 2015; T. Lyseyko, personal communication, April 27, 2016).

It is important to emphasize that in the institutions where our study was conducted, the quality of the caregiving environment was relatively good in comparison to the majority of the childcare institutions in Ukraine. The quality of the rearing environment of the institutions tends to be worse for older children and much worse for children with disabilities, and it can be expected that the impact on their developmental outcomes may be more significant.

In fact, according to the latest statistics, in Ukraine every 3 days, one child raised in institutional care dies due to sickness or accident (Presidential Commissioner for Children's Rights, 2016). Those children who survive and remain in institutional care until their graduation leave with the luggage of physical, emotional, cognitive, and social difficulties caused by early adversity and institutional upbringing, and they also face the challenging task of finding their way in the outside world, from which they were isolated while growing up.

9 Conclusion and Recommendations

In this chapter, we treated the problem of child institutionalization and its persistence in a broader context of collective and historical trauma that continues to affect individuals, communities, and Ukrainian society in general. We hypothesize that, in Ukraine, historical trauma along with imposed ideological convictions of the past promoting institutional care and undermining family systems and values, as well as current hardships, has caused and continue to sustain the widespread phenomenon of social orphanhood and child institutionalization. Therefore, along with the efforts geared toward the transition from institutional to family-based care, working through the traumatic experience; introducing systemic interventions for collective and historical trauma at national, community, family, and individual levels; changing mentality; and strengthening families and communities should be an integral part of deinstitutionalization efforts.

Our empirical studies demonstrate that children infected by HIV appear to thrive better in their multiple-problem families than healthy children in relatively good institutions. For vulnerable children deprived of parental care and/or infected by HIV, mother's or caregiver's continuous presence and sensitive care is crucial and may ameliorate environmental and child-related adversities. Therefore, efforts should be made to prevent child abandonment and to support vulnerable families in their parenting role through the development of the community-based Early Childhood Intervention services. For those children who nevertheless end up in an institution and have little chance of being adopted or placed in family-based care, the rearing environment must be optimized and regularly monitored. Given that adequate physical and medical care is provided, it can be achieved by ensuring stability and improving the quality of caregiving.

The timing of such interventions is of great importance. Because (structural) neglect and traumatic experiences during the first year of life may have long-term or even permanent detrimental impact on children, interventions should be introduced at the earliest possible stages of life, and children under the age of three should not be placed in institutional care.

Questions for Discussion

1. Although the evidence of the harmful effect of institutional care is well documented, scientifically proven, and widely recognized, millions of children across the world continue to live in institutional care. Which factors may cause and sustain the widespread phenomenon of the institutional placement of children?
2. How can the phenomenon of "social orphanhood" be explained and prevented?
3. What may be more beneficial for the development of the child – a well-functioning institution or his or her own dysfunctional family and why? Should countries invest their resources in the improvement of the quality of existing residential institutions for children?

References

Aviezer, O., Van IJzendoorn, M. H., Sagi, A., & Schuengel, C. (1994). "Children of the dream" revisited: 70 years of collective child-rearing in Israeli kibbutzim. *Psychological Bulletin, 116*, 99–116.

Bailey, H., Semenenko, I., Pilipenko, T., Malyuta, R., Thorne, C., & Ukraine European Collaborative Study Group (2010). Factors associated with abandonment of infants born to HIV positive women: Results from a Ukrainian birth cohort. *AIDS Care, 22*(12), 1439–1448. Retrieved from http://doi.org/10.1080/09540121.2010.482127

Bakermans-Kranenburg, M. J., Dobrova-Krol, N. A., & Van IJzendoorn, M. (2012). Impact of institutional care on attachment, disorganization and insecurity of Ukrainian preschoolers: Protective effect of the long variant of the serotonin transporter gene (5HTT). *International Journal of Behavioral Development, 36*, 11–18.

Bakermans-Kranenburg, M. J., & Van IJzendoorn, M. H. (2009). No evidence for orphanages being 'not so bad'. Comments to Whetten et al. (2009). A comparison of the wellbeing of orphans and abandoned children ages 6–12 in institutional and community-based care settings in 5 less wealthy nations. *PLoS One, 4*(12), e8169. doi:10.1371/journal.pone.0008169. Posted 24 Dec 2009.

Balakireva, O. M., Chernin, I. M., Hmelevska, O. M., Nychyporenko, S. V., Kalashnikova, T. M., Bondar, T. V., & Klymenko, Y. M. (2010). *Analitychnyi zvit: Zhyttievyi shliah vypusknykiv internatnykh zalkadiv, dytiachykh budynkiv simeynogo typu ta pryiomnukh simei.* [Analytical report: The live journey of orphanage alumni and children growing up in family-type and foster homes]. Kyiv, Ukraine: Oleksandr Yaremenko Ukrainian Institute of Social Research.

Ball, A. M. (1994). And now my soul is hardened. In *Abandoned children in Soviet Russia, 1918–1930*. Berkeley, CA: University of California Press.

Ball, J. (2010). Indigenous fathers' involvement in reconstituting "circles of care". *American Journal of Community Psychology, 45*, 124e138.

Barel, E., Van IJzendoorn, M. H., Sagi-Schwartz, A., & Bakermans-Kranenburg, M. J. (2010). Surviving the Holocaust: A meta-analysis of the long-term sequelae of genocide. *Psychological Bulletin, 136*, 677–698. doi:10.1037/a0020339.

Barone, L., Dellagiulia, A., & Lionetti, F. (2015). When the primary caregiver is missing: Investigating proximal and distal variables involved in institutionalised children's adjustment. *Child Abuse Review*. doi:10.1002/car.2365.

Bezo, B., & Maggi, S. (2015a). Living in "survival mode:" Intergenerational transmission of trauma from the Holodomor genocide of 1932–1933 in Ukraine. *Social Science & Medicine, 134*, 87–94. doi:10.1016/j.socscimed.2015.04.009.

Bezo, B., & Maggi, S. (2015b). The intergenerational impact of the Holodomor genocide on gender roles, expectations and performance: The Ukrainian experience. *Annual Psychiatry Mental Health, 3*, 1030.

Bilson, A., & Carter, R. (2008). *Strategy development for the reform of the state care system for children deprived of parental care living in state care institutions*. A report for UNICEF Ukraine. UNICEF. Retrieved September 2, 2016, from http://www.unicef.org/ceecis/BilsonCarterReportFinal.pdf

Bowlby, J. (1951). *Maternal care and mental health, World Health Organization monograph no. 2*. Geneva, Switzerland: WHO.

Bowlby, J. (1997). *Attachment and loss: Vol. 1: Attachment*. London, UK: Pimlico.

Bradley, R.H., Whiteside, L., Caldwell, B.M., Casey, P.H., Kelleher, K., & Pope, S., ... Cross, D. (1993). Maternal IQ, the home environment, and child IQ in low birth weight premature children. *International Journal of Behavioral Development, 16*, 61–74.

Braitstein, P. (2015). Institutional care of children in low- and middle-income settings: Challenging the conventional wisdom of Oliver Twist. *Global Health: Science and Practice, 3*, 330–332. Retrieved from http://doi.org/10.9745/GHSP-D-15-00228

Brave Heart, M. Y. H. (2003). The historical trauma response among natives and its relationship with substance abuse: A Lakota illustration. *Journal of Psychoactive Drugs, 35*, 7–13.

Bronfenbrenner, U. (1970). *Two worlds of childhood*. New York, NY: Russell Sage Foundation.

Browne, K., Hamilton-Giachritsis, C., Johnson, R., & Ostergren, M. (2006). Overuse of institutional care for children in Europe. *British Medical Journal, 332*, 485–487.

Carp, E. W. (2006). Two cheers for orphanages. *Reviews in American History, 24*, 277–284.

Cicchetti, D., & Valentino, K. (2006). An ecological transactional perspective on child maltreatment: Failure of the average expectable environment and its influence upon child development. In D. Cicchetti & D. J. Cohen (Eds.), *Developmental psychopathology (2nd ed.): Risk, disorder, and adaptation* (Vol. 3). New York, NY: Wiley.

Conquest, R. (1986). *The harvest of sorrow: Soviet collectivization and the terror-famine*. New York, NY: Oxford University Press.

Dixon, J. (1982). The community-based rural welfare system in the Peoples Republic of China – 1949–1979. *Community Development Journal, 17*, 2–12.

Dobrova-Krol, N. A. (2009). *Vulnerable children in Ukraine: Impact of institutional care and HIV on the development of preschoolers*. Dissertation. Leiden, Netherlands: Mostert and van Ouderen.

Dobrova-Krol, N. A. (2014). *Rannee vmeshatelstvo: Kluchevie aspekti i mezhdunarodniy opit*. [Early childhood intervention. Main principles and international experience]. UNICEF. Retrieved September 14, 2015, from http://www.unicef.org/ukraine/ukr/Early_Intervention_Concept_RUS.pdf

Dobrova-Krol, N. A., Van IJzendoorn, M. H., Bakermans-Kranenburg, M. J., Cyr, C., & Juffer, F. (2008). Physical growth delays and stress dysregulation in stunted and non-stunted Ukrainian institution-reared children. *Infant Behavior and Development, 31*, 539–553.

Dobrova-Krol, N. A., Van IJzendoorn, M. H., Bakermans-Kranenburg, M. J., & Juffer, F. (2010a). The importance of quality of care: Effects of perinatal HIV-infection and early institutional rearing on preschoolers' attachment and indiscriminate friendliness. *Journal of Child Psychology and Psychiatry, 51*, 1368–1376.

Dobrova-Krol, N. A., Van IJzendoorn, M. H., Bakermans-Kranenburg, M. J., & Juffer, F. (2010b). Effects of perinatal HIV-infection and early institutional rearing on social cognitive development of children in Ukraine. *Child Development*, *81*, 237–251.
Dozier, M., Kaufman, J., Kobak, R., O'Connor, T. G., Sagi-Schwartz, A., Scott, S., & ... Zeanah, C. H. (2014). Consensus statement on group care for children and adolescents: A statement of policy of the American Orthopsychiatric Association. *The American Journal of Orthopsychiatry*, *84*(3), 219–225. doi:10.1037/ort0000005.
Dunstan, J. (1980). Soviet boarding education: Its rise and progress. In J. Brine, M. Perrie, & A. Sutton (Eds.), *Home, school and leisure in the Soviet Union* (pp. 110–141). London, UK: George Allen & Unwin.
Ellman, M. (2000). The 1947 Soviet famine and the entitlement approach to famines. *Cambridge Journal of Economics*, *24*, 603–630.
Evans-Campbell, T. (2008). Historical trauma in American Indian/Native Alaska communities: A multilevel framework for exploring impacts on individuals, families, and communities. *Journal of Interpersonal Violence*, *23*, 316e338.
Ferris, M., Burau, K., Constantin, A. M., Mihale, S., Murray, N., Preda, A., ... Kline, M.W. (2007). Influence of institutionalization on time to HIV disease progression in a cohort of Romanian children and teens. *Pediatrics*, *120*, E1476–E1480.
Ganson, N. (2006). *Famine of victors: The Soviet hunger of 1946–1947 in historical and global perspective*. Available from ProQuest Dissertations & Theses Global. Retrieved August 20, 2016, from https://search-proquest-com.ezproxy.leidenuniv.nl:2443/docview/305281528?accountid=12045
Gornostay, P. P. (2014). Kollectivnie travmi i nazionalniy kharakter. [Collective traumas and the national character]. *Psychologichne Konsultuvnnya i Psychotherapia*, *1–2*, 145–157.
Gorshkova, E. A. (1995). Sirotskie priyuti v Rossiyskoy imperii. [Foundling homes in the Russian empire]. *Pedagogika*, *1*, 117–120.
Gouroff, M. (1829). *Essai sur l'histoire des enfants-trouvés, depuis les temps les plus anciens, jusqu'à nos jours; servant d'introduction aux Recherches sur les enfants-trouvés et les enfants illégitimes en Russie, et dans le reste de l'Europe*. [Essay on the history of foundlings, from the most ancient times until our days; serving as an introduction to research into foundlings and illegitimate children in Russia, and in the rest of Europe]. Paris, France: Au Bureau des Connaissances Usuelles.
Gunnar, M. R. (2001). Effects of early deprivation. In C. A. Nelson & M. Luciana (Eds.), *Handbook of developmental cognitive neuroscience* (pp. 617–629). Cambridge, MA: MIT Press.
Hacsi, T. A. (1998). *Second home: Orphan asylums and poor families in America*. Cambridge, MA: Harvard University Press.
Hartmann, H. (1958). *Ego psychology and the problem of adaptation*. New York, NY: International Universities Press, Inc..
Harwin, J. (1996). *Children of the Russian state: 1917–95*. Aldershot, UK: Avebury.
Haskell, L., & Randall, M. (2009). Disrupted attachments: A social context complex trauma framework and the lives of aboriginal peoples in Canada. *Journal of Aboriginal Health*, *5*, 48–99.
Khrushchev, N.S. (1956, February 15). Otchetnyi doklad Tsentral'nogo Komiteta Kommunisticheskoi Partii Sovetskogo Soyuza XX s'ezda partii. [Summary report of the Central Committee of the Communist Party of the Soviet Union to the XXth Party congress]. *Pravda*.
Kukuruza, A., Skrypka, N., Roshkovich, I., Kalandyak, O., Kryvonogova, O., Dobrova-Krol, N., & Bloemkolk, F. (2015). *Early childhood development and disability in Ukraine: Lessons learned and future recommendations*. Report prepared for Europe and Central Asia Region, Human Development Unit, World Bank.
Langmeier, J., & Matejeek, Z. (1984). *Psykhicheskaya deprivatsiya v detskom vozraste*. [Mental deprivation in childhood]. Prague, Czech Republic: Avizenum.

Lopatchenko, I. M. (2014). Sutnist socialnogo siritstva ta yogo profilaktika v derzhavnomu upravlinni. [The essence of social orphanhood and its prevention in the state policy]. *Teoriya ta Praktika Derzhavnogo Upravlinnya, 45*, 1–9.

Lunacharsky, A. V. (1991). Rech na Vserossiyskoy konferentsii detdomov, 15–20 noyabrya 1927 g. [Speech at the All-Russian Conference of the Children's Homes. November 15–20, 1927]. In Hrestomatiya (Ed.), *Lishennie roditelskogo popechitelstva* (pp. 51–54). Moskva, Russia: Prosveschenie.

Maercker, A., & Hecker, T. (2016). Broadening perspectives on trauma and recovery: A socio-interpersonal view of PTSD. *European Journal of Psychotraumatology, 7*, 29303. doi:10.3402/ejpt.v7.29303.

Magocsi, R. (2010). *A history of Ukraine: The land and its people*. Toronto, Canada: University of Toronto.

Mathews, E., Rosenthal, E., Ahern, L. & Kurylo, H. (2015). *No way home: The exploitation and abuse of children in Ukraine's orphanages*. Report by Disability Rights International. Retrieved July 12, 2016, from http://www.bettercarenetwork.org/sites/default/files/No%20Way%20Home%20-%20The%20Exploitation%20and%20Abuse%20of%20Children%20in%20Ukraine's%20Orphanages.pdf

McCall, R. B. (2013). The consequences of early institutionalization: Can institutions be improved? – Should they? *Child and Adolescent Mental Health, 18*, 193–201.

McKenzie, R. B. (1996). *The home: A memoir of growing up in an orphanage*. New York, NY: Basic Books.

Miller, L. C. (2005). The handbook of international adoption medicine. In *A guide for physicians, parents, and providers*. Oxford, UK: Oxford University Press.

Miller, L. C., Chan, W., Litvinova, A., Rubin, A., Tirella, L., & Cermak, S. (2007). Medical diagnoses and growth of children residing in Russian orphanages. *Acta Paediatrica, 96*, 1765–1769.

Nelson, C., Zeanah, C. H., Fox, N. A., Marshall, P. J., Smyke, A. T., & Guthrie, D. (2007). Cognitive recovery in socially deprived young children: The Bucharest Early Intervention Project. *Science, 318*, 1937–1940.

Oslon, V. N., & Holmogorova, A. B. (2001). Zameschauschaya professionalnaya semya kak odna is modeley resheniya problemi sirotstva v Rossii. [Professional foster family as one of the solutions of the problem of orphanhood in Russia]. *Voprosi psikhologii, 3*, 79–90.

Pullan, B. (1989). *Orphans and foundlings in early Modern Europe: The Stenton Lecture 1988*. Reading, UK: University of Reading.

Ransel, D. R. (1988). *Mothers of misery: Child abandonment in Russia*. Princeton, NJ: Princeton University Press.

Rutter, M., Kumsta, R., Schlotz, W., & Sonuga-Barke, E. (2012). Longitudinal studies using a "natural experiment" design: The case of adoptees from Romanian institutions. *Journal of the American Academy of Child & Adolescent Psychiatry, 51*(8), 762–770.

Rutter, M., O'Connor, T. G., & The English and Romanian Adoptees (ERA) Study Team. (2004). Are there biological programming effects for psychological development? Findings from a study of Romanian adoptees. *Developmental Psychology, 40*, 81–94.

Sagi-Schwartz, A., Van IJzendoorn, M. H., & Bakermans-Kranenburg, M. J. (2008). Does intergenerational transmission of trauma skip a generation? No meta-analytic evidence for tertiary traumatization with third generation of Holocaust survivors. *Attachment & Human Development, 10*, 105–121. doi:10.1080/14616730802113661.

Seelye, K. Q. (1997, December 20). Orphanage revival gains ground. *The New York Times*, p. 8.

Shamai, M. (2016). *Systemic interventions for collective and national trauma: Theory, practice and evaluation*. New York, NY: Routledge.

Shao Chuan, L. (1989). *Changes in China: Party, state and society*. Lanham, MD: University Press of America.

Sidorenko, O. (2013). Socialno-psychologichniy portret vypisknikiv internatnih zakladiv. [Psychosocial portrait of the graduates of residential care institutions]. *Teoretichni i Prikladni Pproblemi Psychologii, 3*, 248–255.

Stolee, M. K. (1988). Homeless children in the USSR, 1917–1957. *Soviet Studies, 40*, 64–83.

The President's Commissioner for Children's Rights. (2013). *Zvit pro zdiysnennya Upovnovazhenym Prezydenta Ukrayiny z prav dytyny monitorynhovoho doslidzhennya stanu funktsionuvannya zakladiv dlya ditey-syrit ta ditey, pozbavlenykh bat'kivs'koho pikluvannya, ditey, yaki ne mayut' neobkhidnykh umov dlya vykhovannya ta navchannya v sim"yi, ditey z osoblyvymy potrebamy, efektyvnist' vykorystannya takymy zakladamy byudzhetnykh koshtiv, spryamovanykh na zabezpechennya yikh diyal'nosti.* [Report on the implementation of the President of Ukraine Commissioner for Children's Rights Monitoring study of the functioning of institutions for orphans and children deprived of parental care, children who do not have the necessary conditions for education and training to families of children with special needs, the effectiveness of such establishments the budget aimed at ensuring their activities]. Retrieved July 20, 2016, from http://sirotstvy.net/upload/iblock/ced/cedc372c32a73ce1ef14c8b25cdb44e0.pdf

The Presidential Commissioner for Children's Rights. (2016). *Monitoringove doslidzhennya funkzionuvannya systemi internatnih zakladiv ta zakladiv sozialnogo zahisty ditey.* [Monitoring study of functioning of the system of institutional care and social protection of children]. Retrieved July 28, 2016, from http://www.president.gov.ua/storage/j-files-storage/00/19/29/17d0ed24dde1279b11273ebe4f05d0ed_1455184778.pdf

Tobis, D. (2000). *Moving from residential institutions to community-based services in Eastern Europe and the former Soviet Union*. Washington, DC: The World Bank.

Ukrainian Institute of Social Studies. (2001). *Causes of institutionalization of young people leaving public care and their future prospects*. Kiev, Ukraine: UNICEF.

UNAIDS. (2007). *Children and AIDS: A stocktaking report*. Retrieved February 15, 2008, from http://data.unaids.org/pub/Report/2007/20060116_stocktaking_report.pdf

UNAIDS. (2015). *Ukraine: Country Progress Report*. Retrieved August 17, 2016, from http://www.unaids.org/sites/default/files/country/documents/UKR_narrative_report_2015.pdf

UNICEF. (2010). *Child poverty and disparities in Ukraine*. Ukrainian Centre for Social Reforms: Kiev, Ukraine.

UNICEF. (2012). *Children under the age of three in formal care in Eastern Europe and Central Asia: A rights-based regional situation analysis*. Geneva, Switzerland: UNICEF.

UNICEF. (2015). *Situation analysis of children in Ukraine*. Kiev, Ukraine: UNICEF.

United Nations Office of the High Commissioner Human Rights. (2012). *The rights of vulnerable children under the age of three: Ending their placement in institutional care*. Geneva, Switzerland: OHCHR. Retrieved from http://www.europe.ohchr.org/Documents/Publications/Children_under_3__webversion.pdf

Van IJzendoorn, M. (2008). *Opvoeding over de grens. Gehechtheid, trauma en veerkracht.* [Parenting across borders. Attachment, trauma and resilience]. Amsterdam, Netherlands: Boom Academic.

Van IJzendoorn, M. H., Bakermans-Kranenburg, M. J., & Sagi-Schwartz, A. (2003). Are children of Holocaust survivors less well-adapted? A meta-analytic investigation of secondary traumatization. *Journal of Traumatic Stress, 16*, 459–469.

Verkhovna Rada. (2006). *Pro Holodomor 1932–1933 rokiv v Ukraini.* [On Holodomor in Ukraine in 1932–1933]. Law from 28.11.2006 No 376-V. Retrieved August 29, 2016, from http://zakon3.rada.gov.ua/laws/show/376-16?zahyst=4%2FUMfPEGznhhAMY.Zi691C5hHI4ags80msh8Ie6

Whetten, K., Ostermann, J., Whetten, R. A., Pence, B. W., O'Donnell, K., Messer, L. C., …, The Positive Outcomes for Orphans (POFO) Research Team. (2009). A comparison of the wellbeing of orphans and abandoned children ages 6–12 in institutional and community-based care settings in 5 less wealthy nations. *PLoS One, 4(12)*, e8169. doi:10.1371/journal.pone.0008169.

World Bank. (2009). *An avoidable tragedy: Combating Ukraine's health crisis, lessons from Europe.* Health and demography series. Kyiv: World Bank.

Chapter 12
Divergent Developmental Pathways of Children and Adolescents Reared in Long-Term Residential Protective Care in Turkey

Nese Erol, Zeynep Simsek, Abdullah Oskay, and Kerim Münir

We are half of an apple
the other half is our huge world
We are half of an apple
the other half is mankind
You are half of an apple
I am the other half
you and me!

(Nazim Hikmet, 1949)

1 Introduction

Despite remarkable progress in reducing childhood mortality globally, the majority of the estimated number of 41,000 homicide deaths involving children and adolescents 15 years of age and under is related to abuse and neglect. This figure includes

N. Erol (✉)
Department of Child & Adolescent Psychiatry, School of Medicine, Ankara University, Ankara, Turkey
e-mail: erol@medicine.ankara.edu.tr; profdrnese.erol@gmail.com

Z. Simsek
Faculty of Health Sciences, Istanbul Bilgi University, Istanbul, Turkey
e-mail: zeynep.simsek9@gmail.com

A. Oskay
Hayat Sende Association for Children Under Legal Protection, Ankara, Turkey
e-mail: abdullahoskay@gmail.com

K. Münir
Division of Developmental Medicine and Department of Psychiatry, Boston Children's Hospital, Harvard Medical School, Boston, MA, USA
e-mail: kerim.munir@childrens.harvard.edu

A.V. Rus et al. (eds.), *Child Maltreatment in Residential Care*,
DOI 10.1007/978-3-319-57990-0_12

all types of physical and/or emotional ill-treatment, sexual abuse, neglect which results in potential harm to the victims' survival, as well as growth and development (WHO, 2016). To date, research shows that the effects of abuse and neglect during childhood years cascade throughout the lifespan, with costly consequences not only for affected individuals and their families but also for their communities and for society at large.

Children's experiences of long-term consequences of such adverse exposures vary significantly, depending on the severity, chronicity, and timing of abuse or neglect, as well as the salient protective factors present in their lives. Studies have examined several psychosocial and environmental stressors for child abuse and neglect. They include poverty, physical/mental health problems of a family member, deficient parenting skills, violence, single parent status, having a nonbiological parent, hyperresponsiveness to child-related stimuli, unrealistic expectations of children, poor stress management, low social supports, and social isolation (Finkelhor, 1994; Kessler et al., 1997).

Children and adolescents abandoned by their families and reared in long-term residential protective care institutions can in turn be exposed to varying degrees of neglectful and abusive practices and living conditions that also contribute to their psychological and physical ill-health. This is a fundamental concern since residential protective care is also viewed as a remedy but more often itself serves as a major contributory cause of the persistence of childhood neglect and abuse. Converging evidence from research and human rights analyses categorically cannot condone national policies that permit parents to surrender their offspring to institutional care. A policy of institutional protective care of children facing adversity therefore cannot be consistent with the standard of the best interests of the child nor can it be concordant with the child rights principle inherent in Article 3 of the Declaration of the United Nations Convention on the Rights of the Child (Beckett, Bredenkamp, Castle, & ERA, 2002; Cicchetti & Toth, 2000; Erol et al., 2004, 2005, 2007, 2008; Erol and Şimşek 2007, 2008; Goldfarb, 1943; Keil & Price, 2006; MacLean, 2003; Roy, Rutter, & Pickles, 2000; Spitz, 1945; Tizard & Hodges, 1978; UNHR, 1990; Vorria, Rutter, Pickles, Wolkind, & Hobsbaum, 1998; Wolff & Fesseha, 1998; Yörükoğlu, 2003).

Many parents and families living in low- and middle-income countries (LMICs) continue to struggle to cope with rapid social change. They face great disparities in education and income, as well as social crises such as displacement and migration that in turn contribute to family disruption, mental illness, and exposure to violence and terrorism. These salient factors lead to children and adolescents being more likely to be placed in institutional care due to parental burden and abandonment, as well as exposure to specific abuse or neglect. Although research has highlighted the negative impact of institutional care on infant, child, adolescent, as well as adult life, there has been a rather slow paradigm shift from institutional- to family-based care systems in LMICs.

2 History of Child Welfare System in Turkey

The services available for children and adolescents under protection in Turkey have a unique history dating back to 1863 with the provision of humanitarian care, housing, nutrition, education, and vocational training of orphaned youth introduced by the governor of Niş, Mithat Pasha. The "Darülaceze" administration was opened in Istanbul in 1886 to care for a range of needs and problems of orphaned youth after the Russian–Ottoman War (1877–78). The population of Turkey at this time was 10 million. As the orphanage movement grew rapidly and solutions offered based on volunteerism did not prove to be sufficiently effective, state-based institutions were eventually established. The first example of such institutions was "Darülhayr-ı Ali" (1903–09) which looked after about 400 children. Later on "Darü'l Eytam's" (orphanages) were founded in 1914 to care for as well as educate the orphaned youth of the Balkan Wars and World War I. These institutions served approximately 16,000 children and adolescents in the Ottoman Empire. "Darülhayr-ı Ali" and "Darü'l Eytam's" were replaced by "Himaye-i Etfal Cemiyeti," meaning Child Protection Agency in Istanbul. The aims of this agency included the care and education of children in general, their protection from addictions, organization of recreational activities for them, and provision of opportunities for play and socialization. In 1917 Children's Guest Houses were opened for the children gathered from the World War I zones, and these homes provided care and protection for 2027 children between 1917 and 1922. An underlying premise of these humanitarian foundations was a sense of regard for the children as being the offspring of martyrs who served the country and who therefore deserved to be cared for with dignity and respect. The Child Protection Agency carried out two main services. First, it established a house to give children vocational training in farming. Second, it offered mother-infant health services, free of charge, in various cities (Cavusoglu & Acar, 2004; Erol et al., 2005).

A branch of the Child Protection Agency was founded in Ankara in 1921, and the agency continued establishing a nationwide organizational network to provide services for mothers and children under the auspices of the newly founded Republic of Turkey in 1923, with a population of 13 million citizens at the time of founding. The agency took on the formal status of a public welfare foundation under the name of Turkish Child Protection Agency (Turkiye Cocuk Esirgeme Kurumu) in 1937. The aims of the Turkish Child Protection Agency included a broad range of activities: establishing children's homes and orphanages; providing food, clothing, and financial aid for the children of low-income families; supporting the education of poor children; placing foster children in families; paying and supervising foster families; supplying job opportunities for children capable of working; providing childbirth services; paying the health expenses of orphans; and building play grounds. The agency housed infants and preschoolers in foundations called "Mother's Lap." When the residents of these foundations reached 7 years of age, they were transferred to boarding schools. As the numbers housed by these foundations outgrew their capacity in 1930, some orphans were placed in poor families who were allocated supportive payments. With the closure of boarding schools in 1931 in cities, older children began to be housed in Mother's Lap foundations that led to overcrowding. The services were later consolidated under the Children's Homes, Compassion Homes, and Orphanages (residential care houses) in 1939 at which time the national population reached 17 million (Cavusoglu & Acar, 2004; Erol et al., 2005).

Following a long interval of status quo, the Turkish Child Protection Agency was faced with severe financial difficulties following the coup d'etat in 1980. It was closed down in 1981 by an act of the National Security Board, and all its responsibilities were handed over to the Ministry of Health and Social Support. In 1983 the Social Services and Child Protection Administration (Sosyal Hizmetler ve Çocuk Esirgeme Kurumu-SHCEK) became a state-based organ under the authority of the Ministry of Health and Social Support with the population of the country reaching 48 million citizens (Cavusoglu & Acar, 2004; Erol et al., 2005).

Since 1991, the SHCEK has been directly governed under the Prime Ministry. Until recently, the primary mission of the child protection system in Turkey was residential care in crowded orphanages. According to the 2000 census, the national population had reached 65 million, and 38.4% of the Turkish population was aged 18 years and under. As per records of the Turkish Social Services General Directorate in December 2005, there were approximately 20,000 children and adolescents in the age group 0–18 years living under orphanage care (General Directorate of Social Services, 2005). About 92% of these youngsters were placed in institutions, 4% in foster care, and a small number were adopted, often by extended family (Simsek et al., 2007). In lieu of the lack of foster care and adoption services as a matter of social policy, the reasons for the increasing number of children being placed in institutional care in Turkey included the continuing financial inability of parents to care for their children and/or lack thereof of parenting skills to care for them, parental unwillingness to rear children with frank disabilities, and loss of parental rights because of abuse and/or neglect. The orphanages also represented a form of local employment and have been bureaucratically maintained. In 2005, Erol and colleagues reported the presence of 95 orphanages for children (0–12 years) and 107 for youth (13–18 years). Abuse and neglect therefore was considered as an important reason among others, for institutional care, with the institutional "culture" primarily concerned with the physical care of children and youth.

3 Inception of Research and Educational Activities Highlighting the Need for Change

A series of evidence-based studies began to identify the prevalence and predictors of emotional and behavioral problems reported among institutionally reared children and adolescents in Turkish orphanages compared with community controls

(Erol et al., 2005, 2010; Şimşek et al., 2007). Ankara University School of Medicine Child Psychiatry Department sponsored symposia and highlighted related publications that served to introduce the fundamentals of evidence-based practice and alternative models to institutional care, highlighting the identification of reactive attachment difficulties, as well as emotional and behavioral disorders in children and youth reared in institutional care. These activities also coincided with the ongoing work at this time under the auspices of the National Mental Health Policy in the aftermath of the Marmara earthquakes (Munir et al., 2004) that led to a heightened interest as well as political will in developing community-based and family-oriented primary mental health services across the country's 81 provinces with the support of the Ministry of Health (Munir et al., 2006).

The symposium on children under state protection (2004) held in Ankara further catalyzed interest in the plight of children under protective care. The Ankara University School of Medicine compiled a book that summarized the related research activities in the Department of Child Psychiatry on effects of institutional care on children and adolescents, as well as the psychological well-being and attachment issues among adult subjects who were faced with rearing children of their own conceived while under institutional care (Erol et al., 2005). During this period, the key Turkish investigators participated in the Fogarty International Center/National Institute of Mental Health-sponsored D43 research and education program at the Boston Children's Hospital under various opportunities to learn about organizational and educational aspects of family-oriented protective childcare and mental health services in the United States. In 2005, the Foster Care and Adoption Association and Infant Mental Health Association established in Turkey provided university-based researchers, advocates, and families a medium to regularly address issues of common interest related to clinical services as well as social and economic problems faced by families adopting and fostering children. During the subsequent decade, an important groundwork was established. By 2015, the success stories and voices of foster and adoptive parents as well as the children and youth that had been reared in the orphanages began to be heard all over the country, highlighted by various television, newspaper, and social media outlets. The parent groups were particularly empowered to share their problems on social media. The national population by that time had reached 80 million citizens.

An epidemiological study undertaken by the General Directorate of Family and Social Services and the Turkish Statistical Institute regarding family life that collected data on 12,280 households with a total of 24,647 persons, 18 years and older, was a key threshold. The results showed that 82.8 percent of the participants were not aware of foster care practice (Gurcan, 2008).

These activities led to the National Foster Care, Adoption and Mental Health Symposium held in Ankara/Turkey in 2007 with the participation of professionals, advocates, members of Family and Social Policies Ministry, as well as families and children. An important result of this meeting was the impetus for the establishment of volunteer "ambassadors" in the provinces promoting the formation of provincial foster family networks.

Based on the dissemination of the various cross-sectional and clinical research findings on the psychosocial, emotional, and behavioral effects of institutional care, national scientific and advocacy symposiums and family meetings were launched with increasing media interest. This led to the formation of the governmental initiatives on “Reuniting of Children with Their Families” and the “Support Within the Family” both with goals to reduce the number of children living in institutional care and increase their inclusion within their families. These programs had a particular emphasis at the outset on children 3 years of age and under. Increased socioeconomic support for vulnerable families and children, as well as social protection services, would provide families opportunities to remain intact, consistent with the UNICEF message (UNICEF, 2015).

4 Shift from Institutional to Family-Based Care

Turkey has witnessed an important policy shift from institutional to family-based care as a result of renewed socioeconomic policies and the development of foster care nationally through convergence of evidence-based research, increased awareness, and national advocacy. In less than a year (from 2012 to 2013) the number of children under 3 years of age housed in institutions was substantively reduced. Figure 12.1 present care data between 2011 and 2015 by the Ministry of Family and Social Policies. As noted in these figures, large institutional care was decreased through rapid systemic change, including a policy of reunification with biological parents with allocation of economic benefits, and transition to residential care in smaller settings, children’s homes, as well as foster care (Ministry of Family and Social Policies, 2016).

More recently the goal of the Ministry of the Family and Social Policies has been to further improve aspects of the current child welfare system in Turkey, by strengthening families and promoting foster care and adoption services nationally and by

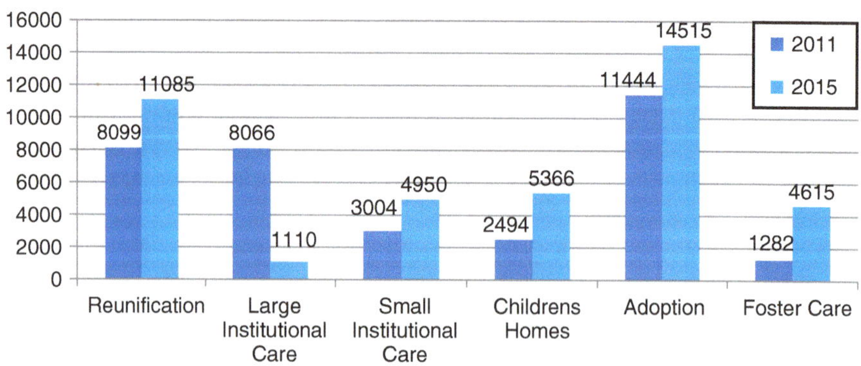

Fig. 12.1 Number of children under state protection models in 2011 and 2015

enhancing training of child welfare staff and foster parents. The overarching objective is the establishment of safe and stable environments for children (Ministry of Family and Social Policies, 2016).

5 Risk and Protective Factors on Children's Development

5.1 Children 0–6 Years in Residential Care

Children's experiences of residential care vary enormously depending on factors such as biological, demographic (age, gender), family, residential characteristics, and social and cultural factors that contribute to a supportive climate. Infants and toddlers (0–3 years) in institutional care without positive and stable relationships particularly are at risk of harm in terms of reactive attachment disorder, insipient developmental delay, neural atrophy, and emergence of discrete mental disorders across their lifespan (NSPCC, 2016; Yağmurlu et al., 2005). The neglect and damage caused by early deprivation can be considered equivalent to violence (Browne et al., 2005).

Figure 12.2 compares children, 0–6 years (mean age 34 months), living in institutional care (n = 154) with community control children within biological families (n = 286; mean age in each group 34 months), with equal gender distribution. Their development was assessed using the Ankara Development Screening Inventory (Savasır et al., 1998).

These young children in institutional care were four times more likely than controls to have development delay in all subscales (see Fig. 12.3) as well as deficits in terms of their sense of basic trust and severe attachment disturbances. The children in institutional care were notably deprived of responsive caregiving including limitations in eye contact and physical touch (Erol, 2004).

This is consistent with findings by Schore (2001) that both child abuse and neglect generate a high level of stress that is pathogenetic to the immature brain, with neglect having an even greater devastating effect on development than the former. Indeed, most of the problems were a natural consequence of being brought up in overcrowded care without any opportunities for forming selective attachments which would help the children to feel special and enable them to develop consistent relationships and enable them to regulate their emotions on a developmental trajectory that would promote healthy cognitive, emotional, and social development. The children's inability to take care of any belongings and take others' possessions without asking for permission was likely related to the fact that none of them had any personal clothing items or toys. Hitting and shouting at peers and aggression seem to be associated with a compulsion to repeat their traumatic experiences by victimizing others.

Over the years, a significant part of the problem was the quality of the institutions throughout the country. The social climate and the environmental stimulation

Fig. 12.2 Gender distribution by residential care and biological family care (%)

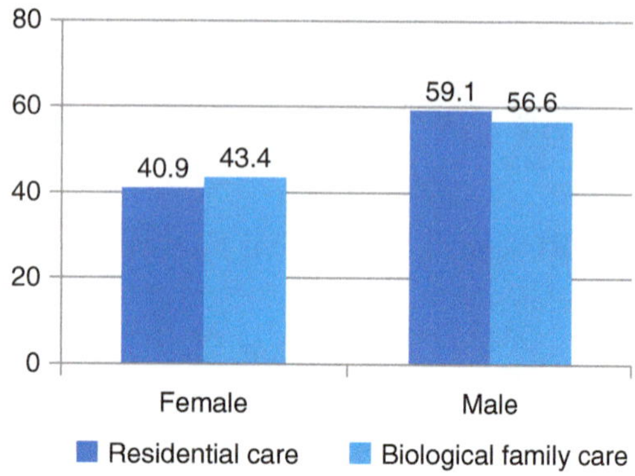

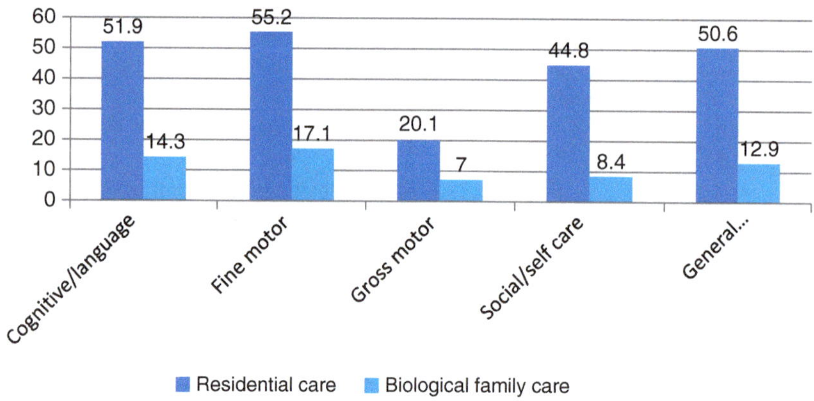

Fig. 12.3 Prevalence of developmental delay by residential vs. biological family care (%)

were directly insufficient, in particular with differential impact on the preschool age group. In an institutional-based pilot study in 2003, we observed that some of the 3–4-year-olds were unable to recognize their own photograph presented to them by asking, "Who is she/he?" They recognized each other and knew each other's names. We noted that there were no mirrors in the residence that children could use to see and recognize their own faces, since the mirrors used by staff were quite high for the children's height (Erol, 2004).

Vignette 1 and 2 presents the results of growing in institutional care, especially without one-to-one sensitive caregiver and child maltreatment from clinical cases of the first author.

Vignette 1

A 5-year-old boy reared in an institution and adopted when he was 4 years of age wanted to buy chewing gum to give to children residing there during his visit to the same institution. When the adoptive parents asked why he chose chewing gum and not cookies, he replied, "No one can take chewing gum from our mouths, it belongs to us and it never disappears or melts." When this example was presented to a young adult group reared in institutions, one of them noted, "We need to make sure that, like a chewing gum, we can find something that does not disappear, that belongs to us, I think that is love. When we were in the orphanage we needed something that is our own."

Vignette 2

Sara was emotionally, physically, and sexually abused by an uncle when she was 3 years and 7 months of age. At 4 years of age, after her medical treatment, she was referred to the Department of Child Psychiatry outpatient clinic at Ankara University by the residential care personnel for assessment of the impact of her traumas. Sara's mother had committed suicide by hanging; in her suicide note left for her husband, she specifically requested that her daughter be given to the care of her maternal grandmother. Sara's father was unable to take care of the kids and was living with his own mother in a village where there were no schools. Sara was therefore sent to her maternal grandmother. Sara's two older brothers were sent to a children's home under the Directorate of Family and Social Policy; her younger brother was given to kinship care. During her maternal grandmother's care, Sara was sexually abused by her maternal uncle and subsequently also emotionally and physically abused by her grandmother. She was thrown down the stairs and threatened to be dropped from a balcony in an attempt to murder her. Sara was saved by a neighbor's complaint to the authorities and rescued by the police. She was sent to a hospital where she required surgical treatment including a colostomy. Both her uncle and grandmother were tried by the court, found guilty, and jailed. Sara was adored by her doctors and nurses during her 3 months' hospital stay. She was discharged to a residential children's home; she shared a room with four other children. Residential care staff was not told of her story. Sara herself was never told clearly that her mother was dead but instead given explanations such as "she is in heaven" and that "she is an angel." Sara had differing caregiver staff in various locations at the children's home. Her caregivers were otherwise kind, warm, and loving. In one of her therapy visits at the university hospital clinic, Sara was asked to describe "Someone special that you can share your feelings with," she could not respond. In a play therapy session when Sara was presented with a figure that symbolized her uncle, she put it in the middle of the wild animal figures and stated, "These animals will prevent him from causing harm to other children." Sara continued in therapy with her psychologist; asked if she wanted anything at the end of summer vacation she added, "I would like to go on top of the wings of a ladybug and fly to be near you."

Ayaz et al. (2012) aimed to examine the prevalence of mental disorders in institutionalized children between the ages of 3–5 years. The authors investigated the factors associated with mental disorders and compared these findings with data from a community sample of children raised in their biological families in Kocaeli. Children were assessed using the DSM-IV-R diagnostic criteria, a sociodemographic form, and the Early Childhood Inventory. Results showed that children reared in institutional care had higher rates of mental disorders. Furthermore, the symptom severity of attention deficit hyperactivity disorder, reactive attachment disorder, oppositional defiant disorder, and pervasive developmental disorder (equivalent to autism spectrum disorder or subtypes) was higher than among the community sample. Age, time spent with father, duration of institutionalization, number of siblings, and number of hospital admissions because of physical symptoms and presence of abuse before institutional care were all determined to be predictive of psychiatric symptoms. Studies from across the world highlight the high prevalence of mental health problems among children in institutional care compared to those in the community. These studies also endorse that the mental health problems are a product of both the institutionalized children's experiences before care and the impact of living in the care system (Browne et al., 2005).

These findings are consistent with the observation that the quality of children's attachment relations is fundamental to their development and should be of primary concern to all those working with young children in general as well as those under care. Sensitive, stable relationships and placement stability are protective factors of mental health for children in care. For infants and young children under care, the impact of trauma, compounded by placement instability, places them at greater risk for mental health problems and other poor outcomes across their lifespan unless intervention is early and evidence based. Within the context of stable and supportive relationships, challenges such as meeting new people create healthy stress for young children that in turn forge good brain development. But "toxic stress" for young children caused by trauma, abuse, and neglect disrupt the architecture and chemistry of the brain (Shonkoff et al., 2012). The brain can become severely damaged in these early developmental stages under the influence of salient toxic exposures with lifelong consequences. Stable relationships really matter, but many children who are in care get moved from one placement to the next or returned to a home that cannot support them well. Significant adversity impairs development in the early years of life, and the more adversity a child faces, the greater the odds of a developmental delay with impairments in their emotional as well as adaptive and cognitive functioning. Risk factors associated with maltreatment have a cumulative impact with studies showing that children exposed to as many as six or more additional risks face a 90–100% likelihood of having one or more delays in their adaptive, cognitive, language, and/or emotional development (ION & NRC, 2014). Global developmental delay as well as borderline intellectual functioning is common in children who have been neglected with significant adaptive as well as cognitive functioning difficulties (Munir, 2016a, 2016b). Neglect and unhealthy stimulation, such as abuse, derail a child's development (Knudsen, 2004). Experiences of stability, loving attachments, and nurturing have an exceptional effect on the recovery of the developing brain. A stable and loving placement for a young child in care can undo neural damage caused by neglect. When infants and young children who have suffered neglect and abuse are placed with loving carers, with or without familiar family figures, they demonstrate healthy brain development that is comparable to peers not in care (Zeanah, 2000).

There is evidence that clinical treatment and service intervention approaches that promote resiliency through the parent-child relationship are the most effective vehicles to recovery from trauma because parental functioning predicts both child resiliency and child response to trauma. Berument (2005) aimed to develop an intervention program involving environmental enrichment and caregiver training to improve the language and cognitive development of infants and young children residing in institutional settings in Turkey. Results indicated that institutional care quality was significantly improved in the intervention institutions, but remained unchanged in the control institutions. Furthermore, while the cognitive and language developmental gap of infants and toddlers in the control group increased, the gap declined slightly for the infants and children in the intervention group. For the preschool age group, the general development scores in the intervention group increased, but those of the control group children decreased. The intervention program was therefore effective in increasing the care quality in orphanages and had a positive effect on the language and cognitive development of infants and preschoolers.

5.2 *Children 6–18 Years in Residential Care*

We examined the prevalence of emotional and behavioral problems and associated factors in children and adolescents aged 6–18 years in residential care compared with a nationally representative age-matched sample raised by their biological families (Erol & Simsek, 2000; Erol et al., 2010; Simsek et al., 2007, 2008). The study included 674 children and adolescents aged 6–18 years selected from the national Directorate's residential care centers ("orphanages") using a stratified probability cluster sampling. A sociodemographic information form and the ASEBA Child Behavior Checklists (CBCL), Teacher's Report Form (TRF), and Youth Self-Report (YSR) form were used for data collection (Achenbach & Rescorla, 2001; Dumenci et al., 2004). The mean ages of the youth were 14.6 ± 2.0 years in the institutionalized sample and 14.4 ± 2.1 years in the community care sample. There were no significant differences in the mean ages and gender distribution of the institutional and community care adolescents ($p > 0.05$). The mean admission age to the institutional unit was 90.3 ± 42.2 months (range 1–180 months). Among the institutional youth, 51.9% had lived with their parents, and 7.4% had lived with their relatives prior to admission to the institutional unit, with 34% having previously lived in other institutions prior to referral to the present facility.

About 72% of the children from a stable family background had been admitted to an orphanage unit primarily because of family disruption, parental separation, or divorce (71.7%), poverty (13.2%), 6.9% were abandoned baby, and 5.4% of the children were admitted because of physical or sexual abuse. In fact, 35.2% of the youth had gone through inter-institution transfers more than two times. Mean duration of institutional care was 39.8 ± 31.1 months (range 1–168 months). The majority of the children (74.8%) had been transferred between institutions. It was evident from data that children experience many placements and they were not receiving the support they needed for their success. Furthermore, repeated placements increased the likelihood of children developing multiple problems ultimately needing more intensive and high cost care.

Almost 68.9% of the children had a mother or father, or both. The presence of parental mental disorders was assessed from case records compiled at the time of the children's admission into the orphanage; 22.9% of the parents had a history of mental disorder. Nearly 70% of the children continued to have regular contact with their parents or close relatives, visiting them, spending vacations with them, or having telephone contact with them.

According to teacher interviews, 22.8 percent of orphanage staff reported any participation in school meetings. Table 12.1 presents the prevalence of problem behaviors by YSR, CBCL, and TRF for institutional and community care samples.

The total problems overall were higher by YSR than by caregiver/parent (CBCL) and teacher informants (TRF). The prevalence of total problems by youth, teacher, and caregiver/parent reports was 47%, 23.2%, and 18.3% institutional sample compared to 10.1%, 11%, and 9% community sample, respectively. All differences were significant at $p < 0.01$. The mean internalizing problems scores by youth, teacher, and caregiver/parent reports were 40.1%, 15.6%, 6.2% institutional sample compared to 11.5%, 8.9%, and 9.9% for the community sample, respectively. On externalizing problems, the mean scores by youth, teacher, and caregiver/parent reports were 41.9%, 22.7%, and 21.4% for institutional sample compared to 10.9%, 9.3%, and 6.9% for the community sample, respectively.

The youths in institutional care reported far more internalizing problems than evident by caregiver or teacher assessments. Raising awareness among caregivers and teachers of children's distress and how to identify warning signs of internalizing problems should be an important consideration in planning primary prevention as well as specialty mental healthcare treatment. In terms of utilization of specialty mental health services, even though the prevalence of problem behaviors was high among adolescents in institutional care, only 2.4% in fact received any specialty mental health services.

6 Predictors of Behavioral Problems

Protective factors related to family, intellectual capabilities, and social support were found to be significantly associated with the problem behaviors (Table 12.2). The results were consistent with those of previous studies that indicate risk of psychopathology to be lower among children who maintain contact with a parent or a parental figure, obtain social support within the orphanage, and/or improve their competence to effectively adapt, overcome challenges, and gain achievements (competent performance) within one or more domains in the orphanage (e.g., developmental, social competence, academic achievement) (Masten & Coatsworth, 1998; Rutter, 1990). Two other protective factors included regular contact between teachers and orphanage staff and appropriate task involvement such as sports and folk dances. There is now widespread agreement that effective collaboration between orphanage social care staff and school teachers at all levels is central to decreasing problems. For example, through close cooperation between orphanage staff and teachers,

Table 12.1 Prevalence of internalizing, externalizing, and total problems by residential care and community sample according to gender and age (%)

	Internalizing		Externalizing		Total problem	
	Residential care	Family	Residential care	Family	Residential care	Family
CBCL/6–18 (care givers/parents)						
Girls (6–11 aged)	7.0	9.4	18.8	5.1	19.5	8.7
Girls (12–18 aged)	7.3	14.4	19.7	3.9	14.6	7.1
Boys (6–11 aged)	6.1	7.0	27.3	10.8	21.8	11.9
Boys (12–18 aged)	3.6	8.9	16.7	7.4	15.5	7.9
Total	**6.2**	**9.9**	**21.4**	**6.9**	**18.3**	**9.0**
	$\chi^2 = 7.102$, $p = 0.001$ CRR = 0.6; 0.3–0.9 (95%)		$\chi^2 = 122.94$, $p = 0.001$ CRR = 3.7; 2.9–4.7 (95%)		$\chi^2 = 43.687$, $p = 0.001$ CRR = 2.3; 1.8–2.9 (95%)	
TRF/6–18						
Gils (6–11 aged)	12.1	10.9	20.6	5.9	17.8	8.6
Girls (12–18 aged)	23.7	10.6	15.3	4.5	23.7	5.8
Boys (6–11 aged)	13.3	8.6	32.8	12.5	29.7	14.4
Boys (12–18 aged)	9.6	5.3	19.2	11.3	17.3	13.1
Total	**15.6**	**8.9**	**22.7**	**9.3**	**23.2**	**11.0**
	$\chi^2 = 17.050$, $p = 0.001$ CRR = 1.7; 1.3–2.3 (95%)		$\chi^2 = 66.46$, $p = 0.001$ CRR = 2.5; 2.0–3.2 (95%)		$\chi^2 = 46.16$, $p = 0.001$ CRR = 2.1; 1.7–2.6 (95%)	
YSR/11–18						
Girls (11–15 aged)	38.3	10.1	40.7	9.7	49.6	9.4
Girls (16–18 aged)	47.4	13.8	28.6	11.7	50.0	12.0
Boys (11–15 aged)	33.3	10.6	42.9	9.8	42.0	9.3

(continued)

Table 12.1 (continued)

	Internalizing		Externalizing		Total problem	
	Residential care	Family	Residential care	Family	Residential care	Family
Boys (16–18 aged)	45.2	13.9	48.7	14.7	42.9	11.3
Total	**40.1**	**11.5**	**41.9**	**10.9**	**47.0**	**10.1**
	$\chi^2 = 46.706, p = 0.001$ CRR = 3.4; 2.9–4.1 (95%)		$\chi^2 = 119.48, p = 0.001$ CRR = 3.9; 3.2–4.6 (95%)		$\chi^2 = 310.21, p = 0.001$ CRR = 4.6; 3.9–5.5 (95%)	

CRR crude relative risk

Table 12.2 Results of multiple regression model explaining predictors for total problems score

Variables	*B*	*t*	*p*	95% *CI*
Age	−1.573	−2.374	0.018	(−2.87)–(−0.30)
Gender (male)	3.542	0.987	0.324	(−3.52)–(10.6)
Age at first admission	−.127	−2.397	0.017	(−.23)–(−.023)
Reason for admission (abuse)	18.001	2.266	0.024	(2.37)–(13.36)
Moves between orphanages	6.162	1.541	0.124	(1.71)–(14.03)
Died or unknown parents	5.970	1.396	0.164	(−2.45)–(14.32)
Regular contact with parents/relatives	−11.370	−2.478	0.014	(−20.2)–(−2.36)
Regular contact between teachers and orphanage staff	−12.87	−2.385	0.018	(−23.53)–(−2.22)
Appropriate task involvement	−20.83	−4.191	0.001	(−30.6)–(−11.02)
Positive characteristics of close friends	−9.628	−1.731	0.085	(−20.60)–(1.35)
Stigmatization	38.645	2.667	0.008	(9.06)–(11.23)
Fatalistic beliefs	14.672	2.997	0.002	(1.51)–(6.98)
Perceived social support	−14.73	−3.284	0.001	(−23.54)–(−5.91)
Total competencies	−4.109	−13.673	0.001	(−4.70)–(−3.52)

$R = .780$; $R^2 = .726$; $F = 6.642$; .001*; Durbin-Watson* = 1.912

difficulties can be identified at an earlier stage so that appropriate additional supports can be provided and the risk of psychopathology reduced (Erol et al., 2010; Simsek et al., 2008).

One of the factors we identified (Erol et al., 2010) included stigmatization with expressed negative attitudes toward the children because they lived in orphanage care – by peers at school as well as others in their social environment. This exerted an important adverse influence for the emergence of emotional and behavioral problems. Prior research also shows that stigmatization associated with mental illness adds to the public health burden of mental illness. Stigmatization leads to loss of social status and ensuing discrimination triggered by negative stereotypes about people labeled as abnormal (Link & Phelan, 2001). Such stigma impedes recovery by eroding the individual's social status, social networks, and self-esteem thus contributing to poor outcomes such as increased isolation, feelings of hopelessness, and psychological symptoms (Ritsher et al., 2003). It is inevitably very important for all social services staff to acknowledge that stigmatization and its associated prejudice are not only a rights violation but also are a real risk factor for the development of children and adolescents in orphanage care.

A possibility that children admitted for financial convenience and/or family disruption factors may have had less adverse experiences during their period of early family care was further examined. Thus, if their early family relationships were good, it might be expected that these youngsters would be more likely to maintain positive family ties during their period in institutions. With respect to this study question, we found that emotional abuse and neglect had a substantial negative effect on the emergence of emotional and behavioral problems in affected children. This finding is consistent with previous research documenting that maltreatment during childhood leads to higher incidence of physical, emotional, behavioral, as well as cognitive problems (Cicchetti & Toth, 2000; De Bellis, 2001; Manly, Kim, Rogosch, & Cicchetti, 2001).

Abuse and neglect of children may take many forms, from a lack of care for their physical needs, through a failure to provide consistent love and nurturance, to overt hostility and rejection. It is likely that children and adolescents in orphanage care were exposed to full range of such early experiences. As expected, the duration of institutional care was correlated with problem behaviors; the children who spent a longer period of time in institutional care exhibited higher severity of problem behaviors. This finding is also consistent with prior studies (Ames, 1997; Beckett et al., 2002; Fisher et al., 1997; Marcovitch et al., 1997).

Previous research has highlighted that having a parent with a mental disorder and associated psychosocial adversity and parenting problems frequently precede a child's admission to orphanage care (Quinton & Rutter, 1984). Nevertheless, our findings support Vorria and colleagues' (1998) observations that parental mental disorder was unrelated to any of the behavioral problems in children in this study. This may reflect the psychosocial adversity and parenting problems among these families that lead to institutionalization in Turkey, irrespective of any identifiable parental mental disorder.

The discontinuation of any orphanage care notwithstanding the results of this study had immediate ethical and practical implications for improvement of intervention conditions for children and adolescents who experience multiple forms of deprivation and who continue their care in orphanages. The identification of risk and protective factors regarding the emotional and behavioral health of children in orphanage care can directly assist social workers, psychologists, and other care staff in identifying essential priorities. The children and adolescents in orphanage care are clearly at risk for developing a variety of emotional and behavioral problems – i.e., it's not necessarily the conditions that precede their placement but the very nature of the care environment within such institutions that also contribute to poor mental health outcomes. For this reason, in order to eliminate the stigma and discrimination these youth face, there is a need for more intensive, multifaceted interventions, preferably including identified parents or relatives, other caregivers, including classroom teachers. We recommended that these involve the addition of parental training programs; encouragement of enhanced and regular contact between children and their families, relatives, and classroom teachers; social skills training and problem solving skills training programs; and increased supports for improving their competencies. This study identified the importance of including parents, caregivers, and classroom teachers in the prevention of youth mental health problems. The development of such methods will increase the efficacy of parents or relatives as team members in residential care settings as well as the implementation of required early interventions. Nonetheless, child welfare and social workers face multiple barriers as they attempt to include parents, teachers, and trusted caregivers as members of the care teams. In the absence of policies that eliminate institutional care, there is a need to promote innovative collaborations that include therapeutic recreation spaces, appropriate milieu activities, as well as parent-child support and school-child support groups.

The study also underscored the effects of fatalistic beliefs as being powerful predictors of adolescents' emotional and behavioral problems. Previous research also examined the effect of fatalism, the belief in external control over life chances, as a risk factor in particular for development of adolescent depression. The higher rate of self-reported internalizing problems in terms of affective, anxiety, and somatic concerns by adolescents support the hypothesis that the youth felt helpless over their life chances and control over their lives, otherwise externally unrecognized by key informants. It has been hypothesized that adolescents who demonstrate greater fatalism would be at higher risk for emotional and behavioral problems (Roberts et al., 2000). Erol and Sahin (1995) examined children's fears in terms of their age, gender, and socioeconomic characteristics using the "Fear Survey Schedule for Children (FSSC)." The most prevalent 10 fear items were examined: fears related to death and separation from parents had the highest rank, with religious fears (e.g., violating a religious edict, fear of hell and devil) mentioned often by children in the lower SES group.

Caman and Ozcebe (2011) aimed to assess the distribution of psychological symptoms and their association with the level of physical activity in adolescents living in orphanages in Ankara. Female gender, nonparticipation in school or work, dissatisfaction with school, lack of contact with family, chronic disease, chronic medication use, sleep problems, regular tobacco use, chronic disease in the family, and low quality of life were associated with increased risk for mental disorders. Adolescents who were physically active had a lower frequency of tobacco, alcohol, and other drug usage; lower depression scores; and higher quality of life scores than their less active counterparts.

The child welfare system, and policy makers as well as mental health practitioners should also ensure safe and stable social care environments for children and adolescents. In order to create high-quality safe environments and child-friendly care models at the policy level, the child welfare systems must scrutinize potential carers, organize training programs, evaluate care systems, maintain high standards of staff conduct, and provide the necessary support and advocates to strengthen children's rights and promote their well-being.

7 Reintegration Back into Families of Origin

We examined problem behaviors of 6–18-year-old youth who have been moved from institutions to their biological parents (n = 37) compared with age-matched youth in institutional care (n = 65) and those who stayed within families with governmental financial support (n = 81) (Sacan et al., 2014). A sociodemographic information form, CBCL, TRF, and YSR were used for data collection. The youth who had been moved from institutions to their biological families had higher problem scores than those who stayed within their biological families with governmental financial support as well as those who were in institutional care. A move out of institutional to biological family care, however desirable, requires adequate planning. Among biological families, 40.5% willingly accepted their children, and 24.3% were reluctant to do so. Among those youth who were reintegrated, 10.8% had to be returned back to institutional care. The youth, as well as their biological family caregivers, experienced significant reintegration difficulties if not sufficiently prepared and supported. The United Nations Convention on the Rights of the Child emphasizes the importance of child participation in decision-making process in matters affecting their life. Deinstitutionalization is not a one-way process but a complex dynamic developmental trajectory that entails managing ensuing change that affects the lives of children, as well as their families and other caregivers.

8 Foster Care and Adoption

Ustuner, Erol, and Simsek (2005) examined and compared the emotional and behavioral problems among children and adolescents aged 6–17 years reared in foster family care (n = 39) with similarly aged-matched control samples raised by biological parents (n = 62) and those reared in residential care (n = 62). A sociodemographic information form, CBCL, TRF, and YSR were used for data collection. According to the information provided by parents, caregivers, and teachers, the prevalence of problem behaviors was 9.7% based on parent reports, 12.9% based on foster family reports, and 43.5% based on caregiver reports in residential care. When the total problem scores were compared based on care systems, significantly higher total problem scores were obtained in youth in residential care ($p < 0.05$). However, no significant differences were found on the total problem scores for those in foster care compared with youth in biological families. Since the prevalence of mental health problems is particularly high among youth in residential care, in the absence of available integration in biological families, encouraging foster parenting and putting standards in place is likely to be highly beneficial. The training of foster families on mental health problems should therefore be an important priority.

Altınoglu-Dikmeer, Erol, and Gencoz (2014) examined emotional and behavioral problems associated with attachment security and parenting style in "adopted and nonadopted children" in Turkey. The study aimed to investigate and compare emotional and behavioral problems in Turkish adoptees and nonadopted peers raised by their biological parents. The study included 61 adopted children (34 females, 27 males) aged 6–18 years and 62 age- and gender-matched nonadopted children (35 females, 27 males). Parents rated their children's problem behaviors using the Child Behavior Checklist/6–18, temperament characteristics using the School Age Temperament Inventory, their own personality traits using the Basic Personality Traits Inventory, and their parenting styles using the Measure of Child Rearing Styles. Children rated their parents' availability and reliability as attachment figures using the Kerns Security Scale and parenting styles using the Measure of Child Rearing Styles. Adolescents aged 11–18 years self-rated their problem behaviors using the Youth Self-Report. Group differences and correlations were analyzed. Results showed that there were nonsignificant differences in all scale scores between the adopted and nonadopted groups. The age of the children at the time of adoption was not associated with problem behaviors or attachment relationships. On the other hand, the findings indicated that as the age at which the children learned they had been adopted increased, their emotional and behavioral problems increased. Thus, adoption alone could not explain the problem behaviors observed in the adopted children; the observed problem behaviors ought to be considered within the context of the developmental processes.

9 Adults Reared in Institutional Care

Ustun and Erol (2008) examined adults reared in residential care. The authors posited that growing up in an institution has negative outcomes both during childhood and adolescence and might have long lasting negative effects during adulthood. On the contrary, some studies had emphasized that institution-reared adults were not destined to experience high rates of adversity and that certain factors might promote resiliency. There was no previous study in Turkey directing attention to the outcomes of adults reared in institutions. Thus, the objectives of this study were to examine the emotional and behavioral problems, romantic adult attachment styles, traumatic experiences, and current stress level of adults reared in institutions compared to those reared in families. A total of 28 adults who had grown up in institutional care were compared to 28 matched family-reared subjects. The Demographic Information Form, Young Adult Self-Report (YASR) (18–59), Traumatic Stress Symptom Checklists, and Relationship Scales Questionnaire were used. The results showed that institution-reared adults reported experiencing significantly more past traumatic events, but no significant differences were found between family- and institution-reared adults in terms of current stress level, romantic attachment styles, and emotional and behavioral problems.

The findings could be explained by sampling characteristics. For instance, Stein (2008) proposed that three outcome groups can be identified among youth leaving care: "moving on," "survivors," and "victims." In this regard, consistency of relational stability and relational continuity with the biological family are important assets that ameliorate the stress experienced during the years spent in institutions and in adaptation to new challenges and responsibilities of adult life after leaving care.

In the Ustun and Erol (2008) study, 53.6% of institution-reared adults had positive feelings and thoughts about their institutions, whereas 42.9% of them had negative feelings and thoughts. Results were discussed considering the possible protective factors for the institution-reared adults that might help them to experience positive psychological outcomes such as having a certain job, a good education, and having friends. The risk of psychopathology might be lesser in children remaining in contact with a parent or a parental figure, obtaining social support, and improving their competencies in the orphanage (Masten & Coatsworth, 1998; Rutter, 1990). The results need to be interpreted in the context of such institutions in Turkey that may not be representative and generalizable across other settings.

Despite the Ustün and Erol (2008) study, in Turkey there remains no follow-up system for individuals leaving care; furthermore, no prior studies reported on how people cope after discharge. Additional studies are needed both to replicate the results with larger sample sizes and in order to provide assessment of the institution-reared adults with different levels of social and psychological functioning.

Nonetheless, the issues underlined herein are not confined to Turkey but represent a global concern affecting millions of youth facing abandonment, homelessness, as well as threatening and dangerous living conditions. The transition across the lifespan to adulthood and to parenthood presents ongoing challenges for these individuals. There is a need for global research collaborations in unique LMIC contexts to understand and address various conditions and trajectories facing youth in institutional care.

10 Examples of Interventions

Primary interventions should be focused on prevention of early marriages, planned and safe parenthood programs by primary health and social care services, and infant-toddler-preschool child- and youth-focused collaborative programs with participation of relevant ministries, universities, and NGOs. Secondary and tertiary preventions should be focused on alternative family-based models such as foster care and adoption and creating aftercare programs aimed at preventing maltreatment and increasing the resiliency of these individuals.

10.1 Promotion of Children's Early Psychosocial Development Through Primary Healthcare Services

Preventive action with emphasis on the psychosocial health of the children is of great importance and falls within the priorities set by the World Health Organization, especially since the adoption by the member states of the "Health for All by the year

2000" program and the evaluation of its goals. The program had been implemented with collaboration of Ministry of Health, Primary Health Care General Directorate Mental Health Department, Ankara University School of Medicine Child Psychiatry Department, and World Health Organization in Turkey. The pilot study was started in 1992. After this implementation, it had been conducted in nine provinces between 1995 and 1999. The aim of the program was to develop training for primary health-care workers (PHCWs) to improve their ability to assess factors relevant to children's psychological development and to provide preventive approaches to foster their development, building on family strengths. The focus was on the period from pregnancy to the end of the children's second year of life. The program has been evaluated in terms of (a) its impact in terms of training on both the PHCWs' knowledge and attitudes with regard to infant behavior and development and on PHCWs' use of a semi-structured interview and (b) the effect of the intervention on maternal well-being, infant language development and behavior, home environment, and mother-infant interactions (Erol, Şimşek, & Ertem, 1997). This model is now disseminated through a train-the-trainer model in Turkey within the Ministry of Health.

10.2 Let's Break the Social Walls Project

Let's Break the Social Walls project was implemented by the Hayat Sende Gençlik Akademisi ("Life Is Yours" Hayat Sende Youth Academy) established in 2007 by the youth leaving institutional care by the first and third authors. The project was conducted from September 2013 through April 2014 with the support of the Sabancı Foundation Social Development Grant Program. The project's aim was to remove any negative labels in the media usage with the implementation of "Correct Dictionary" in reference to youth in institutional care, with promotion of usage of positive words that could reduce prejudice and increase acceptance among public attitudes. The academy launched a comprehensive communication campaign to address prejudices toward youth in state institutions with outreach to 30,000 people through presentations through formal and social media channels. To enhance project awareness, additional events were organized including bicycle and skate tours in the capital Ankara. Accompanying press releases were issued to publicize the events and to provide a media message to emphasize "No to labelling in any aspect of life" and "Not to aide but share in success!"

10.3 Education Without Stigma Project

The Sabanci Foundation project also analyzed the challenges confronting youth under state protective care with an innovative "Education Without Stigma" project that targeted the education system in Turkey. This program was implemented between 2014 and 2015 by the Hayat Sende Youth Academy along with project partners (Agenda Child Organisation, Teacher Academy Foundation, Ankara, Istanbul, and Denizli Foster Family Association). The overall aim of the Education Without Stigma project was to keep the youth living in protective care included in the formal education system in Turkey, to evaluate struggles regarding stigma in areas of education and training, to study the problems, and to look for possible solutions. An overarching goal was to increase participation in education with a contribution by all shareholders in order to fight against stigma. The program also enhanced the youth's access to their rights and educational services especially with teachers working in the field. Topics of discussion in training sessions included ethical principles on social inclusion and distributive justice, as well as specific capacity building regarding attachment awareness, effects of neglect and abuse, as well as frequent moves between orphanages and schools. The project included an initial literature review on stigma and social inclusion, followed by series of focus groups that included youth raised under state protection, field case workers in the child protective system in Turkey, adoptive and foster families, and teachers as well as school personnel. The project emphasized building empathy; use of media as a tool to enhance public awareness; addition of new courses in the curriculum to improve access and social participation of youth reared under protective care, thus bringing them into the forefront and making them visible to raise their voice, guiding them to reach a helping hand in solving problems; encouraging volunteerism; role modeling; and building advocacy to achieve "education without stigma" in Turkish society. The program reached 1200 teachers and was adopted by the Ministry of Education to be implemented nationwide.

10.4 Project Pomegranate Arils

The Project Pomegranate Arils was initiated in 2009 with the cooperation of the Ministry of Family and Social Policies and Boyner Holding and its subsidiaries and with the support of the United Nations Population Fund, the General Directorate of Child Services, and the Human Management Association of Turkey. In 2013, the initiative was continued through collaboration with the Family Health and Planning Foundation of Turkey (TAPV). The project objective was to provide support to young women aged 18–24, who were raised in orphanages and subjected to social and economic exclusion: in order for them to continue their education, bolster their personal development, and prepare for the job market by improving job-seeking skills. From 2009 through 2012, 162 young women from across Turkey completed a two-week educational program and received a year of mentorship support. A group of mentors provided the women with social and economic guidance and helped them in overcoming problems associated with gender discrimination. Some 51% of the young women who participated in the project became employed, 33% continued their education, and 16% are active job seekers.

11 Implications for Improving Children's Care

Persons reared in institutional care settings face a challenging journey. Although Turkey is no exception, the country has clearly made significant strides in recent years to help children, adolescents, and adults to overcome otherwise permanent obstacles that have long hindered their optimal development and participation in society. The activities described in this chapter provide an encouraging repertoire of interdisciplinary, collaborative, evidence-based efforts with ensuing important public policy and attitudinal changes. This is an example where evidence-based work has provided an important impetus for development of partnerships across health-care, social protection, and education sectors. A key achievement has been the development of adoption and foster care networks both nationally and provincially. Our initial research had focused on understanding of the epidemiological dimensions of the problem of institutionally reared persons including the operant risk and protective factors. We subsequently have moved on to building a developmentally informed preventive strategy to increase awareness, improve screening and early diagnosis, and provide interventions in order to reduce the adaptive, cognitive, emotional, and behavioral burdens faced by institutionally reared persons. The lifespan perspective and partnership between social welfare and primary care services (in terms of both psychosocial and physical care) has also been a major accomplishment.

Additionally, the work of the mental health Gap Action Plan (mhGAP) by the World Health Organization has made important contributions globally in scaling up tangible evidence-based interventions in LMICs. The mhGAP is currently increasingly emphasizing child and adolescent mental health as well as child development perspectives as major approaches. In the absence of family and community-centered services that are urgently needed, caregiver training and support remain a critical future step. Preventive mental health interventions that improve problem solving skills and decrease fatalistic beliefs among adolescents reared in institutional care are important nodal points given their protective effects. Both tobacco and alcohol use were additional negative predictors of mental health in particular among adolescents reared in institutional care. Our results support research findings that suggest that substance use and dependence are associated with behavioral problems; this finding holds true for both high-income and low- and middle-income settings. Further, importance of proximal relationships with parents/parental figures in mitigating the impact of abuse and neglect and occurrence of cognitive, emotional, behavioral, as well as physical problems cannot be understated.

Finally, the work on child protective services and transition from institutional to family care services in Turkey has had a unifying effect at the operational level between various governmental agencies, universities, and NGOs and has led to increased awareness and policy changes that take into consideration not only the primary prevention of abuse and neglect but also an appreciation of the negative impact of institutional care, as the problem, and not the solution.

We propose the following recommendations for improving children's care under protective services:

Primary Prevention Measures

- Elimination of poverty
- Prevention of early marriages
- Provision of comprehensive family planning, as well as pre- and postnatal and maternal child health services
- Support teams comprised of midwifery, nursing, psychology, and social services with enhanced training in prevention of abuse and neglect as well as identification of risk of child abandonment
- In the absence of biological parents, identification of family members/relatives to enable the children's sense of belonging within their communities

Secondary Prevention Measures

- Provision of professional community-based family care protective models including foster and adoption services under circumstances where the children's reunification with their biological families is neither feasible nor warranted.
- Provision of residential children's home services with explicit measures to support their socialization and community integration when foster and adoption services may not be available.

Tertiary Prevention Measures

- Implementation of care standards in residential children's home services with continuous oversight of children's physical, psychological, and social well-being in the context of identified risk factors.
- Early identification of attachment, cognition, emotion, and behavior problems and concurrent monitoring of children's psychological and physical well-being with access to appropriate referral and evidence-based interventions.
- Attention to children's individual developmental characteristics as well as areas of need for provision of personalized care and inclusiveness of children as much as possible in their care decisions.

Questions for Discussion

1. In addressing problems of abuse and neglect of children, how can we organize a well-coordinated community-based approach promoting their engagement in safe, stable, nurturing, and stimulating family life and "home" environments?
2. How can we strengthen child protection models based on innovative epidemiological evidence-based perspectives in effecting public social policy change?
3. What kind of positive and culturally informed strategies, awareness campaigns, can be implemented to ensure the adoption of evidence-based models in child protection services by professionals beyond social services and healthcare, including education, law, as well as by communities and society at large? How can such ethical, sociocultural values be nurtured?

Acknowledgments We gratefully acknowledge, in part, the support of the Fogarty International Center and National Institute of Mental Health/NIH (grants D43TW005807 and D43TW009680 at Boston Children's Hospital) at various phases of the work and preparation of manuscript (NE, ZS, KM).

References

Achenbach, T. M., & Rescorla, L. A. (2001). *Manual for the ASEBA school-age forms & profiles*. Burlington, VT: University of Vermont, Research Center for Children, Youth, and Families.

Altınoğlu-Dikmeer, I., Erol, N., & Gençöz, T. (2014). Emotional and behavioral problems associated with attachment security and parenting style in adopted and non-adopted children. *Turk Psikiyatri Dergisi, 25*(4), 234–243.

Ames, E. W. (1997). *Development of Romanian orphanage children adopted to Canada*. Final report to the Human Resources Development Office, Ottawa, Canada.

Ayaz, M., Ayaz, A.B., Basgul, S.S., Karakaya, I., Gulen Sismanlar, S., Yar, A., … Dikmen, S. (2012). Prevalence of mental disorders and associated factors in institutionalized 3–5 year old children. *Turkish Journal of Psychiatry, 23*(2), 1–7.

Beckett, C., Bredenkamp, D., Castle, J., & The English and Romanian Adoptees (ERA) Study Team. (2002). Behavior problems associated with institutional deprivation: A study of children adopted from Romania. *Journal of Developmental and Behavioral Pediatrics, 23*, 297–303.

Berument, S. K. (2005). Environmental enrichment and caregiver training to support the development of birth to 6-year olds in Turkish orphanages. *Infant Mental Health Journal, 34*(3), 189–201. doi:10.1002/imhj.21380.

Browne, K.D., Hamilton-Giachritsis, C.H., Johnson, R., Agathonos, H., Anaut, M., Herczog, M., … Zeytinoglu, S. (2005). *Mapping the number and characteristics of children under three in institutions across Europe at risk of harm*. European Commission Daphne Programme in collaboration with the World Health Organization Regional Office for Europe & The University of Birmingham. Birmingham, UK: University of Birmingham.

Caman, O. K., & Ozcebe, H. (2011). Adolescents living in orphanages in Ankara: Psychological symptoms, level of physical activity, and associated factors. *Turkish Journal of Psychiatry, 22*(2), 93–103.

Çavuşoğlu, T., & Açar, F. (2004). Mithatpaşa ve Islahhaneler. Sosyal Hizmet Sempozyumu 2004: *Türkiye'de Sosyal Hizmet Uygulamaları İhtiyaç ve Sorunlar*. 4–6 Kasım 2004, Alanya. Başkent Üniversitesi Sağlık Bilimleri Fakültesi Sosyal Hizmetler Bölümü, Bildiri Özetleri, 35.

Cicchetti, D., & Toth, S. (2000). Developmental processes in maltreated children. In D. Hansen (Ed.), *46th annual Nebraska symposium on motivation: Motivation and child maltreatment* (pp. 85–160). Lincoln, NE: University of Nebraska Press.

De Bellis, M. (2001). Developmental traumatology: The psychobiological development of maltreated children and its implications for research, treatment, and policy. *Development and Psychopathology, 13*, 539–564.

Dümenci, L., Erol, N., Achenbach, T. M., & Simsek, Z. (2004). Measurement structure of the Turkish translation of the Child Behavior Checklist using confirmatory factor analytic approaches to validation of syndromal constructs. *Journal of Abnormal Child Psychology, 32*(3), 337–342.

Erol, N. (2004). Yuvalar, sorunun mu yoksa çözümün mü parçası?. Koruma Altındaki Çocuklar Sempozyumu 2004, Ankara Üniversitesi Çocuk Ruh Sağlığı ve Hastalıkları Anabilim dalı Yayınları, yayın no:9. Ankara Üniversitesi Basımevi.

Erol, N., & Sahin, N. (1995). Fears of children and the cultural context: The Turkish norms. *European Child and Adolescent Psychiatry, 4*(2), 85–93.

Erol, N., & Şimsek, Z. (2000). Mental health of Turkish children: Behavioral and emotional problems reported by parents, teachers and adolescents. In N. Singh, J. P. Leung, & A. N.

Singh (Eds.), *International perspectives on child and adolescent mental health* (pp. 223–247). Oxford, UK: Elsevier Science Lt.

Erol, N., & Simsek, Z. (2007). Korunma Gereksinmesi Olan Çocuklar: Kurum Bakımı ve Koruyucu Aile Sistemi". Çocuk ve Ergen Ruh Sağlığı Hastalıkları, A.S Aysev ve Y.I Taner (Eds.), Janssen-Cilag, İstanbul, Turkey, pp. 963–985.

Erol, N., & Simsek, Z. (2008). Evlat Edinme ve Ruh Sağlığı. Çocuk ve Ergen Psikiyatrisi Temel Kitabı. F. Ç.Çetin ve ark (Eds). Hekimler Yayın Birliği, Ankara, Turkey, 748–762.

Erol, N., Şimşek, Z., & Ertem, İ. (1997). Önleyici Çalışmalar: Anne-baba-bebek ilişkisini güçlendirme ve çocuğun psikososyal gelişimini Temel Sağlık Hizmetleri yoluyla destekleme projesi. Farklılıkla Yaşamak: Aile ve Toplumun Farklı Gereksinimleri Olan Bireylerle Birlikteliği. In N. Karancı (Ed.), *Türk Psikologlar Derneği Yayınları* (Vol. 13, pp. 113–137). Ankara, Turkey: Şelale Matbaacılık.

Erol, N., Simsek, Z., & Munir, K. (2010). Mental health of adolescents reared in institutional care in Turkey: Challenges and hope in the twenty-first century. *European Child & Adolescent Psychiatry, 19*(2), 113–124. doi:10.1007/s00787-009-0047-2.

Erol, N., Şimşek, Z., & Üstüner, S. (2005). *Çiçekli Dünyamda Elimi Yalnız Bırakma; Dünyada ve Türkiye'de Çocuk Koruma Sistemleri; Kurum Bakımı, Koruyucu Aile ve Evlat Edinme*. Ankara, Turkey: Ümit Matbaacılık.

Finkelhor, D. (1994). The international epidemiology of child sexual abuse. *Child Abuse & Neglect, 18*, 409–417.

Fisher, L., Ames, E. W., Chisholm, K., & Savoie, L. (1997). Problems reported by parents of Romanian orphans adopted to British Columbia. *International Journal of Behavioral Development, 20*, 67–83.

Goldfarb, W. (1943). The effects of early institutional care on adolescent personality. *Journal of Experimental Education, 12*, 106–129.

Gurcan, A. (2008). Türk toplumunda koruyucu aile ve evlat edinme hizmetlerine ilişkin bakış açısı ve yaklaşımı. Koruyucu Aile, Evlat Edinme Hizmetleri ve Ruh Sağlığı; (Foster Care and Adoption Services and Mental Health) Prof. Dr. Mualla Öztürk anısına XX.sempozyum sunumları (N. Erol, Ed.), 15–16 Şubat, 2007. Ankara Üniversitesi Basımevi, (pp. 29–40). (in Turkish).

Hikmet, N. (1949). You and me. In: Nazim Hikmet Selected Poems. Parachiya – Unity Publication, Calcutta, India, 1952, (p. 58). (original English translation by Massess & Mainstream) https://www.scribd.com/doc/21635233/16093525-Nazim-Hikmet-Selected-Poems

IOM (Institute of Medicine) and NRC (National Research Council). (2014). In A. C. Petersen, J. Joseph, & M. Feit (Eds.), *New directions in child abuse and neglect research*. Washington, DC: National Academies Press.

Keil, V., & Price, J. M. (2006). Externalizing behavior disorders in child welfare settings: Definition, prevalence, and implications for assessment and treatments. *Children and Youth Services Review, 28*, 761–779.

Kessler, R. C., Davis, C. G., & Kendler, K. S. (1997). Childhood adversity and adult psychiatric disorder in the U.S. National Comorbidity Survey. *Psychological Medicine, 27*, 1101–1119.

Knudsen, E. I. (2004). Sensitive periods in the development of the brain and behavior. *Journal of Cognitive Neuroscience, 16*(8), 1412–1425.

Link, B. G., & Phelan, J. C. (2001). Conceptualizing stigma. *Annual Review of Sociology, 27*, 363–385.

MacLean, K. (2003). The impact of institutionalization on child development. *Development and Psychopathology, 5*, 853–884.

Manly, J., Kim, J., Rogosch, F., & Cicchetti, D. (2001). Dimensions of child maltreatment and children's adjustment: Contributions of developmental timing and subtype. *Development and Psychopathology, 13*, 759–782.

Marcovitch, S., Goldberg, S., Gold, A., Washington, J., Wasson, C., Krekewich, K., & Handley-Derry, M. (1997). Determinants of behavioral problems in Romanian children adopted to Ontario. *International Journal of Behavioral Development, 20*, 17–31.

Masten, A., & Coatsworth, J. D. (1998). The developmental of competence in favorable and unfavorable environments: Lessons from research on successful children. *American Psychologist, 53*(2), 205–220.
Ministry of Family and Social Policies. (2016). Statistics, 2011–2015 data. Retrieved from http://cocukhizmetleri.aile.gov.tr/data/544e2899369dc318044059c3/aralik%20ay.pdf
Munir, K., Ergene, T., Tunaligil, V., & Erol, N. (2004). A window of opportunity for the transformation of national mental health policy in Turkey following two major earthquakes. *Harvard Review of Psychiatry, 12*(4), 238–251.
Munir, K. M. (2016a). Analysis of service and legislative frameworks in Turkey across the lifespan. In L. I. Rubin, J. Merrick, D. E. Greydanus, & D. R. Patel (Eds.), *Health care for people with intellectual and developmental disabilities across the lifespan* (3rd ed.pp. 529–535). Dordrecht, Switzerland: Springer International Publishing.
Munir, K. M. (2016b). The co-occurrence of mental disorders in children and adolescents with intellectual disability/intellectual developmental disorder. *Current Opinion in Psychiatry, 29*(2), 95–102.
Munir, K. M., Ergene, T., Dag, I., Erol, N., & Aker, T. (Eds.). (2006). *The Republic of Turkey National Mental Health Policy*. Ankara, Turkey: The Republic of Turkey, Ministry of Health Directorate of Primary Health Care.
NSPCC (National Society for the Prevention of Cruelty to Children). (2016). *Looking after infant mental health: Our case for change. A summary of research evidence*. London, UK: NSPCC.
Quinton, D., & Rutter, M. (1984). Parents with children in care. Current circumstances and parenting skills. *Journal of Child Psychology and Psychiatry, 25*, 231–250.
Ritsher, J. B., Otilingam, P. G., & Grajales, M. (2003). Internalized stigma of mental illness: Psychometric properties of a new measure. *Psychiatry Research, 121*, 31–49.
Roberts, R. E., Roberts, C. R., & Chen, I. G. (2000). Fatalism and risk of adolescent depression. *Psychiatry-Interpersonal and Biological Processes, 63*(3), 239–252.
Roy, P., Rutter, M., & Pickles, A. (2000). Institutional care: Risk from family background or pattern of rearing? *Journal of Child Psychology and Psychiatry, 41*(2), 139–149.
Rutter, M. (1990). Psychosocial resilience and protective mechanisms. In J. Rolf, A. S. Masten, D. Cicchetti, K. H. Nuechterlein, S., & Weintraub (Eds). Risk and protective factors in the development of psychopathology (pp. 651–682). New York, NY: Cambridge University Press.
Sacan, S., Artan, I., Erol, N., & Simşek, Z. (2014). Problem behaviors of 6–18 year old children who have been moved from institutions to their biological parents. NWSA-Qualitative Studies Status: Original Study. ISSN: 1306-3111/1308-724X. NWSA ID: 2014.9.2.E0019. Accepted: April 2014. E-Journal of New World Sciences Academy.
Savasır, I., Sezgin, N., & Erol, N. (1998). *Manual for the Ankara Developmental Screening Inventory*. Ankara, Turkey: Turkish Psychological Association. (Ankara Gelişim Tarama Enventeri El Kitabı).
Schore, A. N. (2001). The effects of early relational trauma on right brain development, affect regulation, and infant mental health. *Infant Mental Health Journal, 22*, 201–269.
Shonkoff, J.P., Garner, A.S., Siegel, B.S., Dobbins, M.I., Earls, M.F., McGuinn, L.,… Wood, D.L. (2012). The lifelong effects of early childhood adversity and toxic stress. *Pediatrics, 129*(1), 232–246. doi:10.1542/peds.2011-2663.
Simsek, Z., Erol, N., Oztop, D., & Munir, K. (2007). Prevalence and predictors of emotional and behavioral problems reported by teachers among institutionally reared children and adolescents in Turkish orphanages compared with community controls. *Children and Youth Services Review, 29*, 883–899.
Simsek, Z., Erol, N., Oztop, D., & Ozcan, O. O. (2008). Epidemiology of emotional and behavior problems in children reared in orphanages: A national comparative study. *Turk Psikiyatri Dergisi, 19*(3), 235–246.
Spitz, R. (1945). Hospitalism: An inquiry into the genesis of psychiatric conditions in early childhood. *Psychoanalytic Study of the Child, 1*, 54–74.
Stein, M. (2008). Resilience and young people leaving care. *Child Care in Practice, 14*(1), 35–44. doi:10.1016/j.childyouth.2005.05.005.

Tizard, B., & Hodges, J. (1978). The effect of early institutional rearing on the development of eight-year- old children. *Journal of Child Psychology and Psychiatry, 19*, 99–118.

UNHR (United Nations Human Rights Office of the High Commissioner). (1990). *Convention on the Rights of the Child*. Retrieved from http://www.ohchr.org/en/professionalinterest/pages/crc.aspx. Accessed 11 Nov 2016.

UNICEF. (2015). *Compendium of promising practices to ensure that children under the age of three grow up in a safe and supportive family environment*. Geneva, Switzerland: UNICEF Regional Office for Central and Eastern Europe and the Commonwealth of Independent States.

Üstün, B., & Erol, N. (2008). *Yetiştirme yurdu deneyimi olan genç yetişkinlerin ve çocukların duygusal ve davranışsal sorunları. Ankara Üniversitesi Sosyal Bilimler Enstitüsü.* Ankara, Türkiye: Uygulamalı Psikoloji Anabilim Dalı.

Üstüner, S., Erol, N., & Şimşek, Z. (2005). Koruyucu aile bakımı altındaki çocukların davranış ve duygusal sorunları. *Çocuk ve Gençlik Ruh Sağlığı Dergisi, 12*(3), 130–140.

Vorria, P., Rutter, M., Pickles, A., Wolkind, S., & Hobsbaum, A. (1998). A comparative study of Greek children in long term group care and in two-parent families: I. Social, emotional, and behavioral differences. *Journal of Child Psychology and Psychiatry, 36*(4), 1633–1644.

Wolff, P. H., & Fesseha, G. (1998). The orphans of Eritrea: A five-year follow-up study. *Journal of Child Psychology and Psychiatry, 40*, 1231–1237.

World Health Organization. (2016). *Child maltreatment* (Fact sheet). Retrieved from http://www.who.int/mediacentre/factsheets/fs150/en/

Yagmurlu, N., Berument, S. K., & Celimli, S. (2005). The role of institution and home contexts in theory of mind development. *Applied Developmental Psychology, 26*, 521–537. doi:10.10167/j.aadev.2005.06.004.

Yörükoğlu, A. (2003). Koruma altındaki çocuklar ve hakları. *Çocuk ve Gençlik Ruh Sağlığı Dergisi, 10*(3), 148–150.

Zeanah, C. H. (2000). Disturbances of attachment in young children adopted from institutions. *Journal of Developmental & Behavioral Pediatrics, 15*, 215–220.

Chapter 13
Experiences of Victimization by Peers and Staff in Residential Care for Children at Risk in Israel from an Ecological Perspective

Shalhevet Attar-Schwartz

We are acutely mindful that the first principle undergirding therapeutic residential care must be "primum non nocere": to first, do no harm. Thus, our strong consensus is that "Safety First" be the guiding principle in the design and implementation of all therapeutic residential care programs.

Whittaker et al. (2016, p. 96).

1 Introduction

Young people in public care are considered to be a vulnerable group. Many of them have been removed from home because of their parents' inability to provide them with a safe and nurturing environment (Barter, 2011; National Council for the Child, 2012). Out-of-home care settings are intended to provide young people with a rehabilitative experience in a safe, secure environment, and there is an expectation that these settings will protect them from further maltreatment (Hobbs, Hobbs, & Wynne, 1999). Unfortunately, the emerging evidence about victimization experiences against young people by peers and staff in public care paints a disquieting picture of the scale of such phenomena (e.g., Barter, Renold, Berridge, & Cawson, 2004; Gibbs & Sinclair, 2000; Hobbs et al., 1999; Rus et al., 2013, 2017). Examining the victimization of children in care is critical in helping child welfare professionals develop policies and programs to protect these young people (Attar-Schwartz, 2011, 2014).

S. Attar-Schwartz (✉)
School of Social Work and Social Welfare, The Hebrew University of Jerusalem, Mount Scopus, 9190501 Jerusalem, Israel
e-mail: shalhevet@mail.huji.ac.il

A.V. Rus et al. (eds.), *Child Maltreatment in Residential Care*,
DOI 10.1007/978-3-319-57990-0_13

This chapter summarizes the results of an Israeli study based on the reports of 1324 Israeli adolescents, aged 11–19, on their victimization experiences while in residential care. The study addressed these research questions: (1) What is the prevalence of peer (physical, sexual, verbal, and relational) and staff (physical and verbal) victimization of Israeli adolescents in residential care settings? (2) What characteristics of the adolescents are linked with such victimization? (3) What characteristics of the residential care facilities are linked with such victimization? While exploring the latter two questions, the study was guided by a social-ecological paradigm (Bronfenbrenner, 1979), which offers a framework for integrating the various factors associated with experiences of victimization among youth. This paradigm describes victimization in care as an interplay among several relevant systems, such as child, family, institution, and culture.

2 What's Out There Today? Established Research and Practice

This chapter presents the findings of a large-scale study conducted in Israel of verbal and physical staff violence (Attar-Schwartz, 2011) and physical, sexual, indirect, and verbal victimization by peers (Attar-Schwartz, 2014; Attar-Schwartz & Khoury-Kassabri, 2015; Khoury-Kassabri & Attar-Schwartz, 2014) of adolescents in residential care facilities for children at risk. This section provides a brief overview of some of the international and Israeli existing literature on staff and peer victimization in public care (or in other settings for children) and introduces some of the characteristics of the Israeli residential care system.

2.1 What Do We Know About Victimization by Staff and Peers in Public Care?

Although many large-scale studies examine staff maltreatment (e.g., Hyman, Zelikoff, & Clarke, 1988; Khoury-Kassabri, 2006; Kim et al., 2000; Youssef, Attia, & Kamel, 1998) and peer victimization (e.g., Benbenishty & Astor, 2005; Crick & Grotpeter, 1995; Mishna, 2012; Olweus, 1993; Ostrov & Keating, 2004; Smith, Kwak, & Toda, 2016) in settings such as schools, there are few empirical studies of staff maltreatment and victimization by peers in out-of-home care. The few studies that exist, however, paint a worrisome picture.

There is evidence that maltreatment of children and youth in public care is prevalent and a serious problem. Young people in state care are involved in official maltreatment reports and police investigations much more often than young people from the general population (e.g., Benedict, Zuravin, Brandt, & Abbey, 1994; Bolton, Laner, & Gai, 1981; Hobbs et al., 1999; Rindfleisch & Rabb, 1984). For example, Hobbs et al. (1999) examined pediatricians' reports of physical and sexual abuse among children in foster care or residential care in the United Kingdom. They found that foster children are seven to eight times more likely than children in the general population to be assessed and reported as victims of abuse. Children in residential care are six times more likely. A study examining the outcomes of 569 US alumni (ages 20–33) who had been placed in foster care as children found that one-third (32.8%) of the sample reported some form of maltreatment by a foster caregiver or other adult in the foster family during their foster care experience (The Northwest Foster Care Alumni Study; Pecora et al., 2005). Rus et al. (2013) conducted a study based on a representative sample of approximately 1400 institutionalized Romanian children aged 7–20 years. In their study, about 40% of the children reported that they had been severely punished, including being beaten, by staff. Of these, 7.7% said that they had been severely punished once, and 32% reported having been severely punished many times.

Studies of peer violence among young people in care also show that adolescents in RCSs are highly victimized (Barter et al., 2004; MacLeod, 1999; Morris & Wheatley, 1994; Rus et al., 2017; Sekol & Farrington, 2009). For example, in their study of 71 young people in 14 children's homes in England, Barter et al. (2004) found that over half of the young people (53.5%) reported having been physically victimized by peers during their stay in residential homes. A similar trend was found in another British study (Gibbs & Sinclair, 2000), where a considerable portion of the young people (43.9%) had been bullied in their RCS. However, Gibbs and Sinclair (2000) used a general subjective question about bullying that did not differentiate between various types of bullying.

There is evidence that sexual harassment and abuse by peers is prevalent among young people in care (e.g., Farmer & Pollock, 1998; Freundlich, Avery, & Padgett, 2007; Green & Masson, 2002; Sinclair & Gibbs, 1998), especially among those in RCSs (Green & Masson, 2002; Kendrick, 2011; Morris & Wheatley, 1994; Spencer & Knudsen, 1992). For example, Gibbs and Sinclair (2000) interviewed 223 young people in 48 RCSs across the United Kingdom and found that 44% of them reported having been bullied during their time in care. They also found that 7% of the males and 23% – nearly a quarter – of the females reported that someone had tried to take sexual advantage of them after they had moved into the children's homes. Gibbs and Sinclair (2000), however, relied exclusively on a subjective, one-item, generalized question about having been sexually harassed, rather than on questions about specific sexually harassing behaviors. The researchers themselves acknowledged that this may have led to uncertainty among the young people about what constitutes sexual harassment by peers and that therefore their data might contain inaccuracies due to underreporting. Barter et al. (2004) found, on the other hand, that reports of unwanted sexual behaviors by peers among young people in UK children's homes were low (see also Sekol & Farrington, 2009), but their study included incidents of coercive sexual behaviors and severe abuse such as rape, which one might expect to be less frequent than the more common, less severe behaviors included in the current study (see Attar-Schwartz, 2009a).

The few existing studies of peer violence in care generally focus on physical and sexual violence. Less severe but more common forms of violence, such as verbal violence (e.g., cursing at and name calling) and indirect violence (e.g., gossiping, spreading rumors, and social exclusion), have received considerably less attention in research and in the public care policy agenda and practice (for a discussion, see Attar-Schwartz & Khoury-Kassabri, 2015). There is compelling evidence, however, that victims of these forms of violence can suffer serious consequences, such as long-lasting emotional harm and social maladjustment. Extreme cases, such as suffering continuous social exclusion, can lead to suicidal thoughts and behavior (Archer & Coyne, 2005; Barter, 2003).

Studies examining verbal and indirect forms of violence among young people in care have found that verbal insults are common but are often taken for granted as a normal aspect of residential life and go ignored and unchallenged by staff. For example, Barter et al. (2004) found that among young people in UK children's homes, nearly all (61 of the 71 young people or 86%) of the young people interviewed had experienced some form of verbal violence such as name calling. In their study of 643 young people from 22 Croatian institutions, Sekol and Farrington (2009) found that 55% of all residents from children's homes (including community residential homes, state residential homes, and children's homes) and 40% of residents from correctional homes reported at least one experience of indirect victimization. Verbal violence was reported by about a third (33.6%) of the residents in children's homes and by a similar number (30.1%) of the residents in correctional homes.

The absence of a comprehensive picture of the prevalence or types of maltreatment and peer victimization that youth experience in care (Stein, 2006) is mainly due to definitional confusion and the lack of any central mechanism for reporting investigations (Benedict et al., 1994; Kendrick, 1997). In addition, existing studies of victimization by peers and staff use varying methodologies and populations, which does not allow for a valid comparison of their findings. They are often based on unrepresentative, small-scale samples (e.g., Agathonos, 1983; Barer, 1998; Barter et al., 2004; Benedict et al., 1994; Benedict, Zuravin, Somerfield, & Brandt, 1996; Gibbs & Sinclair, 1999, 2000; Green & Masson, 2002; Groze, 1990; Hargrave, 1991; Sekol, 2013) and retrospective samples (e.g., Freundlich et al., 2007; Gibbs & Sinclair, 1999; Hobbs et al., 1999). Some of the studies are based on general, subjective questions about being victimized in the RCS (e.g., Gibbs & Sinclair, 2000; Rus et al., 2013). The catch-all, subjective nature of these questions may have led to different understandings for different respondents and might have made it difficult to understand the actual nature of the behavior being asked about (Barter, 2011; Barter et al., 2004).

Much of the existing research on both peer violence and staff violence in care relies on secondhand reports by adults, such as the children's social workers, or on administrative data and official investigation records (e.g., Attar-Schwartz, 2008, 2009b; Barter, 1998; Benedict et al., 1994, 1996; Freundlich et al., 2007; Groze, 1990; Poertner, Bussey, & Fluke, 1999; Rosenthal, Motz, Edmonson, & Groze,

1991) and does not include the perspectives of the residents themselves. Relying on such data creates inaccurate estimates of victimization in public care because of underreporting (Barter et al., 2004; Stein, 2006). This data usually only includes extreme cases, such as severe physical or sexual violence, in which the abuse is reported to an authority and has been evaluated as serious enough to warrant further inquiry (see Barter, 2011). This data may therefore exclude victimizing behaviors that are less extreme and more common, but which do not reach formal investigation.

In Israel, little is known about maltreatment of at-risk youth by staff in RCSs, and the study described in this chapter is the first one to describe children's experiences of victimization while in residential care for children at risk. Several studies, published in the past decade, used large-scale, representative samples of Israeli students to examine staff use of violence (e.g., Benbenishty, Zeira, & Astor, 2000; Khoury-Kassabri, 2006) and victimization by peers (e.g., Attar-Schwartz & Khoury-Kassabri, 2008; Benbenishty & Astor, 2005) in Israeli schools. Davidson-Arad and Golan (2007) conducted one of the only studies to investigate victimization of youth in settings other than schools in Israel. They focused on youth in correctional facilities for juvenile delinquents and found that about a third of the residents (35%) reported experiencing some form of verbal maltreatment by staff at least once in the month prior to the survey and approximately one quarter (28%) reported experiencing physical maltreatment in that period. They also found that more than three quarters (76%) of the youth had experienced at least one act of verbal violence by one of their peers in the facility; however, fewer adolescents reported incidents of sexual harassment (32%) and physical violence (16%) at the hands of their peers.

The study outlined in this chapter is guided by an ecological contextual perspective (Bronfenbrenner, 1979; Fulcher, 2001; Whittaker, 1978), which suggests that in order to understand children's development and behavior, one should consider influences from various aspects of their lives. This ecological framework is particularly useful for understanding the complex issues of victimization and for developing sensitive and effective intervention and prevention programs (Barboza et al., 2009; Nesmith, 2006). Although this contextual perspective may appear obvious, there are extremely few studies that use this framework to assess risk factors for violence in RCSs (for exceptions, see Rus et al., 2013, 2017). Existing studies often examine only a limited range of factors, mainly focused on the child's demographic characteristics such as the gender and age. Previous studies (e.g., Benedict et al., 1996; Davidson-Arad & Golan, 2007; Poertner et al., 1999; Sekol & Farrington, 2009; Spencer & Knudsen, 1992) too frequently overlook the experiences of youth in RCSs and institution-level factors and their association with children's experiences of violence. The current study examined various forms of victimization by peers and by staff in RCSs by both child-level (including factors such as gender, age, adjustment difficulties, self-efficacy, and perceptions of the RCS climate) and institution-level (including size, structure, type of care, and ethnic affiliation of the institution) correlates. What follows is a description of the main characteristics of the Israeli residential care system for children at risk.

2.2 *Residential Care for Children at Risk: The Israeli Context*

Unlike many other Western countries (King, 2013), the majority of children in public care in Israel are placed in residential care, with only about 25% in foster care (Service for Children and Youth, 2014). In 2014–2015, for example, 9143 children and adolescents lived in out-of-home care for children at risk. About 75% of these children were placed in RCSs. The rest were placed with foster care families (National Council for the Child, 2014; Service for Children and Youth, 2014) under the aegis of the Ministry of Social Affairs and Services. The unique status of public care in Israel compared to other Western countries is usually explained by Israel's unique historical-ideological circumstances of nation building, in particular the need to absorb massive waves of immigrants, including the arrival of thousands of Holocaust orphans after World War II (Jaffe, 1978). Residential care in Israel was also a tool for socialization and acculturation of youth, and residential facilities were considered (especially the youth agricultural villages) elite institutions, which yielded some of the important leaders in Israel. These circumstances explain to some extent the present legitimacy and acceptability of child residential care in Israel (Dolev, Ben-Rabi, & Zemach-Marom, 2009; King, 2013). There is also a strong lobby for residential care in Israel. The gatekeepers' perception of residential care facilities is of institutions that provide high-quality care with a concentration of services and expertise in a single location (King, 2013). According to King (2013), the absence of visible severe abuse and scandals in residential care facilities in Israel also contributes to the stability of the system by preventing large-scale shocks to the system.

In Israel, the Ministry of Social Affairs and Services appoints an interdisciplinary decision committee to make decisions about placing at-risk children in public care. The committee can refer the child to a foster care family, which is not the focus of the current chapter, or to a residential care setting. There are three main types of residential care settings in Israel for children at risk: rehabilitative, therapeutic, and post-hospitalization (Dolev, Benbenishty, & Timar, 2001; Service for Children and Youth, 2014). Rehabilitative settings serve young people with satisfactory developmental potential who have been removed from their homes because of their parents' critical inability to cope with their developmental, emotional, and/or educational needs. Therapeutic residential care settings are designed to treat young people with extreme family problems, personal needs, and adjustment difficulties (see review in Attar, 2006). The current study focuses on children from rehabilitative and therapeutic settings; it does not include children from post-hospitalization placements, which serve youth who suffer from severe psychiatric problems.

In Israel, rehabilitative and therapeutic RCSs use a variety of institutional structures to accommodate at-risk children. The most common residential care setting structure is the traditional group institution, which cares for large numbers of children who reside in small groups. Each group of children has a social worker, as well as social-educational carers, who work in rotational shifts. In the familial setting, married couples with biological children care for small numbers of children at risk (up to 10). All family units in the facility share administrative, cleaning, and general support services. There are several other types of settings, including hybrid institutions, that combine residential groups and family-like units in the same structure (Attar-Schwartz, 2009b, 2014).

In Israel, Arab schools generally serve the Arab population and Jewish schools the Jewish population. Similarly, residential care for young people at risk is divided into Arab and Jewish institutions. The study described here is the first to compare levels of victimization between Arab and Jewish youth in public care. Studies of Israeli schools have consistently found that Arab students suffer more sexual, verbal, and physical maltreatment by staff than Jewish students (Khoury-Kassabri, 2006, 2009). They also show higher levels of severe physical victimization (such as being stabbed or receiving a beating that results in needing medical treatment; Benbenishty & Astor, 2005) and indirect aggression (such as being excluded from a group) (Attar-Schwartz & Khoury-Kassabri, 2008) than Jewish students. However, Jewish students have reported more experiences of verbal violence than Arab students (e.g., Attar-Schwartz & Khoury-Kassabri, 2008), and no significant difference has been found between Arab and Jewish schools in their rates of moderately severe sexual victimization by peers (Attar-Schwartz, 2009a) or moderate physical victimization (see Benbenishty & Astor, 2005).

There are many sociocultural and socioeconomic differences between Jews and Arabs in Israel. Arabs in Israel are a minority group characterized by rates of poverty and unemployment that are higher than those of the Jewish majority, and fewer public funds are spent on social services for the Arab population than on those for the Jewish population (Haidar, 2005; Hareven, 2002). Schools with lower socioeconomic status have been found to have higher rates of maltreatment by staff (Khoury-Kassabri, 2006).

In addition, traditional collectivist, patriarchal, authoritarian family values are prevalent among the Arab population in Israel, whereas the Jewish population is generally more liberal and Westernized (Haj-Yahia, 2000). Jewish society in Israel tends to have a less authoritarian attitude toward child rearing (Khoury-Kassabri, 2010). Some research has found that attitudes toward parents' use of psychological and corporal punishment are more acceptable among the Arab population than among the Jewish population. Accordingly, the use of psychological and corporal punishment is more common among Arab parents than among Jewish parents in Israel (Khoury-Kassabri, 2010; Khoury-Kassabri & Straus, 2011). Arab teachers also tend to use more corporal punishment than Jewish teachers (Benbenishty et al., 2000; Elbedour, Assor, Center, & Maruyama, 1997). School violence researchers in Israel also suggest that clear gaps remain between Arab and Jewish students in levels of maltreatment by school staff, even when controlling for socioeconomic status (e.g., Khoury-Kassabri, 2006). The study presented in this chapter compares levels of staff and peer victimization in Arab and Jewish RCSs.

3 The Social Climate Study: Research Findings on Youth Victimization by Peers and Staff in Israel

The findings described here are part of the Social Climate Survey, which examined the adjustment of youth in Arab and Jewish child welfare RCSs (i.e., rehabilitative and therapeutic settings) in Israel, as well as the social climate of the institution and safety issues. The study was based on the reports of 1324 adolescents aged 11–19 residing in 32 RCSs and on the reports of the directors of the RCSs on the characteristics of their institutions (see Attar-Schwartz & Khoury-Kassabri, 2015 for more details). The current chapter focuses on the youths' reports of verbal maltreatment by staff, including behaviors such as cursing, name calling, mocking, and insulting, as well as physical maltreatment by staff, such as kicking and punching. It also includes their reports of various forms of peer violence, including physical violence; moderately severe sexual violence, such as unwanted touches, gestures, comments, peeping, and kissing; and verbal and indirect violence, including gossiping, spreading false rumors, and deliberately ignoring or socially excluding. It also identifies some of the multilevel correlates of these types of victimization.

3.1 *Sample*

The sampling frame was derived from a list provided by the Ministry of Social Affairs and Services of 45 RCSs with more than 20 residents in the relevant age group (11–19). Three RCSs in remote villages were excluded from the sample because their inclusion would have demanded special resources. As a result, 42 RCSs were contacted for this study. Of these, seven opted not to participate in the study (17.9%), and three ultraorthodox Jewish RCSs were excluded because their directors asked for significant revisions to the questionnaire (7.14%). The response rate of the RCSs was 76.19%. The sample is broadly representative of the age, gender, ethnic affiliation, and treatment type of adolescents residing in rehabilitative and therapeutic care settings in Israel (Attar, 2006; Attar-Schwartz, 2009b; National Council for the Child, 2010). The study's sample included 1324 adolescents aged 11–19 from 32 RCSs. The mean age of the sample was 14.06 years ($SD = 3.11$); 54% of respondents were male. Most of the RCSs included in this study were Jewish (75%), and the rest were Arab. Approximately 60% of the RCSs were group institutions; the rest were settings with familial elements (see definitions above). About two thirds (62.5%) of the RCSs were rehabilitative; the rest were therapeutic. Each RCS serviced an average of 102 youth of all ages ($SD = 65.34$).

3.2 Data Collection

Information was collected from the adolescents through an anonymous, structured, self-report questionnaire. Letters were sent to the directors of the sampled RCSs requesting assistance in collecting data. Each director also received a letter to be sent to the parents or guardians outlining the purpose of the study and providing contact information in case of questions. Each parent or guardian was asked to return a slip if they did not want their child to take part in the study. The adolescents were told that they were free to withdraw from the study at any time for any reason. The questionnaire was administered by trained research assistants, who visited the facilities to administer the questionnaire to all residents between the ages of 11 and 19 who were on the premises and available at the time. The adolescents completed the questionnaires in the RCS. Given the sensitive nature of the questions, the RCS staff was asked not to be present in the room when the youth were filling out the questionnaires, and the researchers assured the participants that their responses would remain confidential. On completing the questionnaire, the adolescents received a sheet listing child welfare agencies and services they could contact if they felt distress or in need of help from outside the RCS. In addition, the directors were asked to provide some organizational details about their RCSs through structured self-report questionnaires. Questionnaires, procedures, consent forms, and instructions were reviewed by the Ethics Committee of the Hebrew University of Jerusalem.

3.3 Measures

Arab adolescents completed the questionnaires in Arabic; Jewish adolescents completed them in Hebrew. The questionnaire included several measures that originated from English-language scales (e.g., the Revised Social Climate Scale, Colton, 1989), which were translated into Hebrew and Arabic. To enhance the compatibility of the Hebrew and Arabic versions, the authors followed common procedures, enlisting experts familiar with the Hebrew and Arabic languages, as well as the two cultures, to back-translate and discuss the surveys.

3.3.1 Dependent Variables: Victimization by Staff and by Peers

All dependent variables in this study were drawn from Benbenishty and associates' (2000) translation and adaptation of the California School Climate Survey (Furlong et al., 2005) measures into Hebrew and Arabic. It was slightly adapted to the population of young people in RCSs. Below is a description of the items included in each dependent scale.

Physical and Verbal Victimization by Staff

The questionnaire presented adolescents with a list of aggressive behaviors and asked them to indicate whether, within 1 month of the survey, they had been victims of aggressive behavior perpetrated by a staff member in their RCS. The questionnaire defined "staff" as any adult who works or volunteers in the institution, including social workers, direct caregivers, home parents, directors, psychologists, volunteers, and administrative staff. *The physical maltreatment subscal* ($\alpha = 0.74$) was composed of four items that asked whether the respondent had been (1) grabbed or shoved, (2) pinched, (3) slapped, or (4) kicked or punched by a staff member who wanted to hurt him or her. *The verbal maltreatment subscale* included two items ($\alpha = 0.62$): (1) whether a staff member had cursed at the respondent and (2) whether a staff member had humiliated, insulted, or ridiculed him or her. Respondents were assigned one point for each specific behavior they had reportedly experienced at least once in the month prior to the survey. Scores for the physical maltreatment subscale ranged from zero to four physical violent behaviors by a staff member toward the adolescent; scores on the verbal maltreatment subscale ranged from zero to two of such behaviors. It should be noted that physical maltreatment by staff served also as an explanatory variable in the examination of the various forms of victimization by peers.

Physical Victimization by Peers

Adolescents were presented with a list of aggressive physical behaviors and were asked to indicate whether they had been victims of any of these behaviors perpetrated by a peer in their RCS in the preceding month (responding options: 1 = *never*, 2 = *once or twice*, 3 = *three times or more*). The measure included four items indicating whether in the previous month adolescents had been (1) grabbed or shoved, (2) kicked or punched, (3) seriously hit by others, or 4) hit with an object (stick, stone, chair, etc.) deliberately to hurt ($\alpha = 0.79$). The subscale was based on the mean of items, therefore ranging from 1 (*never physically victimized*) to 3 (*victimized more than three times by all listed behaviors*).

Sexual Victimization by Peers

The study included experiences of moderately severe unwanted and unwelcome sexual behaviors by peers but did not include rape and attempted rape (for more details, see Attar-Schwartz, 2014). Adolescents were asked to indicate whether other residents in the RCS had subjected them to any of the eight sexually aggressive behaviors in the month prior to the survey by answering yes or no to each item. The scale consists of the following eight items ($\alpha = 0.75$): (1) a fellow resident tried to kiss you without your consent; (2) sexually insulting things about you were written on walls or spread as rumors; (3) a resident peeped at you while you were in the bathroom or the shower; (4) a resident touched or tried to touch you in a sexual manner when you did not want it; (5) a resident tried to hit on you or made sexual remarks that you did not want; (6) a resident took or tried to take off part of your clothes without your consent; (7) a resident/residents imposed peer pressure on you or threatened to spread rumors about you if you did not consent to their sexual demands; and (8) a resident touched you against your will on an intimate part of your body and threatened to hurt you if you did not consent to his or her demands. To create the sexual victimization subscale, respondents were assigned one point for each behavior they reported experiencing at least once in the month prior to the survey. Scores for this scale ranged from 0 to 8 sexually aggressive behaviors perpetrated by fellow residents.

Verbal and Indirect Victimization by Peers

Adolescents were presented with a list of aggressive behaviors and were asked to indicate how many times they had been victimized by their peers in the RCS in the month prior to filling out the questionnaire: *never*, *once or twice*, or *more than three times*. *The verbal victimization subscale* ($\alpha = 0.65$) consisted of the following two items: (1) a fellow resident cursed at you and (2) a fellow resident mocked, insulted, or humiliated you with words. *The indirect victimization subscale* ($\alpha = 0.82$) included behaviors intentionally aimed at damaging social relationships or feelings of peer acceptance of the victims (Crick, Casas, & Mosher, 1997; Crick & Grotpeter, 1995; Mishna, 2012; Ostrov & Keating, 2004). It consisted of the following four items: (1) a resident gossiped about you or said mean and unpleasant things about you behind your back; (2) a fellow resident told lies or spread false rumors about you; (3) a resident tried to convince other residents not to speak with you or not to be your friend; and (4) you were ignored or excluded from a group of other residents or deliberately left out of things. Both subscales were based on the means of the items, therefore ranging from 1 (*never verbally/indirectly victimized*) to 3 (*victimized more than three times by all listed verbal/indirect violent behaviors*).

3.3.2 Individual-Level Correlates

This chapter summarizes the findings from various analyses examining peer and staff violence against children in RCSs in Israel. A number of the adolescents' individual-level correlates, such as age, gender, and adjustment difficulties, were examined in relation to all of the various types of victimization. Other individual-level factors, such as the adolescents' self-efficacy and their perception of the friendliness at their RCS, were examined only in relation to certain victimization types.

Background Characteristics

Adolescents were asked to report on their gender and age.

Adjustment Difficulties

The adolescents' adjustment difficulties were assessed, for most analyses, by a total difficulties measure derived from the self-report version of the Strengths and Difficulties Questionnaire (SDQ; Goodman, 1997) for 11–17-year-olds, which was translated into Hebrew and Arabic by professionals (www.sdqinfo.com). The SDQ is a three-point Likert-type scale (0 = *not true*, 1 = *somewhat true*, 2 = *certainly true*) measuring four types of difficulty: hyperactivity, emotional symptoms, conduct problems, and peer problems, as well as prosocial behavior (Goodman, 1997). The total difficulties score ($\alpha = 0.75$) was calculated by summing the summative scores for the various difficulty subscales (each including five items): hyperactivity, emotional symptoms, conduct problems, and peer problems. The score for this scale ranged from 0 (*no reported adjustment difficulties*) to 40 (*high level of adjustment difficulties*). It should be noted that the adjustment difficulties scale was used for all analyses presented here, except for the findings of the staff maltreatment (see Attar-Schwartz, 2011), which used two specific subscales: emotional symptoms ($\alpha = 0.67$) and hyperactivity ($\alpha = 0.64$).

Self-Efficacy

The study included two subscales derived from the Self-Efficacy Questionnaire for Children (SEQ-C; Muris, 2001): (a) *social self-efficacy* ($\alpha = 0.75$), which included eight items relating to an adolescent's perceived capability for peer relationships and assertiveness (e.g., "How easily can you tell other children that they are doing something that you don't like?") and (b) *emotional self-efficacy* ($\alpha = 0.77$), which included eight items pertaining to the adolescent's perceived capability of coping with negative emotions (e.g., "How well do you succeed in cheering yourself up when an unpleasant event has happened?"). Each item was scored on a five-point scale (1 = *not at all*; 5 = *very well*). Each subscale was created by computing the mean score of the items. A high score indicated a high level of self-efficacy.

Perceived RCS Social Climate

Adolescents' perceptions of the social climate at their RCS were examined using the Revised Social Climate Scale (RSCS; Colton, 1989). The Original Social Climate Scale was devised by Heal, Sinclair, and Troop (1973) to assess how delinquent boys in community homes perceive their social environments. Colton (1989) modified the scale so that it could be applied to residential and foster care settings for at-risk youth. The scale involved simple statements about the social environment in the institution, which respondents rated as either *true* (1) or *false* (0). The RSCS consists of five subscales: caretaker support, strictness, satisfaction, youth behaviors, and youth friendliness. The questionnaire included the three that were assessed to be most relevant to this study. *The caretaker support subscale* included 10 items ($\alpha = 0.79$) that examined the extent to which the adolescent perceived the RCS staff to be interested, warm, and supportive (e.g., "You usually talk to the staff if you have a personal problem"). The summative score of the subscale ranged from 0 (*not supportive at all*) to 10 (*very supportive*). The *strictness subscale* included 8 items ($\alpha = 0.63$) that examined young people's perceptions of their authority relationship with the staff (e.g., "You get into serious trouble if you don't obey the rules here"). The summative score of the subscale ranged from 0 (*not strict at all*) to 8 (*very strict*). Finally, *the child friendliness subscale*, which was included in some of the analyses, included seven items ($\alpha = 0.65$) that examined the degree to which the young people in care perceived each other as friendly (e.g., "Kids rarely help each other here"). The summative score of the child friendliness subscale ranged from 0 (*not friendly at all*) to 7 (*very friendly*).

Perceived Residential Care Setting Policy Against Violence

The scale of the adolescents' perceptions of the RCS policy against the use of violence was based on five items from the California School Climate Survey (Furlong et al., 2005), which was slightly modified by Benbenishty and associates (2000) to make it culturally relevant to Jewish and Arab youth in Israel. Adolescents were asked to rate their level of agreement with five statements ($\alpha = 0.85$) about their opinions of the policies and procedures in place at the RCS to limit violence (e.g., "The rules against violence in my institution are clear"). Possible responses to these items ranged from *strongly disagree* (1) to *strongly agree* (4). The resulting index was based on the average score of the items.

3.3.3 RCS-Level Correlates

To assess whether the care environment was linked to victimization by staff and by peers, this study included four RCS-level correlates as reported by the directors: type of care, institutional structure, size, and ethnic affiliation. The measure of *RCS type* referred to the type of care provided (rehabilitative or therapeutic). The measure of *RCS structure* indicated whether the RCS was arranged as a traditional group setting, as a collection of familial units, or as a mixed familial-group setting. *Institution size* was measured as the overall number of youth of all ages residing in the RCS. *Ethnic affiliation* identified the RCS as either Arab or Jewish institutions. In Israel, as mentioned above, Arab youth are almost never placed in Jewish settings and vice versa.

3.3.4 Analytic Plan

The study employed hierarchical linear modeling (HLM), a technique that allows the investigation of data organized hierarchically on more than one level (Raudenbush & Bryk, 2002). In this study, adolescents were nested within RCSs. The level-1 model captures the relationships of the individual youth-level characteristics to victimization by peers and staff; the level-2 model captures the relationships of RCS-level variables to such victimization. The HLM method provides separate estimates of the variance in victimization explained by the adolescents' characteristics and by the RCS features.

3.4 Results, Discussion, and Conclusions

3.4.1 Descriptive Statistics

The adolescents average score of adjustment difficulties was 14.02 (*SD* = 6.37). On average, the adolescents considered their RCS staff to be somewhat supportive (*M* = 6.03, *SD* = 2.97, on a 10-point scale ranging from *not supportive* [0] to *very supportive* [10]) but also moderately strict (*M* = 4.62, *SD* = 2.14, on an 8-point scale ranging from *not strict at all* [0] to *very strict* [8]). They considered their RCSs to be child friendly on a moderate level (*M* = 4.37, *SD* = 1.98; on a 10-point scale ranging from *not friendly at all* [0] to *very friendly* [8]). Adolescents showed agreement on a medium to high level that the policy in their RCS against violence was fair and consistent (*M* = 3.04, *SD* = 0.80, on a scale ranging from *low perception of RCS policy aimed at reducing violence* [1] to *high perception* [4]). Youth showed a medium to high level of perceived social efficacy (*M* = 3.66, *SD* = 0.70) and of emotional self-efficacy (*M* = 3.34, *SD* = 0.84); both scales ranging from 1 (*not at all*) to 5 (*very well*). Below are the descriptive statistics of the dependent variables in the current study, namely, the experiences of victimization by peers and staff.

Physical and Verbal Victimization by Staff

About one in four of the adolescents (24.7%) reported having been victims of at least one act of physical maltreatment by staff during the month prior to the survey, and approximately a third (29.1%) reported at least one act of verbal maltreatment in that time. More specifically, approximately one-third of the adolescents (29.9%) reported that a staff member had mocked, insulted, or humiliated them verbally, and 15% of the adolescents reported having been cursed at by a staff member. About one in five of the adolescents (19.2%) reported that a staff member had grabbed or shoved him or her deliberately at least once in the prior month, and about 16% of the adolescents reported that a staff member had pinched them. Approximately 12% of the adolescents reported that a staff member had slapped them, and a similar number (11.1%) reported that a staff member had kicked or punched them with the intention to hurt them. These findings show that even in a society where corporal punishment is illegal, physical maltreatment by residential care staff clearly takes place (see a discussion in Attar-Schwartz, 2011).

Physical Victimization by Peers

The results show that adolescents in Israeli RCSs are highly exposed to victimization by peers. Most participants (56%) reported having been exposed to at least one act of physical violence at the hands of a peer during the previous month. Approximately 45% reported having been grabbed or shoved, and 38.6% reported having been kicked or punched by a peer at least once during the last month. Approximately a third of the participants (29.1%) reported that they had been hit with an object deliberately to hurt, and one in five reported that they had been seriously beaten.

Sexual Victimization by Peers

Around 40% of the adolescents surveyed reported having been a victim of at least one act of peer sexual violence in the month prior to the survey. Nearly one in five of the sampled adolescents (17%) reported that they had been peeped at in the bath or shower at least once in the prior month, and a similar rate (16.6%) reported that sexually insulting things about them had been written on walls or spread as rumors. About 15% (14.6%) of the adolescents reported that a fellow resident had tried to kiss them without their consent. Similar numbers reported that a resident had touched or tried to touch them in a sexual manner when they did not want it (14.1%) and that a resident had tried to hit on them or made unwelcome sexual remarks (13.7%). Approximately 7% of the adolescents reported that a resident had taken or had tried to take off their clothes without their consent, and a similar proportion (6.4%) reported that one or more residents had pressured them, for example, by threatening to spread rumors about them, if they did not consent to their sexual demands. Slightly less than 5% of the adolescents (4.5%) reported that a resident had touched or tried to touch an intimate part of their bodies without their consent and had threatened to hurt them if they did not consent to his or her demands.

Verbal and Indirect Victimization by Peers

Nearly three quarters (73.4%) of the adolescents reported having been a victim of at least one act of verbal violence by a peer in the month prior to the survey. More specifically, about three in four respondents (75.5%) reported having been cursed at, and more than half (54.9%) reported that they had been verbally mocked, insulted, or humiliated at least once in the month prior to the survey. Approximately two thirds of the adolescents (62.4%) reported having experienced at least one act of indirect violence at the hands of a fellow resident in the month prior to the survey. More than half of the adolescents reported that a resident had gossiped about them and said mean things about them behind their back (54.9%) or that a resident had lied or spread false rumors about them (50.4%). In addition, 37% of the adolescents reported that a resident had tried to convince other residents not to speak to them or not to be their friend, and 30.4% reported that they had been ignored, excluded from a group, or left out of things on purpose.

These findings, showing worrisome levels of victimization in RCSs, are consistent with studies from other countries that show that violence in public care is common among youth and staff (e.g., Barter, 2008; Green, & Masson, 2002; Kendrick, 2011; Farmer & Pollock, 1998; Rus et al., 2013, 2017; Sinclair & Gibbs, 1998; Spencer & Knudsen, 1992). However, a comparison of the rates of victimization in RCSs in other countries could be misleading, as mentioned above, because of methodological differences in sampling procedures and target populations, the events the young people were asked to report on, and varying time frames, ranging from the child's entire stay in the RCS to 1 month prior to the child answering the questionnaire (for further discussion, see Khoury-Kassabri & Attar-Schwartz, 2014; Monks et al., 2009). A high incidence of staff maltreatment and peer victimization plays a critical role in creating the atmosphere of an RCS, which can negatively impact a resident, regardless of whether he or she is the direct victim. A negative, intimidating atmosphere can prevent the institution from carrying out its basic mission to protect and nurture youth (Groze, 1990).

Multilevel Correlates of Victimization by Peers and by Staff

The study described here examined RCS contextual variables, such as the RCS cultural affiliation and size, that may be associated with victimization by staff and by peers. This investigation assumed that RCSs differ in regard to the victimization that youth experience from RCS staff and fellow residents (see also Rus et al., 2013). Fully unconditional models (i.e., models with no independent variables) were employed to test that assumption. The fully unconditional model provided useful preliminary estimates on the extent of variance in victimization within RCSs and also across RCSs. According to this model, the RCSs in this study varied by 18.9% in the reports of staff physical maltreatment (χ^2 [31] = 280.374, $p < .001$) and by a lower, but still not to be ignored, 6% in the reports of staff verbal maltreatment (χ^2 [31] = 280.374, $p < .001$). It was also found that 9.98% of the reports of verbal victimization by peers (χ^2 [31] = 151.29, $p < .001$), 6.76% of the reports of indirect victimization by peers (χ^2 [31] = 108.79, $p < .001$), 11.48% of the reports of physical victimization by peers (χ^2 [31] = 188.175, $p < .001$), and 4.68% of the reports in sexual victimization (χ^2 [30] = 82.169, $p < .001$) by peers were accounted for by variance across RCSs in adolescents' reports of their experiences. Because of this variance, a two-level analysis was conducted. The variance between institutions in levels of staff maltreatment and victimization by peers emphasizes the importance of investigating multilevel correlates in relation to victimization by peers and staff in residential care facilities for children at risk (see Attar-Schwartz & Khoury-Kassabri, 2015; Rus et al., 2013). The results presented below summarize the findings of a series of multilevel analyses examining the contribution of youth-level and RCS-level correlates to the various measures of victimization.

3.4.2 Adolescent-Level Correlates

The current study finds that certain adolescents were found to be more likely than others to experience various types of victimization by peers and by staff.

Gender

The findings show that there were no differences between girls and boys in verbal victimization by staff (see also Davidson-Arad & Golan, 2007). Boys reported statistically significant more experiences of physical maltreatment by staff than girls, which is in line with previous studies that show that boys run a greater risk of being physically maltreated by staff (Barter, 2003; Benedict et al., 1996; Davidson-Arad & Golan, 2007; Hobbs et al., 1999; Rus et al., 2013). This finding might also reflect other studies' findings that boys are involved in more aggressive behaviors and discipline confrontations with staff (see, e.g., Attar-Schwartz, 2008; Benbenishty et al., 2000). There are a number of possible explanations for this finding, including the possibility that staff might feel that physical intimidation is more effective than verbal intimidation at enforcing discipline among boys. They might also potentially believe that girls are the weaker sex and therefore require gentler punishment (Youssef et al., 1998).

There were no differences between boys and girls in experiences of verbal victimization by peers, but boys suffered more experiences of physical victimization by their peers (see also Attar-Schwartz, 2008; Glisson, Hemmelgarn, & Post, 2002). On the other hand, boys reported fewer experiences of indirect victimization by peers than girls (see also Monks et al., 2009; Sekol & Farrington, 2009). Gender differences in violence can, at least partly, be interpreted in terms of sexual selection theory (see a discussion in Attar-Schwartz & Khoury-Kassabri, 2008), which explains the different strategies used by males and females to damage the status and reputation of others (Monks et al., 2009; Pellegrini & Archer, 2005). Direct aggressive behavior, such as physical violence, has been found to be more often used by boys and against boys. It is associated with aims that are important for boys, concerning dominance and position within the hierarchy of the peer group (Block, 1983; Crick, 1997; Crick et al., 1997; Scheithauer, Hayer, Peterman, & Jugert, 2006). Girls, on the other hand, are more likely than boys to use more covert, indirect, aggression as a means to achieving social goals, such as maintaining status, power, and popularity in peer groups. These goals have been found to have special value for girls in the context of their psychosocial development within the peer group (Crick, 1997; Leaderbeater, Boone, Sangster, & Mathieson, 2006; Zahn-Waxler & Polanichka, 2004). The insignificant gender gaps in experiences of peer-to-peer verbal, direct, violence, found in the current study, however, cannot be explained by those assumptions and are inconsistent with some previous research findings (e.g., Attar-Schwartz & Khoury-Kassabri, 2008). Other studies have found similarly insignificant gender gaps in verbal victimization by peers among young people in public care (e.g., Davidson-Arad & Golan, 2007). Because of this inconsistency, the meaning and stability of these findings should be further explored in future research.

Age

The study found that although age was insignificantly linked with staff maltreatment, experiences of physical, verbal, and indirect victimization by peers decreased as children's ages increased (see also Attar-Schwartz & Khoury-Kassabri, 2008; Borg, 1999; Gibbs & Sinclair, 2000; Nansel et al., 2001). Several factors might explain this decrease. One common explanation posited by researchers and theorists relates to the association between aggression and cost-benefit considerations. For example, Cillessen and Mayeux (2004) found that the positive associations between popularity and aggression among school students declined from grades 5 to 9. It has also been suggested that younger children have not yet acquired the social aggressiveness skills needed to effectively deal with and discourage aggressive behaviors directed toward them (Smith, Madsen, & Moody, 1999).

Emotional and Behavioral Adjustment Difficulties

Consistent with prior research, this study found that adolescents with more adjustment difficulties (i.e., emotional symptoms and hyperactivity) reported more experiences of maltreatment by staff (see also Benedict et al., 1996; Hobbs et al., 1999; Youssef et al., 1998). Youth in out-of-home care represent a population particularly at risk for psychosocial, health, and developmental difficulties. These characteristics may be important factors in maltreatment by staff (Benedict et al., 1996; Hobbs et al., 1999). For example, according to Hobbs et al. (1999), caregivers often struggle to cope with the demands of these emotionally vulnerable youth, whose maladjusted behavior and patterns of communication may be misinterpreted. For example, staff may interpret a behavior as inappropriate and bizarre in the context of the youth's new environment, but the behavior may be totally adjusted to the abusive context from which he or she came. Maltreatment often can be triggered by difficult behaviors, and the caregiver may perceive the physical assault as a reasonable disciplinary method for controlling adolescents' behavior (Youssef et al., 1998). Despite the complex problems and difficulties exhibited by youth in care, residential care staff in many countries, including Israel (see Attar, 2006, for review), are untrained and lack the knowledge to deal effectively with such behaviors. Placement of youth in such settings creates the risk that they might be maltreated again (Groze, 1990; Hobbs et al., 1999).

The findings also show that adolescents with adjustment difficulties experienced higher levels of all types of victimization by peers (see also Gibbs & Sinclair, 2000). It seems, therefore, that adolescents with more adjustment difficulties are more susceptible to violent experiences and should be identified as a high-risk group deserving special resources. Because this study employs a cross-sectional design and cannot establish a causal direction of relationships among variables, the possibility of reverse causation should be examined in future studies. That is, the measured adjustment difficulties could have existed before the victimization or arisen as a consequence of it, and surely adjustment difficulties could be worsened by experiences of victimization (see Attar-Schwartz, 2011, 2014). Future studies should adopt longitudinal designs to establish causality.

Self-Efficacy

The findings reveal that perceived social self-efficacy was insignificantly linked with verbal victimization by peers (self-efficacy was not examined in regard to peer sexual victimization or staff maltreatment) but was negatively associated with levels of physical and indirect victimization by peers. Emotional self-efficacy was insignificantly linked with physical, verbal, and indirect victimization by peers. Social self-efficacy pertains to children's ability to deal with social challenges (Bandura, Pastorelli, Barbaranelli, & Caprara, 1999). Adolescents with little belief in their social abilities might be less assertive when faced with a violent act. They may have little belief in their ability to be accepted by others and may suffer from feelings of social maladjustment and loneliness. These characteristics could account for the increased risk of these adolescents to be physically, indirectly, and sexually victimized (Andreou & Metallidou, 2004; Crick & Grotpeter, 1995; Kokkins & Kipritsi, 2012). Because of the cross-sectional design of this study, however, causal interpretations should be exercised with caution. Longitudinal studies in the future could help establish causality.

Physical Maltreatment by Staff

In this study it was found that exposure to experiences of physical maltreatment by RCS staff is linked with greater exposure to all the types of peer victimization examined. Rus et al. (2017) similarly found that children in Romanian institutions who reported previous abuse by a staff member were more likely to be aware of exploitation in the RCS or to be victims of further exploitation themselves than those who did not report previous abuse. This finding can be interpreted in light of Bandura's cognitive-social learning theory (1982), which asserts that individuals (in this case, the perpetrators) learn certain behavioral patterns, such as using violence, through observation, role modeling, and reinforcement (e.g., Baldry, 2003; Monks et al., 2009). Assuming this theory, children might turn to violence to solve problems and conflicts when they observe the adults in their environment doing so, especially toward those who are seen to be the targets of adult violence (Geving, 2007; Lewis, Romi, Qui, & Katz, 2005). These young perpetrators of violence might also believe that, by appearing to collude with the adult perpetrators against the same victims, they will be immune to punishment by the adults: a circular situation that perpetuates violence against victims (Khoury-Kassabri & Attar-Schwartz, 2014).

Social Climate of the Institution

Adolescents who perceived the staff as stricter and less supportive reported more experiences of physical and verbal maltreatment by staff. Strictness and support were insignificantly linked with other forms of peer victimization, except for physical victimization by peers, which was linked positively to staff strictness. One possible interpretation for this finding is that the perception of staff as strict and less supportive might decrease young people's tendency to seek help, including in cases of peer victimization and staff maltreatment, resulting in an increase of exposure to violence. These hypotheses should be further tested in future research.

One possible explanation for the insignificant link that was found between adolescents' perception of strictness and lack of support from the RCS staff and experiences of indirect and verbal victimization by peers is that when it comes to subtle, more moderate, violence, there is evidence that even professionals in schools and in public care, who are aware of verbal and indirect aggressive incidents, do not identify those behaviors as victimization but rather see them as an integral part of the children's lives, expecting the children will resolve the issue on their own. These assumptions can lead to nonintervention (Barter et al., 2004; Mishna, 2012). As a result, adolescents might be made to feel that they are expected to deal with such situations on their own or that they are not actually forms of violence, so they therefore do not seek support in such cases, even if support is available in other aspects of their lives in the RCS (Barter et al., 2004). This may explain why this factor has no significance in explaining the variance among youth in RCSs in experiences of indirect and verbal peer violence (see Attar-Schwartz & Khoury-Kassabri, 2015). These possible interpretations, and the insignificant links found also between staff support and strictness and sexual victimization by peers, should be examined in future research.

The degree to which the young people in care perceived each other as friendly was found to be negatively linked to indirect and verbal victimization by peers (this aspect was not examined with regard to other aspects of victimization). This finding is consistent with previous studies that found that one of the most important factors in experiences of intimidation and violence among peers in RCSs is the peer culture and group dynamics (Barter et al., 2004; Sekol, 2013). This finding emphasizes the need to examine peer violence in RCSs from a wider contextual social perspective that includes peer behaviors and cultures (see Barter, 2011 for further discussion) and to focus intervention and prevention efforts in that direction.

Perceived RCS Antiviolence Policy

A key finding of the study is that levels of physical and verbal victimization by staff and levels of peer sexual victimization are negatively linked to young people's perceptions of the RCS's antiviolence policy. The clearer, fairer, and more consistent the adolescent felt the policy was, the fewer reported incidences of peer sexual victimization and staff verbal and physical victimization there were (this aspect was not examined with regard to other forms of victimization). It might be that youth who perceive the RCS antiviolence policy as positive may feel that their RCS does not tolerate any form of violent behavior. They may feel encouraged to be aware of their rights and to be able to distinguish behaviors that are acceptable from those that are not (Attar-Schwartz, 2011, 2014; Barter et al., 2004). Having a clear, fair, and consistent policy can be seen as an important aspect of creating a safe environment for children in care.

3.4.3 RCS-Level Correlates

Guided by an ecological contextual framework and using a multilevel analysis method, the study also found several RCS-level characteristics that correlated to an increased risk of victimization by peers and by staff in the RCS. The present study is consistent with other studies addressing violence experiences among youth in public care (e.g., Barter et al., 2004; Rus et al., 2013) in showing that levels of peer and staff victimization vary significantly across RCSs, depending on various institutional factors.

Ethnic Affiliation of the RCS

This study found more reports of staff physical maltreatment in Arab RCSs than in Jewish RCSs. This finding is consistent with studies of the Israeli educational system (e.g., Khoury-Kassabri, 2006). However, our study did not determine the various factors responsible for this finding. Some research suggests that differences between Arabs and Jews in Israel, and specifically differences in socioeconomic status, sociocultural norms, and sociocultural beliefs, may be relevant in explaining this finding (Benbenithy & Astor, 2005). As mentioned above, much of the Arab society in Israel is generally seen to be characterized by traditional, patriarchal, authoritarian values (Haj-Yahia, 2000). In contrast, the Jewish society is generally seen to be characterized by more Westernized, liberal values (Minkulincer, Weller, & Florian, 1993). Youth in Arab RCSs belong to an ethnic group whose cultural norms generally include greater tolerance toward corporal punishment (Khoury-Kassabri, 2010; Khoury-Kassabri & Straus, 2011). Acting in loco parentis, staff in Arab RCSs may discipline youth as they think parents would (Youssef et al., 1998), that is, by using corporal punishment. In addition, Arabs in Israel are a minority group characterized by rates of poverty and unemployment that are higher than those among the Jewish majority. Arabs also receive lower expenditures of public funds for health, education, and social services than those received by the majority (Haidar, 2005). Moreover, previous studies have found that staff maltreatment is more prevalent in the schools of communities with lower socioeconomic status (Benbenishty & Astor, 2005).

Economic and social factors also have been found to contribute to ethnic variation in aggression. Following the frustration-aggression theory, some argue that racial inequality leads to frustration, which leads in turn to aggression and violence (Berkowitz, 1989; Russell, 1994). Caregivers in a system characterized by lack of resources may therefore face many difficulties, may find it challenging and stressful to cope effectively with the difficult behaviors and needs exhibited by youth in care, and thus may resort to the use of violence. These assumptions find support in the parental child abuse literature, which connects parental stress, lack of adequate support, lack of resources, and child maltreatment (e.g., Parton, 1985). Studies in Israel found that differences between levels of maltreatment in Jewish and Arab schools were greatly reduced when analyses controlled for school socioeconomic status but that the differences remained statistically significant (e.g., Khoury-Kassabri, 2006). Therefore, both cultural and socioeconomic factors may contribute to high rates of maltreatment among Arab youth in RCSs in Israel. The possible links between ethnic affiliation and maltreatment should be examined empirically in future research.

The study shows, however, higher levels of verbal and sexual peer violence among youth from Jewish compared with Arab institutions. Lower rates of verbal victimization in Arab RCSs are consistent with findings in Israeli schools (Attar-Schwartz & Khoury-Kassabri, 2008) and might be associated with the collectivist, traditional values held by many in the Arab community (Dwairy & Achoui, 2006). Among the Arab population, cursing another person or his or her family is often considered to be an act of severe humiliation that has the potential to lead to serious sanctions and conflicts between clans. More control and supervision might therefore be placed on verbal violence and might help to explain why this form of victimization is less prevalent among Arab youth in RCSs (Attar-Schwartz & Khoury-Kassabri, 2008).

The finding that there were more reports of sexual victimization among adolescents from Jewish RCSs than among adolescents from Arab RCSs is inconsistent with some studies of Israeli schools, which showed that Arab students reported more sexual victimization (e.g., Attar-Schwartz, 2009a). This inconsistency might be explained by differences between children in schools and at-risk children in public institutional care, but additional research is needed in order to understand sexual victimization in and across Israeli Arab and Jewish youth in care. Future studies should address the motives and consequences of such behavior in each cultural group. The insignificant link between indirect peer victimization, moderate physical peer victimization, verbal staff victimization, and cultural affiliation, and the interpretations suggested here, should also be replicated in future studies.

Overall Number of Children in the RCS

Institution size – the overall number of children of all ages in the RCS – was found to be positively correlated with levels of physical maltreatment by staff. However, it was not found to be linked to the other types of victimization examined in this study. Greater institution size being linked to more physical maltreatment may raise concerns about the burdens placed on staff in larger RCSs. Large numbers of children may create higher levels of noise, less personal space and privacy, and more interpersonal friction, violence, and bullying, all of which can damage the sense of intimacy and care in the institution (Barter et al., 2004; Gibbs & Sinclair, 1999).

No significant links were found between the other victimization types and the number of children in the RCS, which is consistent with other studies in Israel linking emotional, social, and behavioral outcomes of children in Israeli residential care with institution size (e.g., Attar-Schwartz, 2008). The overall number of children in the care setting might not be very informative per se. For example, large RCSs may be divided into several subgroups, creating smaller, more protective, and intimate environments (see Barter et al., 2004). Alternatively, the limitations of large RCSs can be mitigated by a low child-to-caregiver ratio (Attar, 2006). Future studies should examine RCS size in the context of a broader set of organizational variables, which can combine to explain the effects of various aspects of the RCSs on children's status.

Type of Care

Institutions providing more intensive, therapeutic care for children reported more experiences of physical maltreatment by staff and sexual victimization by peers than rehabilitative institutions. Therapeutic RCSs provide care for youth with more troubled backgrounds and poorer psychosocial functioning than those youth in rehabilitative settings (see Attar-Schwartz, 2008). In keeping with the finding that maltreatment by staff and peer victimization are positively linked with adolescent adjustment difficulties, youth in therapeutic RCSs are found here to have much higher levels of reported physical maltreatment and sexual victimization by peers than their counterparts in rehabilitative settings. This finding suggests that staff maltreatment and peer victimization of youth in care are commonly associated with a high concentration of those regarded as the most troublesome clients (Holder, Nabinger, Lund, Costello, & Morton, 2003; Sinclair & Gibbs, 1998).

RCS Structure

No significant links were found between RCS structure and verbal and indirect victimization by peers or verbal maltreatment by staff. However, reports of physical and sexual victimization by peers and physical victimization by staff were found to be higher in traditional group settings than in settings with familial elements (such as familial clusters or mixed familial-group settings). This finding is consistent with Rus et al. (2013), who found that children in traditional group placement centers for school-aged children had greater odds of being severely punished by staff than those in family- or mixed-type settings. It is possible that in familial placements, the likelihood of maintaining strong relational bonds is higher. Adolescents in such settings may receive more encouragement to report victimization and may seek help more than their counterparts in other settings, which in turn may reduce the probability of their being victimized (Attar-Schwartz, 2011, 2014; Khoury-Kassabri & Attar-Schwartz, 2014). It is also possible that settings with familial elements allow more effective monitoring of peer violence than traditional group settings (Barter et al., 2004).

4 How Can This Knowledge Improve Children's Care?

The findings presented in this chapter show that peer violence and staff maltreatment are pervasive safety concerns among young people in RCSs in Israel. Clearly, stronger mechanisms are needed to ensure the safety of young people in RCSs, and safety issues should be placed high on the public and professional agenda (Barter, 2011; Freundlich et al., 2007). Yet RCSs in Israel and other countries frequently lack strategic approaches to tackle victimization experiences by staff and peers (Attar-Schwartz, 2014; Barter, 2011). This considerable problem calls for systematic planning of prevention and intervention programs to change RCS environments so that various types of victimization are clearly defined, controlled, and no longer tolerated (e.g., Barter, 2011; Gibbs & Sinclair, 1999; Stein, 2006).

Antiviolence prevention and intervention programs should not only focus on more overt, severe violent behaviors such as physical and sexual violence but should also be tailored to address the more common forms of violence outlined in this chapter, such as indirect and verbal violence (see Attar-Schwartz & Khoury-Kassabri, 2015). Targeting these behaviors is critical given their high occurrence and their documented detrimental consequences for children's outcomes.

Using an ecological-contextual perspective, this study revealed the need to address peer and staff violence in RCSs from a holistic point of view, intervening at the personal level with both victims and perpetrators, as well as at the institutional level, identifying the various RCS contexts in which victimization occurs more frequently (see also Rus et al., 2013). Accordingly, interventions should be directed at the entire RCS community (children, staff, directors, and, if possible, parents) rather than only at a selected group of violent or victimized young people or staff. Yong people, staff, and directors need to work together to create a structured and safe everyday living environment that offers constructive opportunities while creating clear guidelines for acceptable and tolerable behaviors (Barter et al., 2004).

The findings seem to suggest a pressing need for improved regulation, registration, and inspection in RCSs (Attar-Schwartz, 2011, 2014; Stein, 2006). It would be helpful for staff members to receive ongoing training to help them understand the backgrounds of the youth entering care as problematic past experiences can make youth afraid to develop trusting and close relationships. Such training should identify the behavioral consequences of young people's experiences, as well as ways to deal effectively with young people of all backgrounds in care (Gill, 1996; Hobbs et al., 1999; Youssef et al., 1998).

Given the widespread nature of physical, sexual, verbal, and indirect victimization by peers in RCSs, it might be beneficial to establish a system of continuous monitoring of peer victimization in RCSs. In addition, specific steps involving all RCS partners should be developed to undertake close supervision of young people in care and to help build positive expectations of accepted behavior (Barter, 2011). There is also a need to develop respectful and nurturing interactions between children and caregivers and among the young people themselves. These steps might help prevent further victimization of children in RCSs, many of whom are removed from their homes because of maltreatment in the first place. Taking these steps might help give these vulnerable young people the opportunity to live and thrive in a safe, healthy, and nurturing environment.

5 Summary

The study found that adolescents in Israeli RCSs are exposed to high levels of peer violence. More than half of the participants (56%) reported that they had been physically victimized by at least one act of physical violence by a peer in their RCS in the previous month, 73% reported having been exposed to verbal maltreatment, 62% to indirect maltreatment, and 40% to at least one act of sexual violence. The adolescents also reported incidences of maltreatment by staff. One in four of the adolescents reported that they had been physically victimized at least once by a staff member, and 29% reported that they had been verbally victimized at least once in the month prior to the survey. This high level of victimization is consistent with the findings of previous studies; however, given the various populations, methodologies, and time frames used in other studies, it might be misleading to compare their findings with those of the study outlined here.

The findings of the present study emphasize the importance of examining the various types of violence to which young people in care can be exposed. Certain ecological correlates act as risk factors for some types of violence but have an opposite or insignificant effect on others. The study highlights the importance of applying an ecological-contextual perspective to the research of correlates of staff and peer-to-peer violence in residential care. They show that adolescent victimization by peers and staff is explained simultaneously by the adolescents' individual characteristics (such as gender, age, and adjustment difficulties) and by the social context (including, e.g., the size of the institution, the type of care) in which the adolescents' development occurs (Kuppens, Gritenes, Onghena, Michiels, & Subramanian, 2008; Rus, Parris, Cross, & Purvis, 2010; Rus et al., 2013). Given the vulnerability of young people in RCSs, many of whom experienced maltreatment prior to being placed in public care, it is critical to find ways to protect them from further harm while in the care setting. Knowing which factors may increase a child's risk of being victimized by peers and staff must be an essential part of designing and implementing interventions to deal with violence in out-of-home facilities.

Questions for Discussion

- Based on the findings presented in this chapter, can you plan an intervention program to address peer and staff victimization in residential care settings for children at risk? Specify the target population and the specific steps needed to put this program into action.
- This study explored several youth-level and institutional-level correlates of youth victimization in care. Can you suggest additional correlates that might be important for predicting victimization?
- This study looked at a number of specific forms of staff and peer victimization. Can you think of other forms of institutional abuse not included in this study that seem important to explore? Can you suggest ways to measure these types of maltreatment?

References

Agathonos, H. (1983). Institutional child abuse in Greece: Some preliminary findings. *Child Abuse & Neglect*, *7*, 71–74.

Andreou, E., & Metallidou, P. (2004). The relationship of academic and social cognition in behavior in bullying situations among Greek primary school children. *Educational Psychology*, *24*, 27–41.

Archer, J., & Coyne, S. M. (2005). An integrated review of indirect, relational, and social aggression. *Personality and Social Psychology Review*, *9*, 212–230.

Attar, S. (2006). *Child, family, and institutional correlates of the psychosocial and educational functioning of children in rehabilitative, therapeutic, and post-hospitalization residential facilities* (Unpublished doctoral dissertation). Hebrew University of Jerusalem.

Attar-Schwartz, S. (2008). Emotional, behavioral and social problems among Israeli children in residential care: A multi-level analysis. *Children and Youth Services Review*, *30*(2), 229–248.

Attar-Schwartz, S. (2009a). Peer sexual harassment victimization at school: The roles of student characteristics, cultural affiliation and school factors. *American Journal of Orthopsychiatry*, *79*, 407–420.

Attar-Schwartz, S. (2009b). School functioning of children in residential care: The contributions of multilevel correlates. *Child Abuse & Neglect*, *33*, 429–440.

Attar-Schwartz, S. (2011). Maltreatment by staff in residential care facilities: The adolescents' perspectives. *Social Service Review*, *85*, 635–664.

Attar-Schwartz, S. (2014). Experiences of sexual victimization by peers among adolescents in residential care settings. *Social Services Review*, *88*, 594–629.

Attar-Schwartz, S., & Khoury-Kassabri, M. (2008). Indirect versus verbal forms of victimization at school: The contribution of student, family, and school variables. *Social Work Research*, *32*(3), 159–170.

Attar-Schwartz, S., & Khoury-Kassabri, M. (2015). Indirect and verbal victimization by peers among youth at-risk in residential care. *Child Abuse & Neglect*, *42*, 84–98.

Baldry, A. C. (2003). Bullying in schools and exposure to domestic violence. *Child Abuse & Neglect*, *27*, 713–732.

Bandura, A. (1982). Self-efficacy mechanism in human agency. *American Psychologist, 37*, 122–147.

Bandura, A., Pastorelli, C., Barbaranelli, C., & Caprara, G. V. (1999). Self-efficacy pathways to childhood depression. *Journal of Personality and Social Psychology, 76*, 258–269.

Barboza, G. E., Schiamberg, L. B., Oehmke, J., Korzeniewski, S. J., Post, L. A., & Heraux, C. G. (2009). Individual characteristics and the multiple contexts of adolescent bullying: An ecological perspective. *Journal of Youth and Adolescence, 38*, 101–121.

Barter, C. (1998). *Investigating institutional abuse of children: An exploration of the NSPCC experience*. London, UK: NSPCC.

Barter, C. (2003). *Abuse of children in residential care: Information briefing*. London, UK: National Society for Prevention of Cruelty to children.

Barter, C. (2008). Prioritizing young people's concerns in residential care: Responding to peer violence. In A. J. Kendrick (Ed.), *Residential child care: Prospects and challenges* (pp. 137–151). London, UK: Jessica Kingsley Publishers.

Barter, C. (2011). Peer violence in residential children's homes: A unique experience. In C. P. Monks & I. Coyne (Eds.), *Bullying in different contexts*. Cambridge, UK: Cambridge University Press.

Barter, C., Renold, E., Berridge, D., & Cawson, P. (2004). *Peer violence in children's residential care*. Basingstoke, UK: Palgrave.

Benbenishty, R., & Astor, R. A. (2005). *School violence in context: Culture, neighborhood, family, school, and gender*. Oxford, UK: Oxford University Press.

Benbenishty, R., Zeira, A., & Astor, R. (2000). *Violence in Israel education system: A summary report*. Jerusalem, Israel: The Hebrew University. (Hebrew).

Benedict, M. I., Zuravin, S., Brandt, D., & Abbey, H. (1994). Types and frequency of child maltreatment by family foster care providers in an urban population. *Child Abuse & Neglect, 18*, 577–588.

Benedict, M. I., Zuravin, S., Somerfield, M., & Brandt, D. (1996). The reported health and functioning of children maltreated while in family foster care. *Child Abuse & Neglect, 20*, 561–571.

Berkowitz, L. (1989). Frustration-aggression hypothesis: Examination and reformulation. *Psychological Bulletin, 106*, 59–73.

Block, J. H. (1983). Differential premises arising from differential socialization of the sexes: Some conjectures. *Child Development, 54*, 1335–1354.

Bolton, F. G., Laner, R. H., & Gai, D. S. (1981). For better or worse? Foster parents and foster children in an officially reported child maltreatment population. *Children and Youth Services Review, 3*(1), 37–53.

Borg, M. K. (1999). The extent and nature of bullying among primary and secondary school children. *Educational Research, 41*(2), 137–153.

Bronfenbrenner, U. (1979). *The ecology of human development*. Cambridge, MA: Harvard University.

Cillessen, A. H. N., & Mayeux, L. (2004). From censure to reinforcement: Developmental changes in the association between aggression and social status. *Child Development, 75*, 147–167.

Colton, M. (1989). Foster and residential children's perceptions of their social environments. *British Association of Social Workers, 19*, 217–233.

Crick, N. R. (1997). Engagement in gender normative versus non-normative forms of aggression: Links to social-psychological adjustment. *Developmental Psychology, 33*(4), 610–617.

Crick, N. R., Casas, J. F., & Mosher, M. (1997). Relational and overt aggression in preschool. *Developmental Psychology, 33*(4), 579–588.

Crick, N. R., & Grotpeter, J. K. (1995). Relational aggression, gender, and social-psychological adjustment. *Child Development, 66*, 710–722.

Davidson-Arad, B., & Golan, M. (2007). Victimization of juveniles in out-of-home placement: Juvenile correctional facilities. *British Journal of Social Work, 37*(6), 1007–1025.

Dolev, T., Ben Rabi, D., & Zemach-Marom, T. (2009). Residential care for children "at risk" in Israel: Current situation and future challenges. In M. E. Courtney & D. Iwaniec (Eds.), *Residential care of children: Comparative perspectives* (pp. 72–87). New York, NY: Oxford University Press.

Dolev, T., Benbenishty, R., & Timar, A. (2001). *Decision committees in Israel: Their organization, work processes, and outcomes*. Jerusalem, Israel: JDC-Brookdale Institute. (Hebrew).
Dwairy, M., & Achoui, M. (2006). Introduction to three cross-regional research studies on parenting styles, individuation, and mental health in Arab societies. *Journal of Cross-Cultural Psychology, 37*, 221–229.
Elbedour, S., Assor, A., Center, B. A., & Maruyama, G. M. (1997). Physical and psychological maltreatment in schools: The abusive behaviors of teachers in Bedouin schools in Israel. *School Psychology International, 18*(3), 201–215.
Farmer, E., & Pollock, A. (1998). *Sexually abused and abusing children in substitute care*. Chichester, UK: Wiley.
Freundlich, M., Avery, R. J., & Padgett, D. (2007). Care of scare: The safety of youth in congregate care in New York City. *Child Abuse & Neglect, 31*, 173–186.
Fulcher, L. (2001). Differential assessment of residential group care for children and young people. *British Journal of Social Work, 31*, 417–435.
Furlong, M. J., Greif, J. L., Bates, M. P., Whipple, A. D., Jimenez, T. C., & Morrison, R. (2005). Development of the California School climate and safety survey–short form. *Psychology in the Schools, 42*, 137–149.
Geving, A. M. (2007). Identifying the types of student and teacher behaviors associated with teacher stress. *Teaching and Teacher Education, 23*, 624–640.
Gibbs, I., & Sinclair, I. (1999). Treatment and treatment outcomes in children's homes. *Child and Family Social Work, 4*, 1–8.
Gibbs, I., & Sinclair, I. (2000). Bullying, sexual harassment and happiness in residential children's homes. *Child Abuse Review, 9*(4), 247–256.
Gill, K. (1996). *Going to court: Child witnesses in their own words; A ChildLine study*. London, UK: ChildLine.
Glisson, C., Hemmelgarn, A. L., & Post, J. A. (2002). The shortform assessment for children: An assessment and outcome measure for child welfare and juvenile justice. *Research on Social Work Practice, 12*(1), 82–106.
Goodman, R. (1997). The strengths and difficulties questionnaire: A research note. *Journal of Child Psychology and Psychiatry, 38*, 581–586.
Green, L., & Masson, H. (2002). Adolescents who sexually abuse and residential accommodation: Issues of risk and vulnerability. *British Journal of Social Work, 32*, 68–149.
Groze, V. (1990). An exploratory investigation into institutional mistreatment. *Children and Youth Services Review, 12*, 229–241.
Haidar, A. (2005). Arab society in Israel: Populations, society, economy. *Report*. Jerusalem, Israel: Van Leer Institute. (Hebrew).
Haj-Yahia, M. M. (2000). Wife abuse and battering in the sociocultural context of Arab society. *Family Process, 39*, 237–255.
Hareven, A. (2002). Towards the year 2030: Can a civil society shared by Jews and Arabs evolve in Israel? *International Journal of Intercultural Relations, 26*(2), 153–168.
Hargrave, M. C. (1991). Sexual incidents in residential treatment. *Child & Youth Care Forum, 20*, 413–419.
Heal, K., Sinclair, I., & Troop, J. (1973). Development of a social climate questionnaire for use in approved schools and community homes. *The British Journal of Sociology, 24*, 222–235.
Hobbs, G. F., Hobbs, C. J., & Wynne, J. M. (1999). Abuse of children in foster and residential care. *Child Abuse & Neglect, 23*(12), 1239–1252.
Holder, W., Nabinger, D., Lund, T.R., Costello, T., & Morton, T.D. (2003). *Maltreatment in out-of-home placement: A leadership initiative of the National Resource Center on Child Maltreatment*. Duluth, GA: National Resource Center on Child Maltreatment.
Hyman, I. A., Zelikoff, W., & Clarke, J. (1988). Psychological and physical abuse in schools: A paradigm for understanding post-traumatic stress disorder in children. *Journal of Traumatic Stress, 1*, 243–267.

Jaffe, E. D. (1978). Child welfare in Israel: An overview of institution care, foster home care and adoption. *Jewish Communal Services, 55*, 171–180.
Kendrick, A. (1997). Safeguarding children living away from home from abuse: A literature review. In R. Kent (Ed.), *Children's safeguards review*. Edinburgh, UK: The Scottish Office.
Kendrick, A. (2011). Peer violence in provision for children in care. In C. Barter & D. Berridge (Eds.), *Children behaving badly? Peer violence between children and young people* (pp. 71–84). Chichester, UK: Wiley.
Khoury-Kassabri, M. (2006). Student victimization by educational staff in Israel. *Child Abuse and Neglect, 30*, 691–707.
Khoury-Kassabri, M. (2009). The relationship between staff maltreatment of students and bully-victim group membership. *Child Abuse & Neglect, 33*, 914–923.
Khoury-Kassabri, M. (2010). Attitudes of Arab and Jewish mothers towards punitive and non-punitive discipline methods. *Child and Family Social Work, 15*, 135–144.
Khoury-Kassabri, M., & Attar-Schwartz, S. (2014). Adolescents' reports of physical violence by peers in residential care settings: An ecological examination. *Journal of Interpersonal Violence, 29*, 659–682.
Khoury-Kassabri, M., & Straus, M. A. (2011). Discipline methods used by mothers: The contribution of ethnicity, socioeconomic status, and child's characteristics. *Child Indicators Research, 4*, 45–57.
Kim, D. H., Kim, K. I., Park, Y. C., Zhang, L. D., Lu, M. K., & Li, D. (2000). Children's experience of violence in China and Korea: A transcultural study. *Child Abuse & Neglect, 24*(9), 1163–1173.
King, M.M. 2013. *Stability and change in institutional out-of-home childcare provision* (Thesis submitted in partial fulfillment of the requirements for the degree of MSc in comparative social policy). University of Oxford, Oxford, UK.
Kokkinos, C. M., & Kipritsi, E. (2012). The relationship between bullying, victimization, trait emotional intelligence, self-efficacy and empathy among preadolescents. *Social Psychology of Education, 15*, 41–58.
Kuppens, S., Grietens, H., Onghena, D. M., & Subramanian, S. V. (2008). Individual and classroom variables associated with relational aggression in elementary-school aged children. *Journal of School Psychology, 46*, 639–660.
Leaderbeater, B. J., Boone, E. M., Sangster, N. A., & Mathieson, L. C. (2006). Sex differences in the personal costs and benefits of relational and physical aggression in high school. *Aggressive Behavior, 32*, 409–429.
Lewis, R., Romi, S., Qui, X., & Katz, Y. J. (2005). Teachers' classroom discipline and student misbehavior in Australia, China and Israel. *Teaching and Teacher Education, 21*, 729–741.
MacLeod, M. (1999). The abuse of children in institutional settings: Children's perspectives. In J. M. N. Stanely & B. Penhale (Eds.), *Institutional abuse: Perspectives across the life course* (pp. 44–65). London, UK: Routledge.
Minkulincer, M., Weller, A., & Florian, C. (1993). Sense of closeness to parents and family rules: A study of Arab and Jewish youth in Israel. *International Journal of Psychology, 28*, 323–335.
Mishna, F. (2012). *Bullying: A guide to research, intervention, and prevention*. New York, NY: Oxford University Press.
Monks, C. P., Smith, P. K., Naylor, P., Barter, C., Ireland, J. L., & Coyne, I. (2009). Bullying in different contexts: Commonalities, differences and the role of theory. *Aggression and Violent Behavior, 14*, 146–156.
Morris, S., & Wheatley, H. (1994). *Time to listen*. London, UK: Child-Line.
Muris, P. (2001). A brief questionnaire for measuring self-efficacy in youths. *Journal of Psychopathology and Behavioral Assessment, 23*, 145–149.
Nansel, T., Overpeck, M., Pilla, R., Ruan, W., Simons-Morton, B., & Scheidt, P. (2001). Bullying behaviors among U.S. youth: Prevalence and association with psychosocial adjustment. *JAMA: Journal of the American Medical Association, 285*(16), 2094–2100.

National Council for the Child. (2010). *Children in Israel: Statistical abstract.* Jerusalem, Israel: Israel National Council for the Child. (Hebrew).
National Council for the Child. (2012). *Children in Israel: Statistical abstract.* Jerusalem, Israel: National Council for the Child. (Hebrew).
National Council for the Child. (2014). *Children in Israel: Statistical abstract.* Jerusalem, Israel: Israel National Council for the Child. (Hebrew).
Nesmith, A. (2006). Predictors of running away from family foster care. *Child Welfare, 85*, 585–609.
Olweus, D. (1993). *Bullying at school: What we know and what we can do.* Oxford, UK: Blackwell.
Ostrov, J. M., & Keating, C. F. (2004). Gender differences in preschool aggression during free play and structured interactions: An observational study. *Social Development, 13*, 255–277.
Parton, N. (1985). *The politics of child abuse.* London, UK: Macmillan.
Pecora, P. J., Kessler, R. C., Williams, J., O'Brien, K., Downs, A. C., English, D., … Holmes, K. (2005). *Improving family foster care: Findings from the Northwest foster care alumni study.* Seattle, WA: Casey Family Programs.
Pellegrini, A. D., & Archer, J. (2005). Sex differences in competitive and aggressive behavior. In B. J. Ellis & D. F. Bjorklund (Eds.), *Origins of the social mind* (pp. 219–244). New York, NY: Guilford Press.
Poertner, J., Bussey, M., & Fluke, J. (1999). How safe are out-of-home placements? *Children and Youth Services Review, 21*, 549–563.
Raudenbush, S. W., & Bryk, S. A. (2002). *Hierarchical linear models: Applications and data analysis methods* (2nd ed.). Thousand Oaks, CA: Sage.
Rindfleisch, N., & Rabb, J. (1984). How much of a problem is resident mistreatment in child welfare institutions? *Child Abuse & Neglect, 8*(1), 33–40.
Rosenthal, J. A., Motz, J. K., Edmonson, D. A., & Groze, V. K. (1991). A descriptive study of abuse and neglect in out-of-home placement. *Child Abuse & Neglect, 15*, 249–260.
Rus, A.V., Parris, S., Cross, D., & Purvis, K. (2010). Romanian institutionalized children's privation and Bronfenbrenner's ecological system theory. In *Research, education and development: Symposium proceedings.* Clju-Napoca, Romania: Risoprint Publishing House. DOI: 10.13140/2.1.5000.8004.
Rus, A. V., Stativa, E., Butterfield, M. E., Pennings, J. S., Parris, S. R., Burcea, G., & Wenyika, R. (2017). Peer Exploitation: Findings from a Romanian National Representative Sample of Children Living in Long-Term Residential Centres. *Child Abuse Review.*
Rus, A. V., Stativa, E., Pennings, J. S., Cross, D. R., Ekas, N., Purvis, K. B., & Parris, S. R. (2013). Severe punishment of children in Romanian placement centers for school-aged children: Effects of child and institutional characteristics. *Child Abuse & Neglect, 37*, 1152–1162.
Russell, K. K. (1994). The racial inequality hypothesis: A critical look at the research and an alternative theoretical analysis. *Law and Human Behavior, 18*, 305–317.
Scheithauer, H., Hayer, T., Peterman, F., & Jugert, G. (2006). Physical, verbal, and relational forms of bullying among German students: Age trends, gender differences, and correlates. *Aggressive Behavior, 32*, 261–275.
Sekol, I. (2013). Peer violence in adolescent residential care: A qualitative examination of contextual and peer factors. *Children and Youth Services Review, 35*, 1901–1912.
Sekol, I., & Farrington, D. P. (2009). The nature and prevalence of bullying among boys and girls in Croatian care institutions: A descriptive analysis of children's homes and correctional homes. *Criminology and Social Integration, 17*, 15–34.
Service for Children and Youth. (2014). *The children and youth service: Data on children in residential care in 2013–2014.* Jerusalem, Israel: Ministry of Social Affairs and Services and Brookdale Institute.
Sinclair, I., & Gibbs, I. (1998). *Children's homes: A study in diversity.* Chichester, UK: Wiley.
Smith, P.K., Kwak, K., & Toda, Y. (Eds.). (2016). *School bullying in different cultures: Eastern and Western perspectives.* Cambridge, UK: Cambridge University Press.

Smith, P. K., Madsen, K. C., & Moody, J. C. (1999). What causes the age decline in reports of being bullied at school? Towards a developmental analysis of risks of being bullied. *Educational Research, 41*(3), 267–285.

Spencer, J. E., & Knudsen, D. D. (1992). Out-of-home maltreatment: An analysis of risk in various settings for children. *Children and Youth Services Review, 14*, 485–492.

Stein, M. (2006). Missing years of abuse in children's homes. *Child and Family Social work, 11*, 11–21.

Whittaker, J. K. (1978). Changing character of residential child-care: Ecological perspective. *Social Service Review, 52*, 21–36.

Whittaker, J. K., Holmes, L., del Valle, J. F., Ainsworth, F., Andreassen, T., & Anglin, J. (2016). Therapeutic residential care for children and youth: A consensus statement of the international work group on therapeutic residential care. *Residential Treatment for Children & Youth, 33*, 89–106.

Youssef, R. M., Attia, M. S. E. D., & Kamel, M. I. (1998). Children experiencing violence II: Prevalence and determinants of corporal punishment in schools. *Child Abuse & Neglect, 22*(10), 975–985.

Zahn-Waxler, C., & Polanichka, N. J. (2004). All things interpersonal: Socialization and female aggression. In M. Pullataz & K. L. Bierman (Eds.), *Aggression, antisocial behavior and violence among girls: A developmental perspective* (pp. 48–68). New York, NY: Guilford Press.

Chapter 14
Structural Neglect in Orphanages: Physical Growth, Cognition, and Daily Life of Young Institutionalized Children in India

Femmie Juffer, Marinus H. van IJzendoorn, and Marian J. Bakermans-Kranenburg

(...) the more the social environment in which a human child is reared deviates from the environment of evolutionary adaptedness (which is probably father, mother, and siblings in a social environment comprising grandparents and a limited number of other known families) the greater will be the risk of his developing maladaptive patterns of social behavior.

Bowlby (1982, p. 166).

1 Introduction

Although a substantial number of children reside in orphanages in India (estimated number of 20 million orphans, defined as children who have been abandoned or lost both parents; SOS Villages India, 2011), empirical studies on these institutionalized children are scarce, especially studies on young children (but see Taneja et al., 2002). For example, Escueta, Whetten, Ostermann, O'Donnell, & The Positive Outcomes for Orphans Research Team (2014) included children in institutional care in their longitudinal study on psychosocial well-being and cognitive development of orphans and abandoned children in five low-income countries (Cambodia, Ethiopia, India, Kenya, and Tanzania), but their study started with children aged 6–12 years. Eapen (2009) examined the physical and cognitive development of institutionalized children aged 8–12 years in India. Both studies found significant developmental delays, but we do not know whether these findings can be generalized to younger children in institutional care in India. In our study we examined the physical and

F. Juffer (✉) • M.H. van IJzendoorn • M.J. Bakermans-Kranenburg
Leiden University, Centre for Child & Family Studies,
Wassenaarseweg 52, 2333 AK Leiden, The Netherlands
e-mail: juffer@fsw.leidenuniv.nl; vanijzen@fsw.leidenuniv.nl;
bakermans@fsw.leidenuniv.nl

A.V. Rus et al. (eds.), *Child Maltreatment in Residential Care*,
DOI 10.1007/978-3-319-57990-0_14

cognitive development of children in the age range of 1–6 years in an orphanage in one of the big cities of India, and we observed the daily life experiences of the youngest, most vulnerable group of toddlers.

1.1 Physical Growth

One area of child development that is negatively affected by growing up in institutional care is physical growth. Several studies have shown that institutionalized children suffer from marked delays in weight, height, and head circumference (e.g., Dobrova-Krol, Van IJzendoorn, Bakermans-Kranenburg, Cyr, & Juffer, 2008; Johnson et al., 2010; Miller et al., 2007; Miller, Chan, Comfort, & Tirella, 2005). Lack of appropriate nutrition as well as growth retardation caused by social-emotional deprivation may contribute to the physical growth delays in institutionalized children (Johnson & Gunnar, 2011).

Remarkably, the physical growth delays of institutionalized children recover or disappear when these children are placed in a more nurturing environment (e.g., Van den Dries, Juffer, Van IJzendoorn, & Bakermans-Kranenburg, 2010). In the Bucharest Early Intervention Project (BEIP; Zeanah et al., 2003), children were randomized either to prolonged institutionalization or to foster care to study the effects of institutional care and possible catch-up after removal from the institutional setting. All institutionalized children showed marked growth delays at the start of the study, but the children randomized to foster care showed significant catch-up in weight and height, but not in head circumference, within 12 months (Johnson et al., 2010).

In the same vein, a meta-analysis of internationally adopted children found massive catch-up in weight and height, and somewhat less catch-up in head circumference after placement in an adoptive family, pointing to plasticity of physical growth in early childhood (Van IJzendoorn, Bakermans-Kranenburg, & Juffer, 2007). Before their adoption, internationally adopted children usually live in deprived settings and often in orphanages (Juffer et al., 2011). The drastic change of environment from institutional care to adoptive family care appears to result in significant gains in physical growth.

1.2 Cognitive Development

Several studies have shown that cognitive development of children in institutional care is severely compromised (e.g., Dobrova-Krol, Van IJzendoorn, Bakermans-Kranenburg, & Juffer, 2010). In a meta-analysis including 75 studies in 19 different countries, we found large IQ delays in institutionalized children (Van IJzendoorn, Luijk, & Juffer, 2008). Children growing up in orphanages showed a substantially lower level of intellectual development (average IQ of 84) than children reared in a family (average IQ of 104). The meta-analysis also included an intervention study – introducing a daily brief structured play session as an intervention – in an Indian orphanage (Taneja et al., 2002). The researchers found severe delays in developmental quotient (DQ) in the infants (aged 6 months to 2.5 years) and a remarkable increase after a 3-month intervention period (from a DQ of 66 to a DQ of 90, as assessed with the Bayley Scales of Infant Development).

Recovery of cognitive development has also been demonstrated in children who were moved from a depriving institutional setting to a more nurturing environment, such as a foster or adoptive family. In the BEIP study (see before), the children randomized to foster care outperformed the children who remained in institutional care in IQ (Nelson et al., 2007). Similarly, a comprehensive meta-analysis on the cognitive development of adopted and non-adopted children showed that adopted children scored substantially higher on IQ tests than children who remained in institutional care (Van IJzendoorn, Juffer, & Poelhuis, 2005).

Family care matters for children's cognitive development. In a study on infants adopted from Chinese orphanages versus Chinese foster families, the adopted children with a foster family background outperformed the adopted children with an orphanage background regarding their DQ, measured with the Bayley Scales of Infant Development (Van den Dries et al., 2010). Two months after their adoption (age at adoptive placement between 11 and 16 months), the children from institutional care in China showed an average DQ of 74, whereas the children from foster care in China had an average DQ of 84. Six months after adoption, both groups showed a similar, significant catch-up: the average DQ of the children from institutional care increased from 74 to 84, while the average DQ of the children from foster care increased from 84 to 92 (Van den Dries et al., 2010).

1.3 Daily Life Experiences

Child development is profoundly affected by growing up in orphanages, and the negative impact of institutional care is of course broader than the domains of physical growth and cognitive development. Children's neurobiological and social-emotional development, their well-being and behavioral functioning, and their attachment relationships are also negatively affected by institutionalization (e.g., Bakermans-Kranenburg et al., 2012; Van IJzendoorn et al., 2011). Given the massive body of evidence, one starts to wonder which features of growing up in an orphanage are so detrimental for children's development.

Several studies have provided global or more detailed descriptions of children's daily life in an orphanage, while all studies converge in their view that stable and adequate, consistently sensitive care is largely lacking in institutions (e.g., Dobrova-Krol, Bakermans-Kranenburg, Van IJzendoorn, & Juffer, 2010; Groark, McCall, Fish, & The Whole Child International Evaluation Team, 2011; Groark, Muhamedrahimov, Palmov, Nikiforova, & McCall, 2005; Smyke et al., 2007). Detailed observations of how orphanages in different countries provide child care to young children may shed more light on this issue.

Two studies have used an observational instrument to measure the daily life experiences of young children in orphanages: spot observations in a time use procedure (Daunhauer, Bolton, Cermak, 2005; Tirella et al., 2008). Daunhauer and colleagues used this measure in a Romanian orphanage, and Tirella et al. used it in Russian baby homes. In the current study, we conducted time use spot observations in an Indian orphanage. In spot observations (comparable to time diaries) a target child's activities and whereabouts are recorded on the spot at preset intervals during a period of time (e.g., during one morning) (Daunhauer et al., 2005). These observations are unannounced and nonintrusive to facilitate spontaneous behavior and interactions. In the studies in the Romanian and Russian orphanages, the observers stepped into the children's room every 10 min during 5 h and coded several categories, including whom the target child was interacting with and what the child was doing at that moment. Both studies found indications for suboptimal levels of care in the orphanages, due to a strong focus on daily routines and schedules with few opportunities for human interaction and play (Daunhauer et al., 2005; Tirella et al., 2008).

2 Current Study

In this study we examined the development of young children and their daily life experiences in an orphanage in one of the big cities of India. In this institution young children resided in a large room for toddlers and a smaller room for preschoolers (with no strict age limit, roughly younger/older than 3.5 years). Common group size was 30–35 for the toddlers and 10–15 for the preschoolers. Caregiver-child ratio was 1:6 in the morning and 1:8 in the afternoon and at night. Usually there were no toys available for the toddlers, whereas the preschoolers had access to some play material. The children in the orphanage had been abandoned or relinquished by their birth family; whenever possible children were placed in domestic or international adoptive families. Infants younger than 1 year, children older than approximately 6 years, and children with disabilities resided in other rooms in the orphanage.

We address the following research questions: (1) Do young children in institutional care in this orphanage show delays in physical growth and cognition? (2) Is there any catch-up in physical growth and cognition after staying in institutional care for a year? (3) What are the experiences of young children's daily life in an orphanage? For the last question, we specifically focus on the youngest age group of toddlers.

2.1 Method

2.1.1 Procedure and Participants

We assessed physical growth and cognition in 37 young children. In a subsample ($n = 20$) we repeated these assessments 1 year later to examine possible catch-up growth. In the youngest age group ($n = 20$ toddlers from the total sample of

Table 14.1 Child characteristics and outcome variables in the total sample, the follow-up subsample, and the time use subsample

	Total $N = 37$ (65% female) *M* (*SD*)	Follow-up $n = 20$ (60% female) *M* (*SD*)	Time use $n = 20$ (75% female) *M* (*SD*)
Age at assessment in months	35.11 (16.40)	43.17 (17.03)	25.46 (8.50)
Age at arrival in months	22.64 (18.68)	27.48 (22.49)	16.84 (10.19)
Time in institution in months	12.46 (11.45)	15.69 (13.90)	8.62 (5.99)
Z-score weight	−1.90 (1.21)	−1.58 (0.91)	−2.22 (1.33)
Z-score height	−1.86 (1.50)	−1.71 (1.12)	−2.11 (1.77)
Z-score head size	−1.56 (1.01)	−1.63 (1.02)	−1.55 (0.97)
Developmental quotient	67.73 (13.70)	68.41 (15.76)	65.21 (11.48)

37 children), we examined children's daily living environment with spot observations. The total sample of young children in institutional care consisted of 24 girls (65%) and 13 boys with a mean age of almost 3 years (35 months, range, 13–80 months; see Table 14.1 for child characteristics). All children had been abandoned or relinquished because of unwed motherhood by their birth family. Weight, height, and head circumference were assessed, and tests for cognitive development were administered. Follow-up assessments after about 1 year ($M = 14$ months, $SD = 4$; range 11–24 months) were available for a subsample of 20 children with a mean age of approximately 3.5 years (see Table 14.1). Post hoc, their results on physical and cognitive development were compared with outcomes from a cohort of 18 young children (not included in the current study) assessed with the same measures in a previous year to see whether our findings were replicated. Finally, spot observations of children's daily life experiences were carried out in a subsample of 20 toddlers from the total sample of 37 children (mean age approximately 2 years; see Table 14.1). Each child was observed on 1 day during 5 h, once every 10 min.

2.1.2 Measures

Physical Growth

To measure height, a measuring tape was attached to the wall, and the child was standing next to it, with his or her back to the wall (>2 years; for younger children supine length was measured when they were lying down). To measure head circumference, the measuring tape was wrapped around the widest circumference of the child's head (broadest part of the forehead, above the ears, most prominent part of the back of the head). All outcomes were converted to Z-scores using the World Health Organization Anthro calculator (WHO, 2016). To compute growth Z-scores, a child's individual outcomes were related to the average outcome of children of the same age, resulting in weight-for-age, height-for-age, and head circumference-for-age. Growth data were collected by the WHO Multicentre Growth Reference

Study and included 8500 children from widely different ethnic backgrounds and cultural settings (e.g., India, Norway, the USA). A Z-score describes how many standard deviations the child's growth outcome lies above or below the mean (zero). Mild delays are indicated by Z-scores between -1 and -2. More severe delays are indicated by Z-scores <-2 for weight (underweight), height (stunting), and head circumference (microcephaly) (Miller, 2005).

Cognition

Two nonverbal tests for cognitive development, one for the younger and one for the older children, were administered by trained research assistants. Because the children were not used to sitting at a table, children and research assistants were sitting on the floor during the test procedure. The tests were administered in a separate room with no other children around. If necessary, a caregiver was invited into the room to reassure the child. The caregiver was not allowed to give any help to the child. When the test continued for too long because of inattentiveness, restlessness, tiredness, or distress of the child, the test was administered in two parts (see also Van der Meulen, Ruiter, Lutje Spelberg, & Smrkovsky, 2004).

To examine the cognitive development of the toddlers, the nonverbal version (Ruiter, Hoekstra, Van der Meulen, & Lutje Spelberg, 2005) of the Dutch Bayley Scales of Infant Development-II was administered (Van der Meulen et al., 2004). All children received a score for cognitive development (Mental Developmental Index). The Bayley Scales of Infant Development are widely recommended for testing young children, and the psychometric qualities of the test are sufficient. For the verbal Dutch version of the Bayley-II, internal consistency was 0.79 and test-retest correlation 0.75.

The preschoolers were tested with the Snijders-Oomen Nonverbal Intelligence Test – Revised (SON-R; Tellegen, Winkel, Wijnberg-Williams, & Laros, 2003). The SON-R is a nonverbal intelligence test for children aged 2.5–7 years. The test can be administered without the use of spoken or written language and can therefore be used for children with learning difficulties and for international and cross-cultural research. In the current study, we selected two of the most reliable subtests of the SON-R (comparable with Dobrova-Krol, Van IJzendoorn et al., 2010): a visual-spatial performance patterns subtest and an abstract reasoning analogies subtest (average internal consistency of the subtests was 0.76). Convergent validity of the SON-R with the WISC-R was 0.80 and with the Raven 0.74 (Tellegen & Laros, 1993).

Based on each child's score on the Bayley or the SON-R, a developmental quotient (DQ) was computed, which has a mean of 100 and a standard deviation of 15. The DQ was computed by dividing the developmental or reference age (derived from the norm tables of the Bayley or SON-R) by the chronological age and multiplying this value by 100.

Daily Life Experiences

Daily life experiences were observed in the toddler group by two trained research assistants. During 5 weeks, time use was measured for 20 children, randomly chosen from the 30 children in the toddler group, with spot observations (Daunhauer et al., 2005; Tirella et al., 2008; see Sect. 1). Between 09:00 a.m. and 14:00 p.m., one child was observed during 1 day, by making a spot observation every 10 min. The research assistant stepped into the toddler room, videotaped in a nonintrusive way the part of the room where the target child was at that moment, and after about a minute stepped out of the room and completed the observation form. When the time use observations started, the research assistants had been filming in the toddler room for several days already, so the caregivers and children were used to them (and their small video camera). The caregivers and children were not aware of who the target child was or what the assistant was looking for. During filming, the assistant avoided eye contact or interaction with the children and caregiver(s). The forms were completed in the hallway, outside the toddler room. One child was observed every 10 min during 5 h resulting in 31 spot observations (620 observations for 20 children).

The observations were coded using ten categories:

1. Interaction of the child (no interaction, interaction with caregiver, interaction with peer)
2. Activity of the caregiver (no caregiver present, monitoring group, adult-led activity)
3. Activity of the child (sleeping, routines, meaningful activities, non-meaningful activities)
4. Activity of the group (no group activity, routines, transition, educational activity, others)
5. Place where the child is (floor, crib, bathroom, outside toddler room)
6. Available material (no material, toys in room but not available to child, toys available, other materials available)
7. Vocalization of the caregiver (no vocalization, speaking to adult, speaking to other child, speaking to target child, speaking to group)
8. Tone of the caregiver's voice (neutral; angry, annoyed, or impatient; friendly)
9. Vocalization of the child (no vocalization, child to other child, child to adult, others)
10. Emotional expression of the child (positive, negative, neutral)

The two research assistants were trained in coding using practical experience until their inter-rater reliability was >85% (cf. Tirella et al., 2008). We restricted the analyses to the child's awake time, leaving out the spot observations while the child was sleeping (cf. Daunhauer et al., 2005; Tirella et al., 2008) for the following pertinent categories: (1) interaction of the child, (7) vocalization of the caregiver, (8) tone of the caregiver's voice, (9) vocalization of the child, and (10) emotional expression of the child.

Table 14.2 Correlations between background and outcome variables ($N = 37$)

	Gender	Age study	Age arrival	Time	Z-weight	Z-height	Z-head
Gender	1						
Age study	0.17	1					
Age arrival	0.11	0.80**	1				
Time	−0.06	0.14	−49**	1			
Z-weight	0.32[1]	0.32[1]	0.33*	−0.08	1		
Z-height	0.14	0.12	0.08	0.04	0.40*	1	
Z-head	−0.12	0.07	−0.03	0.14	0.45**	0.15	1
DQ	0.30[1]	0.03	0.03	−0.005	0.44**	0.43*	0.24

Time time in institution, *DQ* developmental quotient
[1] $p<0.10$; $*p<0.05$; $**p<0.01$

2.1.3 Data Analysis

Data were analyzed with the statistical software package IBM SPPP Statistics 21. No outliers ($|z| > 3.29$) were found in the data. Based on the moderate associations between gender and outcome variables (see Table 14.2), we decided to include gender as covariate in the pertinent analyses. For three children outcomes for head circumference were missing. Four children were too passive or too restless to cooperate in the cognitive test. For four other children in the follow-up subsample, cognitive results were available for the first but not for the second assessment (due to the same reasons). We used regression imputation with the background and outcome variables as predictors to impute estimated means. The results were similar with and without these imputations.

With descriptive statistics and *t*-tests, we analyzed physical growth and cognition, and we used repeated measures (M)ANCOVAs to analyze possible recovery of growth and cognition and to compare our outcomes with a replication sample. The time use observational data are reported in percentages of time.

2.2 *Results*

2.2.1 Physical Growth and Cognition

Weight, Height, and Head Circumference

On average, the young children in the orphanage showed moderate delays in weight, height, and head circumference, indicated by average *Z*-scores between one and two standard deviations (*SD*s) below the mean (Fig. 14.1), with no gender differences ($ps > 0.11$).

A substantial number of children showed severe growth delays, indicated by *Z*-scores larger than two standard deviations below the mean. More than a third and

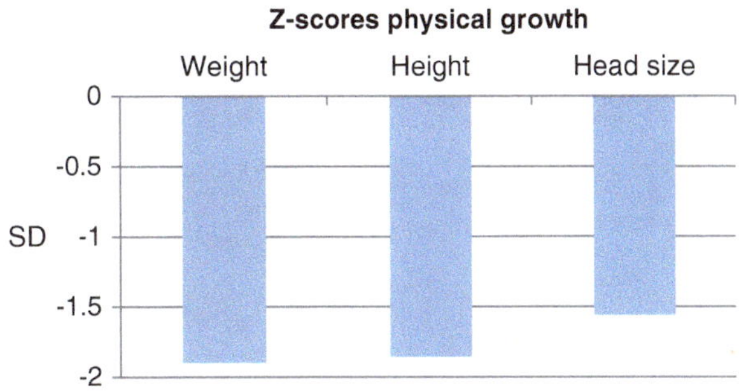

Fig. 14.1 *Z*-scores of weight, height, and head circumference ($N = 37$; see Table 14.1 for mean and standard deviations)

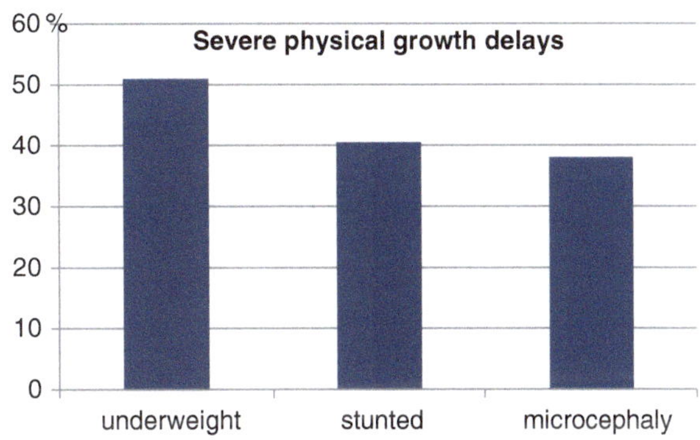

Fig. 14.2 Severe delays in physical growth: 19 children were underweight (51%), 15 had stunted growth (41%), and 14 had microcephaly (38%)

up to half of the children were underweight, had stunted growth, or microcephaly (Fig. 14.2). No gender differences were found ($ps > 0.11$).

Developmental Quotient

Mean developmental quotient of the children in the orphanage was 68 (range 41–97). Girls ($M = 64.74$, $SD = 13.29$) did not differ from boys regarding their developmental quotient ($M = 73.24$, $SD = 13.17$), $t(35) = -1.86$, $p = 0.07$, Cohen's $d = -0.69$.

Scores of 70–85 indicate a mild cognitive delay, while scores above 85 point to normative cognitive development. Scores below a developmental quotient of 70 indicate severe delays in cognitive development. More than half of the children in the study showed severe delays in cognitive development (Fig. 14.3), with no gender differences ($p = 0.45$).

2.2.2 Catch-Up in Institutional Care?

In a subsample we examined possible catch-up in physical and cognitive development, with a first (Time 1) and second assessment (Time 2) after on average 14 months (Table 14.3).

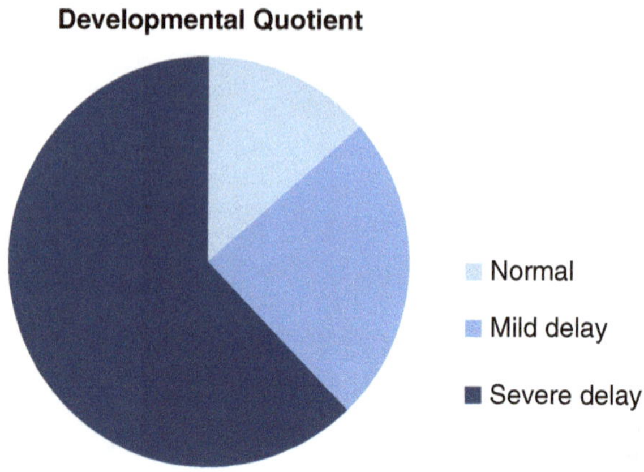

Fig. 14.3 Developmental quotients in the normative range (>85), 5 children (13.5%); mild delays (70–85), 9 children (24.5%); and severe delays (developmental quotients <70), 23 children (62%)

Table 14.3 Physical and cognitive outcomes (n = 20) at Time 1 and Time 2

	Time 1 (*M*, *SD*)	Time 2 (*M*, *SD*)	Correlation T1–T2
Z-score weight	−1.58 (0.91)	−1.84 (1.18)	0.52
Z-score height	−1.71 (1.12)	−1.54 (1.12)	0.89
Z-score head size	−1.63 (1.02)	−1.40 (1.04)	0.84
DQ	68.41 (15.76)	73.90 (15.46)	0.44

Using a repeated measures MANCOVA for the anthropometric indices weight, height, and head circumference with gender as covariate, there was no significant recovery in physical growth, main effect: $F(3, 16) = 0.32$, $p = 0.81$. The interaction of gender with time was not significant ($p = 0.65$), but a main effect of gender was found: $F(3, 16) = 3.78$, $p = 0.03$. Univariate analyses showed that height (but not weight or head size) differed between boys and girls, $F(1, 18) = 5.06$, $p = 0.04$. At Time 1 girls showed a larger average delay in height (−2.14, SD = 1.14) than boys (−1.06, SD = 0.73) (Cohen's $d = -1.28$). At Time 2 girls had an average height Z-score of −1.92 (SD = 1.16) and boys −0.97 (SD = 0.82), showing again larger delays for girls than for boys (Cohen's $d = -1.28$). Summarizing the overall results, there was no catch-up – nor decline – in physical growth after more than 1 year of institutionalization.

Regarding the cognitive outcomes, a repeated measures ANCOVA with gender as covariate showed no difference between the two DQs, $F(1, 18) = 2.55$, $p = 0.13$. Gender nor the interaction between gender and time were significant in this analysis. After a stay of more than a year in the institution, there was no significant catch-up – nor decline – in cognitive development.

Replication of Physical and Cognitive Outcomes?

Post hoc, we compared the Time 1 physical and cognitive findings of the 20 children in the follow-up subsample with thc outcomes of a cohort of 18 children, measured in a previous year. With respect to the background variables of age at study, age at

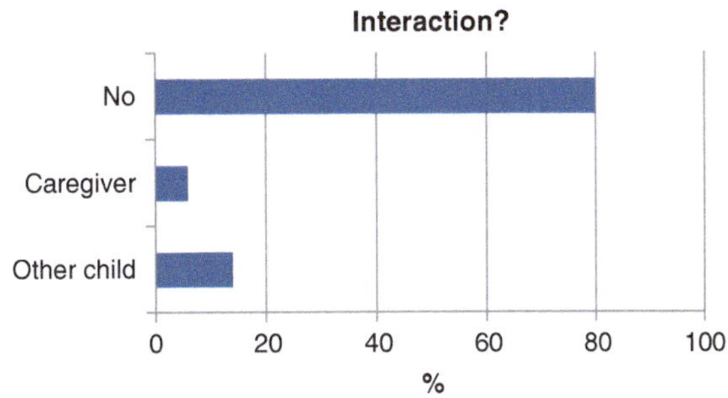

Fig. 14.4 Is the child involved in interaction with peers or caregivers during wake time?

arrival, and time in the institution, these children were very similar to the children in the follow-up study (*p*s of 0.64, 0.99, and 0.47, respectively, and a similar rate of females, 61% vs. 60%). A MANCOVA with gender as covariate revealed no difference in physical growth (weight, height, and head circumference) between the follow-up subsample and the replication sample, main effect: $F(3, 33) = 1.19$, $p = 0.33$ (and no gender effect, $p = 0.23$). Using an ANCOVA with gender as covariate, we found no difference in DQ either, $F(1, 35) = 1.38$, $p = 0.25$ (gender not significant, $p = 0.16$). We conclude that the physical growth and cognitive delays found in the current study could be replicated in a previous cohort of young children growing up in the same orphanage and were thus not exceptional.

2.2.3 Daily Life Experiences in Institutional Care

What are the daily life experiences of children in institutional care? Our observations are reported for the ten categories of the spot observations conducted in the toddler group (see Sect. 2.1).

Is the Child Involved in Interaction?

Most of the time that they were awake, the toddlers were not involved in interaction with a caregiver or peer (80%, Fig. 14.4). Interaction was rare: the target child was interacting with a caregiver only 6% of the time and with another child 14% of the time.

Activity of the Caregiver

Activities and whereabouts of the caregiver who was in charge of the toddler group were also coded. The observations showed that no adult caregiver was present in the room for 23% of the time. When multiple caregivers were present in the room, the behavior of the caregiver who was nearest to the target child was coded. However, often only one caregiver was actually in charge of the group while the other caregiver(s) were busy outside the room (e.g., getting food, cleaning, preparing

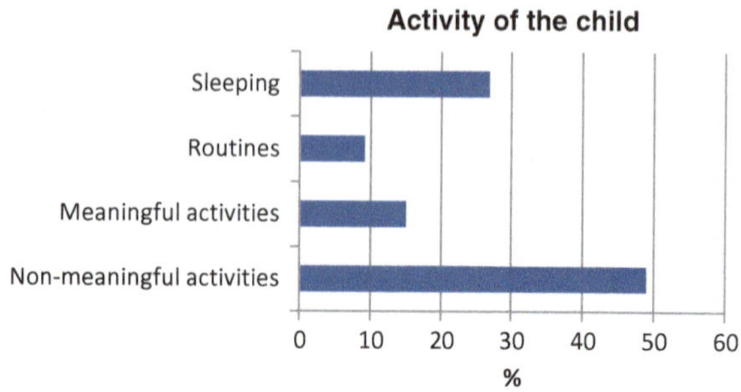

Fig. 14.5 Activity of the child

routines such as bathing time). For a third of the time (33%), the caregiver in charge was monitoring the toddler group, that is, watching the children without active interaction or engagement with them. The caregiver in charge was involved in adult-led activities such as feeding, changing diapers, or playing (with or without the target child) during 44% of the time.

Activity of the Child

During about a quarter of the time, the toddlers were sleeping (Fig. 14.5). The toddlers spent more time on nonmeaningful activities (49%), such as passively sitting or lying, than on meaningful activities (15%) such as playing or motor activities (e.g., crawling). Involvement in routines, including feeding and bathing, was observed 9% of the time.

Activity of the Group

Our observations showed that there was no specific group activity during 21% of the time. Quite some time was spent on the main group activities which were daily routines, such as nap time (32%) or mealtime (13%). For 20% of the time, the toddlers were busy with the transition to the next group activity, for example, when the children had to sit down in a circle to wait for mealtime. In the category "others" (8%), group activities that did not fit in the other categories were coded, such as bathing and toileting. For only 6% of the time, there was an educational group activity, such as playing or singing (Fig. 14.6).

Where Is the Child?

The children of the toddler group were supposed to stay in the same toddler room day and night, except for bathroom routines. The institution did not have a suitable playground outside, and children in the toddler group never went outside the house. Except for three cribs, there was no furniture in the toddler room. All activities took

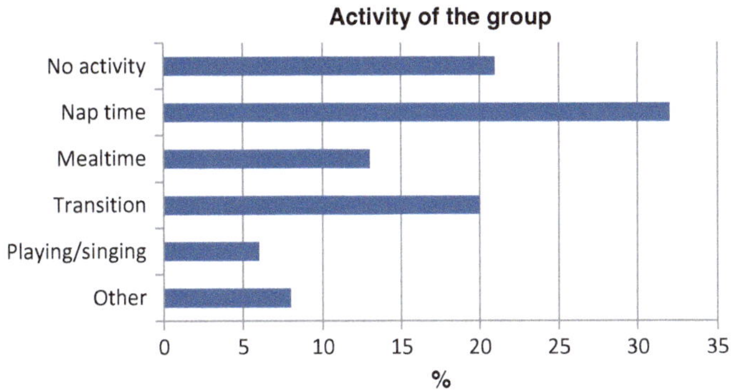

Fig. 14.6 Activity of the group

place in that room, including mealtime and sleeping. Most children slept on the ground: the youngest in a crib and the older toddlers on a sleeping mat that was made available during nap time and during the night. During daytime the youngest toddlers were often put in a crib when they were awake. In those cases the three cribs in the toddler room were used as a playpen (but most of the time without toys). Usually two to three younger toddlers were put in one crib to get them out of the way of the older toddlers. Although the toddlers were supposed to stay in the same room, the most mobile, older toddlers were able to move to places outside the toddler room, such as the preschooler's room or the hallway.

The observations showed that the toddlers were on the floor of the toddler room 57% of the time and in a crib in the toddler room 22% of the time. For 3% of the time they were in the bathroom and for 18% of the time they were in places outside the toddlers room.

Available Material

The observations showed that there was no (play) material at all during two thirds of the time (66%). Alternatively, there were toys in the room, but they were not available for the target child 11% of the time, for example, when other (usually older) children did have toys but did not want to share them. Toys were available for the child 10% of the time. Other materials available for the toddlers included food (5%) and various objects (8%), such as items of clothing and plastic spoons.

Vocalization of the Caregiver

We observed how often the caregiver in charge of the toddler room was vocalizing. We found that they were speaking either to another adult (10% of the time), to another child (21%), to the group in general (2%), or to the target child (1% of the time). For two thirds of the time (66%), the caregiver did not speak at all (Fig. 14.7).

Fig. 14.7 Vocalization of the caregiver (Cg)

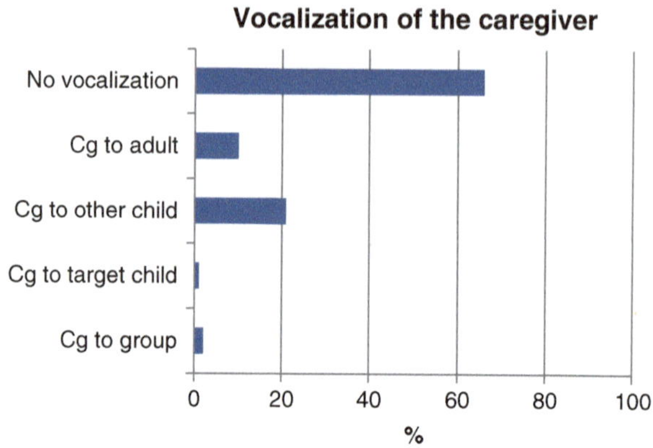

Fig. 14.8 Vocalization of the child

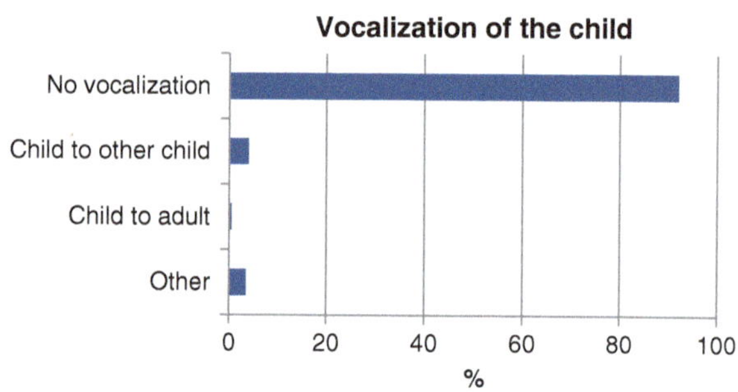

Tone of the Caregiver's Voice

We also coded how the caregiver in charge of the toddler room vocalized. For 66% of the time, the caregiver did not vocalize (see also previous category). The caregiver was vocalizing with a neutral tone during 25% of the time, with an angry, annoyed or impatient tone (6%), and with a friendly tone during 3% of the time.

Vocalization of the Child

The observations showed that children in the toddler group were hardly vocalizing. They were silent and did not speak or babble 92% of the time (Fig. 14.8). The children vocalized to another child 4% of the time and to the caregiver 1% of the time. Other vocalizations (3%) included vocalizing without addressing someone in particular.

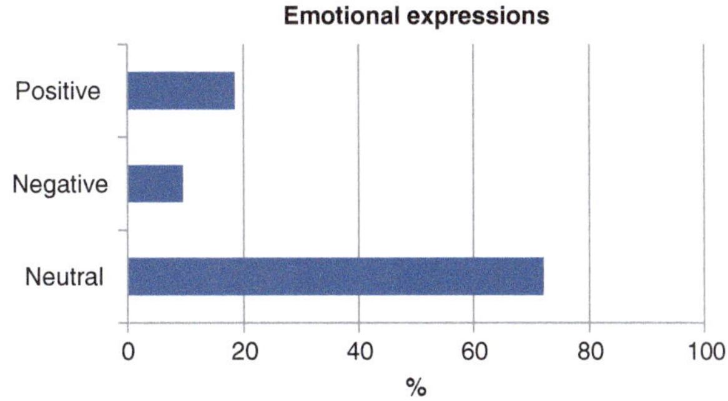

Fig. 14.9 Emotional expressions of the child

Emotional Expressions of the Child

We coded whether the child showed positive, negative, or neutral emotional expressions. Most of the time (72%), the toddlers showed neutral or blank facial expressions (Fig. 14.9). Positive expressions such as smiling, laughing, or looking curious/interested were seen 18% of the time. Negative expressions, including crying or whining, were observed 10% of the time.

3 Conclusion and Discussion

We examined physical growth and cognitive development in 37 young children (1–6 years) in an Indian orphanage, with repeated assessments in a subsample, and extensive observations in another subsample of toddlers. Our findings revealed severe delays in physical growth: 51% of the children were underweight, 41% were stunted, and 38% had microcephaly. Their mean developmental quotient (DQ) was 68, and 62% of the children had a severe delay in cognitive development (DQ < 70). Follow-up assessments and assessments in a replication cohort confirmed the delays in physical and cognitive development with no evidence of recovery (or decline) after more than 1 year of institutionalization.

The observations in the toddler group showed that these children did not interact with a caregiver or peer during 80% of the time. Observations also pointed to compromised child care, including, for example, no adult caregiver present in the room for almost a quarter of the time, practically no educational group activities, caregivers who hardly spoke to the children, and toddlers who were confined to the floor or a (shared) crib day and night in an unfurnished room without toys.

Although our study had a modest sample size of 37 children, the outcomes are strengthened by the follow-up assessments in which we examined whether recovery took place during institutionalization. Also, the main outcomes on physical growth and cognitive development were confirmed in a replication cohort. Finally, the time use procedure resulted in a large number of unique spot observations.

3.1 Delays and Recovery

Our study adds to the vast body of research on the plight of children growing up in institutions. Studies in orphanages in, for instance, Romania, Russia, and Ukraine have shown that child development is affected negatively by institutional care (e.g., Daunhauer et al., 2005; Dobrova-Krol et al., 2008; Groark et al., 2005; Johnson et al., 2010; Miller et al., 2007; Sloutsky, 1997; Smyke et al., 2007; Van IJzendoorn et al., 2011). Our study extends the literature because of its focus on India: empirical research in Indian orphanages is scarce, especially studies on young children growing up in institutional care. Our outcomes converge with the results from two studies in Indian orphanages, both revealing significant delays in older children (6–12 years; Eapen, 2009; Escueta et al., 2014). Based on the current study, we must conclude that such delays are also found in younger children in Indian institutions.

The children in our study did not recover from their physical and cognitive delays after more than 1 year of institutional care. This is in stark contrast to children who are removed from institutions to adoptive or foster family care. Immediate and massive catch-up of developmental delays after children's placement in family care has been noted in a large number of studies and in meta-analyses (e.g., Nelson et al., 2007; Van den Dries et al., 2010; Van IJzendoorn et al., 2007; Van IJzendoorn & Juffer, 2006).

3.2 Stabilization of Delays?

One should of course keep in mind that most children enter institutional care with large delays, because they are orphaned or come from poor, deprived families. Childhood malnutrition is common in India. In a large population study on 1941 children's nutritional status in the slums of Mumbai (India), Das et al. (2012) found high rates of underweight (35%) and stunted growth (47%) in children under 5. Many children in our study came from extremely difficult backgrounds, indicating that they may have had significant delays when they entered institutional care. Adequate child and healthcare facilities may ameliorate at least some of the physical growth delays (e.g., Kapavarapu et al., 2012).

However, in our study there were no signs of catch-up when children were assessed again after more than a year in the institution. Similarly, the correlations between the time the children had been in the institution (on average 12 months) and the anthropometric and cognitive indices were not significant (see Table 14.2). Findings from the BEIP study (see Sect. 1; Nelson, Fox, & Zeanah, 2014) also illuminate the immense differences between children randomized to prolonged institutionalization versus foster care, with the latter children showing remarkable recovery, in contrast to the children who remained in institutional care.

3.3 Daily Life Experiences of Structural Neglect

The spot observations of this study shed a sharp light on the appalling daily experiences of toddlers living in an Indian orphanage. Children clearly miss out on opportunities for interaction and play, while they are left on their own for most of the time. In other words, these children seem to "(...) suffer from 'structural neglect' which may include minimum physical resources, unfavorable and unstable staffing patterns, and social-emotionally inadequate caregiver-child interactions" (Van IJzendoorn et al., 2011, p. 8). The observations in the current study indeed point to experiences of structural neglect and sustained traumatization within a highly regimented, child-unfriendly structure of child care. A larger contrast to sensitive care – perceiving the child's behavior and emotions accurately and responding to what the child needs in an adequate way (Ainsworth, Blehar, Waters, & Wall, 1978; Bowlby, 1982) – is hardly conceivable.

Many factors may contribute to the structural neglect in orphanages. Large groups, suboptimal caregiver-child ratios, high rates of staff turnover, and lack of education in caregivers may be some of the reasons for the insufficient child care. Also, it is hard to change caregiver practices in institutional care (e.g., Groark et al., 2005; McCall, Van IJzendoorn, Juffer, Groark, & Groza, 2011). In Taneja et al.'s (2002) intervention study in an Indian orphanage (see Sect. 1), children clearly profited from a daily structured play intervention. However, in their follow-up study, Taneja, Aggarwal, Beri, and Puliyel (2005) reported that the caregivers lost their interest and returned to their mechanical routine of cleaning and feeding the children. To resume the intervention, a play therapist had to be recruited.

3.4 Recommendation for Practice

Empirical research has convincingly shown that young children's development is seriously jeopardized in institutional care, resulting in profound delays in virtually every area of their functioning (e.g., McCall et al., 2011; Miller, 2005; Rutter, Sonuga-Barke, & Castle, 2010; Smyke et al., 2007; Van IJzendoorn et al., 2011). Our study extends this literature because of its focus on India: studies on young children growing up in institutional care in Indian orphanages are scarce. Based on the empirical evidence, institutional care for young children in India should be replaced by options of family care such as kinship care, foster care, domestic adoption, or – as a last option – international adoption (Bakermans-Kranenburg et al., 2012; Dozier et al., 2014; Forber-Pratt, Loo, Price, & Acharya, 2013; Groza & Bunkers, 2014; Groza et al., 2003; Riley-Behringer, Groza, Tieman, & Juffer, 2014).

Based on our findings and evidence from comparable studies, we conclude that children in institutional care show profound developmental delays, while young children's daily life experiences in orphanages must be qualified as structural neglect. Against the background of the UN Convention on the Rights of the Child, one cannot but conclude that children in orphanages should be taken into good-enough family care as soon as possible to break the cycle of sustained traumatization and enable them to recover from their developmental delays.

Questions for Discussion

1. Taneja's intervention studies (see Sect. 3.3) showed that it is hard to change caregiver practices in institutional care. Reflect on the reasons why it would be difficult to change child care in children's homes, and take into account the empirical evidence on efforts to intervene in institutional care practices (Bakermans-Kranenburg, Van IJzendoorn, & Juffer, 2008; St.Petersburg USA Orphanage Research Team, 2008).
2. Discuss the two options of either improving institutional care or offering good-enough family care to children (kinship care, foster, and adoptive families). Include the perspective of the child's best interest in your discussion.
3. The international organization Better Care Network gives the advice not to volunteer in children's homes (see http://www.bettercarenetwork.org/bcn-in-action/better-volunteering-better-care/activities-and-outputs/orphanage-volunteering-why-to-say-no). How does this advice relate (or not) to the findings of this chapter?

Acknowledgments We would like to thank children and staff of the children's home, and the assistance of Eline Baarda, Reshni Balkaran, Lieneke Jooren, Maartje Luijk, Eva Niemeijer, Lindy Noord, Jolien van der Graaff, Sanneke van der Geest, Vera van Leeuwen, and Janneke van Wingerden. We gratefully acknowledge the support of the Netherlands Organization for Scientific Research (Spinoza, MHvIJ) and the European Research Council (ERC AdG, MJBK), as well as the Gravitation program of the Dutch Ministry of Education, Culture, and Science and the Netherlands Organization for Scientific Research (NWO grant number 024.001.003).

References

Ainsworth, M. D. S., Blehar, M. C., Waters, E., & Wall, S. (1978). *Patterns of attachment. A psychological study of the strange situation*. Hillsdale, NJ: Lawrence Erlbaum.

Bakermans-Kranenburg, M. J., Bunkers, K. M., Dobrova-Krol, N. A., Engle, P., Fox, N. A., Gamer, G., … The Leiden Conference. (2012). The development and care of institutionally reared children. *Child Development Perspectives, 6*(2), 174–180. doi: 10.1111/j.1750-8606.2011.00231.x.

Bakermans-Kranenburg, M. J., Van IJzendoorn, M. H., & Juffer, F. (2008). Earlier is better: A meta-analysis of 70 years of intervention improving cognitive development in institutionalized children. *Monographs of the Society for Research in Child Development, 73*(3), 279–293. doi:10.1111/j.1540-5834.2008.00498.x.

Bowlby, J. (1982). *Attachment and loss. Vol. 1: Attachment* (2nd ed.). New York, NY: Basic Books.

Das, S., Bapat, U., More, N. S., Alcock, G., Fernandez, A., & Osrin, D. (2012). Nutritional status of young children in Mumbai slums: A follow-up anthropometric study. *Nutrition Journal, 11*(100), 1–9. doi:10.1186/1475-2891-11-100.

Daunhauer, L. A., Bolton, A., & Cermak, S. A. (2005). Time-use patterns of young children institutionalized in Eastern Europe. *Occupation Participation and Health, 25*(1), 33–40.

Dobrova-Krol, N. A., Bakermans-Kranenburg, M. J., Van IJzendoorn, M. H., & Juffer, F. (2010). The importance of quality of care: Effects of perinatal HIV infection and early institutional rearing on preschoolers' attachment and indiscriminate friendliness. *Journal of Child Psychology & Psychiatry, 52*(12), 1368–1376.

Dobrova-Krol, N. A., van IJzendoorn, M. H., Bakermans-Kranenburg, M. J., Cyr, C., & Juffer, F. (2008). Physical growth delays and stress dysregulation in stunted and non-stunted Ukrainian institution-reared children. *Infant Behavior and Development, 31*(3), 539–553. doi:10.1016/j.infbeh.2008.04.001.

Dobrova-Krol, N. A., van IJzendoorn, M. H., Bakermans-Kranenburg, M. J., & Juffer, F. (2010). Effects of perinatal HIV infection and early institutional rearing on physical and cognitive development of children in Ukraine. *Child Development, 81*(1), 237–251.

Dozier, M., Kaufman, J., Kobak, R., O'Connor, T. G., Sagi-Schwartz, A., Scott, S., … Zeanah, C. H. (2014). Consensus statement on group care for children and adolescents: A statement of policy of the American Orthopsychiatric Association. *American Journal of Orthopsychiatry, 84*(3), 219–225. doi: 10.1037/ort0000005.

Eapen, D. J. (2009). Institutionalized children: The underprivileged. *International Journal of Nursing Practice, 15*(5), 349–352. doi:10.1111/j.1440-172X.2009.01785.x.

Escueta, M., Whetten, K., Ostermann, J., O'Donnell, K., & The Positive Outcomes for Orphans Research Team. (2014). Adverse childhood experiences, psychosocial well-being and cognitive development among orphans and abandoned children in five low income countries. *BMC International Health and Human Rights, 14*(6), 1–13. doi:10.1186/1472-698x-14-6.

Forber-Pratt, I. A., Loo, S., Price, S., & Acharya, J. (2013). Foster care in India: An exploratory survey of the community perceptions and prospects for implementation of foster care in a developing nation: A study in Udaipur, Rajasthan, India. *Children and Youth Services Review, 35*(4), 694–706. doi:10.1016/j.childyouth.2013.01.002.

Groark, C. J., McCall, R. B., Fish, L., & The Whole Child International Evaluation Team. (2011). Characteristics of environments, caregivers, and children in three Central American orphanages. *Infant Mental Health Journal, 32*(2), 232–250. doi:10.1002/imhj.20292.

Groark, C. J., Muhamedrahimov, R. J., Palmov, O. I., Nikiforova, N. V., & McCall, R. B. (2005). Improvements in early care in Russian orphanages and their relationship to observed behaviors. *Infant Mental Health Journal, 26*(2), 96–109. doi:10.1002/imhj.20041.

Groza, V., & Bunkers, K. M. (2014). Adoption policy and evidence-based domestic adoption practice: A comparison of Romania, Ukraine, India, Guatemala, and Ethiopia. *Infant Mental Health Journal, 35*(2), 160–171. doi:10.1002/imhj.21439.

Groza, V., Kalyanvala, R., Boyer, S., Nedelcu, C., & The Bharatiya Samaj Seva Kendra Research Team. (2003). Indian families adopting Indian children. *Indian Journal of Social Work, 64*(1), 93–113.

Johnson, D. E., & Gunnar, M. R. (2011). Growth failure in institutionalized children. *Monographs of the Society for Research in Child Development, 76*(4), 92–126. doi:10.1111/j.1540-5834.2011.00629.x.

Johnson, D. E., Guthrie, D., Smyke, A. T., Koga, S. F., Fox, N. A., Zeanah, C. H., & Nelson, C. A. (2010). Growth and associations between auxology, caregiving environment, and cognition in socially deprived Romanian children randomized to foster vs. ongoing institutional care. *Archives of Pediatrics and Adolescent Medicine, 164*(6), 507–516.

Juffer, F., Palacios, J., LeMare, L., Sonuga-Barke, E., Tieman, W., Bakermans-Kranenburg, M. J., … Verhulst, F. (2011). Development of adopted children with histories of early adversity. *Monographs of the Society for Research of Child Development, 76*(4), 31–61.

Kapavarapu, P. K., Bari, O., Perumpil, M., Duggan, C., Dinakar, C., Krishnamurthy, S., … Shet, A. (2012). Growth patterns and anaemia status of HIV-infected children living in an institutional facility in India. *Tropical Medicine and International Health, 17*(8), 962–971. doi: 10.1111/j.1365-3156.2012.03022.x.

McCall, R. B., Van IJzendoorn, M. H., Juffer, F., Groark, C. J., & Groza, V. K. (2011). Children without permanent parents: Research, practice, and policy. *Monographs of the Society for Research in Child Development, 76*(4), 1–318.

Miller, L., Chan, W., Comfort, K., & Tirella, L. (2005). Health of children adopted from Guatemala: Comparison of orphanage and foster care. *Pediatrics, 115*(6), E710–E717. doi:10.1542/peds.2004-2359.

Miller, L. C. (2005). *Handbook of international adoption medicine: A guide for physicians, parents, and providers*. New York, NY: Oxford University Press.

Miller, L. C., Chan, W., Litvinova, A., Rubin, A., Tirella, L., & Cermak, S. (2007). Medical diagnoses and growth of children residing in Russian orphanages. *Acta Paediatrica, 96*(12), 1765–1769. doi:10.1111/j.1651-2227.2007.00537.x.

Nelson, C. A., Fox, N. A., & Zeanah, C. H. (2014). *Romania's abandoned children. Deprivation, brain development, and the struggle for recovery*. London, UK: Harvard University Press.

Nelson, C. A., Zeanah, C. H., Fox, N. A., Marshall, P. J., Smyke, A. T., & Guthrie, D. (2007). Cognitive recovery in socially deprived young children: The Bucharest early intervention project. *Science, 318*(5858), 1937–1940. doi:10.1126/science.1143921.

Riley-Behringer, M., Groza, V., Tieman, W., & Juffer, F. (2014). Race and bicultural socialization in the Netherlands, Norway, and the United States of America in the adoptions of children from India. *Cultural Diversity and Ethnic Minority Psychology, 20*(2), 231–243. doi:10.1037/a0035324.

Ruiter, S. A. J., Hoekstra, A. T., Van der Meulen, B. F., & Lutje Spelberg, H. C. (2005). BSID-II-NL, deel III: Niet-Verbale schaal *[BSID-II Dutch version, Part III: Non-Verbal Scale]*. Amsterdam, The Netherlands: Harcourt Test Publishers.

Rutter, M., Sonuga-Barke, E. J. S., & Castle, J. (2010). I. Investigating the impact of early institutional deprivation on development: Background and research strategy of the English and Romanian Adoptees (ERA) study. *Monographs of the Society for Research in Child Development, 75*(1), 1–20.

Sloutsky, V. M. (1997). Institutional care and developmental outcomes of 6 and 7 year-old children: A contextualist perspective. *International Journal of Behavioral Development, 20*, 131–151.

Smyke, A. T., Koga, S. F., Johnson, D. E., Fox, N. A., Marshall, P. J., Nelson, C. A., … The BEIP Core Group. (2007). The caregiving context in institution-reared and family-reared infants and toddlers in Romania. *Journal of Child Psychology and Psychiatry, 48*(2), 210–218. doi: 10.1111/j.1469-7610.2006.01694.x.

SOS Villages India. (2011). See https://www.soschildrensvillages.ca/india-now-home-20-million-orphans-study-finds

St.Petersburg USA Orphanage Research Team. (2008). The effects of early social-emotional and relationship experience on the development of young orphanage children. *Monographs of the Society for Research in Child Development, 73*(3), 1–262. doi:10.1111/j.1540-5834.2008.00483.x.

Taneja, V., Aggarwal, R., Beri, R. S., & Puliyel, J. M. (2005). Not by bread alone project: A 2 year follow-up report. *Child Care Health and Development, 31*(6), 703–706. doi:10.1111/j.1365-2214.2005.00563.x.

Taneja, V., Sriram, S., Beri, R. S., Sreenivas, V., Aggarwal, R., Kaur, R., & Puliyel, J. M. (2002). 'Not by bread alone': Impact of a structured 90-minute play session on development of children in an orphanage. *Child Care Health and Development, 28*(1), 95–100. doi:10.1046/j.1365-2214.2002.00246.x.

Tellegen, P., & Laros, J. (1993). The construction and validation of a nonverbal test of intelligence: The revision of the Snijders-Oomen tests. *European Journal of Psychological Assessment, 9*, 147–157.

Tellegen, P., Winkel, M., Wijnberg-Williams, B., & Laros, J. (2003). *Snijders-Oomen niet-verbale intelligentietest. SON-R 2½-7. Handleiding en verantwoording*. Amsterdam, The Netherlands: Boom.

Tirella, L. G., Chan, W., Cermak, S. A., Litvinova, A., Salas, K. C., & Miller, L. C. (2008). Time use in Russian baby homes. *Child Care Health and Development, 34*(1), 77–86. doi:10.1111/j.1365-2214.2007.00766.x.

Van den Dries, L., Juffer, F., van IJzendoorn, M. H., & Bakermans-Kranenburg, M. J. (2010). Infants' physical and cognitive development after international adoption from foster care or institutions in China. *Journal of Developmental and Behavioral Pediatrics, 31*(2), 144–150. doi:10.1097/DBP.0b013e3181cdaa3a.

Van der Meulen, B. F., Ruiter, S. A. J., Lutje Spelberg, H. C., & Smrkovský, M. (2004). Bayley scales of infant development-II-NL. Handleiding *[BSID-II Dutch version, Manual]*. Amsterdam, The Netherlands: Harcourt Test Publishers.

Van IJzendoorn, M. H., Bakermans-Kranenburg, M. J., & Juffer, F. (2007). Plasticity of growth in height, weight and head circumference: Meta-analytic evidence of massive catch-up after international adoption. *Journal of Developmental and Behavioral Pediatrics*, *28*, 334–343.

Van IJzendoorn, M. H., & Juffer, F. (2006). The Emanuel Miller memorial lecture 2006: Adoption as intervention. Meta-analytic evidence for massive catch-up and plasticity in physical, socio-emotional, and cognitive development. *Journal of Child Psychology and Psychiatry*, *47*, 1228–1245. doi:10.1111/j.1469-7610.2006.01675.x.

Van IJzendoorn, M. H., Juffer, F., & Poelhuis, C. W. K. (2005). Adoption and cognitive development: A meta-analytic comparison of adopted and nonadopted children's IQ and school performance. *Psychological Bulletin*, *131*(2), 301–316. doi:10.1037/0033-2909.131.2.301.

Van IJzendoorn, M. H., Luijk, M., & Juffer, F. (2008). IQ of children growing up in children's homes – A meta-analysis on IQ delays in orphanages. *Merrill-Palmer Quarterly-Journal of Developmental Psychology*, *54*(3), 341–366.

Van IJzendoorn, M. H., Palacios, J., Sonuga-Barke, E. J. S., Gunnar, M. R., Vorria, P., McCall, R. B., … Juffer, F. (2011). Children in institutional care: Delayed development and resilience. *Monographs of the Society for Research in Child Development*, *76*(4), 8–30. doi: 10.1111/j.1540-5834.2011.00626.x.

WHO (2016). *World Health Organization Anthro calculator*. Retrieved from http://www.who.int/childgrowth/software/en/

Zeanah, C. H., Nelson, C. A., Fox, N. A., Smyke, A. T., Marshall, P., Parker, S. W., & Koga, S. (2003). Designing research to study the effects of institutionalization on brain and behavioral development: The Bucharest early intervention project. *Development and Psychopathology*, *15*(4), 885–907. doi:10.1017/s0954579403000452.

Chapter 15
Child Maltreatment and Prevention Practices in Chinese Orphanages

Xiaoyuan Shang and Karen R. Fisher

I read some of the books, and stopped the habit of beating other children. Instead, I began to oppose beating children. I no longer believed beating was an effective way of disciplining them.

Worker and former orphan in a child welfare institution.

1 Introduction

By the end of 2012, around 109,000 children were in the guardianship of child welfare institutions operated by Civil Affairs Departments in China (MCA, 2013). Most of them lived in the institutions, so the extent and prevention of maltreatment in this form of care is a significant policy question. This chapter examines the experience of children in government and nongovernment institutional care based on the authors' empirical research and published and unpublished materials. It addresses the difficult questions about the extent of abuse and neglect within the institutions that are intended to protect them, the types and causes of maltreatment, and how social policy responds to these problems. The chapter examines child protection within child welfare institutions in three respects:

1. It reviews the existing literature and materials from a historical perspective, including cases of child maltreatment reported in the past two decades and the findings about maltreatment from fieldwork for projects conducted by the

X. Shang (✉) • K.R. Fisher
Social Policy Research Centre, University of New South Wales, NSW 2052 Sydney, Australia
e-mail: x.shang@unsw.edu.au; karen.fisher@unsw.edu.au

A.V. Rus et al. (eds.), *Child Maltreatment in Residential Care*,
DOI 10.1007/978-3-319-57990-0_15

authors. A historical perspective is important because the past continues to influence current policies and practices in China.
2. It examines the current policies and practices applied in the child welfare institutions in China. Many of these policies were in response to the reported child maltreatment cases in the past two decades.
3. It examines wider policy changes to which the maltreatment reports contributed. There is a policy shift toward a mixed welfare regime and from institutional to family-based care. This longer-term trend away from institutional care and its associated risks offers the greatest hope for preventing child maltreatment in institutions.

2 Children in Government and Other Welfare Institutions

At the end of 2007, China had about five million children with disabilities (Chen & Chen, 2008), 573,000 orphaned children, and 94,000 children in state care (Shang, 2008b; Beijing Minzheng Xinxiwang, 2014). Most orphans in China are cared for within their extended family. Before 2015, China did not have a child protection system to remove children who were subject to abuse or neglect within their family. Only children without any family connections were eligible for state care, so they were generally children who had been orphaned, without other family members, or left in the care of the state without any way to trace their family members.

Most children living in state care have disabilities for several reasons. Chinese health and welfare systems generally do not provide free support except in some wealthier coastal areas. Some families decide that the only way their child can receive the care they need is if they are left in state care, so they leave their children where they can be found by the state (Shang & Fisher, 2014). Like other countries, alternatives to state care are more likely to be found for children without disabilities. If children come into state care, most are adopted, nationally or internationally, but children with disabilities or infectious diseases are the least likely to have this option (Shang & Fisher, 2014; Shang, 2008a).

2.1 Child Welfare System in China

In China, welfare for disadvantaged children was very limited before 2010. The main support was for children without any known family connections, almost all of which was in the form of institutional care. An international event that influenced improvements in China's child welfare in the 1990s was the BBC investigative documentary, *The Dying Rooms*, about appalling conditions in some Chinese child institutions. The documentary triggered deep concerns from child welfare organizations throughout the world and from the Chinese government (Human Rights Watch, 1996).

In response to this and related investigations (Human Rights Watch, 1996), the state changed policies to allow donations to the welfare institutions and to permit international adoption (Shang & Fisher, 2014; Shang, 2008a). The state also increased funding for state child welfare institutions. Some institutions in poorer cities already had a history of foster care originally for financial reasons. Following the public outcry after *The Dying Rooms,* other major cities including Beijing and Shanghai, also accepted the internationally recognized benefits of family-based foster care as a better alternative to institutional care. Through these practices, foster care also became a method of preventing maltreatment in institutions.

These efforts of international organizations and the Chinese government have since radically changed the way state child welfare operates in China. Changes in policy, funding, and alternative care types have improved the quality and safety of care to children in the guardianship of state welfare institutions (Shang, 2008a). Currently, care for children in the guardianship of the state includes three main forms. The predominant practice remains institutional care, supplemented with formal foster care in the community arranged by the institution, and family-like group care within institutions. Two-thirds of children in state care live in the state child welfare institutions (Beijing Minzheng Xinxiwang, 2014). The remainder lives in foster care arranged by the institution or the local civil affairs department. The guardianship of children living in state care is held by the local state child welfare institution, irrespective of whether they live in the institution or in foster care.

Some nongovernment child welfare institutions also care for children. According to the 2013 survey data of the Ministry of Civil Affairs (MCA), 878 individuals or nongovernment organizations received orphans nationally, including over 500 religious organizations, and cared for 9394 orphans (Xu, 2013). The survey data of the MCA showed the positive contribution of the civil sector in accommodating children but also revealed challenges for the government to protect the safety and interests of the children. Examples are described in this chapter.

2.2 *Defining Child Maltreatment in China*

The definition of maltreatment in each country is based on the local history, culture, and custom. In Chinese institutions, neglect is more common than other forms of maltreatment due to regulations about standards, although the findings in this chapter demonstrate a wide range of maltreatment. Unfortunately, even neglect results in serious harm or death for some children in care. The Chinese government does not have a legal definition of child maltreatment, so in this research, we shall use an international definition.

The International Society for the Prevention of Child Abuse and Neglect (ISPCAN) compared definitions of child abuse from 58 countries and found some commonality in what were considered abusive behaviors to children (Bross, Miyoshi, Miyoshi, & Krugman, 2000). The WHO Consultation on Child Abuse Prevention (1999: p. 15) drafted the following definition:

> Child abuse or maltreatment constitutes all forms of physical and/or emotional ill-treatment, sexual abuse, neglect or negligent treatment or commercial or other exploitation, resulting in actual or potential harm to the child's health, survival, development or dignity in the context of a relationship of responsibility, trust or power.

3 Past Maltreatment in Institutions

The Chinese government does not collect data on child maltreatment in institutions. Instead, the rest of the chapter addresses two research questions based on the policy reviews and fieldwork conducted by the authors (Shang, 2008a; Shang & Fisher, 2014, 2016, 2017). Professor Shang has been conducting empirical research about child institutions since the 1990s. The research includes policy analysis and interviews with staff and young people who had grown up in institutions (all names are pseudonyms). They were asked about their experiences of maltreatment in institutions. What was the extent and type of child maltreatment in Chinese institutions? And what were the policy and practice responses to prevent maltreatment institutions?

Past maltreatment included extreme levels of neglect in under-resourced or unregulated state and nongovernment institutions, practices in institutions that would now be considered maltreatment, and physical and emotional abuse reported by children and young people who grew up in institutional care.

3.1 Neglect in Child Welfare Institutions

In the 1990s, the mortality rate and living conditions of children in Chinese state child welfare institutions shocked the world through the BBC documentary (Human Rights Watch, 1996). Many abandoned children, mostly healthy girls, who were living in state child welfare institutions, died of poor care or lack of medical treatment. At that time, the death rate was 50–72% in some welfare institutions (Human Rights Watch, 1996).

The high mortality rate was due to policy decisions that provoked increases in the number of children in state care. Before 1992, the policy of state child welfare institutions was to prioritize domestic adoption for most of the children in their care. As a result, only a few thousand children lived in the care of state in the 1980s. However, at the end of the 1980s and early 1990s, the strict application of the family planning policy permitted each family to have one child for urban residents and two for rural residents. Parents who gave birth and kept any children above the quota would be fined heavily, which sharply increased the number of abandoned children in certain areas. At the same time, changes to the Adoption Law in 1992 set much stricter criteria for domestic adoption.

With these two policy changes, institutions in some parts of China became responsible for a larger number abandoned children yet fewer adoptive families were eligible to accept them. These institutions did not have adequate financial or staff resources to care for these babies, which resulted in many babies dying from a lack of adequate care and medical services. For example, an institution director told Professor Shang that during that time, the institution accepted nearly 1000 babies each year. At the peak, she saw 11 abandoned babies at the front gate of her institution at the same time, and she had no means to find enough space or staff to care for any of them. Policy responses to these extreme pressures are described later in the chapter.

In addition to neglect in state institutions, neglect in nongovernment institutions was also revealed, including recent problems. An example was in Lankao, Henan, Province in 2013, where seven children died in a fire. One woman and an adult with disabilities cared for seven children and young people aged between 7 months and 20 years, most of whom had disability support needs. Although responsibility for the tragedy was widely debated, it was clear that serious neglect was the reason they died. The nongovernment care was run by an individual woman who had no legal guardianship and had raised more than 100 orphans since 1986. Local authorities were in the practice of referring newly found children to her care, despite the obvious risk that her facility did not meet any minimum safety standards for raising children in group care (China Youth Newspaper, 2013). The event led to practice change to more strictly follow the policy that prohibits this type of informal care facilities from taking in children (Shang & Fisher, 2017).

3.2 *Institutional Practices of Maltreatment*

In addition to the gross neglect risking death described above, some accepted practices within institutions would now also be considered maltreatment. Some of them have been addressed by subsequent policy and practice change. Two examples here are naming practices that removed the identity of children and forced sterilization of girls and young women with disabilities.

Until the 1980s, most state institutions named children in state care with politically related surnames or numbers. The family name of most of the children when they came into care was unknown because they were anonymously left at the gate of the institution or found by a member of the community. In these circumstances, many institutions gave them a nationalistic family surname when they entered state care, such as Dang (Party, implying they were children of the Communist Party), Fu (Welfare), or Guo (Country). At the time, the practice of naming them this way was intended as an honor, but the effect was to label the children as orphans without families, attracting stigma during their childhood and adulthood. In addition, some children, especially children with disabilities, were also only called by a nickname rather than their real given first name, or they were only named with a number instead of a given name.

The young people in the authors' research recounted how during their teenage years, the surname Dang was a source of shame, because it indicated they were raised in an institution rather than a family (Shang & Fisher, 2017). They tried to evade acknowledging the origins of their surname, by claiming it was a different "Dang" surname. In contrast to children growing up in their family environment, they viewed their surname as a source of shame. For example, Jin, a young man who grew up at the welfare institution and still lived there said:

> While speaking to my clients [at the massage clinic], they might ask me "Doesn't the surname of 'Dang' suggest children raised at Child Welfare Institution?" But I do not want them know I was an orphan, and I just say that there is a traditional Chinese family name 'Dang', because I do not want them to view me as pitiful.

The practice of naming children with numbers started to cease in the 1980s in the better institutions. However, the practice of naming children with Dang, Fu, or Guo still continues in some parts of China. For example, children in state care in Beijing were not given a usual Chinese surname until 2012. In the 2010s, more institutions stopped the practice, with the expectation that the Ministry of Civil Affairs (MCA) would otherwise have to regulate against it (Heilongjiang News, 2012). These changes are consistent with more recent Chinese government attempts to uphold children's rights, including that the names of children should not include the elements of discrimination, birth defects, political or religious meanings, or that could trace back to their identity as abandoned or orphaned children (Heilongjiang News, 2012).

The second example of institutionalized maltreatment was forcibly sterilizing girls and young women with disabilities. In 2005, the media reported that two girls with disabilities were sterilized in the state child welfare institution in Nantong. The investigation and court action against the institution director revealed that this had been a common practice since 1980s (Nanfang Dushibao, 2005). The legality and ethics of the practice were debated during the court action. The lawyer for the institution argued that the practice was accepted internationally, their disabilities meant that the girls could not look after themselves, they felt pain during their periods, and they would not be able to marry, so the operation was in their interests and should be an accepted practice. The court decision was that the girls were seriously harmed by the practice and the director of the institution was found guilty (Dongfang Zaobao, 2005).

3.3 *Physical and Emotional Abuse in Institutions*

The young people who had grown up in institutions also spoke about maltreatment during their childhood, which included violence, loss of relationships, and discrimination (Shang & Fisher, 2017). Many of the young people said they had experienced violence living in an institution. They said the violence took place when they were young and no longer happened once they grew up, because when they were bigger, they could fight back.

At a focus group, while talking about whether they experienced physical violence from institution staff, all the children became agitated and said they had been beaten or scolded by staff. They said that when they refused to help the workers with the chores, they were beaten and ordered to stand on their knees outside or run outside in the rain as a punishment. They said these forms of physical punishment were used because officially physical punishment was prohibited. A young woman named Ming said that once she would not help a worker do chores and just stayed on the bed, ignoring her requests. The woman kept urging her, and she quarreled with the woman, until the worker kicked her painfully. When a teacher at the institution heard the story, she sent her to be checked by the doctor.

Luo, a 23-year-old man, had lived in an institution when he was very young, then moved to foster care where he had many positive memories. His said his worst experience in institutional care was being denied breakfast as punishment:

> When I was young, I used to be denied breakfast if I wet the bed. Somehow I kept wetting the bed, and the teachers refused to give me food. But older children offered me some food.

Such maltreatment experiences affected their emotional development as observed by the researchers, including strongly self-protective behavior and violence and abusive name-calling toward each other and the workers. For example, Zhong, a 26-year-old man, spoke about being physically punished in childhood, which led to him beating other children:

> The staff disciplined us strictly … sometimes improperly. They might beat or physically punish children. Some children even had broken bones or other physical injuries … Shortly after we arrived at the welfare institution they disciplined us in a harsh way in order to effectively control us. The physical punishment was severe, and the impact on children was negative. For example, children were denied dinner or were beaten or scolded … So we were both bullied by older children and disciplined by the woman staff, facing dual pressures. In a word, we were not very happy there.

Zhong said he too used to beat younger children, replicating his own experience as a younger child. But he said that when he was influenced by a teacher, he stopped beating younger children:

> We had a teacher … who bought educational books, particularly books written by American or UK education experts. I read some of the books, and abandoned the habit of beating other children. Instead, I began to oppose beating children. I no longer believed beating was an effective way of disciplining them.

Formal foster families managed by welfare institutions are also prohibited from physically punishing children; otherwise they become disqualified from caring for a foster child. No young people who had grown up in foster care mentioned being physically punished in their foster family. Instead, the worst experiences of young people who had lived in foster families were associated with lost affectionate relationships with the families, particularly when they were forcibly removed from the family, with whom they had formed family-like relationships. Some children were transferred back to the welfare institutions from the foster families due to policy requirements for their later care.

One example was Hen who was aged 23 years at the time of the research. He had moved between institutional care, foster care, and back to institutional care. At the age of 14 years, Hen was transferred from the foster family where he had lived since he was 4 years old, back to the institution. Initially, Hen was not accustomed to the institutional environment. Everything in the institution was unfamiliar, and he felt the loss of his family. He vividly described the contrast:

> Previously, all my family members sat around table, having dinner. But now [at the institution] a group of children sit in row, having a small dinner and stopping even if we do not feel full. At the beginning, I felt very strongly homesick, but I never told the other children about my bad feelings. My parents visited me several times, but the stipulation of the institution prohibited frequent visiting. One year, they picked me up to celebrate the Spring Festival at home … All in all, everything started over. I felt like a chess piece placed by others at will.

This feeling of loss when relationships were broken by administrative decisions was also shared by young people who had grown up in family groups within institutions. In one institution, all the young people in care participating in the research grew up in small family groups and treated each other as siblings within the group. Li, a 21-year-old man, recounted that when a younger child he looked after at the welfare institution was adopted internationally, Li never saw the child again. He said he would always feel pain from this loss:

> In my childhood, some older children were charged to look after younger children. I looked after a child much younger than me. He made a strong impression on me. But he was taken out of the country … He was basically brought up by me, and I was responsible for his clothing and dinner. So I felt heartbroken when he was taken away.

These examples give a flavor of the types of direct and indirect child maltreatment in child institutions in China, many of which are likely to have been repeated in the lives of other children in institutional care. Most of the examples are from past experiences. Evidence about recent or current maltreatment is not available due to the poor accountability and closed environment of Chinese government and non-government child institutions.

4 Policy Changes to Protect Children in Institutions

Since these reports of maltreatment, the Chinese government has responded with various policy changes to improve the quality of support for children not in the care of their family, whether in state or nongovernment care. The main changes are about resources, supervision, and functions of institutions and the development of family-based care as an alternative to institutional care.

4.1 Redressing Policy Neglect

Many maltreatment cases reported from the past 20 years were the result of policy neglect, in the form of insufficient resources or marginalizing the rights of children in care. The high mortality rate reported in the 1990s was due to insufficient financial and staff resources for institutions, in combination with their responsibility for more children. Resources for staffing and facilities increased in the 2000s, which remedied the worst of these conditions. Perversely in some areas, the new resources also encouraged the re-institutionalization of children to justify the continued operation of the institution. An example was the distressed young man, Hen above, forced to return to the institution, after he had the benefit of living in foster care during the time when the institution had relied on foster care to stretch the limited financial resources.

In the past two decades, the concept of child rights has gradually gained greater acceptance in China, both within the government and in the wider community. Some common practices in the institutions became unacceptable when seen through a children's rights framework, such as the naming, forced sterilization, and physical punishment described earlier by the young people.

More broadly, the Chinese government has accepted a shift toward a mixed welfare system, which has the effect of spreading responsibility for alternative care of children without known family members. It means that financial support for welfare institutions can be shared between government and other sources. For example, in the past, state institutions could not accept donations, but now they are encouraged to seek them from local donors and businesses (Shang, 2001). In addition, state institutions can now contract with nongovernment organizations to care for children, whereas in the past such nongovernment organizations were merely tolerated by ignoring their presence (Shang, 2008a). Similarly, some institutions are now accepting a small number of self-funded children with disabilities to board at the institution, so that they can receive medical and therapeutic interventions otherwise not available to them (Shang, 2008a).

The purpose of state guardianship and state care are also gradually changing in China. Originally, state care was for children who were orphaned and who did not have known extended families to care for them. As described above, as family planning and adoption became stricter and access to public disability and medical interventions waned during the economic reforms in the 1990s, more children with disabilities were left in state care by their families who did not have other choices to support their children.

In wealthier areas, these policy driven causes for children ending up in state care have decreased as the public health and welfare systems improve; the causes for the deaths of parents have decreased (accidents and illness); domestic adoption laws have improved; and parents can be supported to care for their own children with adequate health and welfare support (Shang & Fisher, 2016). For example from 2010, all children who are orphaned are entitled to income support through a national orphan allowance, which makes it more feasible for children to continue to live with their extended families, where the allowance is implemented (General Office of the State Council, 2010).

The functions of child welfare institutions in richer cities in China are now changing toward that of high-income countries. Institutions continue to hold guardianship for state wards, but they are more likely to arrange national or international adoption or other forms of family-based care for children in their care. In addition, some institutions are providing free or low-cost support to the families of children with disabilities so they are not forced to abandon their children to get the support they need. Other institutions are becoming involved in wider child protection support for children experiencing maltreatment in their families. In the long term, it is foreseeable that institutions will become administrative centers that house few or no children. Examples of this already exist, such as in Daxing, a rural area of Beijing (Shang & Fisher, 2017; Shang, 2008a).

4.2 Care Outside an Institution

A fundamental shift away from maltreatment in institutions has been to avoid institutional care altogether by developing family-based alternatives. Like most countries, the main methods are to reunite the child with their family or arrange permanent adoptive families. These methods have effectively stemmed the increase in the total number of children cared for by the state, as well as the proportion of children in institutions (Shang & Fisher, 2014).

Some children who continue to live in care now also have alternatives such as family group care within the institution, where a housemother cares for a group of children to build sibling-like relationships. Other children live with foster families in the community, supervised by the institution. The Standing Committee of the State Council passed the Opinions on Strengthening Welfare Protection of Orphans 2010, which recognized small group family care and foster care, but it did not position these forms of alternative care as preferred types of care. In 2010, social welfare institutions with foster care accounted for over 50% of all welfare institutions with children. Over 50% of orphans and children with disabilities in these institutions were raised in foster families, and foster care became one of the primary approaches to the care of orphans who were in the guardianship of these institutions. Although institutional care continues to be the dominant type of care and policy makers continue to favor it or family care units over foster care, a gradual process of deinstitutionalization continues.

Three management types of foster care have evolved – rural community-based foster care, urban community-based foster care, and urban discrete foster care. These types of foster care have been adapted to the local needs and resources in these areas. The variation between the types can be explained by differences in policy objectives about social inclusion, the approach to managing risks and harm to the children, and managing costs within a limited budget (Shang & Fisher, 2014).

Among the three types, urban foster care offers the greatest opportunities for social inclusion. In this type, children live in regular urban families, attend local schools, and receive health-care services at local hospitals. Their family and community environment is the same as other children in their community. It contrasts with institutional care, which separates children from the community and incurs a high financial cost. Government control of the risks to children in foster care is more remote when compared to institutional care.

None of the approaches or adaptations completely addresses the disability therapy needs of children with disabilities with high support needs. Some child welfare institutions have professional therapy in rural foster care and professional community-based foster care to respond to the large proportion of children with disabilities requiring alternative care.

In summary, in addition to adoption, depending on the location, children subject to state guardianship might be in alternative care ranging from institutional care to foster care. Family-based care has not yet become a dominant type of care in China. The extent of maltreatment in these different care types upon children's lives as they become young adults has not been examined fully despite the different impact of each type of alternative care on the choices that will be available to them in the future.

5 Future Directions to Prevent Maltreatment in Institutions

The Chinese government's attention to maltreatment in child welfare institutions has changed as it has engaged with international frameworks about children's rights and good practice in alternative care. Three sets of policies have contributed to reducing child maltreatment in institutions. The first set is aimed at preventing children coming into state care through improvements in the health and welfare system that support families to remain intact. These changes have been associated with economic development, which has enabled central and local governments to establish systems and allocate resources to ensuring the safety and support of children in their families.

The second set of policy changes was to prioritize permanent international and domestic adoption for children whose extended family could not be found and implementing foster care for remaining children who are not adopted. The policy effectively reduced the number of children growing up in child welfare institutions, thus reducing the incidence of maltreatment in institutions. The shift from institutional care to foster care is not as widely implemented as would be expected according to international guidelines, due to a lack of central government commitment to family-based care as the preferred form of care and also strong local vested interests in continuing institutional care. Most foster care remains supervised and monitored by the state child welfare institutions. This, in addition to the local community oversight, means that in most cases, the quality of care and the opportunity for maltreatment within foster families are under close scrutiny. The intimate Chinese government and local community structures mean that long-term foster care operates quite differently to programs in most developed countries, with maltreatment less likely to remain unnoticed (Shang, 2008a).

The most recent set of policies regulates alternative care provided by nongovernment child welfare organizations. In the past, these arrangements have tended to be conveniently ignored, but now that a mixed welfare system is more established, the government has begun to encourage them and has responded to public criticism about unregulated quality of care.

Each of these sets of policy improvements is far from complete, particularly the implementation of the policies and changes to local practices to prioritize the interests of children. In addition, problems remain about a lack of mechanisms to monitor staff behavior within institutions, apart from the generalized responsibility of institution management.

6 Summary

The state responsibility for orphans whose families cannot be found historically took the form of institutional care. The number of children in care rose during the implementation of strict policy criteria for family planning, adoption, and dismantling of the communist welfare state in the 1980–1990s. During that time, institutions were severely under-resourced, maltreatment levels were extreme, and children were dying from neglect. Young people who grew up in care also reported physical and emotional abuse from practices such as physical punishment from staff despite rules against it, naming practices, forced sterilization, and loss of relationships from forced shifts between forms of care.

In more recent years, the Chinese government has implemented different types of policies that have the effect of reducing the incidence of maltreatment in institutions. Support for children to live in their families and communities, such as improvements in the health and welfare systems, has had the effect of reducing the reasons they become state wards. If they do become state wards, the policies and practices also preference adoption, and now in some areas, they also prioritize family-based alternative care. The regulations about quality of care from nongovernment carers are more likely to be implemented now, following scandals about the death of children in their care. Outstanding problems are how to implement the policies, particularly replacing institutional care, monitoring the behavior of staff, and ensuring nongovernment carers comply with regulations.

Questions for Discussion

1. In the context of China as a large country with variation in policy implementation, how could we find out if children's experiences of maltreatment have improved?
2. The BBC documentary, *The Dying Rooms*, had a significant role influencing policy and practice change about maltreatment in institutions. Why do you think

it was so influential, and what would you make a documentary about to continue that impact?

3. Children with disabilities are most likely to be in institutional care in China. What additional practices should be implemented to protect them from maltreatment and respond to their needs?

References

Beijing Minzheng Xinxiwang. (2014). The Ministry of Civil Affairs issued "*Management methods of foster care*", the coverage of fostered children increased. Retrieved November, 3, 2016, from http://www.bjmzj.gov.cn/news/root/mtbd/2014-09/111488.shtml?NODE_ID=root

Bross, D., Miyoshi, T., Miyoshi, P., & Krugman, R. (2000). *World perspectives on child abuse: The fourth international resource book*. Denver, Colorado: Kempe Children's Center, University of Colorado School of Medicine.

Chen, X., & Chen, Y. (2008). *The status analysis and strategies of children with disabilities in China*. Beijing, China: Huaxia Press.

China Youth Newspaper. (2013). *Mass media reporting the death of seven orphans in Henan: Abandoned when they are alive, and death because neglection*. Retrieved August, 12, 2016, from http://news.ifeng.com/mainland/special/lankaoqiying/content-3/detail_2013_01/09/20977375_0.shtml

Dongfang Zaobao. (2005). *The court open for the case of Jiangshu Nantong Child Welfare Institution cutting off the uterus of girls*. Retrieved June, 3, 2005, from http://news.xinhuanet.com/health/2005-06/03/content_3041276.htm

General Office of the State Council. (2010). Opinions on strengthening safeguarding for orphans. Retrieved March, 21, 2014, from http://www.gov.cn/zwgk/2010-11/18/content_1748012.htm

Heilongjiang News. (2012). *Harbin Child Welfare Institutions naming children according to one hundred surnames (Baijianxing)*. Retrieved August, 22, 2016, from http://www.hljnews.cn/fouxw_cs/2012-02/07/content_1153543.htm

Human Rights Watch. (1996). *Death by default: A policy of fatal neglect in China's state orphanage*. Retrieved from www.refworld.org/docid/3ae6a85a0.html#_ftn139

MCA, Ministry of Civil Affairs. (2013). *Social Service Development Statistical Communiqué*. Retrieved September, 25, 2014, from http://www.mca.gov.cn/article/zwgk/mzyw/201406/20140600654488.shtml

Nanfang Dushibao. (2005). *Jiangshu Nantong child welfare institution was covered by the scandal of cutting off the uterus of girls, 07/Jun*. Retrieved August, 21, 2016, from http://news.sina.com.cn/s/2005-06-07/09106102921s.shtml

Shang, X. (2001). Moving towards a multi-level and multi-pillar system: Institutional care in two Chinese cities. *Journal of Social Policy*, *30*(2), 259–281.

Shang, X. (2008a). *The system of social protection for vulnerable children in China*. Beijing, China: China Social Sciences Academic Press.

Shang, X. (2008b). *Research on the situations of Chinese orphans*. Beijing, China: Social Sciences Academic Press.

Shang, X., & Fisher, K. R. (2014). *Caring for orphaned children in China*. Lanham, Maryland: Lexington Books.

Shang, X., & Fisher, K. R. (2016). *Disability policy in China: Child and family experiences*. London, UK: Routledge.

Shang, X., & Fisher, K. R. (2017). *Young people leaving state care in China*. Bristol, UK: Policy Press.

WHO, World Health Organisation. (1999). *Report of the consultation on child abuse prevention*. Geneva, Switzerland: WHO.

Xu, J. (2013). Starting from systematic, standardization and specialization, to continuously improve the civil society's ability of raising children, a speech at the seminar of raising children by Chinese civil society. 26 October, Beijing. Retrieved September, 10, 2014, from www.chinacatholic.org/fics/children/26371.html

Chapter 16
Child Abuse and Neglect in Charitable Children's Institutions in Uasin Gishu County, Kenya: A Challenge of Context

Paula Braitstein, Samuel Ayaya, David Ayuku, Allison DeLong, and Lukoye Atwoli

> *A child does not question the wrongs of grown-ups; s/he suffers them.*
>
> Chief Dan George (unknown).

1 Introduction

In a slum of Eldoret, Kenya, Denis, aged 5, and his brother Robert, aged 3, took shelter for months with a stray dog in a pile of dirt into which they had dug a hole to get out of the rain. Their mother abandoned them; their father was an alcoholic and seemed to have forgotten that he had two young children who depended on him. Reported to the local children's authorities, no action was taken until eventually a local orphanage was notified and they came and picked them up. The children were both extremely malnourished, their bellies bloated with worms. Denis had obvious evidence of having been raped, repeatedly.

P. Braitstein (✉)
Division of Epidemiology, Dalla Lana School of Public Health, University of Toronto, 155 College Street, 5th floor, M5T 3M7 Toronto, ON, Canada

College of Health Sciences, School of Medicine, Moi University, Eldoret, Kenya
e-mail: paula.braitstein@utoronto.ca

S. Ayaya • D. Ayuku • L. Atwoli
College of Health Sciences, School of Medicine, Moi University, Eldoret, Kenya
e-mail: ayaya.samuelaluanga@gmail.com; ayukud@gmail.com; lukoye@gmail.com

A. DeLong
School of Public Health, Brown University, Providence, RI, USA
e-mail: adelong@stat.brown.edu

A.V. Rus et al. (eds.), *Child Maltreatment in Residential Care*,
DOI 10.1007/978-3-319-57990-0_16

This chapter is based on a body of research, much of it already published, that seeks to understand optimal and cost-effective care environments for orphaned and vulnerable children and adolescents in the county of Uasin Gishu, in the beautiful western highlands of Kenya. With funding from the United States National Institutes of Child Health and Human Development (NICHD R01HD060478), the Orphaned and Separated Children's Assessments Related to their (OSCAR) Health and Well-Being cohort was established in 2009 and is funded through 2020. The study consists of nearly 2500 orphaned and separated children and adolescents, aged 18 years or less at enrollment into the study. Roughly half are living in 1 of 18 Charitable Children's Institutions (CCIs) in Uasin Gishu, such as orphanages and rescue centers, and half are living in extended (usually biological) family environments in 1 of 6 locations in the county (half rural, half peri-urban). The cohort also includes 100 street-connected children and adolescents who continue to be followed today as a preliminary cohort of young people essentially representing a third model of care: self-care (Kamanda et al., 2013).

Using a combination of previously published and newly analyzed data plus examples from our research and personal experiences, we will reveal that child abuse and neglect in this region are serious and highly prevalent, multifactorial problems. We will illustrate how in this region, and in our study, children living in CCIs are generally healthier and happier than those living with extended family and have no additional risk of experiencing emotional, physical, or sexual abuse or neglect compared to them. We will further highlight the extreme levels of abuse, neglect, and exploitation among street-connected children and youth. Our specific objectives with this chapter are:

1. To describe child abuse and neglect (emotional, physical, and sexual) among orphaned and vulnerable children and adolescents living in Charitable Children's Institutions (CCIs) in Uasin Gishu County, Kenya.
2. To compare the prevalence and incidence of child abuse and neglect (emotional, physical, and sexual) between orphaned and vulnerable children and adolescents living in CCIs with that reported by participants living in family-based environments and street-connected children and youth.
3. To illustrate that child abuse and neglect are major social problems in Kenya and that functional and cost-effective child protection and care mechanisms are urgently required.

2 Historical and Socioeconomic Context

In Kenya, a confluence of events and historical, political, social, environmental, and economic factors have steadily contributed to perpetuating conditions of abject poverty for generations of children growing up in the region. Between 1980 and 1990, the urban population in Kenya doubled, with most of the growth concentrated in Nairobi, the capital, and Mombasa, the second largest city, on the coast. Migration from rural areas to urban centers increased dramatically during this period with poor families being further driven from their homes by landlessness, drought, and unemployment. A sprawling collection of slum settlements spread over the outskirts of Nairobi and other towns and cities. With thousands – now millions – of new urban slum dwellers, including a large number of single-parent households headed by women, the numbers of children living on the streets began to rise dramatically (Ayuku, Kaplan, Baars, & de Vries, 2004).

In the 1990s and most of the 2000s, Kenya was badly hit by the HIV/AIDS pandemic. Still in 2015, an estimated 36,000 people died of AIDS in Kenya, and 1.4 million people are presently living with HIV in Kenya, of whom about half are receiving the lifesaving antiretroviral treatment (though with recently revised treatment guidelines, this number should increase quickly). The AIDS epidemic created many generations of often highly stigmatized orphaned and vulnerable children. According to government estimates, there are approximately 660,000 children who have been orphaned by HIV/AIDS living in Kenya as of 2015 (UNAIDS, 2016).

Today, Eldoret is Kenya's fifth largest city, approximately 350 kilometers northwest of Nairobi. It is the capital of Uasin Gishu County, 1 of the 47 counties of Kenya. In 2010, Uasin Gishu was populated by approximately 900,000 individuals from 202,000 households, of whom about 42% are aged ≤14 years (CRA, 2013, 2017). The majority of the county's population (61%) still reside in rural areas (Kenya Open Data Project, 2011) compared to 68% of the population in the rest of Kenya and 77% in East Africa (UN Habitat, 2008). Approximately 51% of the population in Uasin Gishu live below the Kenyan poverty line (1562 Kenyan Shillings per person per month ~ $16 USD), roughly average in the country (Kenya Open Data Project, 2011). HIV prevalence in the region is almost exactly the national average, at around 5% among adults (National AIDS and STI Control Programme, 2013). Eldoret officially has a population of 289,389 (as of the 2010 population census) (Kenya, 2011). Unofficial estimates put its 2010 population closer to 500,000 mostly in the peri-urban settlements (i.e., slums) around the downtown core. Children below 18 years make up 49% of the population of Kenya, and 62% of the population is below 24 years of age (http://www.unicef.org/kenya/overview_15603.html). The region is largely agricultural and is still considered a breadbasket of Kenya. Eldoret is historically a farming town, a stop on the Mombasa-Kinshasa highway.

Kenya is a country of many contrasts, from its landscape to demographics, but its social and economic inequalities are the most dramatic. It is one of the most unequal countries in all of sub-Saharan Africa. Forty two percent of the population of 44 million lives below the poverty line (UNICEF, 2012a). The Gini coefficient is a common measure of inequality ranging from 0 (reflecting complete equality) to 1 (reflecting complete inequality). The Gini coefficient for Kenya is 0.477, indicating a high level of inequality. The Human Development Index (HDI) is a composite statistic of life expectancy, education, and income per capita indicators. In 2014 Kenya ranked 145th of 188 countries ranked (Jahan, 2015). The children of Kenya are growing up in a time of profound political, economic, environmental, and social transformation. Over 75% of children and adolescents in Kenya experience one or more deprivation of their rights, including limited access to safe water and improved sanitation, education, and health and nutrition services (UNICEF, 2012a). With this background, it is hard to imagine how the poorest manage and especially the children of the poorest. This extreme poverty exacerbates and magnifies family conflict and dysfunction and contributes to alcoholism and its many ill effects.

3 An Epidemic of Orphaned and Vulnerable Children and Adolescents

Global UNICEF estimates put the number of children and adolescents for whom one or both parents are deceased at 153 million; millions more have been abandoned (UNICEF, 2012c). The majority live in low- and middle-income countries such as Kenya where approximately 26% of the 2.5 million orphans have been orphaned by AIDS and two-thirds are adolescents (Lee et al., 2014). Compared to non-orphans, orphaned children and youth are at higher risk of acquiring HIV (Magadi & Uchudi, 2015; Operario, Underhill, Chuong, & Cluver, 2011), experiencing malnutrition (Miller, Gruskin, Subramanian, & Heymann, 2007), other childhood illnesses (Amoako Johnson, Padmadas, & Smith, 2010), and stigma and discrimination (Chuong & Operario, 2012; Cluver & Orkin, 2009; Monasch & Boerma, 2004).

Traditionally in sub-Saharan Africa, orphaned or separated children would be absorbed by the extended family, and the majority of orphans today are still cared for by extended family or in other family-based environments (Goodson & Layzer, 2010; Monasch & Boerma, 2004; UNICEF, 2006). The sheer number of children requiring care, layered on top of preexisting poverty and sociocultural factors (Rose, 2005; Witter, Calder, & Ahimbisibwe, 2004), causes a high caregiver burden (Heymann, Earle, Rajaraman, Miller, & Bogen, 2007; Hosegood et al., 2007; Kidman & Thurman, 2014; Miller, Gruskin, Subramanian, Rajaraman, & Heymann, 2006; Monasch & Boerma, 2004) and prevents families from meeting all caretaking expectations and responsibilities. Grandmothers have been bearing the greatest burden of caring for orphans and are the primary caretakers for approximately half of all orphaned children (Monasch & Boerma, 2004).

Extended families, particularly those headed by grandparents, are not always able to meet the material needs of the orphaned children in their care. A study from Botswana found that one-third of working adults were caring for orphans, but 82% of these were living below US$10 per day (adjusted for purchasing power parity) (Heymann et al., 2007). UNICEF studies in both Malawi and Zimbabwe found that orphans were significantly less likely to have basic material goods compared to other children (defined as a blanket, a pair of shoes, and two sets of clothes) (UNICEF, 2005; UNICEF & Ministry of Public Service Labour and Social Welfare, 2005). Research from western Kenya found that orphaned children, the majority of whom were living with extended family, lacked school fees, food, and access to medical care (Nyambedha, Wandibba, & Aagaard-Hansen, 2003). Many of the caretakers were not capable of providing care because of ill health or old age (Nyambedha et al., 2003). Another study from Botswana found that orphaned children lived disproportionately in the poorest households and were 49% more likely to be underweight (Miller et al., 2007). Double orphans aged 6–10 years were half as likely to be at the correct educational level as non-orphaned children, and orphaned children aged 11–14 were two-thirds less likely to be at the appropriate education level (Bicego, Rutstein, & Johnson, 2003). Across sub-Saharan Africa, orphans are less likely to be enrolled in school than non-orphans (Monasch & Boerma, 2004).

Social and cultural factors can also adversely affect the way an orphaned child is cared for within extended family situations. Inheritance laws and practices may exclude or prevent orphans and widows from being able to inherit land or wealth (Laurel Rose, 2005; Witter et al., 2004). Anecdotal evidence from western Kenya suggests that extended families are reluctant to accept orphans because they do not want to have to include the orphaned child in inheritance plans. In one study, 28% of the orphans were looked after by culturally "inappropriate" categories such as matrilineal kin (Nyambedha et al., 2003). Culture remains a strong driver of choices, preferences, and behaviors in Kenya and elsewhere in sub-Saharan Africa.

Evidence from Mozambique clearly points to discrimination in the intra-household allocation of resources against children who are not the direct biological descendants of the household head in poor households (Nhate, Arndt, Barslund, & Van Den Broeck, 2006). Qualitative research carried out in Malawi and Lesotho found that children who had migrated to another household and who also experienced the death or sickness of a parent reported being given different food from other children in the household, being beaten and overworked, and having received inadequate clothing (Ansell & Young, 2004). Analysis based on 19 Demographic and Health Surveys in 10 sub-Saharan countries found evidence of intra-household discrimination against orphans as manifested by investment in schooling, with orphans having lower enrollment rates than non-orphans in the same household (Case, Paxson, & Ableidinger, 2004). The stigma associated with HIV disease further complicates the care of orphaned children in some settings where stigma is high (Cluver, Gardner, & Operario, 2008; Hamra, Ross, Karuri, Orrs, & D'Agostino, 2005). For orphaned children who are themselves HIV-infected, their chances of being outright rejected by extended family are very high (Doring, Franca Junior, & Stella, 2005).

In short, orphaned and otherwise vulnerable children and adolescents may live with family who are either unwilling or unable to support them. Many end up on the street just because they have nowhere else to go. Research suggests that girls on the street are more likely to be double orphans (having lost both parents) compared to boys (Sorber et al., 2014). The primary causes of child and youth homelessness in sub-Saharan Africa and globally are poverty, family dysfunction including alcoholism, and child abuse, whether physical, sexual, emotional, or frank neglect (Embleton, Lee, Gunn, Ayuku, & Braitstein, 2016).

There is in essence an epidemic of orphaned and vulnerable children and adolescents in sub-Saharan Africa. Families and communities are stretched, financially and often emotionally as well. Many of the caregivers are grandmothers who have love to give but little else. Many single orphans (one parent dead or essentially absent from the child's life, rendering them a virtual orphan) are children of single mothers, who either don't know their fathers or whose fathers are not at all involved in their lives.

4 The OSCAR Study

The Orphaned and Separated Children's Assessments Related to their (OSCAR) Health and Well-Being Study is following a cohort of nearly 2500 mostly orphaned and separated children and adolescents who were aged 18 years or less at baseline. Roughly half of the cohort are orphaned and separated children and adolescents living in 1 of 300 randomly selected households (HHs) in six rural and peri-urban locations in Uasin Gishu County (location in this context refers to administrative boundaries within the county); half are living in 1 of 18 institutions caring for orphans and other extremely vulnerable children such as those who are abandoned, neglected, or abused (which in Kenya are called Charitable Children's Institutions or CCIs, aka orphanages, shelters, and rescue centers); 100 are street-connected children and youth in Eldoret; and a relatively small but important group are non-orphaned children living in the same participating households and CCIs (usually the biological descendants of the "house parents" or household heads). These non-orphans were included in the cohort so as not to mark the orphans as different within participating households and CCIs. More details about recruitment, enrollment, study procedures, and other aspects of the study can be found elsewhere (Kamanda et al., 2013). The primary objective of this study is to evaluate the physical and mental health outcomes among orphaned and separated children and adolescents living in different care environments and describe the cost-effectiveness of different care environments.

In general, the first phase of the OSCAR study found that orphans living in CCIs in this region seemed to be at least somewhat healthier, happier, and having their basic rights as children respected, compared to those living in extended family environments (Atwoli et al., 2014; Braitstein et al., 2013; Embleton et al., 2014, 2017). At baseline and after adjusting for length of time in their current care environment, children living in CCIs were more likely to have an adequate diet and were less likely to be malnourished compared to children living in the HHs. In contrast the odds of street children in OSCAR being stunted as measured by height for age were six times that compared to children living in CCIs. A higher proportion of adolescents at baseline in OSCAR living in HH (15%) had post-traumatic stress disorder compared to those in CCIs (12%), while street youth had the highest prevalence of post-traumatic stress disorder in the cohort, at 29%.

The second phase of the study is endeavoring to identify what characteristics explain these findings. Clearly there is nothing inherent in an institution that makes it better for children. All the children and young people participating in OSCAR are children and youth facing adversity – if not because of orphan status, then because of poverty and its consequences. Looking into the future, human activity is putting such strain on the natural functions of the Earth that "the ability of the planet's ecosystems to sustain future generations can no longer be taken for granted" (Millennium Ecosystem Assessment, 2005). Our societies face clear and potent dangers that require urgent and transformative actions to protect present and future generations. What current and future generations of youth most need is, and will be, the ability to adapt quickly and adeptly to changing and challenging environments and circumstances – starting with care environments. How can we best support and cultivate resilience and the ability of these young people to adapt and withstand such challenging circumstances? We can leverage this observational information to eventually develop and test innovative interventions that can help children and youth to adapt in their lives in spite of the adversity they face. OSCAR 2.0 is testing various hypotheses, including whether the quality of the relationship between the child and the caregiver, or children's participation in organized sports, religious, or other activities, successfully promotes resilience and better outcomes such as completion of secondary education and HIV-free survival, among many others. We are also measuring the cost-effectiveness of different care environments which we hope will inform governmental and nongovernmental programs, policies, and approaches to supporting orphans, separated, and otherwise vulnerable children and youth.

4.1 Child Abuse and Neglect Among Orphans

To better understand child abuse and neglect among orphans generally, we conducted both qualitative and quantitative systematic reviews of the literature. The qualitative review confirmed the hypothesis that orphaned children were at higher risk of experiencing abuse and neglect compared to non-orphaned children (Morantz, Cole, Vreeman, et al., 2013). Yet, the systematic review and meta-analysis were unable to confirm this (Nichols et al., 2014). These contradictory findings led us to conclude that while the qualitative data suggest a serious problem, the quantitative data were badly limited by inconsistent definitions of abuse, a lack of comparisons with non-orphaned children, and other methodologic and data limitations and weaknesses. In short, the quality of the literature on the topic is actually rather poor.

4.2 Child Abuse and Neglect Among Children Living in Charitable Children's Institutions (CCIs)

Circumstances like those Denis and Robert found themselves in are, sadly, quite common in Kenya and other similar settings. In 2011–2012, we sought to understand the maltreatment experienced by institutionalized children prior to their admission to CCIs in Uasin Gishu and to describe the sociodemographic characteristics, reasons for admission, and factors associated with prior experiences of maltreatment among resident children (Morantz, Cole, Ayaya, Ayuku, & Braitstein, 2013). We undertook a file review of the records for children living in five large CCIs in Uasin Gishu that together comprised 462 children. The average age of children was 6.8 years at admission, 56% were male, and 71% had lost one or both parents. The reasons for admission were destitution (36%), abandonment (22%), neglect (21%), physical/sexual abuse (8%), and lack of a caregiver (8%). The majority of child and youth residents had experienced at least one form of maltreatment (66%) prior to admission: physical abuse (8%), sexual abuse (2%), psychological abuse (28%), neglect (26%), medical neglect (18%), school deprivation (38%), abandonment (30%), and child labor (23%). The most common reason for non-orphans to be admitted was maltreatment (90%), whereas the most common reason for orphans to be admitted was destitution (49%). Girls were 30% less likely, and orphans were >95% less likely to have a history of maltreatment irrespective of whether it was the reason for admission. Children whose primary caregiver had not been a parent and orphans were less likely to have been admitted for maltreatment, while children who were separated from siblings were 62% more likely to have been admitted for maltreatment.

4.3 Child Abuse and Neglect in Different Care Environments

A key aim of the OSCAR study is to understand child abuse and neglect among orphaned and separated children in different care environments. To do this, we use an instrument called the ISPCAN Child Abuse Screening Tool for Children at Home (ICAST-CH) which measures violence against children. It was developed by the International Society for the Prevention of Child Abuse and Neglect (IPSCAN) There are some extra spaces in this in the online version - ? in partnership with UNICEF and the United Nations Secretary-General's Study on violence against children (Table 16.1).

This assessment was implemented in OSCAR with participants aged at least 10 years of age and annually thereafter and is part of an annual battery of questions and assessments called the OSCAR Psychosocial Encounter. It is usually completed by self-report, with clinical psychologists on hand to assist in case of questions, lack of understanding, or emotional distress.

Slightly over half of the adolescent OSCAR participants were aged 10–13 years at baseline, except for street youth, two-thirds of whom were 14–18 years of age. Just over half of the whole adolescent cohort is male, equally divided between CCIs and HHs. The exception is among street youth, of whom 80% were (and still are) male. Overall, 53% of the cohort are double orphans: 33% of participants in HHs, 78% of participants in CCIs, and 74% of street youth. Over 90% of participants at baseline in both CCIs and HHs were attending school, but 90% of the street youth said they were not. Nearly 30% of participants in CCIs had been there for 2 years or

Table 16.1 Adapted IPSCAN questions for OSCAR study

Question stem: Has anyone in your home ever… *Possible responses:* Never, sometimes, many times, yes it has happened but not in the past 6 months
Emotional abuse
Used drugs and/or alcohol and then behaved in a way that frightened you?
Said they wished you were dead or had never been born?
Threatened to hurt or kill you, including invoking evil spirits against you?
Physical abuse
Have you felt that you did not get enough to eat (went hungry) and/or drink (went thirsty) even though there was enough for everyone?
Have to wear dirty, torn clothes that were not warm enough/too warm or sleep on the ground without a blanket even though there were clothes/mattresses/blankets available?
Has anyone in your home hit, beat, or slapped you hard enough to cause injury?
Has anyone in your home burned or scalded you (including putting hot chilies or peppers in your mouth) or choked, smothered, or tried to drown you?
Sexual abuse
Have you ever exchanged sex for money, shelter, food, protection, or anything else?
Made you look at their private parts or wanted to look at yours?
Touched your private parts or made you touch theirs?
Tried or forced you to have sex when you did not want them to?

less, but the rest had been in their same care environment for more than 2 years and many for more than 2 years. In households, 75% of participants had been living in that care environment for their whole lives. Over two-thirds of the street youth had been on the street for more than 2 years.

Having a history of abuse and/or neglect at enrollment into the cohort was common for the whole study population across all three care environments, inclusive of the participating non-orphans. As seen in Table 16.2, 43% of the whole cohort reported having ever experienced any child abuse or neglect. This is incredibly high, even for such a vulnerable population. Excluding from the analysis the non-orphans does not affect the proportions at all of ever experiencing abuse, meaning that there does not appear to be a systematic difference between orphans and non-orphans in terms of whether they have experienced abuse and/or neglect.

Also observed in Table 16.2 is that 31% of the cohort reported ever experiencing emotional abuse, 38% reported ever experiencing any physical abuse, and 15% reported any sexual abuse. We can assume there is underreporting of abuse, especially at baseline, given that most participants are probably already living in their "last resort" scenario and are afraid of the consequences of reporting truthfully. Similarly, in the initial assessments, we expected that participants were likely not trusting of what we would do with the data, so many may have underreported. There may also be underestimates because we have included "missing" as a category in the analysis (8–14% at baseline, data not shown). If one assumes that "missing" has the same levels of abuse as those participants with data, then closer to 50% would have had experienced any abuse at enrollment into the study. Given then, that these

Table 16.2 Child abuse and neglect among participants in Charitable Children's Institutions (CCIs), family-based households (HHs), and street children (SC) in the OSCAR study

	Total	CCI	HH	SC
	$N = 1158$	$n = 448$	$n = 630$	$n = 80$
Any abuse				
Prevalence at baseline	493, 43%	210, 47%	241, 38%	42, 52%
Experienced during follow-up (sometimes, many times)	523, 45%	178, 40%	279, 44%	66, 82%
Cumulative prevalence by end of follow-up	772, 67%	300, 67%	398, 63%	74, 92%
Any emotional abuse				
Prevalence at baseline	360, 31%	144, 32%	178, 28%	38, 48%
Experienced during follow-up (sometimes, many times)	352, 30%	116, 26%	179, 28%	57, 71%
Cumulative prevalence by end of follow-up	612, 53%	230, 51%	310, 49%	72, 90%
Any physical abuse				
Prevalence at baseline	437, 38%	179, 40%	210, 33%	48, 60%
Experienced during follow-up (sometimes, many times)	444, 38%	149, 33%	230, 37%	65, 81%
Cumulative prevalence by end of follow-up	688, 59%	257, 57%	357, 57%	74, 92%
Any sexual abuse				
Prevalence at baseline	179, 15%	58, 13%	98, 16%	23, 29%
Experienced during follow-up (sometimes, many times)	178, 15%	50, 11%	96, 15%	32, 40%
Cumulative prevalence by end of follow-up	339, 29%	108, 24%	187, 30%	44, 55%

Values presented as *n*, %

estimates can be counted as minimums, there is truly a grave problem at hand – and not only in the institutions.

One expects, at baseline, that more children in CCIs would have some history of abuse and/or neglect, and we see this in the baseline prevalence estimate for CCIs of 47%. This supports the earlier findings that child abuse is a major factor in the admission of children to CCIs. More surprising is that nearly 40% of the children in participating family-based households reported having ever experienced any child abuse or neglect, and again this proportion does not change if you exclude the non-orphans. Slightly over half of the street youth reported any abuse history (although a nontrivial number of street youth are missing data on this section of the OSCAR assessment).

We earlier described how there are important differences between the three groups in their gender, age, orphan status, and length of time they had been in that care environment. These factors could impact the findings in a way that affects our interpretation so we need to adjust for them using statistical methods. After adjusting for all these factors plus clustering by household or institution, we find that there is really no difference in the probability of having ever experienced abuse or neglect between participants in CCIs and those in HHs (i.e., odds ratios were close to 1.0). We find, however, that adjusting for these same variables, the odds of having ever experienced abuse were 4.7 times higher for street youth than for participants in the family-based households (Kamanda et al., 2013). This is consistent with a recent systematic review we conducted on causes of child and youth homelessness that child abuse and neglect are responsible for a large number of children who take to the streets in order to survive (Embleton, Lee, et al., 2016). When we look at these data by gender, we again find there are no statistical differences between the CCIs and HHs in the probability that males or females are more or less likely to experience abuse. Similarly, with age, in CCIs and HHs, there are no statistical differences whether the children are younger (10–13) or older (14–18) and their reporting of abuse. However, when we look at street youth and compare them to participants in HHs, we find that in all strata – males, females, younger, and older – the odds are 4.6–5.7 times greater that street youth will have experienced abuse and/or neglect. The odds of female street youth having experienced sexual abuse are 25 times greater compared to females in the HHs – and this latter population is already considered one at very high risk of sexual violence and exploitation (Operario et al., 2011).

What about during the first 2 years of follow-up? As seen in Table 16.2, 44% of the cohort reported experiencing any abuse during this relatively short follow-up period, including about 30% who reported emotional abuse (26–28% in CCIs and HHs, 71% among SC), 38% who reported physical abuse in follow-up (33–37% in CCIs and HHs, 81% among SC), and 15% who reported any sexual abuse (11% in CCIs, 15% in HHs, and 40% among SC). Overall, 40–44% of participants in CCIs and HHs, and 82% of street youth, reported experiencing any new abuse during the follow-up period.

In all three care environments and as is already known from the literature, the risk of abuse is higher for those who have previously experienced it. When we adjust for all the same factors as before plus whether participants reported having experienced any abuse at baseline, we again find no observable differences in the probability of participants in CCIs experiencing abuse during follow-up compared to those in HHs. In contrast, street youth are 4.8 times more likely than participants in the HHs to experience abuse during follow-up. After adjusting for age and other factors, female street youth are 8.5 times more likely than females in the HHs to experience any abuse during follow-up.

Cumulatively, combining data experienced at or prior to baseline and those collected during the follow-up assessments, 67% of the whole cohort has, so far in their young lives, experienced some kind of child abuse. This includes 67% of participants in CCIs, 63% in family-based HHs, and 92% of SC, suggesting child abuse is nearly ubiquitous in this population. At least 90% of SC have experienced emotional and/or physical violence, and over half have experienced sexual violence. Approximately 50% of participants in both CCIs and HHs have experienced emotional abuse, 57% have experienced physical abuse (much of which was likely inflicted as corporal punishment), and 24% and 30%, respectively, in CCIs and HHs, have experienced sexual abuse and/or violence (Ayuku et al., 2004).

5 How Can This Knowledge Improve Children's Care?

These data suggest that there are unacceptably high levels of child abuse occurring among orphaned and separated children and adolescents living in CCIs and among those living with extended family as well. The highest levels of child abuse are occurring among street-connected children and youth. We have seen that a large proportion of the abuse experienced by participants in CCIs took place before they ever actually moved into the CCI. Although there does seem to be unacceptably high levels of abuse occurring in CCIs, it is at least no greater than the equally unacceptable levels of abuse reported by participants in family-based households. Most alarming are the extremely high levels of emotional, physical, and sexual violence experienced by children and adolescents connected to the street.

These data confirm quantitatively what we have previously found through qualitative research, which is the uncovering of profound levels of abuse, exploitation, and violence among street children and youth: emotional, physical, and sexual (Embleton et al., 2015; Embleton, Wachira, et al., 2016; Wachira et al., 2015, 2016). Both boys and girls are raped, often as part of a ritualized process of being accepted as a member of the street youth community. Girls fairly routinely experience gang rape and are often forced to choose between gang rape and agreeing to be in a sexual relationship with an older male street youth, who shares "his vegetables" (street girls are often referred to by male street youth as *mboga wa jeshi* or "soldiers' vegetables") with his friends as he pleases. If a girl fails to conceive and bear a child, a symbol of ownership by a male, she will often experience serious physical and emotional violence at his hands. Both males and females, and especially the latter, frequently engage in transactional sex in order to survive, exchanging their young bodies for food, shelter, safety, and/or money. In spite of the estimated presence of tens to hundreds of millions of street children globally (UNICEF, 2012b) and in spite of the severe abuse and exploitation that they face, very few programs or interventions are available to assist them, especially in low- and middle-income countries, and often those in a position to assist them, such as police officers or healthcare providers, instead take advantage of their vulnerability.

The challenge in understanding and addressing child abuse and neglect among institutionalized children in Kenya is really one of the contexts. The only real social safety net for vulnerable children in Kenya is the extended family, whom, we have seen, against the backdrop of high dependency ratios, widespread and deeply entrenched poverty, rapid urbanization, and the HIV epidemic, are often not well positioned to care for orphaned and separated children, even if they are willing. Child protection and support systems are weak and insufficiently resourced in Kenya, and CCIs are one of the few viable safety nets that exist for children in this country when their families are either unwilling or unable to care for them. The foster care model is not well scaled or utilized in Kenya, largely for the same reasons why families are not always able to care for the children for whom they are, according to traditional and social expectations, responsible for fostering. The foster care systems in Canada, the United States, and elsewhere contribute to poor outcomes for children and youth who pass through them, in terms of education, subsequent contact with the correctional system, physical and mental health, and abuse and neglect. It is not obvious that the foster care systems that exist elsewhere are really a model that should be replicated globally (Lenz-Rashid, 2006; Tyler & Melander, 2010; Zlotnick, 2009; Zlotnick, Robertson, & Wright, 1999; Zlotnick, Tam, & Soman, 2012).

With international support, the Government of Kenya rolled out a cash support program in 2004 called the "Cash Transfer to Orphaned and Vulnerable Children" (CT-OVC) (Bryant, 2009; Mwasiaji, 2015). A mounting body of evidence from Kenya demonstrates that it works (Ayuku et al., 2014; Kilburn, Thirumurthy, Halpern, Pettifor, & Handa, 2016), and the government has expanded the program to support an estimated 259,000 households in 2014 (Mwasiaji, 2015). Enrolled households receive a cash payment of 2000 Kenya Shillings (approximately $20 USD) per month, which is equivalent to approximately 20% of average monthly household expenditure in the region. This is, more or less, the only form of government support to vulnerable households and vulnerable children (Embleton et al., 2014). We found that while a majority of the CCIs in Uasin Gishu received and relied upon charitable donations and had in place several kinds of income-generating projects including schools, farms, and others, well over a third of households caring for orphans in the OSCAR project reported receiving no external material assistance or support, including from nongovernmental or faith-based organizations. Families who reported receiving some external material support indicated that this support mostly came from other family members and, in one-third (due to the sampling strategy of the study), from the government through the CT-OVC program.

Ideally, the cash transfer program should be scaled up further, and the government should work toward ensuring a basic minimum income for all its citizens in order to alleviate poverty and its downstream consequences. It is also likely that this would reduce the flow of children to the streets, because their basic needs would be more likely to be met by their families. Alleviating poverty would have many positive impacts, including enabling extended families to better absorb orphaned and separated children, reducing stress in households, which itself would likely result in less child abuse and neglect, less alcoholism, and fewer absent parents.

We have previously proposed a hierarchy of care models to respond to the crisis of so many orphaned and separated children growing up in Kenya and other low- and middle-income countries today (Embleton et al., 2014). This model demonstrates that the majority of orphans both are (and should be) cared for by the remaining parent and, when that is not possible, with extended family. Our data suggest that to enable families to adequately care for children in the context of widespread poverty, they do need help. Direct financial support is a good start, but more is needed including subsidized education (primary, secondary, postsecondary) of the highest possible standard, parenting and communications skills and psychological support for caregivers and children alike, and free or subsidized alcohol counseling and rehabilitation programs. Nongovernmental and faith-based organizations should be directing a majority of their resources to supporting families in both rural and urban settings, reserving spots in residential facilities to only a minor few for whom family-based settings are not possible. We hypothesize this would, ultimately, be more cost-effective than setting up and operating ever more and larger institutions. Ideally a robust, well-monitored, and financially supported foster care system would be the next level in the hierarchy, but it does not yet exist in Kenya or in many other settings like it. It is likely that supporting older adolescents to take care of themselves and younger siblings as part of the "self-care" model might well be a viable and cost-effective strategy that empowers youth, rather than punishing them.

Given the absence of alternative care strategies in a setting like Kenya, CCIs have become a necessary component of a safety net for children facing extreme adversity. It is absolutely true that institutions caring for children have an abysmal track record in Canada, the United States, Australia, and Eastern Europe. The conditions and events in those places have left a legacy of multi-generational trauma that indigenous communities and others are still trying to cope with today. The historical and regional realities of institutional environments caring for children must be taken seriously and their pitfalls avoided and learned from at all costs going forward. Whether or not this means that institutions are *inherently* bad for children is not necessarily clear. Our data and data from other regions and investigators in low- and middle-income countries suggest that, as indicated in the hierarchy of care environments seen in Fig. 16.1, there may in fact be an important role for CCIs in helping communities to cope and respond to children facing extreme adversity, as countries continue to develop their infrastructure and ability to meet the basic needs of their citizens. Given that a large proportion of the children in CCIs in Uasin Gishu are double orphans and are there because of having experienced extreme abuse and/or neglect, one must ask the question as to what the alternative should be for those children. Returning to the very real and heartbreaking tale of Robert and Denis with which we started this chapter, what would have happened to them if the orphanage had not stepped in? In all probability, they would by now be dead – of abuse and neglect, by their family, by their neighbors, and by local children's authorities.

We must also begin to grapple with another growing and complex reality: that of street-connected children and youth. Their lives prior to coming to the streets were very hard (Embleton, Lee, et al., 2016), and though they may in some ways be better off on the streets than where they were before, their lives on the streets are fraught with violence, abuse, neglect, and exploitation. Until we come to terms with the fact that so many children are essentially bringing themselves up on the streets of Asia, Africa, and elsewhere in LMIC – because of poverty, abuse, and family dysfunction in the home – we will fail to address the broader needs of orphaned, separated, and otherwise vulnerable children and adolescents in the world today.

This discussion would not be complete without mention of corporal punishment. Corporal punishment is still, in spite of its illegal status in Kenyan educational institutions, all too frequent, both in schools and in homes. Public opinion in Kenya favors corporal punishment (caning, spanking, pinching) in the home, and we have previously reported that 78% of family-based care environments in OSCAR reported using corporal punishment for enforcing discipline, with fewer reporting talking with the child (35%) and only 8% reporting the use of scolding (Embleton et al., 2014). The media in Kenya report regularly on children dying in school from being

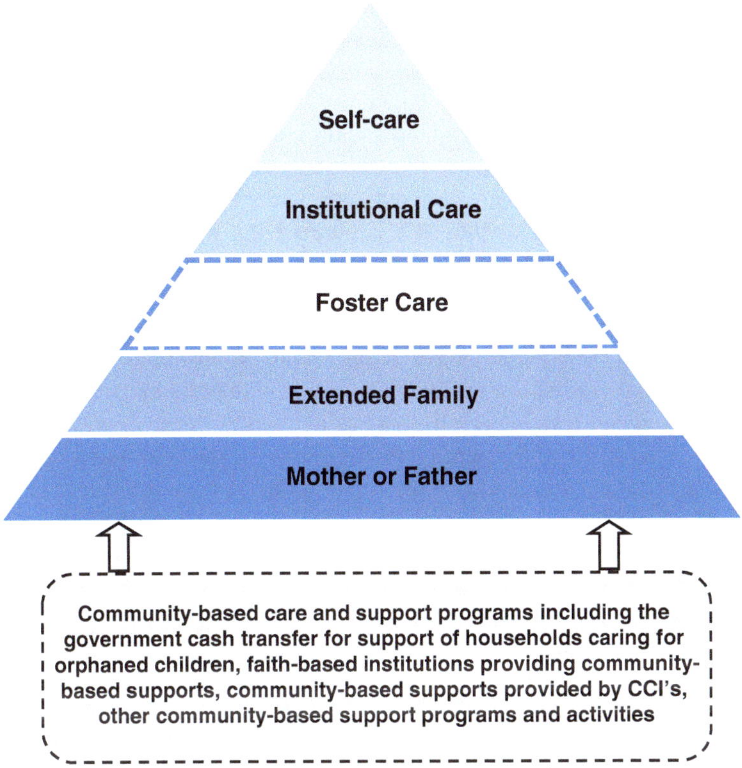

Fig. 16.1 Proposed hierarchy of models of care for orphaned and separated children. Models in *dotted lines* represent opportunities for strengthening family-based care environments

"caned," and it is not uncommon to see physical violence in Kenyan schools – and especially in primary schools (where presumably the children are too small to defend themselves) (UNAIDS, 2016). For corporal punishment in Kenya to reduce and eventually be eliminated, parents, guardians, teachers, and caregivers may need to be taught alternative methods of achieving and enforcing discipline.

6 Summary

The idea for the OSCAR cohort was inspired by observations witnessed "on the ground." Given the overwhelming number of children left orphaned by HIV/AIDS, the optimal care of these and other vulnerable children was (and is still is) a question of great concern. It was a surprise upon visiting the CCIs around Uasin Gishu County that, for the most part, the children seen there were well fed and clothed, laughing, talking, and playful with visitors and with each other. In contrast, during outreach visits with a local HIV-based orphans and vulnerable children program in the same region, the children in those households were usually at least somewhat undernourished, usually wearing dirty and/or well-worn clothing and shoes or not wearing shoes at all, even in the slums which are littered with garbage, broken glass, and human and animal waste. They were mostly very shy, especially around strangers, with titters for smiles and laughter, and those hidden behind their hands, often while turning away. We had expected that the orphanages would be grim and dismal places, with hungry and lonely children sitting sadly in the corners. Instead, we found that the orphaned and vulnerable children living with family in the community, whether urban or rural, appeared far more at risk and often appeared to be actively suffering. Data from the OSCAR cohort at baseline and during a relatively short period of follow-up to date suggests that these observations were accurate. In the context of child abuse and neglect, our data suggest that children living in CCIs are at least at no higher risk of abuse compared to children living with family, while street-connected children and youth are much more likely to experience abuse of all kinds. Over two-thirds of the entire cohort has experienced child abuse, including nearly all of the street youth. This is the single major problem we should be desperately trying to resolve.

The bottom line is that there is no "best solution" magic bullet for children facing adversity, anywhere in the world. We need creative, evidence-based interventions and solutions that support children, families, and communities to care for themselves and for each other. We also need safety nets for children, like Robert and Denis, with no other place to go. As Mr. Julius Yator, Uasin Gishu County Children's Officer, recently said in an OSCAR Community Advisory Board meeting, "Charitable Children's Institutions are unfortunately a necessary evil in our society."

Until better models of care for orphaned and vulnerable children have been developed, tested, and rolled out, we should be cautious about drawing conclusions and developing policies that are premised on the idea that "institutions are bad for children." Standards of care can and should be applied, to families (including foster families) and institutions. Perhaps we unconsciously believe that all families are inherently like the Cleavers and all institutions caring for children are inherently like those in Oliver Twist. We need to create the space for informed dialogue and innovative, creative, locally and culturally appropriate, and cost-effective solutions to emerge. This, ultimately, is what is in the best interests of children.

Questions for Discussion

1. What does an optimal care environment look like for orphaned and separated children and adolescents in sub-Saharan Africa and elsewhere?
2. What are the elements of a care environment that could be cultivated or developed to build and enhance resilience for children and adolescents facing adversity? Are they culturally specific?
3. In the context of weak government infrastructure, widespread poverty, high dependency ratios, and rapid urbanization, how can we decrease child abuse and neglect? In this same context, how can we prevent children and adolescents from having to go to the streets to survive?

Funding Acknowledgments The project described was supported in part by the Eunice Kennedy Shriver National Institute of Child Health and Human Development [R01HD060478]. The content is solely the responsibility of the authors and does not necessarily represent the official views of the Eunice Kennedy Shriver National Institute of Child Health and Human Development or the National Institutes of Health. We gratefully acknowledge the support of the Canadian Institutes of Health Research and Institute of Population and Public Health, for the support of Dr. Braitstein through a Research Chair of Applied Public Health.

References

Amoako Johnson, F., Padmadas, S. S., & Smith, P. W. (2010). Orphanhood and vulnerability: A conduit to poor child health outcomes in Rwanda. *AIDS Care*, *22*(3), 314–323.

Ansell, N., & Young, L. (2004). Enabling households to support successful migration of AIDS orphans in southern Africa. *AIDS Care*, *16*(1), 3–10.

Atwoli, L., Ayuku, D., Koech, J., Hogan, J., Vreeman, R. C., & Braitstein, P. (2014). Impact of domestic care environment on trauma and post-traumatic stress among orphans in western Kenya. *PLoS ONE [Electronic Resource]*, *9*(3), e89937. doi:10.1186/1472-698X-14-9.

Ayuku, D., Embleton, L., Koech, J., Atwoli, L., Hu, L., Ayaya, S., … Braitstein, P. (2014). The government of Kenya cash transfer for orphaned and vulnerable children: Cross-sectional comparison of household and individual characteristics of those with and without. *BMC International Health and Human Rights*, *14*(1), 25. doi: 10.1186/1472-698X-14-25.

Ayuku, D., Kaplan, C. D., Baars, H. M. J., & de Vries, M. W. (2004). Characteristics and personal social networks of the "on" the street, "of" the street, shelter and school children in Eldoret, Kenya. *International Social Work*, *47*(3), 293–311.

Bicego, G., Rutstein, S., & Johnson, K. (2003). Dimensions of the emerging orphan crisis in sub-Saharan Africa. *Social Science & Medicine*, *56*(6), 1235–1247.

Braitstein, P., Ayaya, S., Nyandiko, W. M., Kamanda, A., Koech, J., Gisore, P., … Ayuku, D. (2013). Nutritional status of orphaned and separated children and adolescents living in community and institutional environments in Uasin Gishu County, Kenya. *PLoS ONE [Electronic Resource]*, *8*(7), e70054. doi: 10.1371/journal.pone.0070054.

Bryant, J. H. (2009). Kenya's cash transfer program: Protecting the health and human rights of orphans and vulnerable children. *Health and Human Rights*, *11*(2), 65–76.

Case, A., Paxson, C., & Ableidinger, J. (2004). Orphans in Africa: Parental death, poverty, and school enrollment. *Demography*, *41*(3), 483–508.

Chief Dan George. (unknown). unknown. https://en.wikipedia.org/wiki/Chief_Dan_George

Chuong, C., & Operario, D. (2012). Challenging household dynamics: Impact of orphanhood, parental absence, and children's living arrangements on education in South Africa. *Global Public Health*, *7*(1), 42–57. doi:10.1080/17441692.2011.57414.

Cluver, L., & Orkin, M. (2009). Cumulative risk and AIDS-orphanhood: Interactions of stigma, bullying and poverty on child mental health in South Africa. *Social Science & Medicine (1982)*, *69*(8), 1186–1193. doi:10.1016/j.socscimed.2009.07.033.

Cluver, L. D., Gardner, F., & Operario, D. (2008). Effects of stigma on the mental health of adolescents orphaned by AIDS. *The Journal of Adolescent Health: Official Publication of the Society for Adolescent Medicine*, *42*(4), 410–417. doi:10.1016/j.jadohealth.2007.09.022.

Commission on Revenue Allocation (CRA). (2013). *Kenya County fact sheets: Uasin Gishu County*. Commission on Revenue Allocation, Government of Kenya. Retrieved from http://www.crakenya.org/wp-content/uploads/2013/07/CRA-County-Fact-sheets-2nd-Edition-June-2013.pdf

Commission on Revenue Allocation (CRA). (2017). *Counties: Uasin Gishu*. Retrieved from http://www.crakenya.org/county/uasin-gishu/

Doring, M., França Junior, I., & Stella, I. M. (2005). Factors associated with institutionalization of children orphaned by AIDS in a population-based survey in Porto Alegre, Brazil. *AIDS (London, England)*, *19*(Suppl 4), S59–S63.

Embleton, L., Ayuku, D., Kamanda, A., Atwoli, L., Ayaya, S., Vreeman, R., … Braitstein, P. (2014). Models of care for orphaned and separated children and upholding children's rights: Cross-sectional evidence from western Kenya. *BMC International Health And Human Rights*, *149*. doi:10.1186/1472-698X-14-9.

Embleton, L., Lee, H., Gunn, J., Ayuku, D., & Braitstein, P. (2016). Causes of child and youth homelessness in developed and developing countries: A systematic review and meta-analysis. *JAMA Pediatrics*, *170*(5), 435–444. doi:10.1001/jamapediatrics.2016.0156.

Embleton, L., Nyandat, J., Ayuku, D., Sang, E., Kamanda, A., Ayaya, S., … Braitstein, P. (2017). *Journal of Adolescent Health, 60*(4), 417–424. doi: 10.1016/j.jadohealth.2016.11.015.

Embleton, L., Wachira, J., Kamanda, A., Naanyu, V., Ayuku, D., & Braitstein, P. (2016). Eating sweets without the wrapper: Perceptions of HIV and sexually transmitted infections among street youth in western Kenya. *Culture, Health & Sexuality*, *18*(3), 337–348. doi:10.1080/13691058.2015.1082626.

Embleton, L., Wachira, J., Kamanda, A., Naanyu, V., Winston, S., Ayuku, D., & Braitstein, P. (2015). "Once you join the streets you will have to do it": Sexual practices of street children and youth in Uasin Gishu County, Kenya. *Reproductive Health*, *12*(106), 1–11. doi:10.1186/s12978-015-0090-z.

Goodson, B.D. & Layzer, J.I. (2010). *Defining and measuring quality in home-based care settings* (OPRE research-to-policy, research-to-practice brief OPRE 2011-10d). Washington, DC: Office of Planning, Research and Evaluation, Administration for Children and Families, U.S. Department of Health and Human Services.

Hamra, M., Ross, M. W., Karuri, K., Orrs, M., & D'Agostino, A. (2005). The relationship between expressed HIV/AIDS-related stigma and beliefs and knowledge about care and support of people living with AIDS in families caring for HIV-infected children in Kenya. *AIDS Care*, *17*(7), 911–922.

Heymann, J., Earle, A., Rajaraman, D., Miller, C., & Bogen, K. (2007). Extended family caring for children orphaned by AIDS: Balancing essential work and caregiving in a high HIV prevalence nations. *AIDS Care*, *19*(3), 337–345.

Hosegood, V., Floyd, S., Marston, M., Hill, C., McGrath, N., Isingo, R., … Zaba, B. (2007). The effects of high HIV prevalence on orphanhood and living arrangements of children in Malawi, Tanzania, and South Africa. *Population Studies*, *61*(3), 327–336.

Jahan, S. (Ed.). (2015). *Human development report 2015: Work for human development*. New York, NY: United States.

Kamanda, A., Embleton, L., Ayuku, D., Atwoli, L., Gisore, P., Ayaya, S., … Braitstein, P. (2013). Harnessing the power of the grassroots to conduct public health research in sub-Saharan Africa: A case study from western Kenya in the adaptation of community-based participatory research (CBPR) approaches. *BMC Public Health*, *1391*. doi:10.1186/1471-2458-13-91.

Kenya Open Data Project. (2011). *Kenya open data project*. Retrieved from www.opendata.go.ke/

Kidman, R., & Thurman, T. R. (2014). Caregiver burden among adults caring for orphaned children in rural South Africa. *Vulnerable Children and Youth Studies*, *9*(3), 234–246. doi:10.1080/17450128.2013.871379.

Kilburn, K., Thirumurthy, H., Halpern, C. T., Pettifor, A., & Handa, S. (2016). Effects of a large-scale unconditional cash transfer program on mental health outcomes of young people in Kenya. *The Journal of Adolescent Health: Official Publication of the Society for Adolescent Medicine*, *58*(2), 223–229. doi:10.1016/j.jadohealth.2015.09.023.

Lee, V. C., Muriithi, P., Gilbert-Nandra, U., Kim, A. A., Schmitz, M. E., Odek, J., ... Galbraith, J. S. (2014). Orphans and vulnerable children in Kenya: Results from a nationally representative population-based survey. *Journal of Acquired Immune Deficiency Syndromes*, *66*(Suppl 1), S89–S97. doi: 10.1097/QAI.0000000000000117.

Lenz-Rashid, S. (2006). Employment experiences of homeless young adults: Are they different for youth with a history of foster care? *Children & Youth Services Review*, *28*(3), 235–259. doi:10.1016/j.childyouth.2005.03.006.

Magadi, M. A., & Uchudi, J. (2015). Onset of sexual activity among adolescents in HIV/AIDS-affected households in sub-Saharan Africa. *Journal of Biosocial Science*, *47*(2), 238–257. doi:10.1017/S0021932014000200.

Millennium Ecosystem Assessment. (2005). *Living beyond our means: Natural assets and human well-being. Statement from the board.* New York, NY: Millennium Ecosystem Assessment. Retrieved from http://www.millenniumassessment.org/documents/document.429.aspx.pdf

Miller, C. M., Gruskin, S., Subramanian, S. V., & Heymann, J. (2007). Emerging health disparities in Botswana: Examining the situation of orphans during the AIDS epidemic. *Social Science & Medicine*, *64*(12), 2476–2486. doi:10.1016/j.socscimed.2007.03.002.

Miller, C. M., Gruskin, S., Subramanian, S. V., Rajaraman, D., & Heymann, S. J. (2006). Orphan care in Botswana's working households: Growing responsibilities in the absence of adequate support. American Journal of Public Health, 96(8), 1429–1435. doi: AJPH.2005.072280.

Monasch, R., & Boerma, J. T. (2004). Orphanhood and childcare patterns in sub-Saharan Africa: An analysis of national surveys from 40 countries. *AIDS (London, England)*, *18*(Suppl 2), S55–S65.

Morantz, G., Cole, D., Vreeman, R., Ayaya, S., Ayuku, D., & Braitstein, P. (2013a). Child abuse and neglect among orphaned children and youth living in extended families in sub-Saharan Africa: What have we learned from qualitative inquiry? *Vulnerable Children and Youth Studies*, *8*(4), 338–352. doi:10.1080/17450128.2013.764476.

Morantz, G., Cole, D. C., Ayaya, S., Ayuku, D., & Braitstein, P. (2013b). Maltreatment experiences and associated factors prior to admission to residential care: A sample of institutionalized children and youth in western Kenya. *Child Abuse & Neglect*, *37*(10), 778–787. doi:10.1016/j.chiabu.2012.10.007.

Mwasiaji, W. (2015). *Scaling up cash transfer programs in Kenya*. Nairobi, Kenia: International Policy Center for Inclusive Growth.

National AIDS and STI Control Programme. (2013). *Kenya AIDS Indicator Survey (KAIS) preliminary report*. Nairobi, Kenia: Government of Kenya.

Nhate, V., Arndt, C., Barslund, M., & Van Den Broeck, K. (2006, August). *Orphans and discrimination in Mozambique: An outlay equivalence analysis*. Paper presented at the International Association of Agricultural Economist Conference, Gold Coast, Australia.

Nichols, J., Embleton, L., Mwangi, A., Morantz, G., Vreeman, R., Ayaya, S., ... Braitstein, P. (2014). Physical and sexual abuse in orphaned compared to non-orphaned children in sub-Saharan Africa: A systematic review and meta-analysis. *Child Abuse & Neglect*, *38*(2), 304–316. doi: 10.1016/j.chiabu.2013.09.012.

Nyambedha, E. O., Wandibba, S., & Aagaard-Hansen, J. (2003). Changing patterns of orphan care due to the HIV epidemic in western Kenya. *Social Science & Medicine*, *57*(2), 301–311.doi: S0277953602003593 [pii].

Operario, D., Underhill, K., Chuong, C., & Cluver, L. (2011). HIV infection and sexual risk behaviour among youth who have experienced orphanhood: Systematic review and meta-analysis. *Journal of the International AIDS Society*, *14*(25). doi:10.1186/1758-2652-14-25.

Rose, L. (2005). Orphans' land rights in post-war Rwanda: The problem of guardianship. *Development and Change*, *36*(5), 911–936.

Sorber, R., Winston, S., Koech, J., Ayuku, D., Hu, L., Hogan, J., & Braitstein, P. (2014). Social and economic characteristics of street youth by gender and level of street involvement in Eldoret, Kenya. *PloS One*, *9*(5), e97587. doi:10.1371/journal.pone.0097587.

Tyler, K., & Melander, L. (2010). Foster care placement, poor parenting, and negative outcomes among homeless young adults. *Journal of Child & Family Studies*, *19*(6), 787–794.

UN Habitat. (2008). *The state of African cities: A framework for addressing urban challenges in Africa*. Nairobi, Kenya: UN Habitat.

UNAIDS. (2016). *AIDS by the numbers: HIV/AIDS estimates* (2015). Retrieved from http://www.unaids.org/en/regionscountries/countries/kenya/

UNICEF. (2005). *Report on the pilot survey on orphans and other vulnerable children in Blantyre, Malawi*. Blantyre, Malawi: UNICEF.

UNICEF. (2006). *Africa's orphaned and vulnerable generations: Children affected by HIV/AIDS*. Geneva, CH/Washington, DC: UNICEF. Retrieved from http://www.unicef.org/publications/files/

UNICEF. (2012a). *Kenya at a glance*. Retrieved from http://www.unicef.org/kenya/overview_4616.html

UNICEF. (2012b). *The state of the world's children 2012: Children in an urban world*. New York, NY: UNICEF. Retrieved from http://www.unicef.org/sowc2012/fullreport.php

UNICEF. (2012c). *The state of the world's children: Urbanization*. New York, NY: UNICEF.

UNICEF & Ministry of Public Service Labour and Social Welfare. (2005). *Survey on orphans and other vulnerable children in rural and urban high density Zimbabwe 2004/2005*. Harare, Zimbabwe: UNICEF.

Wachira, J., Kamanda, A., Embleton, L., Naanyu, V., Ayuku, D., & Braitstein, P. (2016). 'Pregnancy has its advantages': The voices of street connected children and youth in Eldoret, Kenya. *PloS One*, *11*(3), e0150814. doi:10.1371/journal.pone.0150814.

Wachira, J., Kamanda, A., Embleton, L., Naanyu, V., Winston, S., Ayuku, D., & Braitstein, P. (2015). Initiation to street life: A qualitative examination of the physical, social, and psychological practices in becoming an accepted member of the street youth community in Western Kenya. *BMC Public Health*, *15*, 569. doi:10.1186/s12889-015-1942-8.

Witter, S., Calder, G., & Ahimbisibwe, T. (2004). *Taking better care? Review of a decade of work with orphans and vulnerable children in Rakai, Uganda*. London, UK: Save the Children. Retrieved from http://www.savethechildren.org.uk/sites/default/files/docs/taking_better_care_1.pdf

Zlotnick, C. (2009). What research tells us about the intersecting streams of homelessness and foster care. *The American Journal of Orthopsychiatry*, *79*(3), 319–325. doi:10.1037/a0017218.

Zlotnick, C., Robertson, M. J., & Wright, M. A. (1999). The impact of childhood foster care and other out-of-home placement on homeless women and their children. *Child Abuse & Neglect*, *23*(11), 1057–1068.

Zlotnick, C., Tam, T. W., & Soman, L. A. (2012). Life course outcomes on mental and physical health: The impact of foster care on adulthood. *American Journal of Public Health*, *102*(3), 534–540. doi:10.2105/AJPH.2011.300285.

Chapter 17
Interaction Competencies with Children (ICC): An Approach for Preventing Violence, Abuse, and Neglect in Institutional Care in Sub-Saharan Africa

Tobias Hecker, Getrude Mkinga, Joseph Ssenyonga, and Katharin Hermenau

"Our children are our future and one of the basic responsibilities is to care for them in the best and most compassionate manner possible".

Nelson Mandela Children's Fund (2016).

1 Introduction

With more than 56 million orphans, Sub-Saharan Africa is the most affected region worldwide regarding the number of orphans needing care (UNICEF, 2014). An orphan is hereby defined as a child under the age of 18, who lost one or both parents

T. Hecker (✉)
Department of Psychology, Bielefeld University, Bielefeld, Germany

vivo international, www.vivo.org, Allensbach, Germany
e-mail: tobias.hecker@uni-bielefeld.de

G. Mkinga
Department of Educational Psychology, University of Dar es Salaam, Dar es Salaam, Tanzania
e-mail: mkingagetrude@gmail.com

J. Ssenyonga
Department of Educational Foundations and Psychology, Mbarara University for Science and Technology, Mbarara, Uganda

Department of Psychology, University of Konstanz, Konstanz, Germany
e-mail: jessenyonga@hotmail.com

K. Hermenau
vivo international, www.vivo.org, Allensbach, Germany

Department of Psychology, University of Konstanz, Konstanz, Germany
e-mail: katharin.hermenau@uni-konstanz.de

A.V. Rus et al. (eds.), *Child Maltreatment in Residential Care*,
DOI 10.1007/978-3-319-57990-0_17

due to death from any cause (UNICEF, 2006). For example, in Tanzania, one in four girls and one in five boys were orphaned in 2009 (UNICEF, 2011). As a result of poverty, political conflicts, and the HIV/AIDS pandemic, the traditional system of care within extended families is overburdened by the rising numbers of orphans (Better Care Network & UNICEF, 2015; Li et al., 2008; Wolff & Fesseha, 1998). Thus, in many Sub-Saharan African countries, childcare institutions, such as orphanages and children's homes, still constitute the most frequently utilized form of providing formal alternative care for children without parents (Rygaard, 2010; Wolff & Fesseha, 1998). Children who are institutionalized are in most cases 5 years or older. Various reasons like poverty, war, and conflict, as well as parental illness or disabilities of the child, can lead to abandonment of the children. Above all, HIV/AIDS is one of the most common reasons for orphanhood and institutionalization in Sub-Saharan Africa (UNICEF, 2006). In most countries, gender distribution of institutionalized children is more or less equal (SOS Children's Villages International & University of Bedfordshire, 2014). Most common are childcare institutions housing large groups of children with very few mostly untrained, female caregivers (SOS Children's Villages International & University of Bedfordshire, 2014). Yet, there has been very little research on the living conditions in African orphanages and other childcare institutions so far. The few studies that have focused on African orphanages have reported a lack of adequate caregiving (Espié et al., 2011; Hermenau et al., 2011; Levin & Haines, 2007; Wolff & Fesseha, 1998, 1999). Besides the lack of educated and competent caregivers, orphans in African countries are additionally confronted with exposure to violent discipline strategies and physical abuse (Hermenau et al., 2011; SOS Children's Villages International & University of Bedfordshire, 2014). Thus, in addition to parental loss, possible maltreatment in the family of origin, and the often unresponsive and distant caregiving in institutional care, orphans are burdened with further experiences of maltreatment in orphanages and other institutional care facilities. Physical and emotional abuse and neglect during childhood are associated with mental health problems and aggressive behavior in children, particularly in those who have been institutionalized early in life (Hermenau, Hecker, Elbert, & Ruf-Leuschner, 2014; Johnson, Browne, & Hamilton-Giachritsis, 2006).

Despite the high risk of maltreatment in institutional care, interventions that focus on the prevention of violence and abuse are rare. We addressed this issue and designed with *Interaction Competencies with Children – for Caregivers (ICC-C)* in institutional care a training workshop that aims at improving care quality and at preventing maltreatment in institutional care, particularly in low-income countries in Sub-Saharan Africa (Hermenau, Kaltenbach, Mkinga, & Hecker, 2015). ICC-C proved its feasibility and showed first promising results in a feasibility study with caregivers in Tanzanian orphanages.

This chapter will give an (1) overview of the current literature on maltreatment and its consequences on the children's development and well-being in African orphanages. Furthermore, we will present arguments that (2) underline the necessity of implementing maltreatment prevention approaches in institutional care. As the main focus of the chapter, we will present (3) with ICC-C an intervention approach in detail that aims at improving care quality and preventing maltreatment in childcare institutions, particularly in countries in which harsh discipline is regarded as culturally accepted and is highly prevalent. The chapter concludes (4) with practical implications and policy recommendations.

2 Maltreatment in African Orphanages

2.1 Institutional Care in Sub-Saharan Africa

The African countries south of the Sahara differ widely in history, culture, language, politics, economics, and social systems. This diversity is also reflected in the welfare systems, child protection systems, and orphan care (e.g., Better Care Network, 2014). In recent years, several organizations and governments have put effort into structuring and formalizing care systems for orphans and other vulnerable children, setting up guidelines in order to strengthen the child protection systems (Better Care Network & UNICEF, 2015; Inter-agency Group on Child Protection Systems in Sub-Saharan Africa, 2012). Formal alternative care encompasses institutional care (private and governmental), foster care in families or communities, and adoption as opposed to informal (i.e., without any official structures and placements) family and kinship care (i.e., care within the extended family or community) (SOS Children's Villages International & University of Bedfordshire, 2014). In general, the efforts support family- and community-based approaches (family and kinship care) and aim to reduce institutional care (Better Care Network, 2015; Better Care Network & UNICEF, 2015). Yet, due to the rising number of orphans, institutional care is still very common in Sub-Saharan Africa. Most institutional care is financed by nongovernmental or religious organizations, a minority of these are state run (Better Care Network & UNICEF, 2015; Chiwaula, Dobson, & Elsley, 2014). In many countries a substantial number of care institutions are unregistered and uncontrolled. The registration rates range from high, for example, in Rwanda and Kenya, to about half in Togo, to very low in Malawi, Tanzania, and Uganda (Better Care Network & UNICEF, 2015; Chiwaula et al., 2014; Walakira, Dumba-Nyanzi, & Bukenya, 2015). Further, Riley (2012) noted that in Uganda more than one third of the childcare institutions were unknown to the officials in districts where they are operating. In addition, the newly introduced registration processes in some countries were reported to be confusing, incomprehensible, or long winded, resulting in many unregistered operating facilities (Better Care Network, 2014; Chiwaula et al., 2014). The high number of unregistered and uncontrolled institutions and the lack of governmental resources make it difficult to collect information and to survey whether a minimum of childcare quality is met. For example, no effective system to monitor institutional care exists in Togo, Tanzania, and Zimbabwe (Better Care Network, 2014; Chiwaula et al., 2014).

Additionally, most countries lack structures that assure adequate training of caregivers. In Malawi, 71% of the caregivers did not undergo any training in childcare. Kenya set standards for caregivers being trained, but the training duration ranged from over a year to only 1 day (Chiwaula et al., 2014). In Tanzania, the governmental social welfare department established an institute to train staff in governmental facilities. However, there were no standards for nongovernmental facilities. The number of staff and the caregiver–child ratio in Tanzanian institutions depended on the funds both in private and governmental institutions. Consequently, many facilities fail to meet standards and have no child protection policy. For example, below 10% of surveyed care facilities in Malawi had a care plan (Chiwaula et al., 2014; SOS Children's Villages International & University of Bedfordshire, 2014). Despite these shortcomings among institutions, sanctions and consequences against unauthorized facilities are mostly not put into action. Although many countries have policy guidelines, which should ensure that competent authorities make placement decisions in the best interest of the child, implementation is often difficult without sufficient resources. For example, in Tanzania, government placements went through a court, but nongovernmental institutions admitted children on their own criteria (Chiwaula et al., 2014). In sum, though in many Sub-Saharan African countries structures exist in which governmental or juridical authorities order placements of children in formal care, these structures are often very weak and do not reach private and unregistered institutions, and it remains in many cases uncertain whether the actions taken are indeed in the child's best interest.

As a consequence of the struggles with controlling institutional care and in awareness of its adverse effects, many countries aim for a complete deinstitutionalization of orphans and other vulnerable children. They plan to transfer children to other formal care settings like formal family or kinship care, foster care, and adoption (Better Care Network, 2015; Better Care Network & UNICEF, 2015). Depending on the country, these forms of care are more or less common (Better Care Network, 2014; Chiwaula et al., 2014). For example, in Ghana and Liberia, formal family care options were underdeveloped and under-resourced (Better Care Network & UNICEF, 2015). In some countries, adoption and even foster care are not common due to cultural customs and attitudes. Again, the lack of resources leads to little data on and monitoring of these formal care settings in many countries (Better Care Network, 2014; Chiwaula et al., 2014; Riley, 2012; Walakira et al., 2015).

Besides the formal care system, many orphans in Sub-Saharan Africa live in informal family or kinship care. The data on and control of informal care is mostly nonexistent because such efforts exceed the capacity of the social welfare system (Better Care Network, 2014; Better Care Network & UNICEF, 2015; Chiwaula et al., 2014). Experts rate the informal care system as the traditional practice in most Sub-Saharan countries, yet it has become overburdened (SOS Children's Villages International & University of Bedfordshire, 2014). Some countries encourage voluntary registration of informal care in order to gather more information and to establish some control for informal care settings. However, most informal care settings are still unknown and un-surveyed. Often no mechanisms are available to protect the children in informal care from abuse and neglect (Better Care Network & UNICEF, 2015).

In summary, countries in Sub-Saharan Africa have started to develop guidelines and monitoring systems. However, weaknesses of governance, and lack of resources and of comprehensive data, still lead to many children living in inadequate care settings. Deinstitutionalization per se may not be the solution to this problem, when institutional care is discontinued without first ensuring sufficient care quality in alternative settings. Thus, because institutional care will remain part of the care system at least medium term, it is of extreme importance to improve the conditions for children in institutional care (Better Care Network & UNICEF, 2015; Chiwaula et al., 2014; McCall, 2013).

3 Prevalence of Abuse and Neglect

Most children in Sub-Saharan Africa, orphans and non-orphans, frequently experience physical and emotional violence (UNICEF, 2014). Though the UN Sustainable Development Goal Nr. 16.2 "end abuse, exploitation, trafficking and all forms of violence and torture against children" has a target for ending all forms of violence against children (United Nations, 2016), only seven (e.g., Benin, Kenya, Togo) of the 54 states in Africa fully prohibit violence against children in all settings. Yet, also in these states prevalence rates of violence against children are still very high, for example, with prevalence rates of physical punishment in the past year of over 50% in Kenya or the Republic of Congo. Overall, one quarter of Africa's children live in the seven states (e.g., Eritrea, Nigeria, Tanzania) that do not prohibit violence against children in any setting (Global Initiative to End All Corporal Punishment of Children, 2016a, 2016b).

Therefore, it is not surprising that research studies repeatedly reported that physical violence and harsh discipline methods (e.g., spanking or beating with objects) and emotional violence (e.g., insulting, humiliating) are highly prevalent in Sub-Saharan Africa (Feinstein & Mwahombela, 2010; Straus, 2010). For example, UNICEF (2014) reported that more than 7 in 10 children between 2 and 14 years of age in Sub-Saharan Africa experience violent disciplining. With more than a quarter of children who experienced severe physical punishment (e.g., hit on the head, face, or ears, or hit hard and repeatedly), worldwide the highest levels of violence against children at home are concentrated in Sub-Saharan Africa. Also school corporal punishment remains widespread in many states in Africa (Global Initiative to End All Corporal Punishment of Children, 2016b). In a recent study in Tanzania, nearly all children reported that they had experienced corporal punishment at some point during their lifetime both in family and school (Hecker, Hermenau, Isele, & Elbert, 2014). Half of the respondents reported having experienced corporal punishment by a family member within the last year. Accordingly, in a national, representative survey in Tanzania, the majority of adolescents (almost 75%) reported exposure to physical violence and one quarter to emotional maltreatment (UNICEF, 2011).

Concerning orphans in different care settings, the findings on childhood abuse and physical punishment are diverse. Qualitative studies have documented cases of the emotional and physical abuse of orphans in community-based care (Morantz, Cole, Vreeman et al., 2013). UNICEF reported from a household-based national survey in Tanzania that approximately 70% of orphans in family or kinship care reported physical abuse and about 30% reported emotional abuse during childhood (UNICEF, 2011). The orphans reported higher rates of emotional abuse but not of physical abuse than non-orphans. Concordantly, child abuse was equally common for orphans and non-orphans in Eastern Zimbabwe (Nyamukapa et al., 2010). A recent meta-analysis of 10 studies from different African countries, such as Zimbabwe, South Africa, Kenya, and Uganda, examined whether orphans in family or kinship care were more likely to experience physical and/or sexual abuse compared to non-orphans in Sub-Saharan Africa. Findings showed that orphans were not more likely to experience physical abuse (OR = 0.96) or sexual abuse (OR = 1.25) compared to non-orphans (Nichols et al., 2014). The authors remarked that their research focused on orphans in family or kinship care and advocated for further research on child maltreatment in institutions.

Moratz, Cole, Ayaya, Ayuku, and Braitstein (2013) carried out a file review in Kenya analyzing the rates of experienced violence and abuse prior to institutional placement. They found that non-orphans were institutionalized more often due to maltreatment than orphans. Orphans reported lower rates of maltreatment prior to institutional placement, as they were mostly institutionalized due to poverty or a lack of suitable caregivers. However, other studies showed that children are not protected from further maltreatment in institutions. The already high rates of maltreatment experienced by children in the general population in Sub-Saharan Africa are often estimated to be even higher in institutional care (Euser, Alink, Tharner, van IJzendoorn, & Bakermans-Kranenburg, 2014; UNICEF, 2014). Concordantly, we found high rates of maltreatment experienced by most of the children in studies in Tanzanian orphanages (Hermenau et al., 2011, 2014). In Benin, children in residential or institutional care reported regular corporal punishment (Chiwaula et al., 2014). In institutional care settings, underqualified and overworked caregivers, in particular, physically maltreat children, frequently use corporal punishment for disciplinary reasons (Chiwaula et al., 2014; SOS Children's Villages International & University of Bedfordshire, 2014). Thus, in addition to possible maltreatment in the family of origin and the often unresponsive and distant caregiving in institutional care, orphans are burdened with further experiences of maltreatment and corporal punishment in orphanages and other facilities of institutional care (Hermenau et al., 2011). Yet, the exposure to violence and other forms of abuse in institutional care have received comparably little attention (SOS Children's Villages International & University of Bedfordshire, 2014).

The Positive Outcomes for Orphans study examined institutionalized and family cared orphans and separated children in five low- and middle-income countries in Sub-Saharan Africa (e.g., Ethiopia, Kenya, Tanzania) and Asia (Gray et al., 2015). Most of the children were institutionalized when they were 5 years or older. Lifetime prevalence by age 13 of any potentially traumatic event, excluding loss of a parent, was 91% in institutionalized children and 92% in children living with extended families. More than half of children in institutions and in family care had experienced physical or sexual abuse by age 13. Prevalence and incidence of potentially traumatic events were high among the surveyed children, but contrary to common assumptions, children living in institutions did not report more potentially traumatic events or more abuse than children living in family care. Gray et al. (2015) concluded that deinstitutionalization would not protect the children from further maltreatment and that protecting orphans and separated children from maltreatment is of high priority, regardless of the setting. They also hypothesized that the risk of maltreatment may be higher for younger children and they therefore need even more protection. We compared Tanzanian children who were institutionalized at birth to 4 years of age with a matched group of children who were institutionalized at 5–14 years of age (Hermenau et al., 2014). Results showed that early-institutionalized children reported more adverse experiences during their time in institutional care and a greater variety of mental health problems than did late institutionalized children. We concluded that adverse experiences in institutional care play an important, but negative, role for early-institutionalized children who instead need protection from these experiences as well as developmentally appropriate and nurturing care from adequately educated caregivers.

When focusing on neglect, however, orphans were generally more likely than non-orphans to go to bed hungry (Makame, Ani, & Grantham-McGregor, 2002), to be underweight (Miller, Gruskin, Subramanian, & Heymann, 2007), and to lack social support and basic needs (Puffer et al., 2012). Consistently, we systematically investigated orphans' experiences of maltreatment, and our findings revealed that orphans reported significantly more experiences of neglect, but not of abuse compared to non-orphans (Hermenau, Eggert, Landolt, & Hecker, 2015). Research on institutional childcare has documented poor caregiver–child ratios and inadequate caregiving as factors increasing the risk of physical and emotional neglect (Hermenau et al., 2011; Johnson et al., 2006).

4 Maltreatment and Mental Health Problems

Prior research, mostly from Western countries, showed that in addition to physical injury, child maltreatment is associated with a number of emotional and behavioral problems that begin in childhood but may last through adolescence and adulthood (Carr, Martins, Stingel, Lemgruber, & Juruena, 2013). Adverse effects of child maltreatment include depression, anxiety disorders, substance abuse, and aggressive or delinquent behavior (Dube et al., 2003; Sugaya et al., 2012). In Tanzania, though a society in which harsh disciplinary methods are culturally normed and highly prevalent, we found a strong relationship between harsh discipline and internalizing as well as externalizing problems (Hecker et al., 2014; Hecker, Hermenau, Salmen, Teicher, & Elbert, 2016). Via internalizing problems, harsh discipline was also indirectly related to impaired cognitive functioning and school performance.

Furthermore, maltreatment has shown to be associated with differential methylation in the genes of the stress response axis (Hecker, Radtke, Hermenau, Papassotiropoulos, & Elbert, 2016). These findings emphasize the detrimental consequences of maltreatment based on both molecular and behavioral grounds.

As a consequence of parental loss, maltreatment in the family of origin, and further maltreatment in institutional care settings, orphans are at increased risk for mental health problems. For example, we found a positive relation between maltreatment and mental health problems in institutionalized children (Hermenau et al., 2011, 2014). Interestingly, the violence that children experienced in the orphanage (vs. the violence that children experienced in the family of origin) was positively correlated with mental health problems.

In a number of studies, evidence has shown that orphans living in African countries in different care settings suffer from more depressive symptoms (Puffer et al., 2012; Unterhitzenberger & Rosner, 2014), more internalizing and externalizing problems (Atwine, Cantor-Graae, & Bajunirwe, 2005; Wild, Flisher, & Robertson, 2011), and greater posttraumatic stress disorder symptom severity than non-orphaned children (Cluver, Gardner, & Operario, 2007; Puffer et al., 2012). Consistently, we found that orphans reported more depressive symptoms, posttraumatic stress symptoms, and aggressive behavior than non-orphans (Hermenau, Eggert et al., 2015). In our study, neglect, abuse, and stigmatization correlated with orphans' internalizing and externalizing problems and neglect and stigmatization with orphans' depression severity. Perceived stigmatization moderated the relationship between neglect and depression (i.e., the relationship was always positive, but it was much stronger when an orphan reported high levels of perceived stigmatization). These findings suggest that maltreatment and perceived stigmatization may play an important role in orphans' psychological distress. In sum, the review of the current literature clearly suggests that maltreatment in institutional care is one important risk factor that is associated with impaired mental health of orphans. Thus, improving the mental health of orphans in institutional care begins certainly with preventing further maltreatment in institutional care.

5 Necessity of Maltreatment Prevention Approaches in Institutional Care

Though a great majority of institutionalized children reported at least one adverse childhood experience during their time in institutional care, the current literature indicates that orphans in institutional care are not generally at higher risk to experience physical or sexual abuse compared to non-orphans or orphans in family or kinship care (e.g., Gray et al., 2015; Nichols et al., 2014). Yet, this is not surprising in countries, in which corporal punishment is legal, highly prevalent, and generally regarded as effective, such as in many countries in Sub-Saharan Africa (UNICEF, 2014). In these countries, the placement in institutional care does not represent a protection from further maltreatment. On the contrary, corporal punishment in institutional care can add to the psychological burden of prior parental loss and possible adverse experiences in the family of origin. Therefore, protecting orphans from maltreatment in institutional care and in other care settings must be a high priority (Gray et al., 2015; SOS Children's Villages International & University of Bedfordshire, 2014).

Furthermore, quality of childcare has been shown to have a crucial impact on children's development and psychological adjustment, particularly for orphans with a history of maltreatment and trauma (Johnson et al., 2006). However, adequate care for orphans is often impacted by unfavorable caregiver–child ratios and in most cases poorly trained, overburdened personnel. This is the status quo in institutional care settings in countries with limited resources and large numbers of orphans, like in many countries in Sub-Saharan Africa (Hermenau et al., 2011; Hermenau, Kaltenbach et al., 2015; SOS Children's Villages International & University of Bedfordshire, 2014).

In a recent systematic review, we investigated the effects of structural interventions and caregiver trainings on child development in institutional environments (Hermenau, Goessmann, Rygaard, Landolt, & Hecker, 2016). The 24 intervention studies reported beneficial effects on the children's emotional, social, and cognitive development. Yet, only four of these studies have been conducted in Sub-Saharan Africa (Espié et al., 2011; Hermenau et al., 2011; Hermenau, Kaltenbach et al., 2015; Wolff, Dawit, & Zere, 1995). Furthermore, very few studies focused on effects of interventions on violence and abuse prevention (Hermenau et al., 2016). Therefore, we argue that it is highly important to develop, implement, and scientifically evaluate interventions that aim at improving care quality and at the same time preventing abuse and neglect in institutional care in Sub-Saharan Africa (Hermenau et al., 2016; SOS Children's Villages International & University of Bedfordshire, 2014).

6 Interaction Competencies with Children: A Preventive Approach for Caregivers Improving Care Quality and Preventing Maltreatment in Institutional Care

6.1 Theoretical Background

The preventive intervention approach *Interaction Competencies with Children (ICC)* aims to improve adult–child relationships and to prevent maltreatment. Following *chronic stress hypothesis* (Johnson & Gunnar, 2011), the typical care environment in an institutional care setting is stressful for children because of the lack of a consistent, warm, sensitive, contingent caregiver, which otherwise would reduce the stressful nature of an insecure environment. Furthermore, ICC is based on *attachment theory* (Bakermans-Kranenburg et al., 2011). As a consequence of parental loss, and the many and varying caregivers, institutionalized children often lack a secure, stable attachment to a caregiver. Attachment theory and chronic stress hypothesis both imply that long-term adverse effects might be avoided if caregiving in the institution were improved (McCall, 2013). Consistently, interventions aiming to improve care quality in institutional care have shown promising results (McCall, 2013). Nevertheless, interventions focusing on both improving care quality and preventing further maltreatment are scarce. Therefore, we expanded the theoretical foundation to elements from social learning, cognitive behavioral, and developmental theories. Besides prevention of neglect through strengthening attachment and bonding, ICC-C in institutional care additionally focuses on the prevention of harsh discipline and other forms of maltreatment. ICC-C has been inspired by the parenting guidelines of the American Academy of Pediatrics (The American Academy of Pediatrics, 1999) and the FairstartGlobal[1] training concept (Rygaard, 2010). As in low-income countries, particularly in Sub-Saharan Africa, the majority of children are institutionalized at the age 5 or older (Gray et al., 2015), we designed ICC-C for caregivers caring for children of preschool to primary school age and early adolescence (4–14 years).

6.2 *ICC Training Workshop for Caregivers in Institutional Care*

ICC-C has been designed as a 2-week training workshop (2 × 5.5 days) for caregivers working in institutional care settings. ICC-C offers a basic introduction to the essential interaction competencies in the work with children focusing mainly on warm, sensitive, and reliable caregiver–child relationships and nonviolent, warm, and sensitive caregiving strategies. ICC-C is guided by the following key principles:

- Participative approach: Trainees are invited to participate actively, to tailor the program, and to develop their own strategies on how to implement the training content in their daily work.
- Practice orientation: Practice units utilize the theoretical foundations to produce practical applications and skills that trainees can use in their daily work.
- Trustful atmosphere: Trainees are encouraged to talk openly about work problems and their own experiences of harsh punishment and maltreatment, with the aim of creating a trusting and open atmosphere assuring confidentiality.
- Sustainability: Sustainability of the training is ensured through intensive practicing, repetition of the new knowledge, self-reflection, and the training component *teamwork and supervision*, described below.

[1] http://www.fairstartglobal.com/

- Teambuilding and new ideas for games: To facilitate teambuilding and to exchange ideas that caregivers can use in their daily work with children, trainers and trainees suggest and play games, sing songs, or dance together.

ICC-C begins with a welcome session in which the expectations, wishes, and concerns of the trainees are explored. Seven core components form the content of ICC-C. They are conducted in the following order:

1. *Child development (3 sessions at 90 min)*: The aim of the first component is fostering empathy and understanding toward the children and enabling trainees to better assess the children's abilities, thus forming age-appropriate expectations. In the beginning, the trainees discuss the needs of children of different ages in a small-group brainstorming. The small groups discuss one of the following questions: *What does a child need to feel happy? What does a child need to be healthy? What does a child need to be good at school? What does a child need to be self-confident? What does a child need to be helpful and cooperative?* The short brainstorming should support the participants to look into the topic of children's needs. A short presentation of topics that came up in the small groups is followed by theoretical input about important steps in the physical, emotional, and cognitive development of children from infanthood to adolescence. The subsequent discussion relates the knowledge about child development to implications for the daily work with children of various ages. A small-group exercise helps trainees to practice forming age-appropriate expectations and caring approaches.
2. *Caregiver–child relationship (4 sessions at 90 min)*: This component aims to point out the importance of secure attachment and bonding as well as elements of how to establish and improve a caregiver–child relationship. In this way, this component aims to reduce or to prevent emotional neglect of the orphans in institutional care. During instruction of theoretical foundations, the importance of secure attachment and bonding for children is emphasized, and possibilities to improve attachment and bonding in institutional care settings are outlined. Subsequently, trainees in small groups elaborate on the implications of being a parental figure and role model for children living in institutional care (e.g., whose parents have died or are unable to care for them). They discuss the following questions in small groups: *Who are important role models in the lives of children? How do children learn from them*? The aim of the small-group discussion is that trainees may realize that children learn more from the caregiver's behavior in daily interaction than from their instructions. In the next unit, communication skills used in a warm, understanding, and sensitive manner are developed together with the trainees and practiced in role-plays. Subsequently, the trainees discuss and practice communicating clear and age-appropriate instructions in small-group discussions and role-plays. In role-plays, different ways of giving instructions are played through (e.g., shouting with a harsh voice, begging and discussion, clear and short instruction with a calm and friendly voice and full attention). By putting the trainees in the shoes of the children, the role-plays

sensitize the trainees to the importance of setting expectations in a realistic and supportive way for the success of the interaction.

3. *Effective caregiving strategies (8 sessions at 90 min)*: This component seeks to provide alternative caregiving strategies in place of harsh discipline and to reduce feelings of helplessness. It starts with a discussion about which caregiving strategies trainees consider useful and effective. As the trainees already have lots of experience in caregiving and working with children, their experiences and views should be valued and integrated in the training workshop. Subsequently, theoretical instruction including discussion of learning theory is used to introduce different strategies to aid in maintaining good behavior and to change misbehavior (e.g., logical consequence, reinforcement systems, privilege removal, behavioral contracts, time-out). Particularly, the role of attention as (unintentional) reinforcement is discussed. In the following units, these strategies are deepened and practiced in small groups using interactive elements such as role-plays. For example, in role-plays trainees practice both how to introduce time-out to the children they work with and how to use time-out in different situations. Reward systems (e.g., chore charts) are developed and adjusted for the use in their particular institutional care setting. Behavioral contracts that may facilitate the modification of certain problem behaviors of particular children are developed based on individual cases. In role-plays, the trainees practice discussing with children the problem behavior, the desired behavior, and the consequences, using the learned communication skills. This unit encompasses several sessions as these nonviolent caregiving strategies are adapted to specific contexts together with the trainees, practiced, and repeated a number of times to include these strategies in the active action repertoire of the trainees. Trainees' ideas about challenges that may occur when implementing new skills in their daily routine are discussed intensively, and potential adaptations that would facilitate implementation are developed together.
4. *Maltreatment prevention (7 sessions at 90 min)*: The aim of this component is to raise awareness of the detrimental consequences of harsh punishment and other forms of child maltreatment. This component is closely linked to the newly learned effective caregiving strategies. ICC-C emphasizes action alternatives as many caregivers use harsh punishment because they lack nonviolent techniques. By developing nonviolent caregiving strategies beforehand, trainees may be more open to question commonly used strategies. At the start of this unit, all trainees are invited to reflect on and share their own experiences of harsh punishment and maltreatment during childhood. First, trainees are invited to reflect individually on their childhood experiences of harsh punishment and maltreatment and the related feelings, but also their experiences of maltreatment in adulthood and related feelings. Trainees should also reflect how their own experiences of harsh discipline and maltreatment affect their own ways of punishing and treating the children they care for or their own children. In the second step, trainees are invited to share their experiences and thoughts with their fellow trainees. To create a trustful atmosphere, trainees agree that all information shared during self-reflection will be confidential and will not be shared with anybody outside

of the workshop. Self-reflection often helps to allow a personal discussion about potential risks and consequences of harsh punishment and other forms of maltreatment that is not so much influenced by societal attitudes. Furthermore, through self-reflection trainees are less likely to feel offended, which will reduce resistance. In the following discussion, common caregiving and discipline strategies in the country and culture are discussed. This also includes a discussion about legal aspects concerning harsh punishment in the home country of the trainees as well as in other countries, in which the use of any form of violence against children is illegal. Instruction in the theoretical foundation points out potential consequences of harsh punishment and other forms of maltreatment on behavioral, emotional, and cognitive development. Subsequently, common myths about corporal punishment are explored and discussed in small groups (e.g., *corporal punishment teaches respect, some children only understand corporal punishment, corporal punishment is time efficient*, etc.). To reinforce a change in attitude, the trainees are invited to reflect on their own use of harsh punishment toward children and their feelings when using harsh punishment. For most caregivers the use of harsh punishment is related to negative feelings. Yet, they are often not aware of these negative emotions. Spending some time for self-reflection may raise their awareness and thus help them to consider nonviolent action alternatives. In small groups and role-plays, trainees develop and discuss ideas, opportunities, and challenges for replacing harsh punishment with nonviolent caregiving strategies in their daily work.

5. *Supporting burdened children (7 sessions at 90 min)*: This component seeks to provide knowledge of common emotional and behavioral problems that children in institutional care may face. It also communicates that burdened children may not misbehave purposely, but rather that it is an expression of psychological problems. Furthermore, this component also aims to reduce the fears and helplessness of caregivers. Common emotional and behavioral problems, such as (traumatic) stress reactions, depression, oppositional and aggressive behavior, bedwetting, delayed development, and being HIV positive, are addressed. Strategies for handling such challenges are introduced and discussed. In small groups the trainees develop ideas and strategies to support particularly burdened children within their institutions. This component also leaves room for the caregivers to describe other common difficulties of at-risk children and to discuss strategies to support these children.
6. *Child-centered institutional care (7 sessions at 90 min)*: The aim of this component is to enable the trainees to realize changes that are possible in their own workplace which may improve the living conditions for children and working conditions for caregivers. In this way, this component aims to reduce or to prevent (emotional) neglect of the orphans in institutional care. Although structural changes are not generally implemented when conducting ICC-C, the importance of an adequate caregiver–child ratio; warm, sensitive, and stable caregiver–child relationship; and family-like groups is explained. In small groups, trainees compare the situations of children in families and in institutional care settings. In many institutional care settings in resource-poor countries, numerous children

live in large groups with few caregivers. Groups are often age homogenously organized, and caregivers are rarely assigned as primary caregiver for specific children. Theoretical instruction emphasizes key elements of institutional care settings that impact children's development, physical, and mental health. Subsequently, together with the trainers, trainees develop ideas about how to change their work environment to make the institutional care setting more family-like. Possible components that may be discussed are assigning each child to a primary caregiver, creating age-heterogeneous subgroups within a large institution and caregivers spending regular quality time with an assigned group of children. In small groups trainees discuss ideas, challenges, and strategies to introduce these key elements into their particular workplace. Furthermore, the importance of daily and weekly structures and schedules, rituals, and rules as a way to make life predictable for the children is introduced and discussed. In small groups, trainees develop ideas and strategies on how to implement the discussed aspects in their work environment. Further, the importance of play for a healthy development is emphasized. This may be increasingly important as in many resource-poor countries education has become a high priority and is seen as a promising approach to break the cycle of poverty, particularly for orphans and other vulnerable children. Therefore, even very young children spend most of their time learning at school or at their home. We stress that learning begins with playing and that for children, playing is more than leisure time and amusement but an important part of their healthy development. Other aspects like safety at home are also introduced and discussed.

7. *Teamwork and supervision (2 sessions at 90 min)*: This component covers improving immediate working conditions and ensuring the implementation of the training contents in the workplace. The importance of a good work atmosphere and supporting colleagues is discussed. Possibilities for peer supervision and where to seek help are discussed together with the trainees.

At the end of the first and second week, one session of 90 min should be used to repeat and highlight what the caregivers have learned and for an open discussion of questions from the group. The intervention ends with a feedback and session, including a farewell ritual.

6.3 Feasibility and First Empirical Evidence of ICC-C

In our recent feasibility study with caregivers in Tanzania (Hermenau, Kaltenbach et al., 2015), the participating caregivers rated the feasibility and effectiveness of ICC-C immediately before, directly after, and 3 months following the intervention. The trainers reported high satisfaction with the implementation of the units, the caregivers' participation, comprehension, and motivation. Consistently, caregivers reported a high demand, good feasibility, and high motivation and acceptance of the intervention. For example, none of the trainees had undergone any training in childcare. Most trainees reported the frequent use of harsh punishment in their daily work with children, and most lacked nonviolent action alternatives to corporal punishment and yelling. But they were highly motivated to participate and had high expectations concerning the usefulness of ICC-C. Most trainees were highly satisfied with the application of the ICC-C training workshop, and all would recommend ICC-C to other caregivers. Three months after the training workshop, trainees reported the frequent use of the ICC-C content in their daily work. Almost all trainees described improvements in caregiver–child relationships, as well as in child behavior. Furthermore, we assessed exposure to harsh punishment and maltreatment, as well as the mental health of all children living in one institution from which all caregivers had been trained. The children were interviewed 20 months before, 1 month before, and 3 months after the training. Children reported a decrease in harsh punishment and physical maltreatment and a decrease in mental health problems. As such, ICC-C seems feasible under challenging circumstances, and our study provides the first glimpses of its effectiveness.

In an earlier study, we implemented a preliminary version of ICC-C in combination with structural changes and a psychotherapeutic treatment (Narrative Exposure Therapy for children; Ruf et al., 2010; Schauer, Neuner, & Elbert, 2011) for trauma-related illness in a Tanzanian orphanage (Hermenau et al., 2011). In response to all, children reported a decline in exposure to harsh punishment and violence by caregivers as well as in PTSD symptoms and related mental health problems. These findings indicate that caregiver training and structural changes may be combined with psychotherapeutic interventions to foster the mental health of heavily burdened and traumatized children.

6.4 Challenges During Implementation

ICC-C is designed to be applicable in low- and middle-income countries and has been particularly developed for its implementation in Sub-Saharan Africa with all its sociocultural similarities and diversities. Through its participative and adaptive approach that considers the particularly background and needs of both the caregivers and the childcare institution, *ICC-C* can be applied in countries with different cultural and socioeconomic background. However, due to limited resources in many of these countries, institutional care settings are often limited to offering only basic provisions of food and shelter and face major difficulties providing sensitive and child-oriented care. For example, unfavorable caregiver–child ratios (e.g., one caregiver caring for 20 or more children) and poorly trained, overburdened personnel rarely allow for sensitive caregiving that will meet the needs of children. Where it is not possible to secure funds necessary to hire more staff, ICC-C can enable caregivers to implement structural changes within the limited opportunities of the particular setting (e.g., creating family-like groups, assigning each child to a primary caregiver, introducing regular meetings within family-like age-heterogeneous groups, etc.). However, the particular circumstances of the institutional care setting determine which and how many of the suggested changes can be implemented.

Many caregivers lack training in childcare as it is often assumed that everyone can raise children. Nevertheless, being a caregiver in African orphanages means raising children who are often burdened with various psychological problems. ICC-C may raise awareness of children's needs and may contribute to improvements in caregiver–child relationships. However, it does not replace long-term and in-depth training in effective child-rearing practices. Rather ICC-C reduces the gap in knowledge between what is required and what exists. Ideally, ICC-C should be implemented on top of a basic education in childcare in order to foster nonviolent caregiving.

It may be that the management of an institution chooses to implement ICC-C without consulting the caregivers. This could result in resistance to actively participate in the training workshop. Caregivers may experience a threat to their self-esteem when outsiders wish to educate them about how to deal with "their" children. Therefore, it is highly important to build trust. It is crucial that trainers adopt an open attitude that acknowledges the difficult work conditions of the trainees and the willingness to collaborate with them. Collegial learning, acceptance of cultural diversity, and empathy are vital here. Teambuilding activities and involving the caregivers and their feedback in the program design help to create an open and trusting atmosphere.

Changing long-standing norms is challenging, especially because the use of corporal punishment and other harsh discipline measures is very common, socially accepted, and generally regarded as effective in Sub-Saharan Africa and many regions throughout the world. Hence, trainees may confront the trainers with strong resistance toward rethinking disciplinary measures. However, involving the trainees in creating the change and formulating their own training may help to promote engagement in the process. Reflections about the caregivers' own experiences of harsh punishment and maltreatment, discussions about consequences of maltreatment for children, and intensive practicing of effective nonviolent caregiving strategies may facilitate a change of attitude regarding harmful discipline and maltreatment.

The support of the management staff of the childcare institution is crucial for achieving long-term sustainability. The management needs to support the ideas that are developed during the implementation of ICC-C and should provide room for peer supervision. Trainees may also become aware of their poor working conditions during ICC-C training. If the management is unwilling or unable to contribute to changes in working conditions, this may reduce the motivation to implement the newly learned strategies and potential structural changes. So, involving the management as well as the caregivers and promoting a dialogue between the different interests is essential to ensure long-term changes.

7 Practical Implication and Policy Recommendation

The demand for a change of policy and for guidelines on alternative childcare in general, and on institutional care in particular, in Sub-Saharan Africa is huge and progress is slow (Chiwaula et al., 2014). Most orphanages in Sub-Saharan Africa are run by nongovernmental organizations, and often there is no overall structure to ensure at least a minimal quality standard (Better Care Network, 2014). We argue that governments need to establish common practices and guidelines that apply to all childcare institutions to ensure a minimum of quality in childcare (Hermenau et al., 2014). Moreover, policies should include an obligation to adequately train caregivers (SOS Children's Villages International & University of Bedfordshire, 2014).

Many countries in Sub-Saharan Africa have signed the United Nations Convention on the Rights of the Child, yet this convention is only a declaration of intent. It remains unclear whether the weak governmental structures, the subordinate governmental priority, the strong societal resistance, or anything else impedes the application of the principles of the UN convention. Yet, fact is that violence against children occurs on a daily basis. That is why more than ever, programs improving caregiving in institutional care in these countries also need to address corporal punishment and maltreatment. An important step is to raise awareness of the consequences of poor and violent caregiving in institutional care among governmental agencies, child welfare systems, and nongovernmental organizations. The common belief still is that providing basic physical needs, such as food and accommodation, and sometimes education equals good caregiving. Policy makers and funding organizations need to become aware that caregiving is more than feeding and housing children and that warm, sensitive, and nonviolent caregiving lays the foundation for a healthy development.

The few scientifically evaluated intervention approaches that aim at improving institutional care settings have some important components in common: they all aim at improving the caregiver–child relationship (attachment and bonding), enriching the caregiving environment through additional stimulation and quality time, and have at least some focus on preventing maltreatment and further harm (Hermenau et al., 2016; McCall & Groark, 2015). When aiming to improve institutional childcare, governmental officials, institutional directors, and caregivers should focus on these core elements. A mandatory adequate caregiver–child ratio for all institutions is needed as orphans need more attention and positive emotional care by their caregivers. Poor caregiver–child ratios contribute to overworked caregivers who are then more likely to react violently toward children who need more assistance, are slower to move or react to instructions, or just try to get the caregivers' attention. Furthermore, overworked caregivers are at higher risk to emotionally neglect orphans due to limited time and capacity.

8 Conclusions

In this chapter we demonstrated once more that maltreatment is common in African childcare institutions and that its consequences have so far not been adequately addressed. While guidelines emphasize family and kinship care, many children in Sub-Saharan Africa remain in institutions. Consequently, a substantial number of children can benefit from improving the care quality in institutions. However, it is important to note that in countries, in which harsh discipline and violence against children are highly prevalent and generally regarded as effective, orphans living in institutions do not report more maltreatment than orphans living in family or kinship care. Also in family and kinship care, often no mechanisms are available to protect children from abuse and neglect (Better Care Network, 2014; Better Care Network & UNICEF, 2015). Therefore, the need for maltreatment prevention includes not only institutional care but also other alternative care settings. Deinstitutionalization can only be a medium- or long-term aim; meanwhile we need to put efforts into fostering nonviolent care in childcare institutions and other alternative care settings (e.g., Better Care Network & UNICEF, 2015; Hermenau et al., 2014; McCall, 2013).

From successful attempts to improve care quality and to prevent maltreatment in institutional care, we can conclude four important implications: (a) broad, theory-based prevention approaches are needed and should be tested using rigorous scientific standards, (b) although basic nutrition, sanitation, safety, and medical care are essential, responsive nonviolent caregiving is crucial to children's healthy development; (c) improving care quality (e.g., adequate caregiver–child ratio, ban of violent discipline, etc.) is more important than the type of care (institutional care vs. family or kinship care); and (d) beyond improving caregiver–child relationships, caregiver trainings in Sub-Saharan Africa (and elsewhere) should also focus on prevention of violence and abuse in institutional care (Hermenau et al., 2016; McCall, Groark, & Rygaard, 2014). With this chapter, we advocate for educating government officials, managers of childcare institutions, and caregivers about the adverse consequences of maltreatment and for training caregivers in nonviolent caregiving strategies to provide them with adequate and nonviolent action alternatives (Hermenau et al., 2014). The prevention of maltreatment in childcare institutions will enable more children in Sub-Saharan Africa and elsewhere to grow up in supportive and nonviolent environments, thereby helping them to develop in a healthy manner (Hermenau et al., 2016).

Questions for Discussion

- Which factors contribute to the high rates of violence and maltreatment in African orphanages? Explain why.
- Which elements of ICC-C may contribute to reduce violence and maltreatment in African orphanages? Explain why.
- Should care quality in institutional care settings be improved or should countries in Sub-Sahara Africa solely focus on deinstitutionalization? Why or why not?

References

Atwine, B., Cantor-Graae, E., & Bajunirwe, F. (2005). Psychological distress among AIDS orphans in rural Uganda. *Social Science & Medicine*, *61*(3), 555–564. doi:10.1016/j.socscimed.2004.12.018.

Bakermans-Kranenburg, M. J., Steele, H., Zeanah, C. H., Muhamedrahimov, R. J., Vorria, P., Dobrova-Krol, N. A., ... Gunnar, M. R. (2011). III. Attachment and emotional development in institutional care: Characteristics and catch up. *Monographs of the Society for Research in Child Development*, *76*(4), 62–91. doi: 10.1111/j.1540-5834.2011.00628.x.

Better Care Network. (2014). *Alternative care assesment in 6 countries (Kenya, Malawi, Swaziland, Tanzania, Zambia, and Zimbabwe)*. Retrieved from http://www.bettercarenetwork.org/library/social-welfare-systems/child-care-and-protection-policies/alternative-care-assessment-in-6-countries-kenya-malawi-swaziland-tanzania-zambia-and-zimbabwe

Better Care Network. (2015). *Country care review Tanzania*. Retrieved from http://www.bettercarenetwork.org/international-framework/country-care-reviews/country-care-review-tanzania

Better Care Network, & UNICEF. (2015). *An analysis of child-care reform in three African countries. Summary of key findings*. New York, NY: Better Care Network and United Nations Children's Fund (UNICEF).

Carr, C. P., Martins, C. M. S., Stingel, A. M., Lemgruber, V. B., & Juruena, M. F. (2013). The role of early life stress in adult psychiatric disorders: A systematic review according to childhood trauma subtypes. *The Journal of Nervous and Mental Disease*, *201*(12), 1007–1020. doi:10.1097/NMD.0000000000000049.

Chiwaula, L., Dobson, R., & Elsley, S. (2014). *Drumming together for change: A child's right to quality care in Sub-Saharan Africa*. Glasgow, UK: SOS Children's Villages International, CELCIS at the University of Strathclyde, and University of Malawi.

Cluver, L. D., Gardner, F., & Operario, D. (2007). Psychological distress amongst AIDS-orphaned children in urban South Africa. *Journal of Child Psychology and Psychiatry, and Allied Disciplines*, *48*(8), 755–763. doi:10.1111/j.1469-7610.2007.01757.x.

Dube, S. R., Felitti, V. J., Dong, M., Chapman, D. P., Giles, W. H., & Anda, R. F. (2003). Childhood abuse, neglect, and household dysfunction and the risk of illicit drug use: The adverse childhood experiences study. *Pediatrics*, *111*(3), 564–572. doi:10.1542/peds.111.3.564.

Espié, E., Ouss, L., Gaboulaud, V., Candilis, D., Ahmed, K., Cohuet, S., ... Moro, M.-R. (2011). Against the odds: Psychomotor development of children under 2 years in a Sudanese orphanage. *Journal of Tropical Pediatrics*, *57*(6), 412–417. doi: 10.1093/tropej/fmq117.

Euser, S., Alink, L. R. A., Tharner, A., van IJzendoorn, M. H., & Bakermans-Kranenburg, M. J. (2014). Out of home placement to promote safety? The prevalence of physical abuse in residential and foster care. *Children and Youth Services Review*, *37*, 64–70. doi:10.1016/j.childyouth.2013.12.002.

Feinstein, S., & Mwahombela, L. (2010). Corporal punishment in Tanzania's schools. *International Review of Education*, *56*, 399–410. doi:10.1007/s11159-010-9169-5.

Global Initiative to End All Corporal Punishment of Children. (2016a). *Corporal punishment of children: Summaries of prevalence and attitudinal research in the last 10 years – Africa*. Retrieved from http://endcorporalpunishment.org/research/prevalence-research/

Global Initiative to End All Corporal Punishment of Children. (2016b). *Prohibiting all corporal punishment of children in Africa: Progress and delay*. Retrieved from www.endcorporalpunishment.org

Gray, C. L., Pence, B. W., Ostermann, J., Whetten, R. A., O'Donnell, K., Thielman, N. M., & Whetten, K. (2015). Prevalence and incidence of traumatic experiences among orphans in institutional and family-based settings in 5 low- and middle-income countries: A longitudinal study. *Global Health, Science and Practice*, *3*(3), 395–404. doi:10.9745/GHSP-D-15-00093.

Hecker, T., Hermenau, K., Isele, D., & Elbert, T. (2014). Corporal punishment and children's externalizing problems: A cross-sectional study of Tanzanian primary school students. *Child Abuse & Neglect*, *38*(5), 884–892. doi:10.1016/j.chiabu.2013.11.007.

Hecker, T., Hermenau, K., Salmen, C., Teicher, M., & Elbert, T. (2016). Harsh discipline relates to internalizing problems and cognitive functioning: Findings from a cross-sectional study with school children in Tanzania. *BMC Psychiatry, 16*, 118. doi:10.1186/s12888-016-0828-3.

Hecker, T., Radtke, K., Hermenau, K., Papassotiropoulos, A., & Elbert, T. (2016). Associations between child abuse, mental health and epigenetic modifications in the proopiomelanocortin gene (POMC): A study with children in Tanzania. *Development and Psychopathology*. doi:10.1017/S0954579415001248.

Hermenau, K., Eggert, I., Landolt, M. A., & Hecker, T. (2015). Neglect and perceived stigmatization impact psychological distress of orphans in Tanzania. *European Journal of Psychotraumatology, 6*, 28617. doi:10.3402/ejpt.v6.28617.

Hermenau, K., Goessmann, K., Rygaard, N. P., Landolt, M. A., & Hecker, T. (2016). Fostering child development by improving care quality: A systematic review of the effectiveness of structural interventions and caregiver trainings in institutional care. *Trauma, Violence, & Abuse*. doi:10.1177/1524838016641918.

Hermenau, K., Hecker, T., Elbert, T., & Ruf-Leuschner, M. (2014). Maltreatment and mental health in institutional care – Comparing early- and late-institutionalized children in Tanzania. *Infant Mental Health Journal, 35*(2), 102–110. doi:10.1002/imhj.21440.

Hermenau, K., Hecker, T., Ruf, M., Schauer, E., Elbert, T., & Schauer, M. (2011). Childhood adversity, mental ill-health and aggressive behavior in an African orphanage: Changes in response to trauma-focused therapy and the implementation of a new instructional system. *Child and Adolescent Psychiatry and Mental Health, 5*(1), 29. doi:10.1186/1753-2000-5-29.

Hermenau, K., Kaltenbach, E., Mkinga, G., & Hecker, T. (2015). Improving care quality and preventing maltreatment in institutional care – A feasibility study with caregivers. *Frontiers in Psychology, 6*, 937. doi:10.3389/fpsyg.2015.00937.

Inter-agency Group on Child Protection Systems in Sub-Saharan Africa. (2012). *Strengthening child protection systems in Sub-Saharan Africa* (Working paper).

Johnson, D. E., & Gunnar, M. R. (2011). IV. Growth failure in institutionalized children. *Monographs of the Society for Research in Child Development, 76*(4), 92–126. doi:10.1111/j.1540-5834.2011.00629.x.

Johnson, R., Browne, K., & Hamilton-Giachritsis, C. (2006). Young children in institutional care at risk of harm. *Trauma, Violence, & Abuse, 7*(1), 34–60. doi:10.1177/1524838005283696.

Levin, K., & Haines, S. (2007). Opportunities for the development of communicative competence for children in an orphanage in South Africa. *Child Care in Practice, 13*(3), 221–237. doi:10.1080/13575270701353564.

Li, X., Naar-King, S., Barnett, D., Stanton, B., Fang, X., Thurston, C., & Turston, C. (2008). A developmental psychopathology framework of the psychosocial needs of children orphaned by HIV. *Journal of the Association of Nurses in AIDS Care, 19*(2), 147–157. doi:10.1016/j.jana.2007.08.004.

Makame, V., Ani, C., & Grantham-McGregor, S. (2002). Psychological well-being of orphans in Dar es Salaam, Tanzania. *Acta Paediatrica, 91*(4), 459–465. Retrieved from http://www.ncbi.nlm.nih.gov/pubmed/12061364

McCall, R. B. (2013). The consequences of early institutionalization: Can institutions be improved? – Should they? *Child and Adolescent Mental Health, 18*(4), 193–201. doi:10.1111/camh.12025.

McCall, R. B., & Groark, C. J. (2015). Research on institutionalized children: Implications for international child welfare practitioners and policymakers. *International Perspectives in Psychology: Research, Practice, Consultation, 4*(2), 142–159. doi:10.1037/ipp0000033.

McCall, R. B., Groark, C. J., & Rygaard, N. P. (2014). Global research, practice, and policy issues on the care of infants and young children at risk: The articles in context. *Infant Mental Health Journal, 35*(2), 87–93. doi:10.1002/imhj.21441.

Miller, C. M., Gruskin, S., Subramanian, S. V., & Heymann, J. (2007). Emerging health disparities in Botswana: Examining the situation of orphans during the AIDS epidemic. *Social Science and Medicine, 64*, 2476–2486. doi:10.1016/j.socscimed.2007.03.002.

Morantz, G., Cole, D., Vreeman, R., Ayaya, S., Ayuku, D., & Braitstein, P. (2013a). Child abuse and neglect among orphaned children and youth living in extended families in Sub-Saharan Africa: What have we learned from qualitative inquiry? *Vulnerable Children and Youth Studies, 8*(4), 338–352. doi:10.1080/17450128.2013.764476.

Morantz, G., Cole, D. C., Ayaya, S., Ayuku, D., & Braitstein, P. (2013b). Maltreatment experiences and associated factors prior to admission to residential care: A sample of institutionalized children and youth in western Kenya. *Child Abuse & Neglect, 37*, 778–787. doi:10.1016/j.chiabu.2012.10.007.

Nelson Mandela Children's Fund. (2016). *Nelson Mandela quotes about children*. Retrieved from http://www.nelsonmandelachildrensfund.com/nelson-mandela-quotes-about-children/

Nichols, J., Embleton, L., Mwangi, A., Morantz, G., Vreeman, R., Ayaya, S., ... Braitstein, P. (2014). Physical and sexual abuse in orphaned compared to non-orphaned children in Sub-Saharan Africa: A systematic review and meta-analysis. *Child Abuse & Neglect, 38*(2), 304–316. doi: 10.1016/j.chiabu.2013.09.012.

Nyamukapa, C. A., Gregson, S., Wambe, M., Mushore, P., Lopman, B., Mupambireyi, Z., ... Jukes, M. C. H. (2010). Causes and consequences of psychological distress among orphans in eastern Zimbabwe. *AIDS Care, 22*(8), 988–996. doi: 10.1080/09540121003615061.

Puffer, E. S., Drabkin, A. S., Stashko, A. L., Broverman, S., Ogwang-Odhiambo, R., & Sikkema, K. J. (2012). Orphan status, HIV risk behavior, and mental health among adolescents in rural Kenya. *Journal of Pediatric Psychology, 37*(8), 868–878. doi:10.1093/jpepsy/jss077.

Riley, M. (2012). *Baseline study: The state of institutional care in Uganda*. Kampala, Uganda: Departments of Youth and Children, Ministry of Gender, Labour and Social Development. Retrieved from http://alternative-care-uganda.org/resources/moglsd-baseline-study-institutional-care-in-uganda-june-2012.pdf.

Ruf, M., Schauer, M., Neuner, F., Catani, C., Schauer, E., & Elbert, T. (2010). Narrative exposure therapy for 7- to 16-year-olds: A randomized controlled trial with traumatized refugee children. *Journal of Traumatic Stress, 23*(4), 437–445. doi:10.1002/jts.20548.

Rygaard, N. P. (2010). Designing the fair start project – A free E-learning and organizational development program for orphanages and foster families in quality caregivning. *Clinical Neuropsychology, 7*(6), 181–187. Retrieved from http://www.clinicalneuropsychiatry.org/pdf/02_rygaard.pdf.

Schauer, M., Neuner, F., & Elbert, T. (2011). *Narrative Exposure Therapy (NET). A short-term intervention for traumatic stress* (2nd ed.). Cambidge, MA/Göttingen, Germany: Hogrefe & Huber Publishers.

SOS Children's Villages International, & University of Bedfordshire. (2014). *From a whisper to a shout: A call to end violence against children in alternative care*. Insbruck, Austria: SOS Children's Villages International.

Straus, M. A. (2010). Prevalence, societal causes, and trends in corporal punishment by parents in world perspective. *Law and Contemporary Problems, 31*, 1–30. Retrieved from http://scholarship.law.duke.edu/lcp/vol73/iss2/2.

Sugaya, L., Hasin, D. S., Olfson, M., Lin, K., Grant, B. F., & Blanco, C. (2012). Child physical abuse and adult mental health: A national study. *Journal of Traumatic Stress, 25*, 384–392. doi:10.1002/jts.21719.

The American Academy of Pediatrics. (1999). In E. L. Schoor (Ed.), *Caring for your school-age child: Ages 5 to 12* (Rev.). New York, NY: Bantam Books.

UNICEF. (2006). *Africa's orphaned and vulnerable generations: Children affected by aids*. New York, NY.: Retrieved from http://www.unicef.org/publications/files/Africas_Orphaned_and_Vulnerable_Generations_Children_Affected_by_AIDS.pdf.

UNICEF. (2011). *Violence against children in Tanzania: Results from a National Survey 2009*. Dar es Salaam, Tanzania: UNICEF. Retrieved from http://www.unicef.org/media/files/VIOLENCE_AGAINST_CHILDREN_IN_TANZANIA_REPORT.pdf.

UNICEF. (2014). *Hidden in plain sight – A statistical analysis of violence against children*. New York, NY: United Nations Children's Fund.

United Nations. (2016). *Open working group proposal for sustainable development goals*. Retrieved from https://sustainabledevelopment.un.org/sdgsproposal.html

Unterhitzenberger, J., & Rosner, R. (2014). Lessons from writing sessions: A school-based randomized trial with adolescent orphans in Rwanda. *European Journal of Psychotraumatology*, *5*, 24917. doi:10.3402/ejpt.v5.24917.

Walakira, E. J., Dumba-Nyanzi, I., & Bukenya, B. (2015). *Child care institutions in selected districts in Uganda and the situation of children in care: A baseline survey report for the strong beginnings project*. Kampala, Uganda: Terres des Hommes Netherlands. Retrieved from http://www.anppcanug.org/wp-content/uploads/research_reports/2015/Baseline_Survey_Report_Full.PDF.

Wild, L. G., Flisher, A. J., & Robertson, B. A. (2011). Risk and resilience in orphaned adolescents living in a community affected by AIDS. *Youth & Society*, *45*(1), 140–162. doi:10.1177/0044118X11409256.

Wolff, P. H., Dawit, Y., & Zere, B. (1995). The Solomuna orphanage: A historical survey. *Social Science & Medicine*, *40*(8), 1133–1139.

Wolff, P. H., & Fesseha, G. (1998). The orphans of Eritrea: Are orphanages part of the problem or part of the solution? *The American Journal of Psychiatry*, *155*(10), 1319–1324. Retrieved from http://www.ncbi.nlm.nih.gov/pubmed/9766761

Wolff, P. H., & Fesseha, G. (1999). The orphans of Eritrea: A five-year follow-up study. *Journal of Child Psychology and Psychiatry*, *40*(8), 1231–1237.

Chapter 18
Why Institutions Matter: Empirical Data from Five Low- and Middle-Income Countries Indicate the Critical Role of Institutions for Orphans

Christine L. Gray, Sumedha Ariely, Brian W. Pence, and Kathryn Whetten

There is nothing so expensive, really, as a big, well-developed, full-bodied preconception.

– EB White (1944).

1 Introduction

Context is critical. Without context or comparisons, the documentation of maltreatment and abuse in institutions that care for orphans can lead to an immediate and understandable conclusion that institutions must be closed to protect children. Without context, such observations suggest that elimination of institutions will answer the question that plagues world leaders, policymakers, and communities: What is the best way to care for our growing population of orphans, such that we prevent neglect and maltreatment, and set them up for a positive, healthy life trajectory?

Asked in isolation, the answers to questions about maltreatment in institutions can result in a seemingly indisputable conclusion that global deinstitutionalization is necessary. Indeed, that is a commonly reached conclusion (Berens & Nelson,

C.L. Gray (✉) • B.W. Pence
Department of Epidemiology, University of North Carolina at Chapel Hill,
Gillings School of Global Public Health, 135 Dauer Drive,
2101 McGavran-Greenberg Hall, CB #7435, Chapel Hill, NC 27599-7435, USA
e-mail: clgray@email.unc.edu; bpence@unc.edu

S. Ariely
Duke Global Health Institute, Duke University, Durham, NC, USA
e-mail: sumi.ariely@duke.edu

K. Whetten
Duke Global Health Institute, Duke University, Durham, NC, USA

Public Policy and Global Health, Duke University, Durham, NC, USA
e-mail: katewhetten@gmail.com

A.V. Rus et al. (eds.), *Child Maltreatment in Residential Care*,
DOI 10.1007/978-3-319-57990-0_18

2015; SaveTheChildren, 2009). The universality and simplicity of this conclusion are highly appealing: it offers a blanket solution for all governments and all communities. However, when these questions are placed in context, different conclusions emerge. The world's orphaned and vulnerable children will still need viable options for quality care. Will they receive it if all institutions are closed?

To understand the context that surrounds the discussion around optimal orphan care structures, we must ask: Why is there a need for institution-based care? What is the alternative? Is maltreatment in institutions worse than in family-based care settings presumed to be the superior care option? What are the long-term outcomes for children in these different settings? What are the critical elements of caregiving that determine child outcomes? If we remove institutions as a care option, are orphaned children better off?

In this chapter, we begin with the historical context that has shaped the global approach to protecting the lives, and the rights, of children. In particular, we briefly recap the formalization of the rights of the child and the multiple care contexts in which modern (post-World War II) institutional solutions for orphan care arose. We then focus on the current context of low- and middle-income countries (LMICs) in sub-Saharan Africa and South/Southeast Asia, drawing on empirical evidence from LMICs, in particular a large, statistically representative study conducted in Cambodia, Ethiopia, India, Kenya, and Tanzania, to inform the discussion. Finally, we describe the need and potential for heterogeneous care options, explore emerging opportunities for intervention, and present areas of needed research to assist leaders, policymakers, and communities in creating quality care options for orphans.

2 Objectives

1. Understand the historical context of the rights and protection of children
2. Describe the current global orphan crisis
3. Summarize the empirical evidence of maltreatment of orphans and vulnerable children in institution-based care compared to family-based care in low- and middle-income countries (LMICs)
4. Describe the context and constraints of orphan care in LMIC
5. Discuss why institutions form an important part of a heterogeneous orphan care structure in LMIC and how research can inform policymakers

3 Historical Context: Existing Literature

Historically, developmental ideas of childhood and religious philosophical notions of child rights have not been static. Instead, childhood can be seen as a social construction in which there are discernible differences even within the same society in how childhood and child rights are defined (James, Jenks, & Prout, 1998; Lancy,

2015). Social class, gender, and labor status all played a role within different cultural groups in defining constructs like developmental maturity, agency, and duties that were important to children's rights. For example, Medieval Europe, while often portrayed as thinking of children as "little adults" like those popularized by French historian Philippe Aries (1962), had models of distinct life stages and church-based laws that defined instances in which children were equal to adults and also distinct from them (Cunningham, 1995; Orme, 2003). Likewise, there was a spectrum of moral, religious, and philosophical codes that defined children's needs, rights, and responsibilities across societies and cultures in the global south (Hsiung, 2007; Kakar, 1979; Kapur, 2015; Wiredu, 1992).

Modern notions of child rights, based largely on an integration of a western philosophical understanding of human nature (Locke, 1693/1995), with judicial reforms, started to shift European social attitudes on human pain, children's developmental needs, and societal responsibilities. Protection-based rights, such as regulating child labor and advancing rights to education, slowly grew as the realities of child exploitation for economic progress jutted against growing cultural awareness of the need to alleviate suffering by adding medical, social, and justice-based improvements. The horrors of World War I, along with continued work by social reformers such as Eglantyne Jebb (Mulley, 2010), Janusz Korczak (Lifton, 2006) and Adam Lopatka (sometimes dubbed "father of the Convention on the Rights of the Child"), helped lead to the League of Nations (1919, later becoming the UN) and the adoption of the Geneva Declaration of the Rights of the Child (1924), which gave for the first time a formal, international focus to responsibilities toward child-specific concerns.

The additional devastation of World War II, rising orphan crises, and mass cross-border social upheavals fostered ongoing international collaborative conversations, leading to current commonly known child-based outcomes such as the UN Fund for Urgency for the Children (1947 and becoming UNICEF), Universal Declaration of Human Rights (1948), Declaration of the Rights of the Child (1959), International Year of the Child (1979), and Convention on the Rights of the Child (1989). The formalization of these organizations and declarations provided a foundation for ongoing critique and negotiations on how best to meet international standards for children as full subjects of human rights and self-determination, how to globally define child rights and responsibilities, and how to measure outcomes (Fass, 2011; Moody, 2015; Sharma, 2015). More recently, growing emphasis on mental health, trauma history, education, and civic context as integral components of child rights has been instrumental in continued advancements in orphan and vulnerable children's care.

The European and American context of care for orphaned and separated children (OSC) and indigent citizens across all ages that resulted from war (civil and international), epidemics (plague, cholera in the 1830s), and social upheaval (industrialization, famine) encompassed a wide variety of solutions that included almshouses, institutions, orphan trains, cross-fostering, formalized family foster care, and community fostering models (Hacsi, 1995, 1997; Johnson, Rolph, & Smith, 2012). These solutions are reminiscent of the multiple care contexts currently existing in LMICs in the global south. Traditional child welfare solutions in the African and Asian context such as community and family fostering have been increasingly besieged with political revolutions, the AIDS epidemic, rising poverty and inequality, climate change, famines, and wars. The current Middle East refugee crises, overwhelming Europe and resulting in permanent refugee camps since 2011, further highlight the need for a variety of programs and options to address the growing groups of OSC and dependent persons. The importance of international and cross-population studies on the mental and physical health outcomes of these groups as they reside, by necessity, in multiple care environments (the street, refugee camps, community and family care, and formal residential care) is critical if we are to come close to adequately addressing the rising displacement of global populations.

4 LMIC Perspectives: Emerging Evidence

As of 2011, over 150 million children ages 0–17 worldwide had been orphaned by the death of one or both parents (UNICEF, 2013). Nearly 100 million, or two-thirds, of the world's orphans are in sub-Saharan Africa or South Asia (UNICEF, 2013). In sub-Saharan Africa alone, 15 million children were orphaned as a result of AIDS (UNICEF, 2013). These numbers do not include the additional millions of children who have been separated from their parents due to circumstances such as war, poverty, or internal displacement. Notably, low- and middle-income countries (LMICs), whose economies are less equipped than more resourced countries to care for the growing numbers of orphans, are disproportionately affected by the orphan crisis. Consideration of the context of LMICs is essential to addressing global orphan care and preventing orphan maltreatment.

4.1 Positive Outcomes for Orphan Study

To identify and understand the characteristics of care associated with improved trajectories for orphans, the Positive Outcomes for Orphans (POFO) study was initiated. The POFO study is a longitudinal cohort following over 3000 orphans and separated children (OSC) from six study sites in five low- and middle-income countries: Battambang District, Cambodia; Addis Ababa, Ethiopia; Hyderabad and Nagaland, India; Bungoma District, Kenya; and Kilimanjaro Region, Tanzania (Whetten et al., 2009).

Inclusion in the POFO study was defined by age and orphan status. All children who were orphaned by one or both parents, or were separated from their parents, and were aged 6–12 at baseline enrollment were eligible for inclusion. Separated children had no expectation of reunification with their parents; most had been abandoned. OSC in the POFO study were randomly sampled from both institution-based care and family-based care. Institutions were defined as residential dwellings where at least five children from at least two different families are cared for by nonrelatives. A two-stage random sampling approach was used to select OSC from each setting (institutional care and family-based care) for the study.

For the institution-based care sample, the study team worked with government officials and community organizations to first enumerate the institutions in each study region. As part of their efforts to identify institution-based care, the local study teams actively sought key informants and ultimately uncovered more orphanages than were previously known. Institutions in each study region were then randomly ordered from the enumerated lists and approached in sequence (Stage 1). Each institution had complete rosters of children, from which up to 20 from each institution were randomly selected until 250 OSC from each region were enrolled (Stage 2). If the number of institutions precluded reaching the targeted 250 children, then the limit of 20 children per institution was relaxed to enable more age-eligible children to participate. In total, 1357 children from 83 institutions were enrolled across the six study sites (Whetten et al., 2009).

The institutions represented in the POFO study encompass a broad range of possible residences in which orphaned children may live, including different sizes, ages of children, caregiver-to-child ratios, religious affiliations (if any), and government vs. non-governmental organization status. Approximately 35% of institutions have less than 25 children, with one housing as few as five, but there are others housing more than 250 children. The children in the POFO study are distributed throughout; about half live in institutions caring for fewer than 100 OSC, and about half live in institutions caring for more than 100 OSC. The heterogeneity of institutions makes describing a "typical" institution difficult. Many are initiated by individuals who see a need in the community. As an example, one governmental institution in Ethiopia was founded by a woman who took in her first child when her neighbor was dying of AIDS and she didn't want the young boy left parentless. She continued taking in children and now runs an institution with 180 children who attend school during the week and do chores and play on the weekends. Most of the financial support comes from local and foreign individuals, but because the government owns the property, the institution is monitored by the government through site visits and routine reporting by staff.

The family-based care sample was selected by first dividing each region into 50 clusters based on administrative or geographic boundaries. In each cluster, up to five children were randomly sampled from available lists or from house-to-house surveys conducted by the study team, until five households with at least one orphaned child meeting the age criterion were identified. If multiple children in the household were eligible for inclusion, the child whose first name came first alphabetically was selected. If there were insufficient numbers of children meeting eligibility criteria in a cluster, then the maximum number of children per cluster was raised to between six and ten. An additional 50 non-orphaned children from each region were sampled for qualitative comparison. Those children were selected from the same geographic clusters used to select the family-based sample.

Family-based care involves a variety of living arrangements, including living with the remaining parent, a relative, or a community member. Family-based care is not regulated by any laws in particular, though in some communities families may receive subsidies or other resources, including opportunities to participate in support groups or to improve parenting skills that facilitate their ability to support the orphaned child.

Baseline data collection began in May 2006–February 2008; start dates varied by study site. A wide range of data including measurements of physical health (e.g., height, weight, body mass index), mental health (e.g., anxiety, cognitive functioning, emotional well-being), risk behaviors, stigma, health-care utilization, social networks, child-caregiver relationships, and potentially traumatic experiences have been tracked annually or semiannually (every 6 months) for 7 years of follow-up.

Several unique features of the POFO study make it a particularly strong cohort from which to draw inferences. POFO is the largest cohort of orphans to be followed longitudinally. In particular, POFO has followed children from multiple low- and middle-income countries who are difficult to reach and to track over time and has retained them for follow-up into late adolescence. Retention in POFO over 7 years of follow-up was approximately 70%. Perhaps most importantly, the design of the POFO study – specifically, random sampling of institutions (or households) and random sampling of children within each setting – enables a scientifically robust mechanism for comparing children in each care setting.

4.2 Key Findings

The seminal findings of the POFO study can be summarized as follows: orphaned children in institution-based care are no worse off than orphaned children placed in family-based care. This result holds true both in terms of physical, emotional, and intellectual well-being outcomes and traumatic experiences, including abuse. A baseline comparison of OSC in both settings showed that OSC in institution-based care have similar BMI-for-age, height-for-age, and caregiver-reported health (measured on a five-point scale) as OSC in family-based care (Whetten et al., 2009). Emotional well-being, measured by the Strengths and Difficulties Questionnaire (Goodman, 1999; Goodman, Meltzer, & Bailey, 1998), indicated that institution-based OSC scored lower (better) than their family-based counterparts. Similarly, institution-based OSC scored higher on memory and general intellectual functioning using the California Verbal Learning Test (Delis, Kramer, Kaplan & Ober, 1987; Kaufman & Kaufman, 2004), respectively. All interviews and measures were administered by highly trained interviewers in the native language of the child. In general, research in LMICs is limited by lack of culturally adaptive well-being measures. However, any bias resulting from lack of cultural adaptation of measures is not expected to differ between family-based and institution-based children and thus should not bias the comparison of children between those groups.

Longitudinal follow-up showed that the baseline observations of well-being measures were maintained over time (Fig. 18.1). After 3 years, there was a negligible difference between institution-based and family-based OSC across outcomes (Whetten et al., 2014). The family-based OSC showed better improvement on some

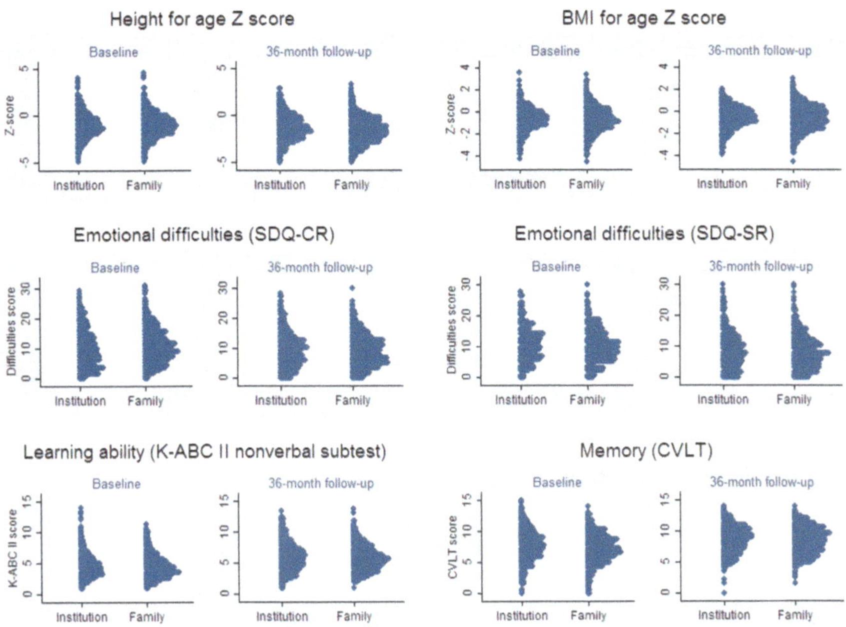

Fig. 18.1 Distribution of child well-being measures at baseline and follow-up, by care setting type (institution based vs. family based). *Blue bars* are dot plots of the well-being measures of individual children at baseline and follow-up, respectively. Each child is represented by one *dot* (Reprinted from Whetten et al., 2014)

measures (sickness in the past 2 weeks, memory) and in essence had caught up to the institution-based OSC at a 3-year follow-up. Importantly, the longitudinal analyses demonstrated that the variation in outcomes at baseline, at 3-year follow-up, and in changes between baseline and follow-up, could not be explained by the different care settings (institution- vs. family-based care). The variation was primarily explained by individual differences in the children and, to a much lesser extent, by the study sites (country regions) and the specific institution or geographically defined community cluster within each site (Table 18.1).

Another key finding in the POFO study was that the prevalence and incidence of potentially traumatic experiences are extremely high among OSC. Using the Life Events Checklist (Elhai, Gray, Kashdan, & Franklin, 2005; Gray, Litz, Hsu, & Lombardo, 2004) to assess trauma experienced by children at least 10 years of age at the time of interview, the POFO study found that over 90% of OSC had experienced at least one trauma beyond the orphaning event of losing a parent (Gray et al., 2015b). By age 13, 50% of institution-dwelling OSC and 54% of family-dwelling OSC had experienced physical or sexual abuse. Over 3 years of follow-up, annual incidence of physical or sexual abuse was higher among OSC in family-based care (19%) than those in institution-based care (13%) (Fig. 18.2). Both boys and girls had similarly high rates of overall trauma and of physical or sexual abuse. Among

Table 18.1 Sample characteristics at baseline, among those retained at 36 months and those lost to follow-up

	N		Unweighted distributions: Mean (SD) or *N* (%)		Weighted difference in means or proportions, confidence interval, and p-value[a]	
	Institution-based	Family-based	Institution-based	Family-based	Institution vs. family	
Panel A. Baseline[b]						
Positive outcomes (higher score is better)						
Caregiver-rated child health (1–5)	957	1263	4.0 (0.7)	3.7 (0.8)	0.38 (0.30; 0.45)	<0.001
Height for age Z score (1 unit = 1 SD))	978	1280	−1.0 (1.4)	−1.0 (1.3)	−0.09 (−0.19; 0.01)	0.076
BMI for age Z score (1 unit = 1 SD)	975	1280	−0.7 (1.0)	−0.7 (1.2)	0.10 (0.03; 0.18)	0.009
Learning ability (K-ABC II, range 0–20))	984	1285	4.7 (1.9)	4.5 (1.8)	0.19 (0.04; 0.34)	0.013
Memory CVLT, range 0–15))	970	1269	7.7 (2.3)	7.2 (2.2)	0.45 (0.23; 0.67)	<0.001
Negative outcomes (higher score or percentage is worse)						
Emotional difficulties (SDQ-CR, range 0–40)	893	1211	10.0 (6.2)	10.8 (5.5)	−0.60 (−1,08; −0.12)	0.014
Emotional difficulties (SDQ-SR, range 0–40)	228	326	10.5 (5.5)	10.2 (5.6)	0.03 (−0.39; 0.46)	0.874
Diarrhea/fever/cough in last 2 weeks	958	1269	194 (20.2%)	505 (39.8%)	−21% (−24%; −17%)	<0.001
Panel B. Difference between baseline and follow-up[c]						
Positive outcomes (higher score is better)						
Caregiver-rated child health (1–5)	957	1263	0.2 (0.9)	0.5 (1.1)	−0.30 (−0.39; −0.22)	<0.001
Height for age Z score (1 unit =1 SD))	978	1280	−0.4 (1.0)	−0.6 (1.0)	0.23 (0.16; 0.31)	<0.001
BMI for age Z score (1 unit = 1 SD)	975	1280	0.1 (0.9)	0.2 (1.0)	−0.10 (−0.18; −0.03)	0.005
Learning ability (K-ABC II, range 0–20))	984	1285	1.3 (2.2)	1.2 (2.2)	−0.09 (−0.24; 0.06)	0.244
Memory CVLT, range 0–15))	970	1269	0.9 (2.8)	1.2(27)	−0.34 (−0.57; −0.12)	0.003
Negative outcomes (higher score or percentage is worse)						
Emotional difficulties (SDQ-CR, range 0–40)	893	1211	−0.7 (8.4)	−1.7 (7.3)	1.15 (0.52; 1.77)	<0.001
Emotional difficulties (SDQ-SR, range 0–40)	228	326	− 1 – 4 (7.7)	−1.8 (7.5)	0.28 (−0.34; 0.90)	0.377
Diarrhea/fever/cough in last 2 weeks	958	1269	−18 (−1.9%)	−304 (−24.0%)	21% (17%; 26%)	<0.001

Panel C. 36-month follow-up						
Positive outcomes (higher score is better)						
Caregiver-rated child health (1–5)	957	1263	4.2 (0.6)	4.2 (0.7)	0.07 (0.02; 0.12)	0.005
Height for age Z score (1 unit =1 SD)	978	1280	−1.4 (1.3)	−1.6 (1.3)	0.14 (0.05; 0.23)	0.002
BMI for age Z score (1 unit = 1 SD)	975	1280	−0.6 (1.0)	−0.5 (1.1)	0.00 (−0.08; 0.08)	0.981
Learning ability (K-ABC III, range 0–20)	984	1285	5.9 (2.1)	5.7 (1.9)	0.10 (−0.08; 0.27)	0.265
Memory (CVLT, range 0–15)	970	1269	8.6 (2.1)	8.5 (2.1)	0.11 (−0.04; 0.26)	0.160
Negative outcomes (higher score or percentage is worse)						
Emotional difficulties (SDQ-CR, range 0–40)	893	1211	9.3 (5.5)	9.1 (5.1)	0.55 (0.12; 0.97)	0.011
Emotional difficulties (SDQ-SR, range 0–40)	228	326	9.1 (5.3)	8.5 (5.1)	0.31 (−0.18; 0.80)	0.209
Diarrhea/fever/cough in last 2 weeks	958	1269	176(18.4%)	201 (15.8%)	1% (−2%; 3%)	0.542

Reprinted from Whetten et al., (2014)

[a]Weighted difference accounts for age and sex differences in the distribution of children across study sites and differential rates of attrition between baseline and follow-up

[b]Baseline values include only those children who were not later lost to follow-up

[c]Difference represents child-level changes between baseline and follow-up

CVLT California verbal learning test, *SDQ-CG* strengths and difficulties questionnaire, caregiver report, *SDQ-SR* SDQ, self report

doi:10.1371/journal.pone.0104872.t002

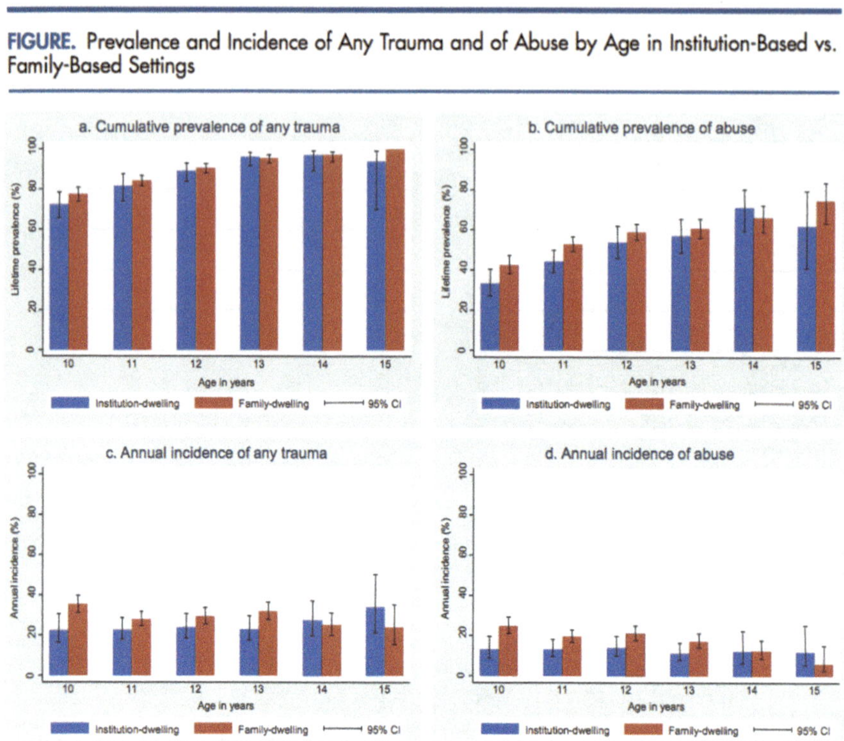

Fig. 18.2 Prevalence and incidence of any trauma and of abuse by age in institution-based vs. family-based settings (Reprinted from Gray et al., 2015b)

those in institution-based care, 14% of boys and 12% of girls had experienced abuse; among those in family-based care, 20% of boys and 19% of girls had experienced abuse (Gray et al., 2015a).

The findings in the POFO study are consistent with other studies in LMICs. A separate study of OSC in Kenya specifically used the Convention on the Rights of the Child framework to assess how different models of care (institution-based or family-based care) upheld the basic rights outlined in the framework (Embleton et al., 2014). Similar to POFO, children were sampled from orphanages or other institutions (all referred to as charitable children's institutions, or CCIs), as well as from family households caring for orphaned children. The study assessed key articles of the framework, including the right to know and be cared for by the child's parents; the right to information; the right to protection from physical or mental abuse, maltreatment, or exploitation; the right to health; the right to a reasonable standard of living; the right to education; and the right to protection from economic exploitation or work that may be injurious or interfere with education. In general, improvements are needed in both CCIs and family-based care to fully uphold the rights of children. Still, children in CCIs were more likely to have basic material needs met, to have a higher standard of living (e.g., pumped water), and to have greater access to books. The use of corporal punishment, though against the Kenyan Constitution, was much more likely to be used in families than in CCIs, where caretakers were more likely to discuss poor behavior, withhold privileges, or assign extra chores to address misbehavior.

In a meta-analysis of 42 studies from 19 countries on the intelligence quotient (IQ) of children growing up in orphanages compared to children placed in foster families, children in orphanages were shown to have lower IQs by 20 points (van IJzendoorn, Luijk & Juffer, 2008). However, in three of the four countries ranking lowest on the Human Development Index, a ranking of life expectancy, education, and per capita income, there were no differences in IQ between children in orphanages and those in family-based care. Caregiver-to-child ratio (only measured among those in orphanages) was not associated with smaller or larger delays in IQ. However, institution-based children with the best caregiver-to-child ratio (maximum of three caregivers per child) did not significantly lag their family-based peers, suggesting that those in smaller groups may not have different IQ developments than their family-based peers. Children assessed before the age of 2 had more delays than those assessed after age 2; a similar result was found for age 4. Delays were only observed for the youngest children, though many studies were missing age at entry data and those studies with missing data had large effect sizes.

While the focus of this chapter is LMICs, it is worth noting that the largest survey of orphanage alumni conducted in the United States showed orphanage alumni achieved higher education and income and reported better attitudes about life than the general population (McKenzie, 1997). The survey was conducted on approximately 1600 orphans from nine homes in the South and Midwest United States, suggesting that the parity of institution-based care and family-based care in terms of well-being outcomes may not be unique to LMICs.

4.3 Context for Maltreatment

It may seem counterintuitive that maltreatment could occur with equal (or greater) frequency in family-based settings as in institution-based settings. Certainly, families and family care environments are essential elements of orphan care. Why might family-based settings have equal or higher prevalence and incidence of trauma, particularly of abuse?

For context, it is not uncommon in many parts of Africa for children to live with extended family, often for the opportunity to advance their education in a more urbanized area (Daniel & Mathias, 2012). Education is a core value and desire, viewed as essential to improving welfare for oneself and one's family. The children may help their "foster" family with household chores and/or the rural family from which they came may send food to help support the foster family (Madhavan, 2004). This voluntary system is viewed as mutually beneficial. However, the current orphan crisis, partly a function of the AIDS epidemic, has created an obligatory environment of fostering orphaned children of relatives without the reciprocal support provided in the voluntary context. Increasingly, families and caregivers in LMIC are facing economic constraints that compromise their ability to care for the orphans in their communities. They simply cannot absorb the number of children in need, particularly given the high probability that they are impoverished themselves.

This reality has manifested in several troubling trajectories for orphaned youth. In one study in Tanzania, rural orphans who did not have adequate family care were interviewed about their lives (Daniel & Mathias, 2012). They fell into two groups: those who were trafficked while being promised an education and those who gave up schooling to head the household for themselves and their siblings. Those trafficked (all girls) were taken to more urban areas by family or neighbors, where they expected to be able to go to school. Instead, they were all forced to work long days, were not allowed to contact their family, were not allowed to attend school, and were not paid for their labor. Many were physically abused; several were raped. Telling an adult generally resulted in shame or worse treatment. Because they had no wages with which to purchase even a bus ticket, and were restricted from reaching out to other relatives or friends, they were at the mercy of encountering a kind and trustworthy neighbor or tenant who could help. Similar phenomena have been described by others who have documented that child fostering can result in child trafficking if the child is deprived of basic rights, including health services, education, and protection from abuse and excessive labor (Blagborough, 2008; Evans, 2005; Koda, 2000; Ochanda, Akinyi, & Wakinya, 2011).

In the child-headed households, the children tried to attend school, but ultimately could not keep up with both school and farming chores (Daniel & Mathias, 2012). This is consistent with a separate study of double orphan-headed households in Uganda (Dalen, Nakitende, & Musisi, 2009). Among the 43 child heads of household interviewed, the reasons varied as to why children remained on parents' property despite having no adult caretakers. Some were refused help from relatives; some were afraid relatives would take their property; and some couldn't trace their relatives. In general, siblings actively sought to stay together rather than being split among relatives. While shelters housing these children differed greatly, most needed at least some repair and children were often sharing one bedsheet or blanket. None of the children interviewed could afford fish or meat; most were routinely hungry. Stress over the lack of basic needs was substantial. Going to school precluded ensuring crops or property were kept safe, and most siblings worked to support the family and could not afford the school fees, even with subsidies from relief organizations. Children reported falling behind in school, not being able to keep up with friends, and feeling the stigma and often, ostracization, from the community. Few had someone to talk to about their situation, and they desired to be more included in the community; such social relationships are essential for their long-term physical and emotional health trajectories (Berkman, 2000; Berkman & Syme, 1979; Prince et al., 2007). Those with stronger self-esteem and greater initiative lived in villages with more supportive chairmen and community members.

4.4 *Family and Caregiver Burden*

Even under more ideal conditions in which the orphaned child is not trafficked or heading the household, recent studies have documented the caregiver burden that strains the family economy, the caregiver's ability to meet family needs, and the caregiver's physical and mental health. One study of caregivers was conducted in Botswana at three hospitals/clinics in three different locations representing the city/village population distribution in the Botswana census (large capital city of Gaborone, medium-sized city of Lobatse, small town of Molepolole) (Heymann et al., 2007). All 1033 respondents were working adults waiting to see a health-care provider for themselves or for an adult or child they were accompanying. More than one-third (37%) of respondents were providing care for at least one orphan; nearly half of those (46%) were caring for more than one orphan. Orphan caregivers and non-orphan caregivers were similar in terms of number of hours per day worked, number of jobs, etc. However, those caring for orphans reported significantly more difficulty meeting caregiving responsibilities, finding reliable child care, helping with homework, and offering emotional support to the children. Orphan caregivers were also significantly more likely to lose pay or take unpaid leave to meet caregiving needs and reported more financial difficulties and shortages of water, food, shelter, and transportation. Those providing care to orphans living outside the home were more likely to receive community help than those caring for orphans in their homes (over half compared to less than 20%). The authors excluded institutional care as an option, citing that out-of-family placement "is viewed by policymakers as the worst of all possible alternatives." They conclude that shifts in workplace policies are needed to support extended family care, as well as improved surveillance on policies and services to assess the impact on both orphaned and non-orphaned children in overburdened households.

In a similar study conducted in South Africa, 40% of orphan caregivers reported high levels of burden using a standard caregiving measure (Kidman & Thurman, 2014). Many caregivers (19%) were also caring for sick family members, partly due to the AIDS epidemic, and 23% suffered from chronic illness themselves. The most commonly reported caregiving concern was feeling they could do a better job for the orphaned child quite frequently or always (83%). Nearly a quarter (23%) were stressed quite frequently/always about caring for the orphaned child and meeting other works or household demands, and 17% reported their own health frequently suffered because of their involvement with orphaned children. Food insecurity was the greatest predictor of caregiver burden; household income was also significantly associated. In general, this study highlights the economic vulnerability of orphan caregivers, as well as the potential for overwhelming burden among those with chronic illness themselves.

4.5 Orphan Stigma

The emergence of the AIDS epidemic brought much attention to the existing orphan crisis in sub-Saharan Africa. As researchers, health-care providers, and aid workers began observing the stigmatization of orphaned children due to fear of the disease, studies began documenting the AIDS-related stigma faced by orphaned children (Campbell et al., 2014; Chi, Li, Zhao, & Zhao, 2014; Cluver, Gardner, & Operario, 2008; UNICEF, 2004, 2006). However, the independent stigma of being an orphan in LMIC remains relatively undocumented. One qualitative study, however, was conducted in the POFO study sites. Five focus groups of 7–9 participants each were conducted with village elders, social workers, caregivers, and other community stakeholders to understand the nature of orphan-specific stigma (Whetten et al., under review). For one question, the adult participants were asked to imagine what life would be like if they were orphaned, specifically about living situations; all had negative responses, such as this one:

> My life will be worse than a street dog. Once death rituals of my parents are over, then I will be taken by one or other relative for some time and later leave me in some hostel and made me to run away from their home.

When asked about differences between orphaned and non-orphaned children, respondents said the orphaned children were thought of and treated as different than others in the household:

> Within the family, an orphaned child is special, not supposed to get tired, have no privileges, orphans get less food because they have no rights, he/she cannot complain when work is assigned.

The responses were similar in nature regardless of the country. While the questions posed were hypothetical questions (rather than reported experiences), they reflect the attitudes and observations of influential stakeholders in communities caring for orphaned children. The shared agreement of these views indicates that stigma toward and differential treatment (including abuse) of orphaned children may be common practice as it often was historically worldwide. These findings help elucidate why maltreatment has been observed in family-based care as or more frequently as it is in institution-based care. Furthermore, stigma is known to be associated with poor outcomes such as depressive symptoms and difficulties with peer relationships (Campbell et al., 2014; Chi et al., 2014).

4.6 Asking Different Questions

It is important to discuss how the findings described here differ from other findings highlighting maltreatment in institutions. The two most commonly cited studies on institutional care are the Bucharest Early Intervention Project (BEIP) and the

English and Romanian Adoptees (ERA). BEIP was a randomized trial of Romanian orphans living in orphanages known for severe abuse and neglect. Children were randomly assigned to remain in institutional care or moved to foster care; an additional never-institutionalized group was also followed. Results from the trial showed worse cognitive development, physical growth, emotional functioning, attachment, and neural development among the children who remained in the institutions compared to those moved to foster care or those who were never institutionalized (Drury, Gleason et al., 2012; Drury, Theall et al., 2012; McGoron et al., 2012; Merz, McCall, & Groza, 2013; Nelson et al., 2007). The English and Romanian Adoptees (ERA) study similarly examined outcomes of children reared in Romanian orphanages (described as ranging from "poor to abysmal") (Rutter et al., 2007) but adopted into families in the United Kingdom (UK). To control for the possible effects of adoption, the comparison group was UK children adopted into UK families. Several studies of this population showed that cognitive outcomes, attachment formations, and neurological imaging were worse in the Romanian adoptees who experienced severe institutional deprivation than the UK adoptees who experienced no deprivation and that longer duration of deprivation yielded worse outcomes (Beckett et al., 2006; Mehta et al., 2009; O'Connor et al., 2003; Rutter et al., 2007). Importantly, the BEIP and ERA studies were primarily focused on early deprivation beginning in infancy. Both the BEIP trial and the ERA study were seminal in their documentation of the effects of early deprivation, as well as in the possibility for improvement when young children were placed into better care.

Importantly, however, neither the BEIP nor the ERA reflected random samples of institutions or institutions representing the range of conditions observed in current institutional orphan care. Thus, the conclusions of these studies are limited to Romanian children who as infants entered orphanages known for severe deprivation. The BEIP compared children remaining in settings known for their severe deprivation to those transitioned to families who were vetted by the BEIP personnel and supported by trained social workers who had weekly consults for the life of the project with experienced psychologists. Broadly, the BEIP studies were designed to answer the question "Can we improve the trajectory of children exposed to terrible deprivation during infancy if they are moved into families supported by trained social workers, as compared to children left in deprived environments?"

The ERA study compared the Romanian orphans adopted into families in the United Kingdom to UK children adopted into UK families. The UK children were all infants under 6 months; the Romanian children were ages up to 42 months. Presumably, any linguistic adjustments for the older Romanian children who would be shifting languages were accounted for in cognitive assessments. Since both groups had experienced adoption, poor outcomes were attributed to the early deprivation experienced. While some of the ERA studies used age-stratified random sampling to select the Romanian adoptees, selection was still restricted to the severely deprived Bucharest institutions. Broadly, the ERA studies were designed to answer the question "If all children are adopted by UK families, are outcomes in Romanian children who experienced severe deprivation during infancy the same as UK children who did not experience deprivation during infancy?"

In contrast, the POFO study enumerated the institutions in six regions in five countries and then randomly sampled from among those institutions. Among the randomly sampled institutions, age-eligible (6–12 years at baseline) children were randomly sampled for inclusion in the study. Similarly, to identify a statistically representative sample of orphans living in family care in the same regions, 50 geographic clusters in each study region were defined, and study teams randomly sampled five households caring for orphans and selected the age-eligible child whose name came first alphabetically. Broadly, the POFO study was designed to answer the question "On average, are outcomes among orphaned children in institution-based care the same as outcomes among orphaned children in family-based care?"

The distinction in the questions is important because the question determines the inference that can be made. While the BEIP and ERA studies enable conclusions about trajectories after interventions following early severe deprivation in institutional care, compared to those who did not receive the intervention or to those who never experienced early deprivation, they do not enable conclusions about "average" institution-based care compared to "average" family-based care for orphans. The POFO study's design of random sampling of children within randomly sampled institutions and randomly sampled families does enable conclusions comparing the two settings. Importantly, the POFO study also focused on children ages 6–12, rather than on infants. While deprivation during infancy is particularly damaging, 95% of orphans are children over 5 years of age, not infants (UNICEF, 2008). The aforementioned meta-analysis on institutional care also noted that institutional care at later ages was less important for IQ differences than institutional care during infancy (van IJzendoorn, Luijk, & Juffer, et. al., 2008).

5 The Role of Institutions: One Size Does Not Fit All

In summary, empirical evidence elucidates several important considerations in the care of orphans. First, LMICs have the greatest number of orphans and greatest need for care solutions. Second, emerging evidence from studies designed to compare settings indicates so far that institution-based care is no worse than family-based care in terms of physical and mental health outcomes for orphans in LMICs and that while maltreatment is prevalent in both settings, it is somewhat higher in family-based care than in institution-based care. Third, prevention of child-headed households and child trafficking is critical. Fourth, educational access is essential. Fifth, families in LMICs are increasingly overextended economically and emotionally because of the orphan crisis. Sixth, and finally, stigma of orphans in LMICs is severe and contributes to acceptability of orphan maltreatment.

While the setting of care (institution vs. family) does not seem to influence outcomes, the care received does matter. At least two studies, one in St. Petersburg, Russia, and one in Tanzania, have conducted trials to assess the effects of caregiver training on outcomes among orphans in institutions (Hermenau, Kaltenbach, Mkinga, & Hecker, 2015; McCall et al., 2013). In the St. Petersburg study, caregivers and children were randomly assigned to groups in which the caregiver was provided training (or not). Results indicated sustained, long-term improvement in outcomes among children assigned to caregivers who had received caregiver training, compared to children whose caregivers received no training, suggesting the possibility for improvement in caregiving. Similarly, the Tanzania study trained caregivers in an institution by emphasizing the importance of the child-caregiver relationship, strategies for handling poor behavior, and detriments of corporal punishment; they compared child outcomes over time, and reports of maltreatment dropped significantly from baseline.

Better understanding of the varieties of group care and institutions is needed. The structure, organization, and daily routine, among other predictors, may be essential in understanding what quality care looks like in institutions that create positive outcomes for orphans. Different structures may be beneficial to different children, depending on their histories, needs, or other predictors. These factors remain unstudied.

Among the critical factors for many orphans is separation from siblings. Gong et al. (2009) showed that sibling separation resulted in substantial anxiety, anger, and depression among orphans in both group care and family care (Gong et al., 2009). Keeping siblings together should be a key consideration in placement of orphans within family or institutional care.

The essential elements of quality caregiving also need more research, for both institution- and family-based care. Characteristics of caregivers who influence positive trajectories for orphans can inform both appropriate hiring in institution-based care and placement in family-based care. Given the findings that much of the variation in child outcomes in the POFO study was determined by individual differences (Whetten et al., 2014), it would be prudent to know whether specific caregiver characteristics were more or less helpful to children with specific characteristics. Such knowledge would inform strategies for caregivers in both institutional and family settings.

Quality orphan care additionally requires addressing the substantial trauma most orphans have faced; recent trauma-focused cognitive-based therapy interventions have indicated promising results (Murray et al., 2014; O'Donnell et al., 2014). These interventions would be appropriate for orphans in all care settings.

Support of families where reintegration with a biological parent or family fostering occurs is essential. Caregivers report substantial burden in caring for orphans, but at least one study documented that caregivers who are in a support group report more positive feelings toward the children for whom they are caring as well as less social marginalization and better family functioning (Thurman, Jarabi, & Rice, 2012). Such support programs may also contribute to reducing stigma and could potentially be augmented to directly address orphan stigma. As indicated in the Heymann study (2007), family support includes identifying workplace policies and conditions that facilitate caregivers being available to children with health needs.

Finally, models that allow children to have the safety and support of a group home or institution while simultaneously having interaction with their parents or living relatives need to be explored. The need for institution-based care often arises from severe economic constraints or inability of parents to properly care for their children. Integrated models that leverage the stability of an institution with the opportunity to experience at least some of the emotional support of a parent need to be tested.

6 Summary

World leaders and policymakers agree that, by definition, children are vulnerable and that it is a global imperative to ensure their basic rights are met, including the rights to education and protection from abuse. These rights have been most recently formalized in the 1989 Convention on the Rights of the Child. Further, the growing orphan crisis has warranted global attention to providing quality care options for orphaned or separated children (OSC) to safeguard their rights and their futures. LMICs in sub-Saharan Africa and South Asia are home to two-thirds of the world's orphans. In LMICs, evidence from a large longitudinal cohort of orphans, designed using two-stage random sampling to be statistically representative of both institution-based and family-based orphan populations, has shown no differences in well-being between orphans in institution-based and family-based care settings. These findings hold for numerous outcomes, including physical health, emotional well-being, cognitive functioning, and maltreatment (physical or sexual abuse).

These findings in the POFO study are consistent with other studies in LMICs. Context is critical: existing poverty, combined with wars, disease epidemics, and social upheaval, makes extended family care extremely difficult. Orphan caregiving strains the family economy as well as the caregiver's ability to earn additional family income and provide support for the orphan and the other children in the household. Stigma of orphans is entrenched, even among well-meaning community members. What is needed is a variety of care options and substantial resources to support placing each child in the most optimal environment, in recognition of the fact that the ideal (living with one or both parents in a loving, stable environment), by definition, often cannot happen. Support for caregivers and support for and monitoring of continued education in all placements are also critical, as is attention to trauma and stigma faced by orphans and strategies for alleviating both over time.

Questions for Discussion

1. What are some of the advantages and disadvantages of a country-level deinstitutionalization policy?
2. If you were tasked with developing orphan care policy for a low-income country, what would you want to know to create quality care options?
3. How would you develop a program to support families fostering orphaned children (relatives or other children)? How would you focus limited resources to provide that support?

References

Aries, P. (1962). *Centuries of Childhood. A Social History of Family Life, translated from French by Robert Baldick.* Jonathan Cape, Ltd.

Beckett, C., Maughan, B., Rutter, M., Castle, J., Colvert, E., Groothues, C., ... Sonuga-Barke, E. J. (2006). Do the effects of early severe deprivation on cognition persist into early adolescence? Findings from the English and Romanian adoptees study. *Child Development, 77*(3), 696–711. doi: 10.1111/j.1467-8624.2006.00898.x.

Berens, A. E., & Nelson, C. A. (2015). The science of early adversity: Is there a role for large institutions in the care of vulnerable children? *Lancet, 386*(9991), 388–398. doi:10.1016/S0140-6736(14)61131-4.

Berkman, L. F. (2000). Social support, social networks, social cohesion and health. *Social Work in Health Care, 31*(2), 3–14. doi:10.1300/J010v31n02_02.

Berkman, L. F., & Syme, S. L. (1979). Social networks, host resistance, and mortality: A nine-year follow-up study of Alameda County residents. *American Journal of Epidemiology, 109*(2), 186–204.

Blagborough, J. (2008). Child domestic labor: A modern form of slavery. *Children and Society, 22*(3), 179–190.

Campbell, C., Andersen, L., Mutsikiwa, A., Madanhire, C., Skovdal, M., Nyamukapa, C., & Gregson, S. (2014). Children's representations of school support for HIV-affected peers in rural Zimbabwe. *BMC Public Health, 14*(1), 402. doi: 1471-2458-14-402 [pii]10.1186/1471-2458-14-402.

Chi, P., Li, X., Zhao, J., & Zhao, G. (2014). Vicious circle of perceived stigma, enacted stigma and depressive symptoms among children affected by HIV/AIDS in China. *AIDS and Behavior, 18*(6), 1054–1062. doi:10.1007/s10461-013-0649-z.

Cluver, L. D., Gardner, F., & Operario, D. (2008). Effects of stigma on the mental health of adolescents orphaned by AIDS. *Journal of Adolescent Health, 42*(4), 410–417. doi:10.1016/j.jadohealth.2007.09.022S1054-139X(07)00421-1. [pii].

Cunningham, H. (1995). *Children and childhood in western society since 1500*. London, UK: Longman.

Dalen, N., Nakitende, A. J., & Musisi, S. (2009). "They don't care what happens to us." The situation of double orphans heading households in Rakai District, Uganda. *BMC Public Health, 9*, 321. doi:10.1186/1471-2458-9-321.

Daniel, M., & Mathias, A. (2012). Challenges and coping strategies of orphaned children in Tanzania who are not adequately cared for by adults. *African Journal of AIDS Research, 11*(3), 191–201. doi:10.2989/16085906.2012.734978.

Delis, D. C., Kramer, J. H., Kaplan, E., & Ober, B. A. (1987). *California verbal learning test (CVLT)*. San Antonio, TX: Psychological Corporation.

Drury, S. S., Gleason, M. M., Theall, K. P., Smyke, A. T., Nelson, C. A., Fox, N. A., & Zeanah, C. H. (2012b). Genetic sensitivity to the caregiving context: The influence of 5httlpr and BDNF val66met on indiscriminate social behavior. *Physiology Behavior, 106*(5), 728–735. doi: 10.1016/j.physbeh.2011.11.014.

Drury, S. S., Theall, K., Gleason, M. M., Smyke, A. T., De Vivo, I., Wong, J. Y., ... Nelson, C. A. (2012a). Telomere length and early severe social deprivation: Linking early adversity and cellular aging. *Molecular Psychiatry, 17*(7), 719–727. doi: 10.1038/mp.2011.53.

Elhai, J. D., Gray, M. J., Kashdan, T. B., & Franklin, C. L. (2005). Which instruments are most commonly used to assess traumatic event exposure and posttraumatic effects?: A survey of traumatic stress professionals. *Journal of Traumatic Stress, 18*(5), 541–545. doi:10.1002/jts.20062.

Embleton, L., Ayuku, D., Kamanda, A., Atwoli, L., Ayaya, S., Vreeman, R., ... Braitstein, P. (2014). Models of care for orphaned and separated children and upholding children's rights: Cross-sectional evidence from western Kenya. *BMC International Health and Human Rights, 14*, 9. doi: 10.1186/1472-698X-14-9.

Evans, R. (2005). Social networks, migration, and care in Tanzania: Caregivers' and children's resilience to coping with HIV/AIDS. *Journal of Children and Poverty*, *11*(2), 111–129.

Fass, P. (2011). A historical context for the United Nations Convention on the rights of the child. *The Annals of the American Academy of Political and Social Science*, *633*(1), 17–29.

Gong, J., Li, X., Fang, X., Zhao, G., Lv, Y., Zhao, J., ... Stanton, B. (2009). Sibling separation and psychological problems of double AIDS orphans in rural China – A comparison analysis. *Child: Care, Health and Development, 35*(4), 534–541. doi: 10.1111/j.1365-2214.2009.00969.xCCH969 [pii].

Goodman, R. (1999). The extended version of the strengths and difficulties questionnaire as a guide to child psychiatric caseness and consequent burden. *Journal of Child Psychology and Psychiatry, 40*(5), 791–799.

Goodman, R., Meltzer, H., & Bailey, V. (1998). The strengths and difficulties questionnaire: A pilot study on the validity of the self-report version. *European Child & Adolescent Psychiatry*, *7*(3), 125–130.

Gray, C. L., Pence, B. W., Ostermann, J., Whetten, R. A., O'Donnell, K., Thielman, N. M., & Whetten, K. (2015a). Gender (in) differences in prevalence and incidence of traumatic experiences among orphaned and separated children living in five low- and middle-income countries. *Global Mental Health. 2015; 2*(3):1–11

Gray, C. L., Pence, B. W., Ostermann, J., Whetten, R. A., O'Donnell, K., Thielman, N. M., & Whetten, K. (2015b). Prevalence and incidence of traumatic experiences among orphans in institutional and family-based settings in 5 low- and middle-income countries: A longitudinal study. *Global Health: Science and Practice.*, *3*(3), 395–404. doi:10.9745/GHSP-D-15-00093.

Gray, M. J., Litz, B. T., Hsu, J. L., & Lombardo, T. W. (2004). Psychometric properties of the life events checklist. *Assessment, 11*(4), 330–341. doi: 11/4/330 [pii]10.1177/1073191104269954.

Hacsi, T. (1995). From indenture to family foster care: A brief history of child placing. *Child Welfare*, *74*(1), 162–180.

Hacsi, T. (1997). *Second home: Orphan asylums and poor families in America*. Cambridge, MA: Harvard University Press.

Hermenau, K., Kaltenbach, E., Mkinga, G., & Hecker, T. (2015). Improving care quality and preventing maltreatment in institutional care – A feasibility study with caregivers. *Frontiers in Psychology*, *6*, 937. doi:10.3389/fpsyg.2015.00937.

Heymann, J., Earle, A., Rajaraman, D., Miller, C., & Bogen, K. (2007). Extended family caring for children orphaned by AIDS: Balancing essential work and caregiving in a high HIV prevalence nations. *AIDS Care*, *19*(3), 337–345. doi:10.1080/09540120600763225.

Hsiung, P. (2007). *A tender voyage: Children & childhood in late imperial China*. Stanford, CA: Stanford University Press.

van IJzendoorn, M. H., Luijk, M. P. C. M., & Juffer, F. (2008). IQ of children growing up in children's homes: A meta-analysis on IQ delays in orphanages. *Merrill-Palmer Quarterly*, *54*, 341–356.

James, A., Jenks, C., & Prout, A. (1998). One child or many? In *Theorizing childhood* (pp. 124–145). Cambridge, United Kingdom: Polity Press.

Johnson, J., Rolph, S., & Smith, R. (2012). *Residential care transformed: Revisiting 'the last refuge'*. Basingstoke, UK: Palgrave MacMillan.

Kakar, S. (1979). *Indian childhood: Cultural ideals and social reality*. New Delhi, India: Oxford University Press (Oxford India Paperbacks).

Kapur, M. (2015). *Psychological perspectives on childcare in Indian indigenous health systems*. New Delhi, India: Springer.

Kaufman, A., & Kaufman, N. (2004). *Kaufman assessment battery for children* (2nd ed.). Circle Pines, MN: American Guidance Services Publishing.

Kidman, R., & Thurman, T. R. (2014). Caregiver burden among adults caring for orphaned children in rural South Africa. *Vulnerable Child and Youth Studies*, *9*(3), 234–246. doi:10.1080/17450128.2013.871379.

Koda, B. (2000). Democratisation of social relationship at the household level: The participation of children and youth in Tanzania. In C. Creighton & C. Omari (Eds.), *Gender, family, and work in Tanzania*. London, UK: Ashgate.

Lancy, D. (2015). *The anthropology of childhood cherubs, chattel, and changelings* (2nd ed.). Cambridge, UK: Cambridge University Press.

Lifton, B. (2006). *The king of children: The life and death of Janusz Korczak*. United States of America: American Academy of Pediatrics.

Locke, J. (1693/1995). *An essay concerning human understanding (great books in philosophy)*. Prometheus Books.

Madhavan, S. (2004). Fosterage patterns in the age of AIDS: Continuity and change. *Social Science & Medicine*, *58*(7), 1443–1454. doi:10.1016/S0277-9536(03)00341-1.

McCall, R. B., Groark, C. J., Fish, L., Muhamedrahimov, R. J., Palmov, O. I., & Nikiforova, N. V. (2013). Maintaining a social-emotional intervention and its benefits for institutionalized children. *Child Development*, *84*(5), 1734–1749. doi:10.1111/cdev.12098.

McGoron, L., Gleason, M. M., Smyke, A. T., Drury, S. S., Nelson 3rd, C. A., Gregas, M. C., ... Zeanah, C. H. (2012). Recovering from early deprivation: Attachment mediates effects of caregiving on psychopathology. *Journal of the American Academy of Child and Adolescent Psychiatry, 51*(7), 683–693. doi: 10.1016/j.jaac.2012.05.004.

McKenzie, R. B. (1997). Orphanage alumni: How they have done and how they evaluate their experience. *Child and Youth Care Forum*, *26*(2), 87–111.

Mehta, M. A., Golembo, N. I., Nosarti, C., Colvert, E., Mota, A., Williams, S. C., ... Sonuga-Barke, E. J. (2009). Amygdala, hippocampal and corpus callosum size following severe early institutional deprivation: The English and Romanian adoptees study pilot. *Journal of Child Psychology and Psychiatry, 50*(8), 943–951. doi: 10.1111/j.1469-7610.2009.02084.x.

Merz, E. C., McCall, R. B., & Groza, V. (2013). Parent-reported executive functioning in postinstitutionalized children: A follow-up study. *Journal of Clinical Child & Adolescent Psychology*, *42*(5), 726–733. doi:10.1080/15374416.2013.764826.

Moody, Z. (2015). The United Nations declaration of the rights of the child (1959): Genesis, transformation and dissemination of a treaty (re)constituting a transnational cause. *Prospects*, *45*, 15–29.

Mulley, C. (2010). *The woman who saved the children: A biography of Eglantyne Jebb: Founder of save the children*. Oxford, England: Oneworld Publications.

Murray, L. K., Skavenski, S., Michalopoulos, L. M., Bolton, P. A., Bass, J. K., Familiar, I., ... Cohen, J. (2014). Counselor and client perspectives of trauma-focused cognitive behavioral therapy for children in Zambia: A qualitative study. *Journal of Clinical Child and Adolescent Psychology, 43*(6), 902–914. doi: 10.1080/15374416.2013.859079.

Nelson 3rd, C. A., Zeanah, C. H., Fox, N. A., Marshall, P. J., Smyke, A. T., & Guthrie, D. (2007). Cognitive recovery in socially deprived young children: The Bucharest early intervention project. *Science*, *318*(5858), 1937–1940. doi:10.1126/science.1143921.

O'Connor, T. G., Marvin, R. S., Rutter, M., Olrick, J. T., Britner, P. A., & English & Romanian Adoptees Study, T. (2003). Child-parent attachment following early institutional deprivation. *Development and Psychopathology*, *15*(1), 19–38.

O'Donnell, K., Dorsey, S., Gong, W., Ostermann, J., Whetten, R., Cohen, J. A., ... Whetten, K. (2014). Treating maladaptive grief and posttraumatic stress symptoms in orphaned children in Tanzania: Group-based trauma-focused cognitive-behavioral therapy. *Journal of Traumatic Stress, 27*(6), 664–671. doi: 10.1002/jts.21970.

Ochanda, R., Akinyi, V., & Wakinya, K. (2011). *A handbook for the organisations working to counter trafficking of women and children in East Africa: A human rights-based approach to trafficking*. Mombassa, Kenya: Koinonia Advisory Research and Development Services.

Orme, N. (2003). *Medievil children*. New Haven, CT/London, UK: Yale University Press.

Prince, M., Patel, V., Saxena, S., Maj, M., Maselko, J., Phillips, M. R., & Rahman, A. (2007). No health without mental health. *Lancet*, *370*(9590), 859–877. doi:10.1016/S0140-6736(07)61238-0.

Rutter, M., Beckett, C., Castle, J., Colvert, E., Kreppner, J., Mehta, M., ... Songua-Barke, E. (2007). Effects of profound early institutional deprivation: An overview of findings from a UK longitudinal study of Romania adoptees. *European Jouarnal of Developmental Psychology*, *4*(3), 332–350.

SaveTheChildren. (2009). *Keeping children out of harmful institutions: Why we should be investing in family-based care?* .Retrieved from http://www.savethechildren.org.uk/sites/default/files/docs/Keeping_Children_Out_of_Harmful_Institutions_Final_20.11.09_1.pdf. Accessed 28 May 2016.

Sharma, B. (2015). Revisiting the United Nations' 1951 convention relating to the status of refugees: A critical analysis of the international refugee law. *Social Development Issues*, *37*(2), 80–94.

Thurman, T. R., Jarabi, B., & Rice, J. (2012). Caring for the caregiver: Evaluation of support groups for guardians of orphans and vulnerable children in Kenya. *AIDS Care*, *24*(7), 811–819. doi:10.1080/09540121.2011.644229.

UNICEF. (2004). *Children on the brink 2004*. Retrieved from http://www.unicef.org/publications/cob_layout6-013.pdf. Accessed 25 June 2015.

UNICEF. (2006). *State of the world's children 2006: Excluded and invisible New York*. Retrieved from http://www.unicef.org/sowc06/pdfs/sowc06_fullreport.pdf. Accessed 25 June 2015.

UNICEF. (2008). *Orphans*. Retrieved from http://www.unicef.org/media/media_45279.html. Accessed 31 May 2016.

UNICEF. (2013). *State of the world's children 2013: Children with disabilities*. Retrieved from http://www.unicef.org/sowc2013/files/SWCR2013_ENG_Lo_res_24_Apr_2013.pdf. Accessed 17 May 2016.

Whetten, K., Ostermann, J., Pence, B. W., Whetten, R. A., Messer, L. C., Ariely, S., … Positive Outcomes for Orphans Research, T. (2014). Three-year change in the wellbeing of orphaned and separated children in institutional and family-based care settings in five low- and middle-income countries. *PloS One, 9*(8), e104872. doi: 10.1371/journal.pone.0104872.

Whetten, K., Ostermann, J., Whetten, R. A., Pence, B. W., O'Donnell, K., Messer, L. C., & Thielman, N. M. (2009). A comparison of the wellbeing of orphans and abandoned children ages 6–12 in institutional and community-based care settings in 5 less wealthy nations. *PloS One*, *4*(12), e8169. doi:10.1371/journal.pone.0008169.

Whetten, R., Whetten, K., Rivenbark, J., Ostermann, J., Thielman, N., O'Donnell, K., Pearson, J., & The POFO Team. "My life would be worse than a street dog": A cross-cultural, qualitative inquiry of orphanhood and stigma. (Under Review)

White, E. (1944). *One man's meat*. New York, NY: Harper and Brothers.

Wiredu, K. (1992). The African concept of personhood. In H. Flack & E. Pellegrino (Eds.), *African-American perspectives on biomedical ethics*. Washington, DC: Georgetown University Press.

Chapter 19
Institutional Care Environments for Infants and Young Children in Latin America and the Caribbean

Afton R. Kirk, Christina J. Groark, and Robert B. McCall

... in serving the best interests of children, we serve the best interests of all humanity. – Carol Bellamy.

(UNICEF, 2005)

1 Introduction

Care for infants and young children in Latin America and the Caribbean is difficult to assess. This chapter provides insights into the reasons for this difficulty as well as what is known about the quality of current care in institutions and its impact on the futures of children who reside there. In addition, recommendations are given for the improvement of care options that have been used in other low-resource countries similar to those in this region.

To understand the potential impact of the relative quality and characteristics of institutional care in Latin America and the Caribbean, it is important to understand the number of children in need of care and the number currently residing in institutional settings in the region. In 2013, 8.4 million children were identified as orphans in Latin America and the Caribbean (UNICEF, 2014). Children are considered to be orphans if they have lost one or both parents. Perhaps of more dire significance is the number of children considered to be double orphans (those who have lost both parents), which was approximately 600,000 in 2004 (The Joint United Nations

A.R. Kirk (✉) • C.J. Groark • R.B. McCall
University of Pittsburgh Office of Child Development,
400 N Lexington Street, Suite LL104, Pittsburgh, PA 15208, USA
e-mail: ark87@pitt.edu; cgroark@pitt.edu; mccall2@pitt.edu

A.V. Rus et al. (eds.), *Child Maltreatment in Residential Care*,
DOI 10.1007/978-3-319-57990-0_19

Programme on HIV/AIDS [UNAIDS], the United Nations Children's Fund [UNICEF], & the United States Agency for International Development [USAID], 2004). Although the need for care is obvious for children who have lost both parents, the potential need also exists for those with one parent remaining, as a substantial number of children in institutions have at least one living parent (estimated at 50–80% in countries outside of the region) (Engle et al., 2011).

Estimates of the number of children receiving care within institutional settings in Latin America (including the Caribbean in many, but not all, documents) range from more than 230,000 to almost 375,000 children (Better Care Network, 2013; RELAF & SOS Children's Villages International, 2010; UNICEF, 2013). The substantial range among estimates is partly associated with which countries keep records and how they define a resident of an institution (Groark, McCall, & Li, 2009). There are 33 nations within Latin America and the Caribbean, but only 27 provide such data (see Table 19.1) (UNICEF, 2013, 2014). Very young children (birth to 3, 4, or 5 years) are represented within those receiving institutional care, with estimates of 8–26 % when national data are available (UNICEF, 2013). According to the Latin American Foster Care Network (RELAF) and SOS Children's Villages International (2010), "there is a lack of reliable data and information relating to this subject" which poses a challenge to understanding the scope of issues relating to children receiving care in this region (p. 13). Table 19.1 demonstrates this challenge as can be seen by the wide discrepancy in numbers depending on data sources. Additionally, it is apparent that the sources are typically organizations that may have a bias in which numbers are selected due to their advocacy missions.

This landscape of institutional care in the region requires a discussion of the quality of care within these institutional environments, the possible reasons children require this type of care, and the potential changes in policy and regulation that influence how children are cared for outside of parental care. These issues provide the rationale to improve the institutions themselves as well as the overall system of care for all children within the region. Although institutional care in these countries may differ in some ways, common depriving characteristics of most traditional institutions across the globe are associated with poor outcomes for children. Thus, improvements need to be made, and we offer suggestions for practice, policy, research, and evaluation to help better support the children requiring care in the Latin American and Caribbean region.

Goals of this chapter will be to discuss:

1. The current happenings within the child welfare space within the region, including potential reasons children require institutional care, recent policy and campaign initiatives that will likely impact future regulations and practice, and the empirical evidence that supports these recent initiatives. This section aims to provide an historical context for the research information.
2. Empirical investigations of institutional contexts in the region, the impact on children receiving this care, and the interventions aimed at improving these settings and child outcomes.

Table 19.1 Number of children in institutions in the region

Country (countries in the region are based on a 2014 UNICEF Report)	Number of children in institutions by country UNICEF (2013)	Number of children in institutions in Latin America by country (RELAF Project, the Latin American Foster Care Network, & SOS Children's Villages International, 2010, p. 16)
Antigua and Barbuda	–	–
Argentina	14,675	The UNICEF study "Deprived of Freedom" done in 2005 found a total of 17,063 children had been taken into care and placed in 642 state and nongovernmental institutions
Bahamas	–	–
Barbados	127	–
Belize	157	–
Bolivia	16,981	10,210 children in institutions, according to UNICEF in February 2010
Brazil	36,929	50,576 children in institutions
Chile	10,342	According to official data there were 12,229 children in institutions in the first quarter of 2010 to "protect their rights"
Colombia	12,925	Of the 38,000 children over the age of 7 in the care of protection agencies, 25,000 are institutionalized
Costa Rica	692	–
Cuba	–	–
Dominica	–	–
Dominican Republic	3030	3200 children below the age of 15 are institutionalized
Ecuador	3300	According to official figures for May 2010 there are 3000 children in nongovernmental institutions and 300 in state institutions
El Salvador	3095	10,042 children in institutions in 2006
Grenada	195	–
Guatemala	5566	5600 children in institutions
Guyana	700	–
Haiti	50,000	187,413 children in institutions
Honduras	12,032	3605 children in institutions
Jamaica	2572	–
Mexico	28,107	29,310 children living in 703 institutions.
Nicaragua	1874	2967 children institutionalized in 88 centers
Panama	2193	–
Paraguay	2573	5000 children in institutions
Peru	19,000	3982 children in institutions according to a CRC report (Initiative for Children) presented to the CRC in 2005
Saint Kitts and Nevis	–	–

(continued)

Table 19.1 (continued)

Country (countries in the region are based on a 2014 UNICEF Report)	Number of children in institutions by country UNICEF (2013)	Number of children in institutions in Latin America by country (RELAF Project, the Latin American Foster Care Network, & SOS Children's Villages International, 2010, p. 16)
Saint Lucia	40	–
Saint Vincent and the Grenadines	–	–
Suriname	3000	–
Trinidad and Tobago	658	–
Uruguay	3994	3273 children institutionalized in 2010–1189 in state institutions and 2084 in nongovernmental institutions
Venezuela	5000	Official figures report 1544 children living in institutions in 2007 (private institutions report a higher figure)
Total	239,757 in Latin America and the Caribbean	374,308 in Latin America

3. The rationale and practical suggestions for a comprehensive child welfare system of care, including a move to family-like options in the community.
4. The rationale and practical suggestions for research and evaluation of the system of care within the region for children without parental care.

2 The Current Landscape

2.1 Reasons for Risk of Losing Parental Care

Children are at risk for losing parental care in this region for a variety of political, economic, social, and cultural reasons (Latin American Foster Care Network [RELAF] and SOS Children's Villages International, 2010). Specifically these reasons include poverty, inequality, internal migration to improvised neighborhoods around large cities, difficulty accessing healthcare, the impact of HIV/AIDS (an estimated 720,000 children in the region were orphaned by AIDS in 2013, UNICEF, 2014), social violence, family breakdown, drug abuse, conflict with the law, domestic violence, child abuse, natural disasters, runaway adolescents, teenage pregnancy, child labor and exploitation, difficulty accessing education, and migration to other countries. RELAF and SOS Children's Villages International (2010) indicate that institutionalization has been the "main response" for children removed from and given up by their families. The institutions include family-type care with small numbers of children, "macroinstitutions" with hundreds of children, "foundling homes" for babies, and variations of these (p. 17). Often a child's mother and father are living but do not have the resources to care for the child, and currently institutionalization is the only option of care.

2.2 Policy and Campaign Initiatives at Play in the Region

A recent Call to Action that may impact the utilization and regulation of institutional care was launched in 2013 to "end the placement of children under three years of age in institutions" (Better Care Network, 2013; UNICEF, n.d., p. 1). This movement was led by the Inter-American Commission on Human Rights (IACHR), the Latin American and Caribbean Chapter of the Global Movement for Children (MMI-CLAC), the Latin American Foster Care Network (RELAF), the United Nations' Special Representative of the Secretary General on Violence Against Children, and UNICEF (UNICEF, n.d.; Better Care Network, 2013). The Call to Action identifies the need to end institutionalization of all children in the region, but in particular those birth to 3 years of age based on the damaging effects that can be caused by institutionalization during the early years of children's development. Aligned with this goal, a communication campaign, Speak Up for Me, was also launched in 2013 (Better Care Network, 2013; RELAF, n.d.). The situation of the region as described by the campaign's website:

- *In the majority of countries in Latin America and the Caribbean there is a disproportionate use of institutionalization observed in children below the age of three, despite the fact that it should be used as a means of last resort.*
- *The little data available shows that this is a serious problem: it is estimated that more than 240,000 girls, boys and adolescents are living in institutions. Amongst them, the most vulnerable are children under three years old.*
- *An early and prolonged institutionalization has serious effects, above all on the youngest children; the cognitive and emotional damage caused by the time spent in an institution can be irreversible.*
  - *Each year a young child spends in an institution, he or she loses four months of development.*
  - *Violence in residential care institutions is six times more frequent than in family based care.*
  - *Sexual violence is four times more frequent than in family based care.*

(speakupforme.org; Inter-American Commission on Human Rights, Latin American and Caribbean Movement for Children, RELAF, Special Representative of the Secretary General on Violence against Children, and UNICEF, n.d.)

The Speak Up for Me campaign calls for states to carry out actions to achieve the goal, including (1) approving legislation to limit the institutional placement of children under 3; (2) providing financial and technical resources to protect children and support families; (3) establishing programs and measures to reunite children with their families or for placement in foster or permanent care environments; (4) developing standards and protocols to prevent family separation; (5) employing public awareness campaigns; and (6) establishing monitoring and evaluation systems for institutions and programs that continue to operate (speakupforme.org). According to RELAF and UNICEF (2013) and RELAF's Technical Cooperation website (relaf.org; RELAF, n.d.), a number of countries in the region have begun this process by introducing a variety of pilot programs, initiatives, events, presentations, and technical workshops in support of alternative care settings and deinstitutionalization, both collectively as a region and within individual countries.

Though the process of deinstitutionalization has been initiated within the region, the numbers of young children who remain in institutional care remain quite large. Although it is difficult to obtain information on the number of children according to age from the aggregate national data in the region, information that is available identifies 26% of children in institutions in Argentina between the ages birth and 5; 25% in institutions in Brazil are between the ages of birth and 5; 12% and 17%, respectively, for children 0–4 years in Guatemala and Panama; and Chile and Uruguay each with 8% of their institutionalized children ages 0–3 years (UNICEF, 2013). The large number of very young children residing in institutions gives rise to the region's Call to Action, which appeals for an end of the institutionalization of very young children based on the detrimental effects of these environments, and the great potential for better quality of care within alternative care arrangements.

2.3 *Empirical Support for Current Initiatives in the Region*

A large body of empirical work supports the goal to end early childhood institutionalization in the region. One component of this work describes the quality and impact of the institutional environments. Although there is variation across institutional settings, there are often common characteristics that can be observed in institutions for infants and young children across the world (Rosas & McCall, 2011; Van IJzendoorn et al., 2011). These common characteristics include (1) large group sizes (9–17 per ward, but up to 70) and a large number of children per caregiver (8:1–31:1, although some have smaller ratios); (2) homogeneity of age and disability status within groups, with children periodically "graduated" to groups based on age; (3) constant changing of caregivers for each child (based on staff turnover and/or discontinuous group assignments and staff scheduling, long shifts with days off in between); (4) children exposed to other inconsistent adults (e.g., volunteers, prospective adoptive parents, medical and behavioral professionals); (5) caregivers with little training, especially on social interaction, and who are largely focused on the routine care of bathing, changing, feeding, and cleaning; and (6) caregivers with a "business-like manner" and a lack of sensitivity, responsivity, and warmth toward the children in their care.

These features are characteristics of *psychosocially depriving* settings, with medical care, nutrition, safety, and sanitation generally acceptable but with caregiver-child interactions being largely deficient (Gunnar, 2001). Settings that are also deficient in medical care, nutrition, safety, and sanitation are considered to be *globally depriving* settings, characteristic of the Romanian orphanages in the early 1990s. However, most institutional environments today do not fall into the category of those globally depriving but can be considered to be psychosocially depriving to at least some degree (McCall, 2011). (See Sect. 3 for a discussion of conditions and care specific to institutions examined in Latin America, which illustrate many of these common characteristics.)

Institutions that have the described common features, while still supporting children's most basic physical needs, lead to a myriad of negative effects for children and their development. Research from around the world indicates that children who are cared for within institutional settings often show substantial delays in cognitive, social-emotional, behavioral, and physical development (Bakermans-Kranenburg et al., 2011; Dobrova-Krol, Van IJzendoorn, Bakermans-Kranenburg, Cyr, & Juffer, 2008; Engle et al., 2007; Gunnar, 2001; Johnson & Gunnar, 2011; Johnson et al., 2010; Smyke et al., 2007; The St. Petersburg-USA Orphanage Research Team, 2008). Children within institutional care are, on average, more than one standard deviation below children who are not institutionalized with regard to their development within each of these domains and also have disturbances in attachment (Rosas & McCall, 2011; Van IJzendoorn et al., 2011). However, as reflected in the Call to Action, institutional environments can put children at early ages at higher risk of longer-term problems dependent on the length of time spent within the institution and the quality of care that is provided. Research on the effects of early institutionalization on later development after children are transitioned to adoptive or foster family care shows that generally the longer the child is in the institution, the greater the likelihood of persistent mental and behavioral problems. But how long is too long in the institution depends on the severity of the institutional environment. In the globally depriving 1990s Romanian orphanages, children adopted after only 6 months had higher rates of longer-term problems; those adopted from the socially-emotionally depriving institutions of Russia had higher rates of longer-term problems after 18 months, and children adopted from the better orphanages of South Korea and China had higher rates of longer-term problems after 24–27 months (McCall, 2013). Many researchers and advocates argue that any deficiency of stable relationships and cognitive stimulation early in the lives of very young children has the potential to disrupt the typical trajectory of children's development.

Empirical research on institutional versus family care is generally consistent. When compared to institutional settings, children do better in family-like settings (including adoptive, foster, and other family-type settings) (The Leiden Conference on the Development and Care of Children without Permanent Parents, 2012). Family settings are more likely to provide sensitive and responsive caregiving from a few consistent caregivers, more cognitive stimulation, and few other children. However, because options do not currently exist for all children to have stable care outside of the institutional setting in the region, and because challenges exist for the development of these more preferable options, improving the conditions and care within institutional environments may be a more practical option at least initially. The following provides a discussion of conditions, care, and child characteristics from empirical examinations particular to Latin America providing rationale for both deinstitutionalization and the essential improvement of remaining institutions specific to this region.

3 Empirical Research, Intervention, and Evaluation in the Region

Generally, research and reports on institutions in Latin America suggest they are similar to traditional institutions in other countries in providing environments that are socially-emotionally depriving. Further, interventions in Latin American institutions have been similar to those elsewhere in attempting to improve the quality of caregiver-child interactions, and they have shown similar effects. This material provides insight into areas of strengths, gaps, and successes that could inform future provision of resources and interventions for the improvement of this region's institutional care environments.

3.1 Characteristics of Institutional Care Settings in Latin America

According to Groark, McCall, Fish, and The Whole Child International Evaluation Team (Groark, McCall, & Fish, 2011), very few empirical examinations have reported the nature of the institutional environment, and this is especially true of institutions in Latin America. What follows are empirical descriptions of a few institutions' organizational structure, overall environment, and caregiver-child interactions as well as children's general behavioral development and problem behaviors. Because of the very small number of institutions involved, generalization to institutions across Latin America is tenuous.

3.1.1 Structural Characteristics

In perhaps the most comprehensive empirical study available, Groark et al. (2011) assessed three somewhat different Central American orphanages. They had groups of 8–10 children, 11–23 children, and up to 50 infants in a single room, with child-caregiver ratios of 8:1–12:1 plus aides (who focused largely on cleaning and serving food). Caregivers worked long shifts (24 continuous hours or 24 h split into two segments often with days off in between shifts). Staff turnover was described as relatively low, but inconsistency in caregiving was produced by sporadic caregiver schedules, frequent substitute caregivers, and periodic "graduations" of children to age-based wards with new caregivers and peers. Because children in these institutions would interact with 6–9 (or more) caregivers over 1 or 2 days, "there is little opportunity to develop a relationship of any kind or even learn consistent consequences to social overtures" (Groark et al., 2011, p. 245). This characteristic is one indication of the institution being *psychosocially depriving*, with caregiver-child interactions being largely deficient based on a lack of continuity and stability in caregiver schedules (McCall, 2011).

3.1.2 The Caregiving Environment

The caregiving environment was assessed within these institutions utilizing the Infant/Toddler Environment Rating Scale (ITERS; Harms, Cryer, & Clifford, 2006), the Early Childhood Environment Rating Scale (ECERS; Harms, Clifford, & Cryer, 2005), and the Caregiver-Child Social-Emotional Relationship Rating Scale (CCSERRS; McCall et al., 2010a).

The ITERS and ECERS assessments measure the quality of the caregiving environment within early care and education environments in the United States. Two of the Central American institutions produced an average ITERS/ECERS score of 1.62, where the highest possible score is 7 and where average scores in US early care and education and Head Start centers are 4.3 and 4.9, respectively, in Pennsylvania in 2002. According to Groark et al. (2011):

> In short, these scores reflect the fact that these wards, while clean, are exceedingly basic in construction with minimum repair of damages, have very limited furniture of any kind, have very few toys which are available only at specified play times, and have a limited organized program of activities other than routine care. Staff receive some administrative and supervisory support, and caregivers talk and listen to children and occasionally display warmth and affection to them, but most interaction occurs during routine caregiving activities. (p. 239)

Another measure employed, the CCSERRS, was designed specifically to assess caregiver-child interactions within the institutional environment. Outcomes on the measure were similar across the three institutions and illustrated that "while caregivers do not express much negative emotion or punishment, neither do they provide much positive affect or affection, they are not particularly animated or expressive, and there is not much caregiver–child interaction" (Groark et al., 2011, p. 241). In addition to the instability of caregivers for children and the large number of children per caregiver, these characteristics constitute a *psychosocially depriving environment*; children's very basic physical needs are adequately met, but their psychological and social needs are not.

3.1.3 Child Development Characteristics

Children's development was assessed within the three Central American institutions described above utilizing the Battelle Developmental Inventory (BDI; Newborg, 2005) and the Children's Problem Behavior Scale (CPBS; Groark et al., 2011). The latter instrument was developed by the authors based on the Child Behavior Checklist (CBCL; Achenbach & Rescorla, 2000), the Infant-Toddler Social-Emotional Assessment (ITSEA; Briggs-Gowan & Carter, 2001), and the authors' experience regarding institutional environments. These assessments of children within the three institutions described above produced mean developmental quotients (DQ) of 58–63, which are approximately two standard deviations below what would be expected of US parent-reared children. The institutionalized children exhibited more indiscriminate friendliness, noncompliance, provocative interpersonal behavior, and aggressive interpersonal violent behaviors than would otherwise be expected (Groark et al., 2011). These developmental characteristics align with the theoretical and conceptual notion that children who lack sensitive, responsive, and stable caregivers have poorer developmental outcomes, even when basic physical needs are adequately met (i.e., a psychosocially depriving environment).

In a separate examination of child characteristics specific to institutions in Chile (Lecannelier, Silva, Hoffmann, Melo, & Morales, 2014), children 2–12 months exhibited psychomotor development comparable to parent-reared children. This result seems to contradict other research on institutionalized children's development. It may be that the institutions in the study did not have time to exert a negative influence or psychomotor development is not influenced as much as other attributes, but the authors also called into question the psychomotor assessment's validity and reliability. More typical of previous findings, 53.2% of the institutionalized children exhibited insecure attachment and behaviors which were more typical of other institutionalized and post-institutionalized children and higher than for parent-reared Chilean children (Lecannelier et al., 2014).

Although these results are from a very few institutions for infants and young children, the characteristics of the institutions and the development of children residing in them are generally similar to empirical studies of institutionalized children from other countries. Some institutions provide very minimal physical facilities and few toys and equipment, but it is likely that the minimal caregiver-child interactions are associated with children's poor development while in residence (McCall, 2011; McCall & Groark, 2015).

3.2 *Intervention and Child Outcomes in Latin American Institutions*

A few separate interventions have been implemented in Latin American institutions, providing information on both the content of the interventions and the effects of these interventions on children's developmental functioning (Groark, McCall, McCarthy, Eichner, & Gee, 2013; Lecannelier et al., 2014; McCall, Groark, Fish, Harkins, Serrano, & Gordon, 2010).

3.2.1 A Social-Emotional Intervention in Chile

A 2-month social-emotional intervention for caregivers of very young children (2–12 months) was implemented in state-run child protection centers and one privately run center in Chile (Lecannelier et al., 2014). The intervention included a "parental sensitivity manual" which focused on the "development and promotion of skills, knowledge, and attitudes adequate to understanding, managing, and assessing the infant's competencies and development." This included basics of competently interacting with very young children (physical and visual contact and verbal interaction) and more complex elements of child engagement, temperament, and attachment (Lecannelier et al., 2014, p. 153). A 1 day face-to-face training on the manual content (including topic areas and activities) was provided to center caregivers, with weekly supervision provided by online, email, telephone, and face-to-face methods.

Although psychomotor development and attachment security were not shown to improve following the caregiver training intervention, significant improvement was observed for children's social orientation, object orientation, activity, and reactivity. Children who exhibited an insecure attachment versus those who had a secure attachment had the same level of performance on social and object orientation. It appears that these improvements in caregiver-child interactions provided additional stimulation to the infants and improved some aspects of their mental development, but perhaps this intervention did not last long enough and the children were not old enough to see effects on attachment. The authors also reasoned that the success of the intervention (particularly for the children with insecure attachment) may lie in the "use of a didactic, practical, comprehensible methodology organized in a manual adapted to the caregivers' sociocultural reality" as well as the optimization of care currently provided by the caregivers rather than imposing work demands external to typical caregiving activities (Lecannelier et al., 2014, p. 157). Based on its success, the intervention is now being implemented across Chile, and in addition this empirical study has become a potential catalyst for the gradual transition from institutionalization in early childhood to specialized foster family care.

3.2.2 A Social-Emotional Intervention in Two Latin American Institutions

An intervention designed and implemented by Whole Child International, a non-profit dedicated to improving institutional and early care, within a Latin American orphanage trained caregivers to provide sensitive and responsive care to children and supported them with technical assistance (observing and coaching) (McCall et al., 2010b). Training was provided 1 week per month for a 12-month period to caregivers of children birth to 8 years and technical assistance for caregivers of children birth to 3 years of age. In addition, structural changes were made, including employment and scheduling patterns for staff, scheduling of caregiving tasks, and the provision of new ward furniture and play materials. Four general principles guided these interventions:

1. Caregiving routines are an important time for interaction between adult and child.
2. Continuity of care is particularly important for children in institutions.
3. Children need freedom of movement to grow and learn.
4. Plentiful, safe, and developmentally appropriate materials must be accessible to children during their waking hours.

Results of the intervention illustrated that the overall caregiving environments as assessed with the ITERS/ECERS improved for both younger and older children's wards and for each individual ward within age groups. Caregiver-child interactions assessed with the CCSERRS showed (1) improvements across all interaction types for the younger age group, (2) improvements during feeding interactions for the older age group, and (3) a higher intervention effect size for the younger age group. This outcome could be expected based on the intervention's principal focus on the birth to 3 age group (McCall et al., 2010b).

Child development also improved. The average improvement for all children was 13.51 total developmental quotient (DQ) points, and there were approximately equal improvements for children of both age groups. Further, the number of children falling below a score of 70 DQ points declined from 82% to 27.8% (McCall et al., 2010b). However, children who transitioned to an older age group during the intervention time period did not show significant improvement, signaling that a change in caregivers and peers dampens the effects of the intervention, a result supported by other works in Russian orphanages (McCall et al., 2012).

A similar intervention was attempted in two other institutions for children with severe disabilities ages 12 months to 10 years. In addition to an emphasis on the quality of caregiver-child interactions similar to the previous intervention, caregivers were given a brief introduction to how to position, handle, and work with children with severe disabilities (Groark et al., 2013). Outcomes of this intervention showed caregivers improved their ability to provide appropriate support for children with severe disabilities and were more sensitive and responsive in their interactions with children. Additionally, children's development improved in the domains of physical growth and behavioral and cognitive competence (Groark et al., 2013). This study showed that improving the warmth, sensitivity, and responsivity of caregiver-child interactions with minimal specialized instruction can improve the development of children with severe disabilities.

Although these are only three studies in Latin America, their results are consistent with interventions conducted elsewhere, especially the very comprehensive intervention in St. Petersburg, Russian Federation (St. Petersburg-USA Orphanage Research Team, 2008). Collectively, improving caregiver-child interactions, by making them more sensitive, warm, and responsive, conducted in an environment that supports such interactions produces improvements in the physical, cognitive, and social-emotional development of young children with and without disabilities (McCall, 2011).

4 Practical Application: Supporting Children's Care and Development

Although organizations, countries, and campaigns are promoting family alternatives to institutional care in Latin America and the Caribbean, many children (including a large number of children under the age of 3) still remain within institutions, many of which are likely to be psychosocially depriving. The task is to develop practice and policy procedures that provide the best possible care for *all* the children.

4.1 The Need for Improvement, Recognized Successes, and Suggested Action

Based on a large body of research from around the world and results from the few studies specifically in Latin America described above, traditional institutional care environments typically provide for children's basic physical needs but not their psychosocial and cognitive needs. More specifically, the quality of caregiver-child interaction and cognitive stimulation is minimal, often consisting of moderate to severe neglect. These psychosocially depriving characteristics were empirically described within several Latin American institutions with concomitant substantial delays in children's physical, social-emotional, and cognitive development (Groark et al., 2011, 2013; Lecannelier et al., 2014). These results constitute the fundamental rationale to develop a better comprehensive system of care.

One part of such a system could be improving the quality of care within institutions. Research from around the world and that reported here by McCall et al. (2010b), Groark et al. (2013), and Lecannelier et al. (2014) in Latin America demonstrate that it is possible to improve institutions with corresponding improvements in children's development. Importantly, these benefits were obtained by training regular institutional staff to interact with children in a normal parental manner, especially while conducting typical routine caregiving duties (e.g., feeding, dressing, bathing) rather than demanding "extra activities" for caregivers. Moreover, at least one study conducted in Latin America (Groark et al., 2013) and one in the Russian Federation (McCall et al., 2013) demonstrated that such an intervention could be maintained for several years with essentially no additional resources.

The issue, then, is not whether institutions can be improved, but should they (McCall, 2013)? In our view, the improvement of institutional environments should be considered as one piece within a more comprehensive effort to improve care for all children within the region, and these improvements should not detract energy, commitment, and financial resources from the development of family alternatives.

4.2 Implications for Practice and Policy

There are other practice and policy implications of the findings discussed above. For example, Latin America and the Caribbean have nongovernmental organizations and awareness campaigns that provide the region with a philosophical foundation to begin building a modern child welfare system. These organizations and individuals are already promoting and piloting services that are supportive and nurturing and can function as the basis of a comprehensive system. Such a system must uphold, above all else, the well-being and rights of children while promoting their health and safety. Modern child welfare services include family care alternatives that protect children from harmful or neglectful care environments and practices. Quality family-like services include a continuum of placements, such as foster and kinship care, domestic and intercountry adoption, family support, and family reunification programs, and they should include institutional care only as the last option.

Although institutional care is considered the last option in this continuum of services, in low-resource countries, such as those within Latin America, professionals recognize that institutions will remain for some time due to war, natural disasters such as earthquakes and hurricanes, financial considerations, social-political circumstances, and parents' inability to provide care due to physical or mental health problems, poverty, disease, and substance abuse. In addition, some children are considered "unadoptable" due to disabilities, age (older teens), and sibling groups (O'Dell, McCall, & Groark, 2015). These professionals recommend that while countries are in the process of developing family alternatives in the community, care in institutions can and should be improved (Groark & McCall, 2011). This has been accomplished successfully by creating smaller groups of children with consistent and fewer caregivers who are trained in areas of child development and by limiting the relocation of children from one group to another based on age or developmental status. Rather, more family-like environments can be created by integrating children into groups by mixed ability and ages and having children stay in the unit over time.

In addition, there are other challenges in creating a modern child welfare system. It is strongly recommended in the literature (McCall & Groark, 2015) that in-country professionals promote solutions that work in their own culture. Such a system generally requires a large initial financial investment that is recouped over time because family care is usually less expensive to maintain than institutional care. To begin the process, there must be political will developed within the general public. This political will is often mobilized through public awareness campaigns that employ politicians, celebrities, and others to act as public advocates in the media. This type of awareness campaign has already been initiated in the region, such as the Speak Up for Me campaign (speakupforme.org).

Next, critical stakeholders in the country must plan and define a system that is focused on the protection of children from abuse, neglect, and a variety of exploitations such as child trafficking and child soldiers. To uphold the infrastructure of such a system, there must be laws and policies that are funded mandates. These must include services provided by well-trained professionals who are supervised, mentored, and given other opportunities to troubleshoot and update their skills.

Finally, these services need to be monitored with quality standards, and children must be evaluated frequently for their continued developmental progress and well-being. In addition, the monitoring must include an assessment of the match between the child's current needs and the services being provided. Children can languish in their initial placement that has long been inappropriate for their current needs without deliberate and frequent monitoring. This is called "gatekeeping" and is a necessary function within a modern system.

Policy efforts in the region must continue to follow what empirical research has shown to be best for children's development by building and mandating the use of strong family-like alternatives to institutional care while improving the quality of care within institutions for children who must remain there. By fully supporting efforts aligned with the Call to Action and by making essential improvements to the remaining institutional care settings, national governments and organizations in the region could lessen the negative impact of developmentally damaging care within institutions.

4.3 Implications for Research and Evaluation

With regard to implications for future research and evaluation, it is crucial for institutional environments maintained within the region and governments to collect and distribute accurate data regarding the number of children within institutional care (and the particular types of care), as well as the ages of children within care and the quality of that care. Inconsistent and partial data on the prevalence of children in various care arrangements makes the tracking of improvements throughout the region difficult. With the Call to Action and initial work to encourage care outside of institutional environments, tracking successes and improvements with accurate and readily available data could provide motivation for continued successes and improvements in the region. Further, empirically examined interventions in institutions are also needed to demonstrate that the interventions have indeed improved children's development and to identify areas needing further improvement.

5 Summary

Although data are inconsistent and difficult to verify, a large number of children are in need of non-parental care in Latin America and the Caribbean for reasons that are many and complex. The institutional environments that have been described as largely psychosocially depriving both specifically in the region and around the world, and the poor child outcomes observed as a result of institutional care, make it imperative to implement policies and practices that have been demonstrated to successfully improve child outcomes. These include (1) creating a continuum of family-like care alternatives outside of the institutional environments, aligned with the recent Call to Action and initiatives underway, and (2) improving the caregiver-child interactions and the environments that support them for those institutions that remain.

Understandably the move toward deinstitutionalization will face challenges and logistical barriers and take years if not decades to accomplish; therefore the improvement of remaining institutions is imperative, with dire consequences if these settings continue to provide care that lacks stable, sensitive, responsive, and stimulating caregiver interactions. As a result of this type of care, children (and particularly those who are very young) are at high risk for poor development across all domains. In considering empirically proven interventions in Latin American institutions (Groark et al., 2013; Lecannelier et al., 2014; McCall et al., 2010b), the implementation of similar interventions across the region can improve caregiver behaviors, care environments, and child outcomes.

Questions for Discussion

1. What is the difference between an institutional care setting that is psychosocially depriving and one that is globally depriving? What are the potential impacts on children's development of these rearing conditions?
2. What are the challenges and the potential positive outcomes for the movement toward deinstitutionalization in the region?
3. What are the potential challenges of implementing successful interventions to improve care in different institutional contexts?

References

Achenbach, T. M., & Rescorla, L. A. (2000). *Manual for the ASEBA preschool forms and profiles*. Burlington, VT: University of Vermont, Department of Psychiatry.

Bakermans-Kranenburg, M. J., Howard, S., Zeanah C. H., Muhamedrahimov, R. J., Vorria, P., Dobrova-Krol, N. A., … Gunnar, M. R. (2011). Attachment and emotional development in institutional care: Characteristics and catch up. *Monographs of the Society for Research in Child Development*, *76*(4), 62–91.

Better Care Network. (2013). *Transforming institutional care*. Retrieved from http://www.bettercarenetwork.org/library/principles-of-good-care-practices/transforming-institutional-care/latin-american-and-caribbean-region-launches-call-to-action-to-end-the-placement-of-children-under

Briggs-Gowan, M., & Carter, A. S. (2001). *Infant-toddler social and emotional assessment (ITSEA) manual*. New Haven, CT: Yale University.

Dobrova-Krol, N. A., Van IJzendoorn, M. H., Bakermans-Kranenburg, M. J., Cyr, C., & Juffer, F. (2008). Physical growth delays and stress dysregulation in stunted and non-stunted Ukrainian institution-reared children. *Infant Behavior & Development*, *31*, 539–553.

Engle, P. L., Black, M. M., Behrman, J. R., Cabral de Mello, M., Gertler, P. J., Kapiriri, L., … The International Child Development Steering Group. (2007). Strategies to avoid the loss of developmental potential in more than 200 million children in the developing world. *Lancet*, *369*, 229–242.

Engle, P. L., Groza, V. K., Groark, C. J., Greenberg, A., Bunkers, K. M., & Muhamedrahimov, R. J. (2011). VIII. The situation for children without parental care and strategies for policy change. *Monographs of the Society for Research in Child Development*, *76*, 190–222.

Groark, C. J., & McCall, R. B. (2011). Improving institutions: Can we? Should we? How? *International Journal of Child and Family Welfare*, *14*, 64–72.

Groark, C. J., McCall, R. B., & Fish, L. (2011). Characteristics of environments, caregivers, and children in three Central American orphanages. *Infant Mental Health Journal*, *32*(2), 232–250.

Groark, C. J., McCall, R. B., & Li, J. (2009). Characterizing the status and progress of a country's child welfare reform. *International Journal of Child & Family Welfare*, *4*, 145–160.

Groark, C. J., McCall, R. B., McCarthy, S. K., Eichner, J. C., & Gee, A. D. (2013). Structure, caregiver–child interactions, and children's general physical and behavioral development in three

Central American institutions. *International Perspectives in Psychology: Research, Practice, Consultation*, *2*(3), 207–224.
Gunnar, M. R. (2001). Effects of early deprivation. In C. A. Nelson & M. Luciana (Eds.), *Handbook of developmental cognitive neuroscience* (pp. 617–629). Cambridge, MA: MIT Press. Retrieved from http://cognet.mit.edu/library/erefs/nelson/n39/abstract.html
Harms, T., Clifford, R., & Cryer, D. (2005). *Early childhood environment rating scale -revised.* New York: Teachers College Press.
Harms, T., Cryer, D., & Clifford, R. M. (2006). *Infant/Toddler environment rating scale.* New York: Teachers College Press.
Inter-American Commission on Human Rights, Latin American and Caribbean Movement for Children, RELAF, Special Representative of the Secretary General on Violence against Children, & UNICEF. (n.d.). *Speak up for me.* Retrieved from http://www.speakupforme.org
Johnson, D. E., & Gunnar, M. R. (2011). Growth failure in institutionalized children. *Monographs of the Society for Research in Child Development*, *76*(4), 92–126.
Johnson, D. E., Guthrie, D., Smyke, A. T., Koga, S. F., Fox, N. A., Zeanah, C. H., & Nelson, C. A. (2010). Growth and associations between auxology, caregiving environment, and cognition in socially deprived Romanian children randomized to foster vs ongoing institutional care. *Archives of Pediatrics and Adolescent Medicine*, *164*(6), 507–516.
Lecannelier, F., Silva, J. R., Hoffmann, M., Melo, R., & Morales, R. (2014). Effects of an intervention to promote socioemotional development in terms of attachment security: A study in early institutionalization in Chile. *Infant Mental Health Journal*, *35*(2), 151–159.
McCall, R. B. (2011). IX. Research, practice, and policy perspectives on issues of children without permanent parental care. *Monographs of the Society for Research in Child Development*, *76*(4), 223–272.
McCall, R. B., Fish, L. A., Groark, C. J., Muhamedrahimov, R. J., Palmov, O., & Nikiforova, N. V. (2012). The role of transitions to new age groups in the development of institutionalized children. *Infant Mental Health Journal*, *33*(4), 421–429.
McCall, R. B. (2013). The consequences of early institutionalization: Can institutions be improved?–should they? *Child and Adolescent Mental Health*, *18*(4), 193–201.
McCall, R. B., & Groark, C. J. (2015). Research on institutionalized children: Implications for international child welfare practitioners and policy makers. *International Perspectives in Psychology: Research, Practice, Consultation*, *4*, 142–159.
McCall, R. B., Groark, C. J., & Fish, L. (2010a). A caregiver-child socioemotional and relationship rating scale. *Infant Mental Health Journal*, *31*(2), 201–219.
McCall, R. B., Groark, C. J., Fish, L., Harkins, D., Serrano, G., & Gordon, K. (2010b). A socioemotional intervention in a Latin American orphanage. *Infant Mental Health Journal*, *31*(5), 521–542.
McCall, R. B., Groark, C. J., Fish, L., Muhamedrahimov, R. J., Palmov, O. I., & Nikiforova, N. V. (2013). Maintaining a social-emotional intervention and its benefits for institutionalized children. *Child Development*, *84*, 1734–1749.
Newborg, J. (2005). *Battelle developmental inventory* (2nd ed.). Itasca, IL: Riverside.
O'Dell, K. E., McCall, R. B., & Groark, C. J. (2015). Supporting families throughout the international special needs adoption process. *Children and Youth Services Review*, *59*, 161–170.
RELAF. (n.d.). *Technical cooperation.* Retrieved from http://www.relaf.org/coop_regionwide_en.php
RELAF Project, the Latin American Foster Care Network, & SOS Children's Villages International. (2010). *Children and adolescents without parental care in Latin America: Contexts, causes and consequences of being deprived of the right to family and community life*. Buenos Aires, Argentina: Latin American Paper. Retrieved from http://resourcecentre.savethechildren.se/sites/default/files/documents/5909.pdf
RELAF & UNICEF. (2013). *Planificano la desinstitucionalización de niñas y niños menores de tres años*. Guía de aportes para la experiencia de las instituciones de cuidado residencial. Retrieved from http://www.relaf.org/materiales/Des_bebes.pdf

Rosas, J., & McCall, R. B. (2011, unpublished manuscript). *Characteristics of institutions, interventions, and resident children's development*. Pittsburgh, PA: University of Pittsburgh Office of Child Development.

Smyke, A. T., Koga, S. F., Johnson, D. E., Fox, N. A., Marshall, P. J., Nelson, C. A., … The BEIP Core Group. (2007). The caregiving context in institution-reared and family-reared infants and toddlers in Romania. *Journal of Child Psychology and Psychiatry, 48*(2), 210–218.

The Joint United Nations Programme on HIV/AIDS (UNAIDS), the United Nations Children's Fund (UNICEF), & the United States Agency for International Development (USAID). (2004). *Children on the Brink, 2004: A joint report of new orphan estimates and a framework for action*. Retrieved from http://www.unicef.org/publications/cob_layout6-013.pdf

The Leiden Conference on the Development and Care of Children without Permanent Parents. (2012). The development and care of institutionally reared children. *Child Development Perspectives*, *6*(2), 174–180.

The St. Petersburg-USA Orphanage Research Team. (2008). The effect of early social-emotional and relationship experience on the development of young children. *Monographs of the Society for Research in Child Development*, *72*, 1–297.

UNICEF. (2005). *A pivotal secade: 1995–2005*. New York: UNICEF.

UNICEF. (2013). *La situación de niños, niñas y adolescentes en las instituciones de protección y cuidado de América Latina y el Caribe*. Retrieved from http://www.unicef.org/lac/UNICEF_Estudio_sobre_NNA_en_instituciones.pdf

UNICEF. (2014, November). *The state of the world's children 2015: Executive summary*. New York: UNICEF. Retrieved from http://www.unicef.org/publications/files/SOWC_2015_Summary_and_Tables.pdf

UNICEF. (n.d.). *A call to action to end the placement of children under three years of age in institutions*. Retrieved from http://www.crin.org/docs/Call%20to%20Action%20-%20Latin%20America%20and%20Caribbean.pdf

Van IJzendoorn, M.H., Palacios, J., Sonuga-Barke, E. J. S., Gunnar M.R., Vorria, Y., McCall, R., … Juffer F. (2011). Children in institutional care: Delayed development and resilience. *Monographs of the Society for Research of Child Development*, *76*, 8–30.

Chapter 20
Experiences and Outcomes of Adults Who Endured Maltreatment as Children in Care in Australia in the Twentieth Century

Elizabeth Fernandez and Jung-Sook Lee

Most participants in this study were denied almost all rights to protection, nurture, learning, health, and wellbeing while growing up in care. Instead, they experienced neglect, abuse, and great trauma. This has clearly had lifelong health and wellbeing impacts.

(Fernandez & Lee, 2017)

1 Introduction

Over the last two decades, the victimization of children through maltreatment in institutions and out-of-home care has been the subject of inquiries in different countries: Australia, Britain, Canada, Denmark, Germany, Ireland, and Norway (Sköld, 2013). Adults who spent their childhoods in care have come forward through public inquiries, truth commissions, and the media to allege physical, emotional, and sexual abuse and neglect while in the care of government, nongovernment, and religious institutions and out-of-home care programs. There has been international concern about the trauma they endured and the significant lifelong impacts.

This chapter reports a national research study which explored the nature and dimensions of institutional child abuse and investigated the impacts of abuse on the

E. Fernandez (✉)
School of Social Sciences, Faculty of Arts and Social Sciences, The University of New South Wales, Sydney, NSW 2052, Australia
e-mail: e.fernandez@unsw.edu.au

J.-S. Lee
School of Social Sciences, Faculty of Arts and Social Sciences,
The University of New South Wales, Sydney, NSW 2052, Australia
e-mail: js.lee@unsw.edu.au

A.V. Rus et al. (eds.), *Child Maltreatment in Residential Care*,
DOI 10.1007/978-3-319-57990-0_20

current health and well-being outcomes of adult survivors who experienced out-of-home care in the twentieth century in Australia. The research draws on the definition of institutional abuse of Wolfe, Jaffe, Jette, and Poisson (2003) which characterizes institutional abuse as the inappropriate use of power and authority to inflict harm, actual or potential, to a child's well-being and development. The study examined a wide range of institutional abuse that encompassed neglect; emotional, physical, and sexual abuse; and other oppressive practices. Key questions explored included: What were the experiences of adults who grew up in care in the twentieth century? How did those experiences influence survivors in their adult lives? A fuller account of this research is reported in Fernandez, Lee, Blunden, McNamara, Kovacs, and Cornefert (2016).

Research participants were care leavers who spent their childhoods in institutions and foster care during the period 1930–1989 and identified as "Forgotten Australians," "Child Migrants," and "the Stolen Generations," respectively. Forgotten Australians are predominantly persons born in Australia who were placed in "care" in the twentieth century. Stolen Generation survivors are Aboriginal and Torres Strait Islander people who were removed from their families under policies that allowed for the forcible removal of Aboriginal and Torres Strait Islander children from the late 1800s to the 1970s (HREOC, 1997). Child Migrants are those children who were born in the United Kingdom, removed from families of origin, and sent to Commonwealth countries, including Australia, since early in the twentieth century.

Auspiced by the University of New South Wales Faculty of Arts and Social Sciences and funded by the Australian Research Council, the research was conducted in partnership with the University of Chicago (Professor Mark Courtney), the University of York (Professor Mike Stein), and six community partners – the Alliance for Forgotten Australians, the Association of Child Welfare Agencies, Berry Street, Relationships Australia, Catholic Care Diocese of Broken Bay, and Micah Projects.

1.1 Care in the Twentieth Century in Australia

During the twentieth century, increasing numbers of children were placed in a range of institutions that were run by the states, religious groups, and other organizations. Although earlier in the twentieth century there was a preference for foster care or "boarding out" children with families as it was called then, "the drift of State children back to institutions increased in the 1930s and 1940s because of a lack of foster families. By the 1940s, most young children needing residential care were placed in institutions" (Senate Community Affairs References Committee, 2004, p. 19). This period was also marked by concern about conditions in institutions, triggering a number of public inquiries (approximately 83 inquiries since 1852).

Once placed in care, children were often forced to undertake arduous work often to the detriment of schooling. This was "justified" in moral terms to instill in them a work ethic, to provide training so they could become "useful" adult members of society, but also fulfilling the labor demands of cash-strapped state and charitable institutions. Regulatory oversight was provided by inspectors; however, as had been evidenced in multiple inquiries, this did not prevent abuse from occurring. Indeed much of the legislation at the time did not actually provide any guidance for dealing with institutional abuse.

The effects of being placed in institutional care were profound and lifelong as the Alliance for Forgotten Australians (AFA) summarizes: "These children suffered from deep and lasting feelings of separation and abandonment. The loss of family, usually including separation from siblings, caused grief, feelings of isolation, guilt, self-blame, and confusion about their identity" (2016, p. 8). It is estimated that over 500,000 Australian children experienced care in institutions, orphanages, or other forms of care during this period, the major cohort being the Forgotten Australians.

Another cohort placed into institutions involved the Child Migrants from the British Isles (and a minority from other parts of British-controlled Europe, such as Malta). The Child Migrants formed a significant population of children in institutional care in Australia in the twentieth century. The extent of child exportation from Britain is documented in the work *Lost Children of The Empire* by Bean and Melville (1989) and publicized through the Child Migrants Trust founded by Margaret Humphreys. It is estimated that 10,000–12,000 children were exported to Australia during and after the Second World War. The vulnerability of Child Migrants to suboptimal care and exploitation is documented (Humphreys, 1996).

The Stolen Generations constitute the third cohort that were separated from kin to enter institutions in significant numbers. The forced removal of Aboriginal children from their families and placement in white families and institutions (Aboriginal specific, state, nongovernment, and religious) is widely documented (Haebich, 2000; HREOC, 1997; Read, 1982; van Krieken, 1991). It is estimated that during the period 1910–1970, between one in three and one in ten Aboriginal and Torres Strait Islander children were removed from their families and communities, equating to 25,000 children forcibly removed from family and culture (HREOC, 1997). The practice of state removal of Aboriginal children was embedded in the context of racist, segregationist, and assimilationist policies of that era. Children were separated from parents using compulsion (court orders) and duress through threats of charges of neglect if the removal was not agreed to (HREOC, 1997). The trauma associated with the severance of parental and family relationships, the added alienation from culture, and the attempted erasure of Aboriginality has had a severe and lasting impact on the Stolen Generations and their descendants. The legacies of the policies that created the Stolen Generations are felt by Aboriginal communities across Australia. Currently Aboriginal children continue to be disproportionately represented in the care system nationally (Australian Institute of Health and Welfare, 2016).

1.2 Public Inquiries, Apologies, and Redress

In Australia, there have been several significant Commonwealth and state inquiries into child removal policies and institutional care of children. The Inquiry into Children in Institutional Care (Senate Community Affairs References Committee, 2004) focused on Australian-born children who were placed into care and the unsafe, improper, and unlawful care or treatment of children in institutions. This produced the Forgotten Australians report, which recommended compensation for victims, and a Royal Commission to investigate criminal sexual assault. The National Inquiry into the Separation of Aboriginal and Torres Strait Islander Children from their Families (HREOC, 1997) investigated the removal of Aboriginal children from families during the assimilationist period 1910–1975, made many recommendations including provision of compensation, and issued a formal apology in the "Bringing Them Home" report. The Inquiry into Child Migration and its report "Lost Innocents: Righting the Record" (Senate Community Affairs References Committee, 2001) focused on the practice of migrating children to Australia in the early part of the twentieth century and contained a number of recommendations. There have also been a number of state-based inquiries, notably the Commission of Inquiry into Abuse of Children in Queensland Institutions (1998–1999) (Commission of Inquiry, 1999).

National and state apologies and redress have also been part of inquiry outcomes. For example, the Stolen Generations were given a belated formal apology on February 13, 2008, and the Forgotten Australians and former Child Migrants on November 16, 2009, to acknowledge their stolen childhoods.

Currently, national concern about children's victimization through sexual abuse while in "care" has led to the establishment of the Australian Government's Royal Commission into Institutional Responses to Child Sexual Abuse, particularly in relation to organizations with responsibility for children in their care. The Royal Commission has held over 5,900 private sessions with individuals and referred 1,700 matters to the authorities including the police. It has recommended a national scheme for victims of child sexual abuse which is expected to be established by 2018 and will offer a direct personal response for those survivors who seek it, options to receive psychological counseling, and a monetary payment to acknowledge the wrongdoing inflicted upon them (Minister for Social Services and Attorney-General, 2016).

1.3 The Care Experience

The phenomenon of housing large numbers of children in institutional care was not unique to Australia but was widespread in Britain, Europe, North America, and other parts of the world (Perry, Sigal, Boucher, & Paré, 2006). Although child welfare systems were intended to safeguard children's well-being, maltreatment in out-of-home care was widely prevalent. There was little understanding of children's emotional needs until the 1960s, nor much understanding of the lasting effect of harsh, physical, sexual, and psychological mistreatment (Commission of Inquiry, 1999). Moreover, the "institutional culture" that characterized the homes created a "depersonalising and punitive living environment in which nobody of any age could thrive" (Penglase, 2005, p. 50). The institutional environment in itself was traumatic, damaging, and harmful (Musgrove, 2013).

Evidence indicates physical needs were unmet and that children were exposed to physical and sexual abuse. The Lost Innocents Report (Senate Community Affairs Reference Committee, 2001) identified eight categories of abuse experienced by care leavers while they were in care: physical assault, depersonalization, psychological abuse, abusive work practices, lack of education, inadequate food and clothing, and a lack of aftercare (pp. 72–73). The Care Leavers Australian Network (2008) found that 83.2% of survey respondents reported being "hit, smacked, or whacked" while in care (2008, p. 7) and 44.5% had experienced sexual abuse while in care. In addition, trauma, resulting from acts of commission and omission, was pervasive in experiences of growing up in suboptimal "care." Retrospective accounts from care leavers allude to the high level of disruption and dislocation experienced while in care, resulting from movements between children's homes, foster families, and placement breakdowns leading to abrupt endings to caregiver and social relationships. Length of time in care has been correlated with persistent socioemotional problems (Ames, 1997; Fries & Pollak, 2004; O'Connor et al., 2000). There are many studies on the effects of disrupted care trajectories on children, such as the effects of the deprivation of stable, consistent relationships that foster emotional learning and social bonds (Rubin, Dwyer, Booth-LaForce, Kim, & Burgess, 2004; Rutter, Quinton, & Hill, 1990).

Several studies have suggested that young people in care systems present a higher level of emotional and behavioral problems than those in the general population (Clausen, Landsverk, Ganger, Chadwick, & Litrownik, 1998; Fernandez, 2008; Meltzer, Gatward, Corbin, Goodman, & Ford, 2003). Evidence of psychological concerns in the clinical range also comes from studies of mental health service utilization (Burns et al., 2004; Stahmer et al., 2005).

Evidence from reviewing studies undertaken overseas (Biehal, Clayden, Stein, & Wade, 1995; Daly & Gilligan, 2010; Pecora et al., 2006; Stein & Carey, 1986) and in Australia (Cashmore & Paxman, 1996; McDowall, 2009) indicates that young adults discharged from care experience considerable material disadvantage, marginalization, and social exclusion. Studies suggest that those who were in care may have poorer outcomes over a range of indicators including eating disorders and personality disorders are mental health problems and substance abuse (Guest, 2012; Rutter & Quinton, 1984), lower emotional and mental well-being generally (Broad, 2005; Buchanan, 1999; Cocker & Scott, 2006), involvement in the criminal justice system (McFarlane, 2008; Narey, 2007; Robson, 2008), lower educational attainment (Connelly & Furnivall, 2013; Goddard, 2000; Jackson & Sachdev, 2001), higher housing instability and homelessness (Dixon, 2008; Robson, 2008), and higher rates of chronic health conditions and morbidity (Kendall-Tackett, 2002).

In summary, it is well established from research that care leavers experience a range of poorer outcomes in adult life generally (Fernandez & Atwool, 2013). While a minority of studies based on limited sample sizes show no or less intensity of detrimental effects, the vast majority of research findings indicate that outcomes are poor across a range of domains, although protective factors can mitigate this (Gilligan, 2007).

International research in recent years has established that childhood adversities are implicated as risk factors in the development of later mental health problems. There is a large body of research that has shown that childhood exposure to physical abuse, sexual abuse, emotional abuse, and witnessing violence are factors that contribute to impaired health in adult life (Buckingham & Daniolos, 2013; Chapman et al., 2004; Edwards, Holden, Felitti, & Anda, 2003; Gilbert et al., 2009; Kaplan et al., 1998; Lueger-Schuster et al., 2014; Springer, Sheridan, Kuo, & Carnes, 2007; Sugaya et al., 2012; Wegman & Stelter, 2009). Previous studies have identified a number of psychological conditions associated with childhood maltreatment including anxiety, depression, post-traumatic stress disorder (PTSD), substance abuse, sleep disorder, and suicide attempts (Afifi et al., 2014; Clemmons, Walsh, DiLillo, & Messman-Moore, 2007; Kaplan et al., 1998; Mullen, Martin, Anderson, & Romans, 1996; Norman et al., 2012; Twaite & Rodriguez-Srednicki, 2004; Widom, DuMont, & Czaja, 2007). Additionally, there is an emerging literature that draws attention to the impact of exposure to multiple and cumulative abuses or polyvictimization in increasing the risk of psychological disturbance including anxiety, depression, PTSD, suicide ideation, and self-harm (Afifi et al., 2014; Edwards et al., 2003; Finkelhor, Ormrod, & Turner, 2007; Ford, Goodman, & Meltzer, 2003; Moore et al., 2015; Nurius, Green, Logan-Greene, & Borja, 2007; Widom et al., 2007; Wright, 2007). An Australian study quantifying the burden of mental disorders attributable to multiple forms of maltreatment concludes that a significant proportion of depressive and anxiety disorders and intentional self-harm is attributable to maltreatment in childhood (Moore et al., 2015).

Childhood maltreatment experienced early in life can further impact on the quality of relationships with family and significant others over the life course (Belt & Abidin, 1996; Colman & Widom, 2004; Savla et al., 2013; Schafer, Ferraro, & Mustillo, 2011; Walker, Holman, & Busby, 2009). Attachment theorists (Bowlby, 1988; Sroufe, 2005) posit that neglectful caregiving and disruption of attachment relationships contribute to insecurity and negative perceptions of self and others, which in turn compromise trust and intimacy in relationships in later life (Egeland & Sroufe, 1981; Savla et al., 2013; Styron & Janoff-Bulman, 1997; Underwood & Rosen, 2011). For example, Savla et al. (2013) conclude from their research that childhood emotional and physical abuse had a cumulative effect on their respondents' personal relationships throughout their life course contributing to psychological and social distance from family in later years.

Against this overview of the historical context of out-of-home care in the twentieth century and trends in the literature that documents the outcomes of care, we proceed to outline the methodology of the study and its findings.

2 Method

2.1 Study Design

This study employed a mixed-methods design to develop a more comprehensive understanding of participants' lives (Doyle, Brady, & Byrne, 2009; Sandelowski, 2000). It included surveys, interviews, and focus groups. Using a convergent parallel design (Creswell & Plano, 2011), quantitative and qualitative research components were run simultaneously with equal priority. From the development of the project to reporting of findings, this research benefited from the active involvement of partner organizations with extensive experience of working with adult care leavers. To complement the expertise and input of the researchers and partners, the project included a critical reference group with representation from researchers, policy makers, and representatives of care leaver organizations (approximately 25% of the membership was Aboriginal and Torres Strait Islander peoples). Ethics approval was obtained from the Human Research Ethics Committee at the University and two community organizations.

2.2 Participants

The target population was people who have lived in child welfare institutions and other substitute care as children during the period of 1930–1989. We used diverse sampling strategies including purposive and opportunity sampling. It was believed that a considerable proportion of people were not involved in organizations that serve care leavers. Therefore, a broad approach for recruitment was taken, including an intensive media campaign and selected advertising, as well as distribution of information through partner organizations and other service providers.

The total number of survey participants was 669. In terms of the cohort, 75.9% were Forgotten Australians, 10% were Child Migrants, 6% identified as members of the Stolen Generations, and 8.1% did not report their group identification. The mean age of survey participants was 61.74 (*SD* = 11.24) (ranging from 27 to 100 years old). More than half (57.4%) were female and 7.8% were Aboriginal or Torres Strait Islander persons. About half of respondents were married (42.7%) or in a de facto relationship (7.7%) at the time of surveys. Participants were from all Australian states and territories, although the majority of participants were from the three most populated states: New South Wales (35.3%), Queensland (28.9%), and Victoria (18.6%). The remaining 17.4% were from five other states and territories. See Table 20.1 for details of demographics.

Participants for interviews and focus groups were chosen to reflect the diversity of care leavers and to capture a range of experiences. The selection criteria included gender, age, indigenous status, education, region, and experiences during and after care (both negative and positive). In-depth interviews were conducted with 92

Table 20.1 Demographics

	n	Frequency	%
Age group	645		
Under 45		40	6.2
45–49		48	7.4
50–54		73	11.3
55–59		118	18.0
60–64		105	18.3
65–69		103	16.0
70–74		85	13.2
75 or older		75	11.6
Gender	658		
Female		378	57.4
Male		280	42.6
Aboriginal status	655		
Aboriginal and Torres Strait Islander		51	7.8
Nonindigenous		563	86.0
Don't know		41	6.3
Relationship status	653		
Married		279	42.7
De facto		50	7.7
Never married single		99	15.2
Separated		43	6.6
Widowed		50	7.7
Divorced		132	20.2

participants. Forty-nine were female (53%) and 44 were male (46%); 12 persons identified as Aboriginal or Torres Strait Islander (13%). In addition, 15 interviews with specialist informants were conducted. Seventy-seven persons participated in 20 focus groups in a variety of locations throughout Australia. Forty-five were female (58%), and 32 were male (45%); ten were identified as Aboriginal or Torres Strait Islander (13%).

2.3 *Instruments*

The survey questionnaire was developed drawing on Australian and international research literature and modified based on feedback from partner investigators and members of the critical reference group which included Aboriginal people. The questionnaire focused on experiences in care, experiences of leaving care, life outcomes after care (education, employment, health, well-being, and relationships), current service needs, and participation in organizations and the Royal Commission into Institutional Responses to Child Sexual Abuse. The questionnaire included two standardized scales: the Kessler Psychological Distress Scale (K10) (Kessler et al., 2002) and the Multidimensional Scale of Perceived Social Support (MSPSS) (Zimet, Dahlem, Zimet, & Farley, 1988). K10 measures nonspecific psychological distress on a five-point scale (ten items) and is widely used worldwide (Andrews & Slade, 2001). Following the Australian Bureau of Statistics (ABS) categorization, K10 scores are grouped as "low" (10–15), "moderate" (16–21), "high" (22–29), and "very high" (30–50). MSPSS is a self-report measure of social support on a seven-point scale (12 items). It has three domains: significant other, family, and friends. These standardized measures offered an opportunity for national and international comparison with general population normative data. The survey questionnaire was designed to include the short form (19 questions) and the long form (110 questions).

The interview guide for care leavers broadly focused on the same issues explored in the surveys. In addition, participants were asked about their coping strategies and resilience, significant events post care to the present, and their views on formal apologies. The interview guide for specialist informants focused on the nature, types, utilization, and values of services provided to the study population. They were also asked about gaps in services, the adequacy of resourcing, and some broader policy issues. The focus group guide covered the same themes; however, less emphasis was given to questions about individual experiences, due to focus groups being collective in nature. The guides used for interviews and focus groups with Aboriginal and Torres Strait Islander peoples were designed to capture their unique experiences in out-of-home care (e.g., cultural deprivation) and were developed in consultation with Aboriginal members of the critical reference group.

2.4 Data Collection

Surveys were conducted from December 11, 2014, to March 31, 2016. When participants directly contacted researchers for paper or telephone surveys, they received a long version of the survey. In the case of telephone surveys, a researcher made a telephone call at the time agreed by participants. When participants completed online surveys, at the end of the short form, they were asked whether they would like to continue the long form online or complete it on paper or over the telephone. When participants opted for the completion on paper or over the telephone, they received the long form by mail and calls were made if needed. Two-thirds ($n = 445$) completed online surveys and one-third ($n = 224$) completed paper or telephone surveys. Total 65.5% ($n = 438$) completed the long form and 34.5% ($n = 231$) completed the short form only.

Interviews usually ran for 45 min to 1 h 15 min. Focus groups usually involved 4–8 people with the optimum number being five persons and typically ran for 1.5 h. For groups of Aboriginal care leavers, an Aboriginal co-facilitator attended and co-facilitated. With the permission of participants, interviews and focus groups were audio recorded and transcribed.

2.5 Data Analysis

Descriptive statistics were examined to understand demographics, care experiences including abuse and neglect in care, and post care outcomes. To better understand the impact of abuse, a two-step cluster analysis was conducted based on the types of abuse experienced while in care, and then clusters were compared on various outcomes. For group comparisons, various bivariate statistical analyses were conducted: t-test, ANOVA, chi-square test, Fisher's exact test, Mann-Whitney U test, and Kruskal-Wallis H test. IBM SPSS Statistics 23 (IBM Corp., 2015) was used for all analyses.

Qualitative data from interviews, focus groups, and open-ended questions of the surveys were analyzed using NVivo software. The coding broadly followed the thematic structure of the interview schedule. In reporting, all study participants have been assigned a pseudonym. Findings from quantitative data and qualitative data were integrated within broad themes. These provided the basis for considering implications and suggestions for practice, policy, and future research to promote well-being of adult care leavers and to improve the current care system.

3 Results

3.1 Care Status

At the time of entry into care, about 52.9% of survey participants were state wards, and they were 6.28 years old on average (ranging from at birth to 17.58 years old). Respondents entered care for various and multiple reasons. The most cited reasons were parents' inability to cope (39.4%), marital problems between parents (36.4%), neglect (27.2%), abandonment (24.6%), domestic violence (24.4%), parental drug and alcohol problems (24.2%), financial difficulties (22.1%), and parental illness (21.2%). Less frequently mentioned reasons included maltreatment, parental death, war, or child's behavioral difficulties. Table 20.2 displays details at entry into care.

Respondents provided additional comments on their perceptions of the circumstances that led to care. One Aboriginal woman commented on the stringent and biased assessments of their family's housing which precipitated her entry to care:

> They said a black woman couldn't bring up white children – my grandmother was black. That's what led up to all this. They said we were neglected children and the house was in a filthy condition. Both those were lies because my grandmother had a perfectly spotless house. ("Hannah")

Another participant recounted parental health circumstances which triggered removal to care:

> My mother had a nervous breakdown, she had shock treatment and she was in and out of hospital. She had 4 children. I was the second eldest. As a result of my father being out in

Table 20.2 Entry into care

	n	Frequency	%
Age at entry into care	612		
Under age 1		72	11.8
1–2		74	12.1
3–5		169	27.6
6–10		178	29.1
11–15		110	18
16 or older		9	1.5
Status at entry	420		
Voluntary placement		83	19.8
State wardship		222	52.9
Don't know		57	13.6
Other		58	13.8
Reasons for placement[a]	467		
Death of parents		68	14.6
Affected by war		64	13.7
Parental illness or disability		99	21.2
Parental drug/alcohol dependence		113	24.2
Domestic violence		114	24.4
Parents' marital problems		170	36.4
Parents' inability to cope		184	39.4
Abandoned by parents		115	24.6
Housing/financial difficulties		103	22.1
Physical maltreatment		84	18
Sexual maltreatment		41	8.8
Emotional maltreatment		91	19.5
Neglect		127	27.2
Child's behavioral difficulties		45	9.6

Note: [a]The total exceeds 100% because participants were able to choose more than one option

> the navy somewhere and her not being able to cope and a few health problems, she collapsed in a big heap and we were shipped off to institutions for the rest of our lives. ("Carl")

In the case of Child Migrants, family poverty and financial imperatives were in some instances implicated in their transfer to care in Australia:

> I've got the letter where (the institution) coerced her into signing it……they said… if you agree to let your sons go to Australia you no longer will have to pay the ten shillings a week to keep them. Well 10 shillings a week in England in 19 bloody 50, it would be like a hundred dollars now or more. ("George")

As illustrated in Table 20.3, the majority of survey participants (84.8%) had experience of being in a children's home or orphanage. Many participants also experienced various types of care: foster care (33.0%), juvenile detention or youth correction facility (25.0%), family group home (11.5%), or others (e.g., residential care, boarding house, psychiatric hospital, or training institution).

Table 20.3 Circumstances in care

	n	Frequency	%	Mean	*SD*	Range
Types of placement experienced	637					
Children's home/orphanage		540	84.8			
Residential care		47	7.4			
Family group home		73	11.5			
Foster care		210	33			
Hostel or boarding house		77	12.1			
Psychiatric hospital/asylum		41	6.4			
Training institution		59	9.3			
Youth correctional facility		159	25			
Other		85	13.3			
Number of placements	394			3.96	3.89	(1–27)
Duration in care	616			8.62	5.01	(0.06–21)
Age at leaving care	396			15.21	3.24	(0.06–22)
Overall satisfaction with care	620			1.92	1.42	(1–6)

Note: SD refers to standard deviation

Participants referred to the regimented and militaristic orientation of institutions. One of them spoke of the depersonalization he experienced:

> When I went in there, I was only a number, and it wasn't until I was 10, 11 years old when I found out, that I had a name. ("Frank")

Research participants commented on the quality and demeanor of staff, their lack of warmth, and inadequate interpersonal skills. One participant commented on his experience of a war veteran employed in his home:

> I mean when you take a sergeant major out of the British Army and put him in charge of an orphanage, he was absolutely brutal. Absolutely brutal. I mean he was just terrible. Nothing good happened there, you know? ("Mark")

On average, respondents experienced 3.96 placements in care (ranging from 1 to 27 placements) and stayed in care for 8.62 years (ranging from 3 weeks to 21 years). While some participants experienced stable care in a single institution, many were subject to frequent placement changes. Meryl described their extreme experience of instability:

> I moved every year as a child from the age of 4, 5, to the age of 13. I moved every year into a different family home. And I was then in, another year, nearly a year in another one, but then I was nearly 5 years and another one, so I know about packing my bags. ("Meryl")

At time of leaving care, they were 15.21 years old on average (ranging from 3 weeks to 22 years[1]). The majority of participants (83%) were dissatisfied with their care experiences (61% very dissatisfied, 15% dissatisfied, and 7% somewhat dissatisfied). The average score of satisfaction with care was 1.92 (*SD* = 1.42) on a six-point scale. See Table 20.3 for details.

[1] One respondent continued staying at the convent as an adult until the age of 31. Therefore, the maximum age in care was set to the next highest value in the data (age 22).

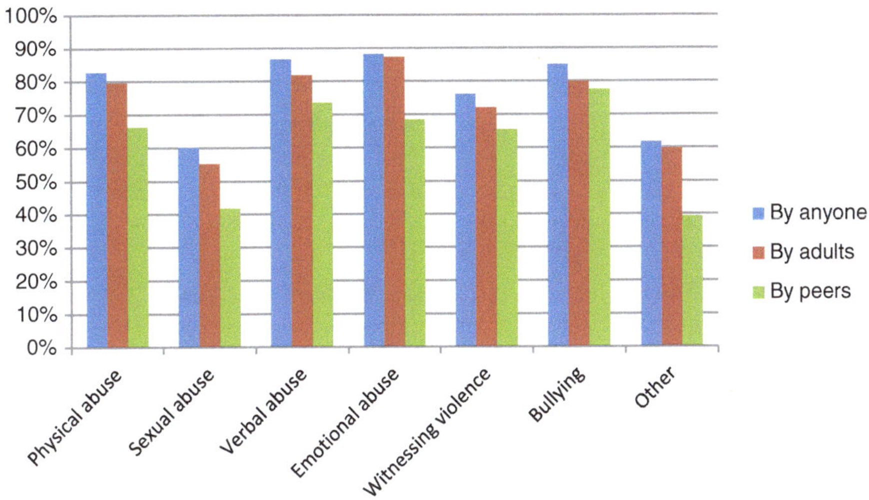

Fig. 20.1 Prevalence of maltreatment in care (*Note*: the sample size varies, $n = 407$ to 418)

3.2 *Maltreatment While in Care*

Maltreatment was prevalent in care as illustrated in Fig. 20.1. The vast majority of survey participants (96.7%) experienced some types of maltreatment in care, and 40.9% reported to have experienced all types of maltreatment in care. The most prevalent type of abuse experienced was emotional abuse (88.2%) and verbal abuse (86.8%). When the source of abuse was asked separately, the most prevalent abuse by adults was emotional abuse (87.3%), followed by verbal abuse (82%). The most prevalent abuse by peers was bullying (77.6%), followed by verbal abuse (73.7%). Sexual abuse was widespread in care, and 60% experienced this form of abuse from someone: 55.3% experienced sexual abuse by adults and 41.8% experienced sexual abuse by peers.

In interviews and focus groups, participants detailed their experience of verbal, physical, emotional, and sexual abuse. Verbal abuse from staff conveyed negative messages to children designed to make them feel worthless and unwanted. This was evident in Janice's account:

> I mean we were told quite often that we were there because nobody wanted us. That we were a blight on society, basically. That we were there because we were no good. That's how we were treated. You know, 'if your own parents don't want you, who the hell else is gonna want you?' And we were told that over and over and over again until you believed it. ("Janice")

Physical abuse was rife and reported by many. Participants rendered accounts of several abusive practices. Bill recalls:

> That (indicating deep scarring on leg) was from [name of the institution]. The Major belted me with a piece of wood. It aches all the time (sixty years later). If I get a rash on it, there's

> a good chance it'll break out again because it's right down on the bone....They put a... rag on my leg and gave me a pair of crutches for 6 months.... ("Bill")

The relentlessness and unpredictability of the culture of violence dominating the home environment gave rise to high levels of mistrust and hypervigilance on the part of participants:

> Now the worst fear wasn't the whipping. The pain after a while, I could stand. It was the fear of not knowing when it was going to happen again. For hours afterwards, I'd stand there shivering with fear because I never knew. ("Michael")

Respondents also recalled the sense of powerlessness experienced in witnessing violence including the physical abuse of their own siblings:

> The hardest thing – you were made to witness the punishment of your siblings. So they would get everyone around to witness. My younger sisters were punished for accidently breaking a toy and so we were all – all the children in the cottage had to stand around and weren't allowed to move. You weren't allowed to say anything. You were not allowed to avert your eyes and they were beating. Just beating and beating. ("Lucy")

Punishment meted out also included solitary confinement:

> It is a criminal offence to take children at the age of 10 and lock them in an isolation room that the windows all boarded up, there's a hole in the door like we call a doggy door that your meals are passed through and there's a mattress on the floor and a metal potty and you're locked in there for 24 hours at the age of 10 years old because you rolled your eyes? ("Simone")

Sexual abuse was pervasive including a spectrum of abuse including sexual assault, inappropriate touching, and voyeurism. Accounts of sexual abuse by staff and visiting professionals were common in both genders. Typically children were silenced, disbelieved, or threatened if they attempted to disclose the abuse. This is evident in the recollections of some respondents in the study:

> I was raped by a priest, only to be flogged by the nuns and told that I was the one that was at fault... there was nothing nice about an orphanage. ("Eliza")

> I didn't know what to do, and they told us to shut our mouth or we'll never ever get released from the home. They had us over a barrel. ("Maxine")

> ...sexual abuse was as common as bricks in a wall (laughs), if someone said they were not in any way sexually active, especially in the governments children's homes, I'm sorry I just have to say that's the perfect children's home, I've never heard of it. ("Shane")

Aboriginal children were cruelly punished for speaking languages other than English or for expressing their culture of origin in other ways (Atkinson, 2002). "Russell" described such punishment:

> [If you spoke language] You'd get a big – you'd get put in a corner with no food. You'd get in trouble– you'd get ah, no blanket, no mattress, just sleep as you are. And the clothes you go on your back. Like they won't give you another clothes til you learn not speak language. ("Russell").

Table 20.4 Abuse clusters based on types of abuse experienced while in care

	All types of abuse (n = 212)	All but sexual abuse (n = 76)	Some or no abuse (n = 128)
Physical abuse	100.0	100.0	43.8
Sexual abuse	100.0	0.0	30.5
Verbal abuse	100.0	93.4	60.9
Emotional abuse	100.0	100.0	61.7
Witnessing violence	100.0	100.0	22.7
Bullying	100.0	100.0	51.6

Note: Numbers are percentages of individuals who experienced each type of abuse in care

Given the fact that many participants experienced multiple types of abuse while in care, we conducted cluster analysis to better understand their experiences of abuse and the impacts of abuse on them. As shown in Table 20.4, three clusters were identified based on types of abuse experienced while in care (note that "other" category was excluded because a small number of participants answered this item). Cluster 1 (51%) experienced all types of abuse, cluster 2 (18.3%) experienced all types but sexual abuse, and cluster 3 (30.8%) experienced some types or no abuse.

3.3 *Lack of Schooling and Child Labor While in Care*

Lack of schooling was another problem experienced while in care. On average, care leavers in this study attended 2.59 schools (0–21 schools). About 70% regularly attended school while in care. Nonetheless, only 19.2% obtained a Higher School Certificate (equivalent to Year 11 or 12), 23.8% obtained an Intermediate School Certificate (equivalent to Year 10), and 56.9% did not obtain any school certificate (see Fig. 20.2).

Survey respondents who did not have a Higher School Certificate reported the reasons for non-completion. Almost half of respondents (46.7%) reported that institutions did not offer the opportunity. Many participants also reported that they could not pay attention at school (36.4%), and there was a lack of encouragement from institutions (39.6%) and teachers (34.6%). See Fig. 20.3 for details.

Participants in this study confronted many challenges in relation to their education while in care – poor in-house schooling, education assuming lower priority in favor of unpaid child labor in the institution, negative and stigmatizing attitudes toward them, and being forced to leave school at minimum school leaving age irrespective of ability and potential. Many males reported being conscripted into farm and other work at the age of 15 years. Luan's experience detailed below was by no means unique:

> What education? My education, my educational potential was like my childhood, stolen, I don't know what I could have been. I had no education. I was taken out of school before I turned 14 and was sent to work on a dairy farm. ("Luan")

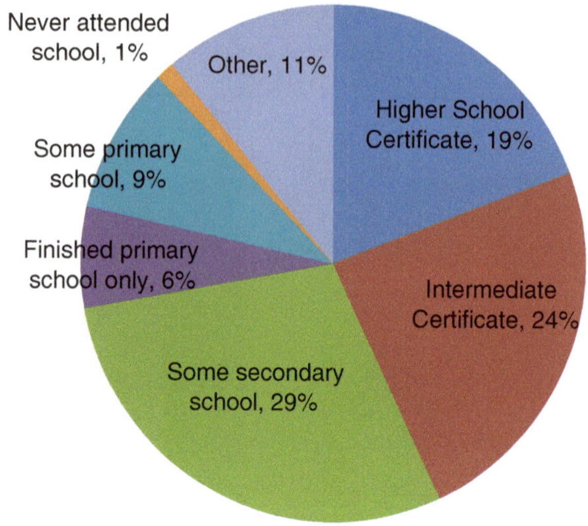

Fig. 20.2 Schooling while in care (*Note*: $n = 650$)

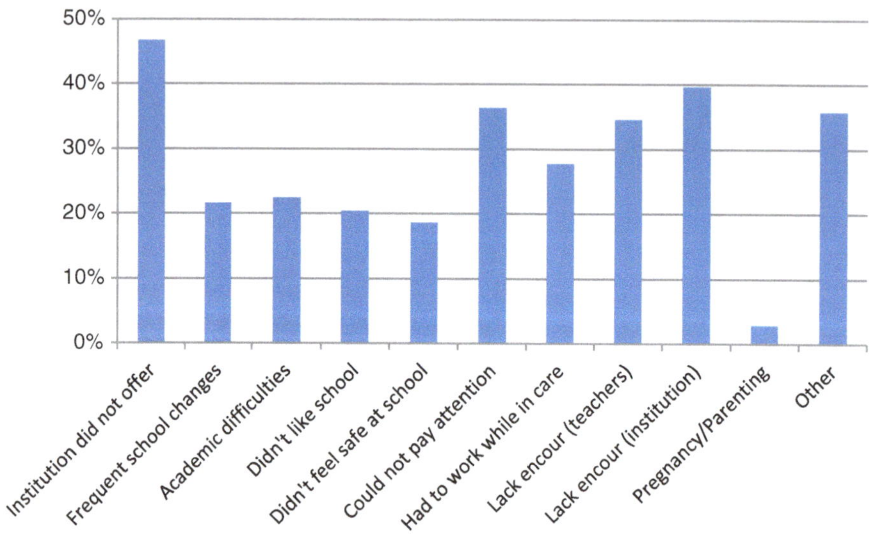

Fig. 20.3 Reasons for not finishing a Higher School Certificate (*Note*: $n = 338$)

Participants were conscious of the stigma attached to being a state ward and the low expectations derived from being perceived as a "home kid" by teachers. One research participant recalls:

> We were never permitted to be called by name. We were all called simply "home kid". We were ostracised by both teachers and students. Our school work and/or homework was never checked as we were told that we were only home kids and not expected to do anything in life other than life on government assistance. ("Anon")

Table 20.5 Hours of working while in care

	Under age 13 (*n* = 222)						At age 13 or above (*n* = 205)					
	All		Paid		Unpaid		All		Paid		Unpaid	
	Fr.	%	Fr.	%	Fr.	%	Fr.	%	Fr.	%	Fr.	%
0 h	41	18.5	210	94.6	48	21.6	27	13.2	162	79	51	24.9
1–10 h	56	25.2	7	3.2	53	23.9	41	20	15	7.3	40	19.5
11–20 h	60	27	2	0.9	60	27	50	24.4	9	4.4	51	24.9
21–30 h	40	18	1	0.5	39	17.6	28	13.7	1	0.5	25	12.2
31–40 h	13	5.9	0	0	12	5.4	36	17.6	14	6.8	23	11.2
41 or more	12	5.4	2	0.9	10	4.5	23	11.2	4	2	15	7.3

Note: Fr. refers to frequency

One relevant issue was working while in care. Under the age 13, 81.5% reported that they did some type of work while in care. Their working hours varied greatly, and the average was 16.24 h per week (0–112 h), and the median was 14 h. Among them, 78.4% did unpaid work, whereas only 5.4% did paid work while in care. At age 13 and above, 86.8% reported that they did some type of work while in care. On average, they reported to work for 22.51 h per week (0–112 h), and the median was 20 h. Among them, 75.1% did unpaid work, whereas 21% did paid work while in care. See details in Table 20.5.

The majority of respondents recalled having to spend substantial time working. Work was particularly gendered with females assigned domestic chores such as cleaning, laundry, and cooking, while males undertook farm and outdoor work. Work was a constant feature of the lives of children in institutions as noted by Ethan:

> Every morning before school you worked, come home and then you worked again until tea time, and you did that Monday to Friday, and then you worked all day Saturday, and on Sunday you're in church all day praying to God and thanking him for the great life you were living! ("Ethan")

Another female referred to her laundry duties which deprived her of play and sleep:

> I never really knew from the age of 10 to just be a little girl. I always had chores. From getting up – this is why I enjoy my sleeps now – 4 o'clock in the morning before anybody got up, I had to have so many uniforms ironed, ironed morning noon and night. Morning before breakfast, after breakfast until going to school. Then lunchtime, iron again until afternoon. Then iron again, at playtime until going to bed. ("Meg")

Work often took precedence over school. Children often worked under cruel and oppressive staff supervision as Eddie recalled:

> There was very little bit of schooling only. You either worked in the orchard, you worked in the farm or you worked in the dairy or you worked in the kitchen. And everyone who was there was allocated a job, so you worked. You had to work and that was all there is about it. And if you didn't work, the guys who were there, the so-called wardens, the people who were supposed to be looking after you would come around and belt you. ("Eddie")

3.4 Factors Related to Abuse and Neglect in Care

Various factors were associated with the experience of abuse and neglect in care. These factors differed by the type and source of abuse and neglect. A higher proportion of male care leavers experienced physical abuse by peers in care, $\chi^2(1, N = 400) = 5.44$, $p = .020$. There was no significant gender difference on physical abuse by adults or sexual abuse by anyone. Respondents who experienced sexual abuse were younger at the time of survey than people without such experiences: $t(346.24) = 2.98$, $p = .003$ for sexual abuse by adults and $t(393) = 2.71$, $p = .007$ for sexual abuse by peers. There was no significant age difference on physical abuse in care. Compared to nonindigenous participants, a higher proportion of Aboriginal persons experienced sexual abuse in care: $\chi^2(2, N = 405) = 11.74$, $p = .003$ for sexual abuse by adults and $\chi^2(2, N = 398) = 17.28$, $p < .001$ for sexual abuse by peers. Aboriginal status was not significantly related to physical abuse in care. See Table 20.6 for details.

On average, survey participants who experienced sexual abuse were about 1 year younger at the time of entry into care than their counterparts: $t(391) = 2.04$, $p = .043$ for sexual abuse by adults and $t(383) = 2.45$, $p = .015$ for sexual abuse by peers. Age at entry into care was not significantly associated with physical abuse in care. Respondents who entered care as state wards were more likely to have had experiences of physical abuse by peers ($\chi^2(2, N = 400) = 13.14$, $p = .001$), sexual abuse by adults ($\chi^2(2, N = 408) = 13.48$, $p = .001$), and sexual abuse by peers ($\chi^2(2, N = 400) = 7.67$, $p = .022$). State wardship at entry into care was not significantly related to physical abuse by adults in care. Overall, respondents who experienced physical and sexual abuse had more placements in care: $t(182.19) = -3.04$, $p = .003$ for physical abuse by adults, $t(365) = -3.91$, $p < .001$ for physical abuse by peers, $t(372.57) = -4.16$, $p < .001$ for sexual abuse by adults, and $t(252.28) = -3.06$, $p = .002$ for sexual abuse by peers. On average, participants who experienced sexual abuse stayed in care 1.2–1.4 years longer: $t(386.95) = -2.49$, $p = .013$ for sexual abuse by adults and $t(387) = -2.91$, $p = .004$ for sexual abuse by peers. The duration in care was not significantly associated with physical abuse in care. Respondents without experiences of physical abuse by peers had more frequent contact with their family than respondents with experiences of physical abuse by peers, $U = 13{,}169$, $p = .006$ with the mean rank of 212 ($Mdn = 3$) for people without the experiences and the mean rank of 180 ($Mdn = 3$) for people with the experiences. Contact with family was not significantly related to physical abuse by adults or sexual abuse by anyone. The percentages of people who did not have anyone helpful in care were higher among people with experiences of physical and sexual abuse in care: $\chi^2(1, N = 362) = 16.21$, $p < .001$ for physical abuse by adults, $\chi^2(1, N = 355) = 10.34$, $p = .001$ for physical abuse by peers, $\chi^2(1, N = 362) = 19.23$, $p < .001$ for sexual abuse by adults, and $\chi^2(1, N = 355) = 12.50$, $p < .001$ for sexual abuse by peers. See Table 20.7 for details.

As shown in Table 20.8, care leavers with a Higher School Certificate were younger at the time of survey than people with an Intermediate School Certificate or

Table 20.6 Demographics related to abuse in care

	Physical abuse by adults			Physical abuse by peers			Sexual abuse by adults			Sexual abuse by peers		
	No	Yes	$t/\chi2$	No	Yes	$t/\chi2$	No	Yes	$t/\chi2$	No	Yes	$t/\chi2$
Gender[a]						5.44^{*}						
Female				61.9%	49.6%							
Male				38.1%	50.4%							
Age at survey[b]							64.2	60.9	2.98^{**}	63.6	60.7	2.71^{**}
ATSI[a]									11.74^{**}			17.28^{***}
Indigenous							3.3%	9.3%		2.2%	11.9%	
Nonindigenous							93.3%	81.8%		92.6%	80.4%	
Don't know							3.3%	8.9%		5.2%	7.7%	

Note: Only significant differences are presented. $^{*}<.05$, $^{**}<.01$, $^{***}<.001$. [a]Chi-square test, [b]t-test. The sample size varies, $n = 395$ to 409

Table 20.7 Care circumstances related to abuse in care

	Physical abuse by adults			Physical abuse by peers			Sexual abuse by adults			Sexual abuse by peers		
	No	Yes	$t/\chi^2/U$	No	Yes	$t/\chi^2/U$	No	Yes	$t/\chi^2/U$	No	Yes	$t/\chi^2/U$
Age at entry[a]							6.7	5.8	2.04^{*}	6.7	5.6	2.45^{*}
Care status at entry[b]						13.14^{**}			13.48^{**}			7.67^{*}
Voluntary				29.3%	15.0%		28.2%	13.7%		22.7%	15.6%	
Wardship				42.9%	58.1%		46.4%	58.1%		47.2%	61.1%	
Other				27.8%	27.0%		25.4%	28.2%		30.0%	23.4%	
Number of placements[a]	3.1	4.3	-3.04^{**}	3.1	4.5	-3.91^{***}	3.1	4.7	-4.16^{***}	3.5	4.8	-3.06^{**}
Duration in care[a]							8.3	9.5	-2.49^{*}	8.4	9.8	-2.91^{**}
Contacts with family[c]						13169^{**}						
Never				19.4%	27.0%							
Less than yearly				17.7%	20.3%							
2–3 times a year				16.1%	20.3%							
Monthly				17.7%	16.0%							
Fortnightly or more				29.0%	16.4%							
Someone helpful in care[b]			16.21^{***}			10.34^{**}			19.23^{***}			12.50^{***}
No one	23.3%	49.5%		32.0%	49.8%		31.5%	54.5%		35.9%	54.8%	
Someone	76.7%	50.5%		68.0%	50.2%		68.5%	45.5%		64.1%	45.2%	

Note: Only significant differences are presented. *<.05, **<.01, ***<.001. [a]t-test, [b]chi-square test, [c]Mann-Whitney U test. The sample size varies, $n = 263$ to 409

Table 20.8 Demographics and care circumstances related to schooling in care

	Schooling status			
	HSC	ISC	NSC	F/H
Age at survey‡	58.61[a]	61.74[b]	62.95[b]	5.77**
Number of placements‡	3.66[a, b]	3.29[a]	4.39[b]	3.06*
Contact with family§				17.64***
Never	20.3%	15.5%	30.6%	
Less than yearly	17.4%	16.5%	21.3%	
2–3 times a year	14.5%	22.3%	19.9%	
Monthly	17.4%	19.4%	14.4%	
Fortnightly or more	30.4%	26.2%	13.9%	

Note: Only significant differences are presented. * <.05, **<.01, ***<.001. HSC refers to a Higher School Certificate, ISC indicates an Intermediate School Certificate, and NSC means no school certificate. ‡Welch ANOVA, §Kruskal-Wallis test. The sample size varies, $n = 388$ to 633

no school certificate, *Welch's* $F(2, 269.38) = 5.77$, $p = .004$. On average, respondents who did not have any school qualification had more placements in care than respondents with a school qualification, $F(2, 387) = 3.06$, $p = .048$. Respondents with a Higher School Certificate or an Intermediate School Certificate had more frequent contact with their family than respondents without any school certificate, $H(2) = 17.64$, $p < .001$ with the mean rank of 218 (*Mdn* = 3) for Higher School Certificate, 222 (*Mdn* = 3) for Intermediate School Certificate, and 174 (*Mdn* = 2) for no school certificate. Other demographics or care experiences did not differ significantly by schooling status.

3.5 *The Effects of Abuse and Neglect in Care*

Respondents provided their own assessment on the impacts of maltreatment in care. The most negatively affected areas while in care were education (3.77), relationship with friends (3.75), and mental health (3.68) in that order. The most negatively affected areas in present life were mental health (3.50), education (3.29), and relationship with partner (3.26) in that order (see Fig. 20.4).

Current well-being reported by participants was compared by abuse cluster and schooling status. In general, compared to care leavers who experienced some types of abuse, care leavers who experienced all types of abuse reported significantly lower levels of current well-being on all nine domains: physical health ($H(2) = 36.82$, $p < .001$), mental health ($H(2) = 44.56$, $p < .001$), relationship with family ($H(2) = 31.79$, $p < .001$), relationship with friends ($H(2) = 35.94$, $p < .001$), financial situation ($H(2) = 43.60$, $p < .001$), personal safety ($H(2) = 36.60$, $p < .001$), coping with stress ($H(2) = 26.85$, $p < .001$), receiving services ($H(2) = 31.02$, $p < .001$), and life in general ($H(2) = 52.91$, $p < .001$).

Care leavers with different levels of schooling significantly differed on five domains of current well-being: physical health ($H(2) = 9.08$, $p = .011$), relationship

Fig. 20.4 Self-assessed impacts of maltreatment in care (*Note*: 1 = not at all, 2 = slightly, 3 = moderately, 4 = considerably, 5 = enormously. The sample size varies, n = 150 to 382)

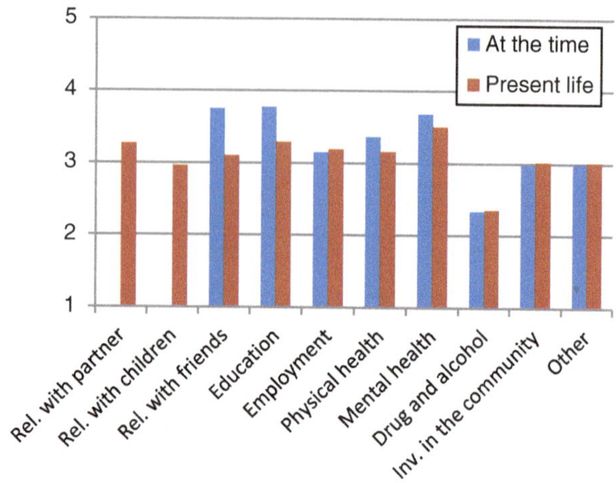

Fig. 20.5 Self-reported physical and mental health by abuse cluster (*Note*: *<.05, ***<.001. The sample size varies, n = 366 to 405)

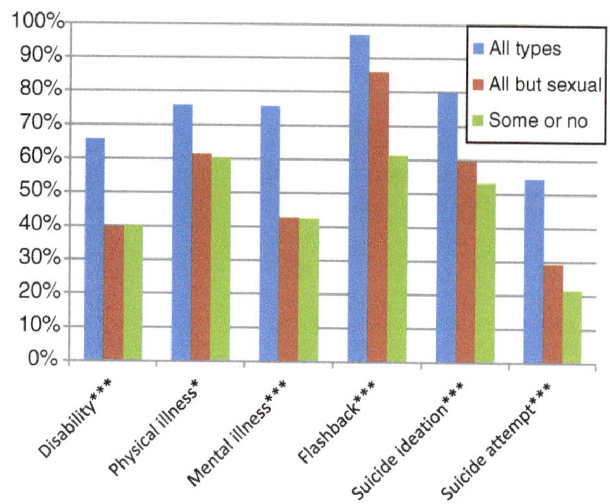

with friends ($H(2) = 11.56$, $p = .003$), financial situation ($H(2) = 14.77$, $p = .001$), coping with stress ($H(2) = 6.17$, $p = .046$), and life in general ($H(2) = 14.03$, $p = .001$). Overall, care leavers with a Higher School Certificate had higher levels, and care leavers without any school certificate had lower levels of well-being on these five domains.

More specifically, survey participants reported on their physical and mental illnesses that require ongoing treatment and suicide-related issues. Among participants, 68.2% had physical illnesses, 51% had a disability, and 59% had mental illnesses. Among participants with mental illnesses, 85.9% considered their mental illnesses were related to their experiences in care. Seventy-six percent reported experiencing flashbacks. Approximately 65% reported experiencing suicidal ideations at some point in their lives, and 39% had attempted suicide.

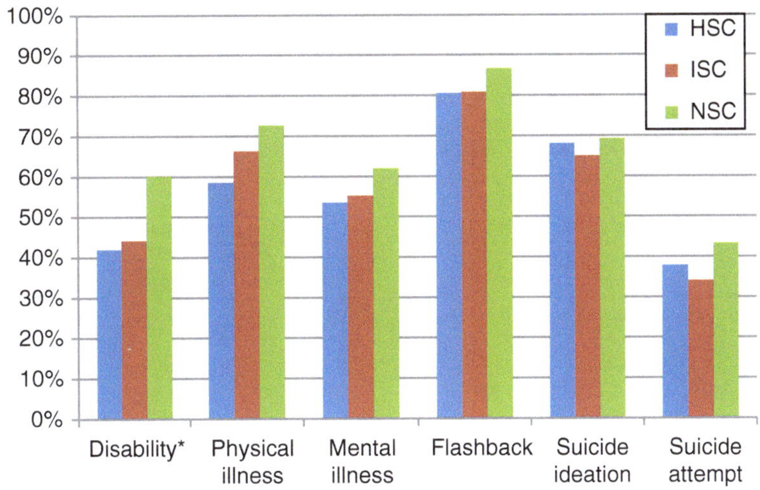

Fig. 20.6 Self-reported physical and mental health by schooling status (*Note*: HSC refers to a Higher School Certificate, ISC indicates an Intermediate School Certificate, and NSC means no school certificate. *<.05. The sample size varies, $n = 366$ to 405)

Self-reported physical and mental health significantly differed by abuse cluster. Compared to care leavers who experienced some types of abuse, care leavers who experienced all types of abuse in care had significantly higher proportion of disability ($\chi^2(2, N = 388) = 25.63, p < .001$), physical illness ($\chi^2(2, N = 405) = 10.90, p = .004$), mental illness ($\chi^2(2, N = 405) = 45.97, p < .001$), flashbacks ($\chi^2(2, N = 366) = 67.75, p < .001$), suicide ideation ($\chi^2(2, N = 383) = 26.53, p < .001$), and suicide attempt ($\chi^2(2, N = 373) = 36.25, p < .001$). Lack of schooling in care was not significantly related to self-reported physical and mental health outcomes or suicide-related issues, except disability status. A significantly higher percentage of respondents without any school qualification reported to have a disability, $\chi^2(2, N = 389) = 10.94, p = .004$. See Figs. 20.5 and 20.6 for details.

When results from a standardized measure of K10 psychological distress was examined, compared to the general community, higher percentages of care leavers in this study reported "very high" (38%) or "high" (21%) levels of psychological distress. For example, when percentage of people in the "very high" distress category is compared, the percentage found in this study is 8.5 times greater than the percentage found in 2007 Household Income and Labour Dynamics in Australia (HILDA) and 14.4 times greater than the percentage found in the National Survey of Mental Health and Wellbeing (NSMHW). However, the level of distress significantly differed by both abuse cluster and schooling status. Compared to people who experienced some types of abuse in care, survey participants who experienced all types of abuse in care reported significantly higher levels of psychological distress, $\chi^2(6, N = 385) = 71.10, p < .001$. Care leavers without any school certificate reported significantly higher levels of psychological distress than care leavers with a school certificate, $\chi^2(6, N = 388) = 16.36, p = .012$. See Figs. 20.7 and 20.8 for details.

Fig. 20.7 K10 psychological distress by abuse cluster (*Note*: K10 refers to the Kessler Psychological Distress Scale (Kessler et al., 2002). $n = 385$)

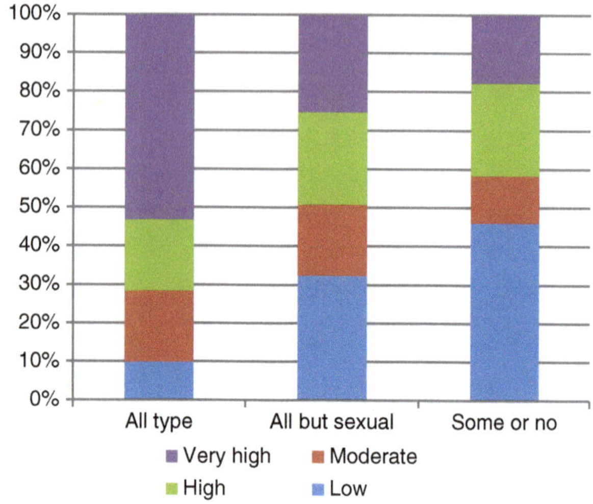

Fig. 20.8 K10 psychological distress by schooling status (*Note*: *K10* refers to the Kessler Psychological Distress Scale (Kessler et al., 2002). HSC refers to a Higher School Certificate, ISC indicates an Intermediate School Certificate, and NSC means no school certificate. $n = 388$)

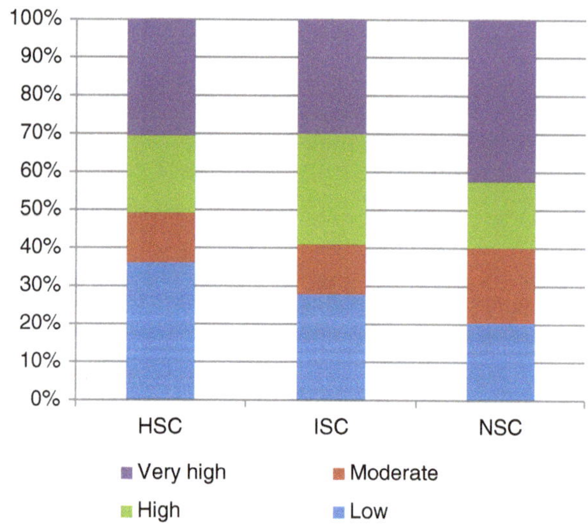

Physical injuries experienced by participants in care were often severe. Participants reported these were rarely addressed appropriately at the time, exacerbating their long-term impacts. Unset broken bones and muscular-skeletal damage, hearing loss and neurological impacts (of untreated ear infections and savage blows to the head), and serious trauma to internal organs (especially from being kicked and punched by physically powerful adults and sometimes as result of violent sexual assault) have resulted in ongoing medical problems:

> My arthritis is very early onset, and my specialist has said it's from the beltings I've had. I've got no cartilage there. I'm 64 years old; my mind sometimes feels like its 30, my body feels like its 80. ("Sylvie")

Chronic pain and illness, the need for regular specialist medical attention, and frequent hospitalizations have been frequently described by participants. Reparative surgeries (rarely completely successful) and a wide range of permanent disabilities, especially mobility issues, are lifelong companions for many participants in this study; premature aging would appear common in this research cohort.

Participants spoke of having difficulty paying for specialists and dental work. Some had to choose or prioritize one treatment over another. Another obstacle to accessing health care was the fear of the institutional hospital environment:

> I had appendicitis and I was in the hospital, and I freaked out. They put me in this room that reminded me a bit of [the Home], and it took everything in me not to run. I just wanted to rip out everything and go. ("Angela")

Ongoing anxiety, depression, flashbacks, dissociation, phobias, mistrust and paranoia, instability of mood, suicidality and self-harm, poor impulse control, and hypervigilance are some of the disturbed mental health phenomena described by participants to the researchers. Those who experienced trauma as children (and, possibly again, in adulthood) have come to realize that PTSD was an underlying condition through counseling and interaction with mental health professionals:

> I went and had counseling and I said I don't understand what is happening and she said you've got post-traumatic stress disorder, you've got this, you've got that. Oh my god. I was patting myself on the back thinking I had survived. Well I haven't survived at all. I've gone through life thinking I've survived. ("Simone")

As a result of childhood trauma and ongoing PTSD, or depression, a significant number of participants experienced suicide ideations, some to the extent of planning it:

> The nightmares started again. Fifteen years ago I tried to kill myself for probably about the third time. I should have died but I didn't. Then I ended up in the mental health system in Western Australia and eventually a psychiatrist said you're suffering from post-traumatic stress disorder because of what they'd done to you as a child. ("Michael")

Relational outcomes also differed by abuse cluster. Respondents who experienced all types of abuse in care reported significantly shorter length in their first relationship, *Welch's* $F(2, 160.23) = 22.26$, $p < .001$, and in their longest relationship, *Welch's* $F(2, 163.20) = 20.66$, $p < .001$. Fisher's exact test also indicated that abuse clusters significantly differed in their self-reported effects of care experiences on their intimate relationships, $p < .001$. Although there was no significant difference on parental status, compared to care leavers in cluster 3 (some or no abuse), significantly higher percentages of care leavers in cluster 1 (all types of abuse) and cluster 2 (all but sexual abuse) reported that their care experiences influenced their children in some ways, $\chi^2(2, N = 302) = 22.90$, $p < .001$. Perceived social support also significantly differed by abuse cluster. Respondents who experienced all types of abuse in care reported significantly lower scores on MSPSS social support scale, $F(2, 387) = 17.42$, $p < .001$. See Table 20.9 for details. Schooling status was not significantly related to relational outcomes.

Table 20.9 Relational outcomes by abuse cluster

	Abuse cluster			
	All types	All but sexual	Some or no	χ^2/F
Duration of 1st relationship[a]	15.14	22.21	28.41	22.26***
Duration of longest relationship[a]	19.54	26.18	31.03	20.66***
Care effects on relationships[b]	98.0%	94.1%	80.3%	
Care effects on children[b]	86.2%	78.0%	59.3%	22.90***
MSPSS: Social support scale[a]	3.6	4.4	4.6	17.42***

Note: ***<.001. [a]ANOVA or Welch ANOVA, [b]Fisher's exact or chi-square test. The sample size varies, $n = 302$ to 389

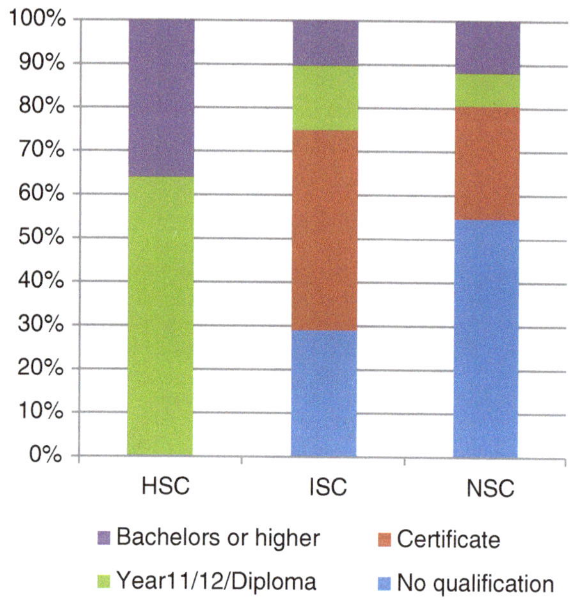

Fig. 20.9 Highest educational and vocational qualification by schooling status (*Note*: HSC refers to a Higher School Certificate, ISC indicates an Intermediate School Certificate, and NSC means no school certificate. *<.05, **<.01, ***<.001. $n = 650$)

Educational and financial outcomes were also compared. The highest educational and vocational qualification[2] did not differ significantly by abuse cluster but differed by schooling status. As expected, the highest education and training qualification significantly differed by schooling in care, $H(2) = 197.96$, $p < .001$, with the mean rank of 523(*Mdn* = 3) for a Higher School Certificate, with the mean rank of 321 (*Mdn* = 2) for an Intermediate School Certificate, and with the mean rank of 261(*Mdn* = 1) for no school certificate. Overall, care leavers with a Higher School Certificate were more likely to have a bachelor's or higher degree than their counterparts. See Fig. 20.9 for details. The levels of income did not differ signifi-

[2]The highest educational and vocational qualification includes schooling and vocational training. When a person has both a HSC and a certificate, a HSC was set to be the highest educational and vocational qualification.

cantly by abuse cluster or schooling status. Nonetheless, the experience of financial hardships significantly differed by abuse cluster, $\chi^2(2, N = 405) = 29.25, p < .001$. Nearly two-thirds of care leavers (65.9%) in cluster 1 (all types of abuse) reported financial hardships, whereas 40.8% and 38.1% of care leavers in cluster 2 and 3 reported financial hardships, respectively. The experience of financial hardships did not differ significantly by schooling status.

For many participants their lived adult experience has been associated with insecure and substandard housing and homelessness. Many participants had experienced housing difficulties: 46% had experienced homelessness, 48% lived in public housing, and 60% had temporary housing at some point in their lives. However, housing outcomes significantly differed by abuse cluster. Respondents who experienced all types of abuse in care were less likely to have had experience of owning a residential property ($\chi^2(2, N = 399) = 16.04, p < .001$) and more likely to have had experiences of living in public housing ($\chi^2(2, N = 410) = 11.80, p = .003$), being homeless ($\chi^2(2, N = 407) = 46.43, p < .001$), and living in temporary housing ($\chi^2(2, N = 409) = 42.17, p < .001$) at some point in their lives. Schooling was significantly related to the experience of owning a property ($\chi^2(2, N = 411) = 7.03, p = .030$) and being homeless ($\chi^2(2, N = 419) = 6.80, p = .033$) but not related to the experience of living in public housing or temporary housing. See Figs. 20.10 and 20.11 for details.

3.6 *Recent Development in Responding to Historic Abuse in Australia*

About 39% of respondents (n = 159) participated in the Royal Commission into Institutional Responses to Child Sexual Abuse. Participants rated their experiences on a ten-point scale (1 = not at all and 10 = very much), and their perceptions were somewhat positive: the opportunity to express their concerns was rated 6.8, and the acknowledgment of their concerns was rated 6.2.

4 Discussion

The lives of most participants in this study were characterized by extreme neglect and abuse while in institutional and other forms of out-of-home care. From the point of entry to care, maltreatment began and continued throughout, even through changes of placement. Transitioning out of care after years of institutionalization was a further traumatic and demoralizing process (Fernandez et al., 2016). To recap, the reasons participants in this study were separated from their primary caregivers and placed in care can be understood at the microsystems and macrosystems levels (Bronfenbrenner, 1979) of individual or family vulnerability, the child rescue model, and assimilationist and racist polices. Removal to care, as is the case today,

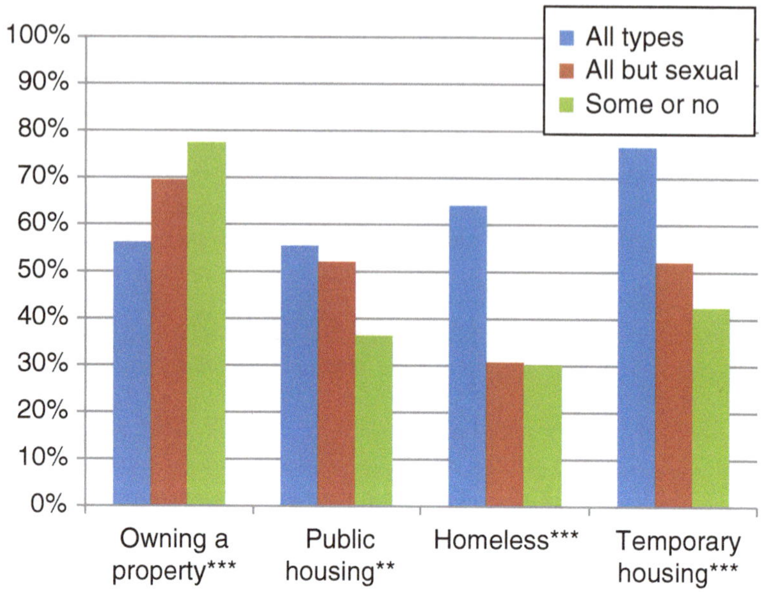

Fig. 20.10 Housing experience by abuse cluster (*Note*: **<.01, ***<.001. The sample size varies, *n* = 399 to 410)

was rooted in structural determinants, especially poverty and disadvantage (Bywaters, Brady, Sparks, & Bos, 2016; Lindsey, 1994; Pelton, 1989, 2015). Lack of welfare programs and early intervention services meant there was no service system safety net to address need in times of family crisis. Placement in care was the only real option available to parents or to child welfare organizations who intervened. As they entered placement, abusive cleansing and depersonalization rituals were frequently inflicted upon new arrivals (Find & Connect, 2016; Musgrove, 2013; Penglase, 2005).

4.1 Maltreatment in the Care Environment

Child neglect was endemic in out-of-home care during the study period along with horrific corporal punishment and emotional and sexual abuse. Very few participants reported evidence of kindness, encouragement, respect, warmth, or any form of physical affection that was not the sinister companion to sexual abuse (Penglase, 2005). This contributed to emotional isolation, anxiety, and sadness that many children experienced during their years in care. In adult life such maltreatment has clearly been a major contributor to serious mental health difficulties and, for many, lifelong psychiatric disabilities that have seriously undermined well-being. For participants overall, the daily regimen of drudgery and hard physical labor limited the scope for normative developmental growth.

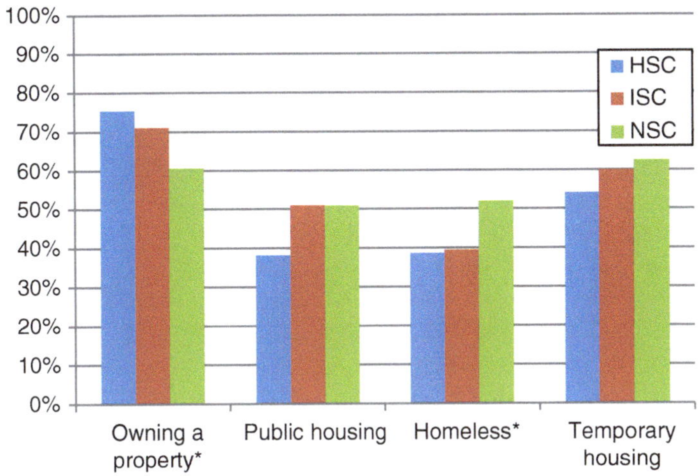

Fig. 20.11 Housing experience by schooling status (*Note*: HSC refers to a Higher School Certificate, ISC indicates an Intermediate School Certificate, and NSC means no school certificate. *<.05. The sample size varies, $n = 411$ to 422)

Every category of abuse was described to the researchers. Physical, emotional, and sexual abuse coexisted and was reported by participants on a scale that is extremely difficult to contemplate. The prevalence of neglect and emotional, physical, and sexual abuse in this study is higher than that identified in the Adverse Childhood Experience (ACE) study in the United States and in current Australian Child Protection statistics (AIHW, 2016). Results in this study are also in line with previous research which has found a high prevalence of multiple and co-occurring types of maltreatment (Finkelhor et al., 2007; McMillen et al., 2005; Witt et al., 2016).

Other forms of neglect that have had long-term deleterious impacts on participants include those of a social, cultural, or intellectual nature. Most study participants experienced a marginalized childhood devoid of fun or play. Aboriginal children were deprived of the opportunity to identify with and understand their culture. They had no chance to know their communities and could not speak their language without being severely punished. See further details in Fernandez et al. (2016).

Findings of this study indicated that the vulnerability to abuse and neglect in care differed by children's characteristics and care circumstances. As examples, we explored physical abuse and sexual abuse by peers and by adults. In this study, participants who were younger at entry into OOHC, were state wards at entry, stayed longer in OOHC, had more placements, did not have or rarely had contact with their families, and did not have anyone helpful in care were more likely to have experienced sexual abuse while in care. Given the racism that prevailed in Australia during the time, it is understandable that Aboriginal children were more vulnerable to various abuses; however, it is unclear why the younger cohort of this study were more vulnerable to sexual abuse in care. Children without a support network outside or inside seemed to be preyed upon by adults and peers. These were children separated from family and society, with no voice, protection, or advocate to support them in a system that supported a culture of silence.

The savage institutional abuse and serious neglect described by participants in this study derived directly from institutional authority figures invested with unfettered power and control. Some staff clearly took absolute advantage of the opportunity the powerful roles afforded them, to prey on vulnerable and traumatized children (Musgrove, 2013). Even when staff were not abusive toward their charges, there were few accounts from participants of receiving any real warmth or even basic respect. Staff did not challenge the status quo nor did they draw official attention to rampant abuse (Senate Community Affairs References Committee, 2004). These harms continue to impact harshly on the lives of victims with intergenerational effects.

The period under study was in an era where screening of recruits, referee reports, and police checks were for the most part not mandatory. Orientation processes, professional qualifications, training programs, practice standards, supervision, and oversight were either negligible or nonexistent. There was effectively little or no oversight or accountability for staff or for organizations until very late in the study period (Senate Community Affairs References Committee, 2004). Even then, monitoring practices seem to have been questionable and limited in scope. Sexual offenders were still often moved from one institution to another rather than being reported to police or even dismissed. This meant that participants often encountered these offenders repeatedly, even with placement changes.

4.2 Educational Neglect

The UN Convention of the Rights of the Child emphasizes the child's right to learn, formally and informally, so that he/she is adequately prepared to take their place in adult society and achieve optimum well-being. It is documented that educational outcomes are associated with employment and financial security (Hook & Courtney, 2011; Jackson & Sachdev, 2001; Okpych & Courtney, 2014), housing (Davison & Burris, 2014; McNamara, 2015; Robson, 2008), physical and mental health (Buchanan, 1999; Dixon, 2008; Fernandez, 2008; Gilligan, 2007; Harvey, McNamara, & Andrewartha, 2016; Stein, 2012), and vulnerability to involvement in the criminal justice system (Narey, 2007). Participants in this study had significantly less education as apparent from the quantitative and qualitative data. Almost half of participants in this study mentioned that institutions did not offer an opportunity for them to continue education until Year 11/12 or equivalent. Compared to the older cohort, the younger cohort in this study had more schooling. This seems to be derived from the increase of the minimum school leaving age in the 1960s. Findings of this study also showed that placement stability and contact with family were relevant to schooling of children in OOHC. A finding that emerged was that many experienced placement instability such that exposed them to changes of schools and disruption of their education. It is known that placement instability significantly influences school attendance, school engagement, and school stability (Sebba et al., 2015; Smith & McLean, 2013; Zorc et al., 2013). Findings of this study confirmed that it was difficult for children to stay engaged and do well at school when they had to move placements and schools. Families who stayed connected to their children were likely to maintain interest in their children's well-being, including education.

Additionally, where schooling was integrated into large institutions, neglect and abuse that characterized the home was manifest within the school. Physical, emotional, and sexual abuse frequently occurred within the classroom. Humiliations were often extreme. In mainstream schools, "homies" were frequently bullied and ostracized. It is theorized that schooling provides the structure and stability that enables individuals toward greater competence and potentially counteracts the effects of adverse experiences in children's care environments. The school environment they experienced did little to ameliorate the victimization they were enduring or provide nurturance and stimulation. In summary, many participants left care without basic life skills and competencies such as literacy and numeracy and were educationally neglected. This is clearly an area for redress.

4.3 *Child Labor as Maltreatment*

Australian "orphanages" were largely modeled on the children's institutions developed in England and Ireland during the nineteenth century (Swain & Hillel, 2010). As the financial sustainability of these institutions depended upon the labor of residents, children were forced to work at the same or similar physical capacity of adults, from a very young age. Such arrangements would have been in direct contravention of the UN Convention on the Rights of the Child (1989). The practices did actually breach child labor laws in place. The large institutions – and later, cottage, foster, and kinship homes – were effectively unregulated and were not held to account. Children were wakened before dawn to draw water, light fires, and milk cows. They carried out arduous work in the fields and endured horrendous conditions in the "Magdalene" laundries and other industrial settings. All domestic work in the institutions, and much of that in cottage and even foster homes, was completed by child laborers under cruel and oppressive staff supervision. Participants in this study have shared extreme examples of this, and their narratives are consistent with earlier evidence (HREOC, 1997; Humphreys, 1996; Senate Community Affairs References Committee, 2004). Children were poorly or almost never remunerated in any way for the work they undertook. Chronic illnesses, injuries, and permanent disabilities are still experienced by this study's participants as a legacy of their engagement in child labor while living in out-of-home care (Senate Community Affairs References Committee, 2004). The legal implications of these Dickensian practices and their shocking legacy have been raised by participants as matters for redress and reparation.

4.4 The Effects of Maltreatment on Adult Outcomes

Child maltreatment has physical and psychological consequences that are immediate and long term (Widom, Czaja, Bentley, & Johnson, 2012). This study generated evidence that the consequences of maltreatment in care extended well beyond their childhoods persisting into late adulthood. The maltreatment experiences of this cohort included multiple subtypes and reported trauma rather than single events, predisposing them to a wider range of symptomatology. While researchers have documented the harmful consequences of maltreatment in its individual and multiple forms, Aber and Cichetti (1984) note the complexities in separating the effects of subtypes of maltreatment. Evidence of the correspondence between experiencing a high number of types of victimization and a higher prevalence of psychological conditions comes from a number of studies (Felitti et al., 1998; Greger, Myhre, Lydersen, & Jozefiak, 2015). In attempting to deal with the complexity of exposure to multiple types of maltreatment, the cluster analysis was conducted to identify specific constellations of abuse subtypes and their respective impacts. This inclusive analysis aligns with the approach advocated by Nurius et al. (2007) and Moore et al. (2015) who emphasize the importance of examining trauma from a cumulative adversity perspective to understand long-term impacts.

The experiences of maltreatment have left indelible marks on participants including lifelong fear, mistrust, low self-esteem, and hypervigilance. Abuse also resulted in horrendous injuries leading to chronic physical illness, serious mental health problems, and a wide range of disabilities. The level of abusive behavior inflicted on participants growing up in cottage homes or in foster or kinship care seems little different in quality or extent from that experienced by the large cohort of children in institutions.

4.5 Health

Physical health of care leavers in this study was perceived to be poorer than the general population. The impact of maltreatment on health and well-being is noted to extend into adult life, the experience of abuse in childhood being implicated in poorer physical and mental health (Chapman et al., 2004; Edwards et al., 2003; Erikson, Egeland, & Pianta, 1997; Fisher et al., 2010; Gilbert et al., 2009; Kaplan et al., 1998; Lueger-Schuster et al., 2014; Radford, Corral, Bradley, & Fisher, 2013; Silverman, Reinherz, & Giaconia, 1996; Springer et al., 2007; Sugaya et al., 2012; Wegman & Stelter, 2009). The adult mental health impacts of trauma experienced as a result of a childhood in "care" have proved to be the most profound impacts on lifelong well-being. Previous studies have also linked childhood maltreatment to a number of psychological conditions such as anxiety, depression, post-traumatic stress disorder (PTSD), and suicide ideations (Afifi et al., 2014; Clemmons et al., 2007; Kaplan et al., 1998; Moore et al., 2015; Mullen et al., 1996; Norman et al., 2012; Twaite & Rodriguez-Srednicki, 2004; Widom et al., 2007). Findings of this study were consistent with findings of previous studies. Compared to participants who experienced some types of abuse, participants who experienced all types of abuse presented significantly worse physical and mental health outcomes. Participants who experience multiple types of maltreatment (see Table 20.4) stood out as having higher proportion of disability, physical illness, mental illness, flash backs, suicide ideation and attempts, and recording significantly higher levels of psychological distress on the K10 standardized measure of psychological distress. Findings related to the effects of educational neglect on health were less consistent. While the maltreatment had stopped after they left care, their impaired functioning as adults suggests the consequences of their exposure to these adverse events in care were difficult to reverse for many.

Many participants described having tried to end their lives and have been hospitalized in a psychiatric facility, often on numerous occasions. For many of the Aboriginal participants, the experience of multiple losses and disrupted identity has had a deleterious impact on their own mental health and in many instances that of their children and grandchildren (Creative Spirits, 2016; HREOC, 1997).

Participants' self-assessments of the most negatively affected areas in their present lives included not only health and education but also relational outcomes. The quality of later intimate and family relationships was also affected by their early victimization. Participants who experienced all types of abuse in care reported significantly shorter duration of their first relationship and their longest relationships. Coherent with attachment theories, researchers have noted that the experience of abusive caregiving can promote negative views of self-worth, constraining relationships of trust and intimacy in later life. Similar to other studies (Colman & Widom, 2004; Lowell, Renk, & Adgate, 2014; Savla et al., 2013; Sroufe & Fleeson, 1986), this research found that early and multiple maltreatment experiences had a cumulative effect on personal relationships, contributing to difficult relationships in their adult lives.

In summary the mental health impacts of trauma experienced in care have led to extreme levels of marginalization, disempowerment, and social isolation for many participants and their peers (Fernandez et al., 2016; Senate Community Affairs References Committee, 2004). Social isolation for Aboriginal participants, who have struggled to locate and reconnect with their families and communities, has often been extreme (HREOC, 1997). For many former Child Migrants, also dislocated from kin on the other side of the world, developing a clear identity has been challenging. Social support networks have also often been difficult to establish after leaving care (Humphries, 1996).

4.6 Education

As noted earlier, very few participants left care with an adequate education. For many, the most rudimentary competencies in literacy and numeracy were lacking. That deficit in formal preparation, together with health and mental health issues and financial disadvantage, has made participation in continuing education enormously difficult. This finding is consistent with existing research on contemporary out-of-home care systems (Courtney et al., 2011; Goddard, 2000; Harvey et al., 2016; Mendes & Snow, 2016; Pecora et al., 2006). Research has established that exposure to adverse childhood experiences undermines learning and academic achievement, impacting adulthood outcomes with respect to education and employment domains (Nurius et al., 2007; Sansone, Leung, & Wiederman, 2012; Zielinski, 2009). Lack of education and training has impeded access to fulfilling paid work for many of this study's participants. A lifetime of unemployment has predictably been the reality for many of this study's participants and a common experience for Forgotten Australians (Senate Community Affairs References Committee, 2004). Long-term unemployment has meant financial hardship and, in many instances, grinding poverty. Aboriginal care leavers are at even greater risk of long-term unemployment and its attendant problems (ABS, 2016). Without rewarding paid employment, participants have been excluded from many of life's most important opportunities for long-term well-being.

4.7 Limitations

Care leavers self-identified and self-selected to participate in this study. Because there is no comprehensive list of care leavers in Australia, it was not possible to use probability sampling strategies. Therefore, the study sample is not representative of all care leavers who lived in child welfare institutions or other forms of institutional care during this period. It is recommended to interpret findings of this study with caution.

Despite extensive efforts made to recruit participants in this study (e.g., media campaign), the number of participants in some states and territories were relatively small. Also, Aboriginal people seem to be underrepresented in this study. However, demographics of this study indicate that this study captured views of care leavers with diverse backgrounds in terms of gender, age, Aboriginal status, education, region, experiences during and after care (both negative and positive), and involvement with care leaver organizations.

Another limitation is that this study is based on self-report, and it may reflect participants' perceptions and recollections. However, self-report measures are widely used in the social sciences and deemed to be best to capture perceptions, feelings, and interpretations that are core interests of social science research.

4.8 Implications for Policy and Services

The legacy of maltreatment in terms of damage to the individual's self-worth and impairment of emotional, cognitive, and social functioning is profound (Erikson et al., 1997) and warrants close attention. Identifying the patterns and consequences of maltreatment of vulnerable individuals who spent their childhoods in public care has important implications for therapeutic, legal, and policy decisions relevant to victimization and trauma. It cannot be overstated that a comprehensive health safety net is urgently needed to support the increasing frailty, illness, and disability within this vulnerable and aging cohort. Audiology, pathology, optometry, dentistry, physiotherapy, occupational therapy, prosthetics, and orthotics are just some of the ancillary health services which participants need on an ongoing basis (Fernandez et al., 2016). These are in addition to their primary health-care needs for ongoing assessment, review, and management of chronic health issues, disabilities, and illnesses. Most also require multiple medications and surgeries. For Aboriginal participants, the risk of type 2 diabetes and renal failure is elevated (Diabetes Australia, 2015; Shaw & Tanamas, 2012), along with hearing loss and vision impairment (Creative Spirits, 2016). Many participants in Fernandez et al. (2016) described frustrations with help-seeking within the health system directly related to injuries sustained during their years in care.

Long-term mental health impacts of trauma associated with abuse in care included flashbacks, anxiety, depression, self-harm, dissociation, and suicidality. Many participants reported that they were in urgent need of ongoing counseling and of specialist psychiatric help (Fernandez et al., 2016). Some have been able to access the public mental health access provisions currently in place but frequently reported that these were inadequate or inappropriate (Fernandez et al., 2016). Such impacts are especially powerful for Aboriginal participants whose profound losses have impacted on their own lifelong mental health and those of subsequent generations. For members of the Stolen Generations, culturally competent services are essential (Creative Spirits, 2016). Services for former Child Migrants must be sensitively attuned to the unique trauma that arises from their experience of separation, loss, and, in most cases, abuse and neglect (Humphries, 1996).

The continuing need for out-of-home care for vulnerable children speaks to the need for professional and public awareness of the damaging and long-term effects of child maltreatment and the need for preventive and rehabilitative interventions.

As children, most participants reported feeling sad, lonely, unstimulated, and socially isolated; many described adulthood similarly (Fernandez et al., 2016). The majority of participants have struggled to reestablish positive connections with family and extended family. Many found friendships and intimate relationships confronting and difficult to sustain; this is consistent with existing research findings (Senate Community Affairs References Committee, 2004). The demands of parenting without positive role models, or a nurturing experience of caregiving in their own childhood to draw upon, have been challenging. Some participants have tragically experienced the removal of their own children on protective grounds or have been forced to place them in care (Fernandez et al., 2016). In some instances participants were subject to the practice of forced adoption as they gave birth to a child while in care, experiencing the grief, loss, and possible retraumatization that subsequent life events may trigger (Fernandez et al., 2016). Others, especially Aboriginal and Torres Strait Islander participants, are currently providing kinship care for grandchildren or the children of other relatives, either formally or informally (Fernandez et al., 2016).

This is clearly enormously courageous combined as it is with a legacy of trauma from their own childhood.

As an aging population, one of the greatest fears expressed by older participants in this study is an anticipation of placement in aged care institutions or settings (Fernandez et al., 2016). For most participants, entry to aged care represents a return to the vulnerability, fear, and disempowerment they experienced as children in that almost all of them experienced abuse and neglect while in care. The findings of this study suggest that to support the needs of aging care leavers, noninstitutional forms of aged care need to be explored, and residential care settings should not replicate the abusive and oppressive aspects they were exposed to as children. Training is needed for social workers and public health practitioners to understand the impact of exposure to neglect and abuse on social, emotional, and psychological problems across the life course. The findings also underline the importance of a comprehensive trauma assessment for this population as they present to adult and aged care services.

5 Conclusion

Based on the findings of this study, it is evident that the rights listed in the United Nations Convention on the Rights of the Child (1989) were breached in Australia's out-of-home care system during the twentieth century. Most participants in this study were denied almost all rights to protection, nurture, learning, health, and well-being while growing up in care. Instead, they experienced neglect, abuse, and great trauma. This has clearly had lifelong health and well-being impacts. For this study's participants, chronic illness, disability, relationship breakdown, homelessness, social isolation, anxiety, and depression were common. Substantial investment is needed in reducing the potential for maltreatment in care and its costs in terms of trauma for children and the health and disability burden in adulthood. Other impacts, for most, include marginalization from educational and work opportunities; this has almost always resulted in financial hardship and often a lifetime of poverty. Lack of a clear identity and a secure sense of belonging are also too frequently the lived experience of participants.

Acknowledgment The authors acknowledge the research assistance of Dr. Hazel Blunden, Dr. Patricia McNamara, Szilvia Kovacs, and Paul-Auguste Cornefert School of Social Sciences, UNSW Sydney.

The funding supporting this research from the Australian Research Council is also gratefully acknowledged.

References

Aber, J. L., & Cichetti, D. (1984). The social-emotional development of maltreated children: An empirical and theoretical analysis. In H. Fitzgerald, B. Lester, & M. Yogman (Eds.), *Theory and research in behavioural paediatrics*. New York: Plenum.

Afifi, T. O., MacMillan, H. L., Boyle, M., Taillieu, T., Cheung, K., & Sareen, J. (2014). Child abuse and mental disorders in Canada. *CMAJ, 186*(9), E324–E332. doi:10.1503/cmaj.131792.
Alliance for Forgotten Australians. (2016). *Forgotten Australians: Supporting survivors of childhood institutional care in Australia*. Available at http://forgottenaustralians.org.au/assets/docs/Booklet/AFA_Booklet.pdf. Accessed 12 Oct 2016.
Ames, E. (1997). *The development of Romanian orphanage children adopted to Canada*. Final report to the National Welfare Grants Program: Human Resources Development Canada. Burnaby, Canada: Simon Fraser University.
Andrews, G., & Slade, T. (2001). Interpreting scores on the Kessler psychological distress scale (K10). *Australian and New Zealand Journal of Public Health, 25*(6), 494–497.
Atkinson, J. (2002). *Trauma trails, recreating song lines: The transgenerational effects of trauma in Aboriginal Australia*. North Melbourne, Vic: Spinifex Press.
Australian Bureau of Statistics (ABS). (2016). Characteristics of employment. *Australia*. Available at http://www.abs.gov.au/ausstats/abs@.nsf/mf/6333.0?OpenDocument. Accessed 8 Sept 2016.
Australian Institute of Health and Welfare (AIHW). (2016). *Child Protection Australia 2014–15*. Child welfare series no. 63. Cat. No. SWS 57. Canberra, Australia: AIHW.
Bean, P., & Melville, J. (1989). *Lost children of the empire*. London: Unwin Hyman.
Belt, W., & Abidin, R. R. (1996). The relation of childhood abuse and early parenting experiences to current marital quality in a nonclinical sample. *Child Abuse & Neglect, 20*, 1019–1030. doi:10.1016/0145-2134(96)00092-0.
Biehal, N., Clayden, J., Stein, M., & Wade, J. (1995). *Moving on: Young people and leaving care schemes*. London, UK: HMSO.
Bowlby, J. (1988). *A secure base: Parent–child attachment and healthy human development*. London, England: Routledge.
Broad, B. (2005). *Improving the health and well being of young people in care*. Lyme Regis, Dorset: Russell House.
Bronfenbrenner, U. (1979). *The ecology of human development: Experiments by nature and design*. Cambridge, MA: Harvard University Press.
Buchanan, A. (1999). Are care leavers significantly dissatisfied and depressed in adult life? *Adoption and Fostering, 23*(4), 35–40.
Buckingham, E. T., & Daniolos, P. (2013). Longitudinal outcomes for victims of child abuse. *Current Psychiatry Reports, 15*(2), 342. doi:10.1007/s11920-012-0342-3.
Burns, B. J., Phillips, S. D., Wagner, H. R., Barth, R. P., Kolko, D. J., Campbell, Y., & Landsverk, J. (2004). Mental health need and access to mental health services by youths involved with child welfare: A national survey. *Journal of the American Academy of Child & Adolescent Psychiatry, 43*(8), 960–970.
Bywaters, P., Brady, G., Sparks, T., & Bos, E. (2016). Inequalities in child welfare intervention rates: The intersection of deprivation and identity. *Child & Family Social Work, 21*(4), 452–463.
Care Leavers Australian Network (CLAN). (2008). A terrible way to grow up: The experiences of institutional care and its outcomes for care leavers in Australia. Bankstown/Sydney, NSW: Care Leavers Australia Network.
Cashmore, J., & Paxman, M. (1996). *Report: Wards leaving care, a longitudinal study*. Sydney, NSW: Department of Community Services.
Chapman, D. P., Whitfield, C. L., Felitti, V. J., Dube, S. R., Edwards, V. J., & Anda, R. F. (2004). Adverse childhood experiences and the risk of depressive disorders in adulthood. *Journal of Affective Disorders, 82*(2), 217–225. doi:10.1016/j.jad.2003.12.013.
Clausen, J. M., Landsverk, J., Ganger, W., Chadwick, D., & Litrownik, A. (1998). Mental health problems of children in foster care. *Journal of Child & Family Studies, 7*(3), 283–296.
Clemmons, J. C., Walsh, K., DiLillo, D., & Messman-Moore, T. L. (2007). Unique and combined contributions of multiple child abuse types and abuse severity to adult trauma symptomatology. *Child Maltreatment, 12*, 172–181.
Cocker, C., & Scott, S. (2006). Improving the mental and emotional well-being of looked after children. Connecting research, policy and practice. *The Journal of the Royal Society for the Promotion of Health, 126*(1), 18–23.

Colman, R. A., & Widom, C. S. (2004). Childhood abuse and neglect and adult intimate relationships: A prospective study. *Child Abuse & Neglect, 28*, 1133–1151. doi:10.1016/j.chiabu.2004.02.005.

Commission of Inquiry. (1999). *Commission of inquiry into abuse of children in Queensland institutions report*. Brisbane, QLD: Commission of Inquiry.

Connelly, G., & Furnivall, J. (2013). Addressing low attainment of children in public care: The Scottish experience. *European Journal of Social Work, 16*(1), 88–104.

Courtney, M. E., Dworsky, A., Brown, A., Cary, C., Love, K., & Vorhies, V. (2011). *Midwest evaluation of the adult functioning of former foster youth: Outcomes at age 26*. Chicago, IL: Chapin Hall at the University of Chicago.

Creative Spirits. (2016). www.creativespirits.org.au

Creswell, J. W., & Plano, C. V. L. (2011). *Designing and conducting mixed methods research*. Los Angeles, CA: SAGE Publications.

Daly, F., & Gilligan, R. (2010). Selected educational outcomes for young people aged 17–19 years in long term foster care in Ireland. In E. Fernandez & P. Barth (Eds.), *How does foster care work: International evidence on outcomes* (pp. 243–257). London: Jessica Kingsley Publishers.

Davison, M. S., & Burris, E. W. (2014). Transitioning foster care youth and their risk for homelessness: Policy, program, and budgeting shortcomings. *Human Welfare, 3*(1), 22–33.

Diabetes Australia. (2015). About diabetes. Available at https://www.diabetesaustralia.com.au/about-diabetes. Accessed 23 Sept 2016.

Dixon, J. (2008). Young people leaving residential care: Experiences and outcomes. In A. Kendrick (Ed.), *Residential child care: Prospects and challenges*. London: Jessica Kingsley Publishers.

Doyle, L., Brady, A. M., & Byrne, G. (2009). An overview of mixed methods research. *Journal of Research in Nursing, 14*(2), 175–185. doi:10.1177/1744987108093962.

Edwards, V. J., Holden, G. W., Felitti, V. J., & Anda, R. F. (2003). Relationship between multiple forms of childhood maltreatment and adult mental health in community respondents: Results from the adverse childhood experiences study. *American Journal of Psychiatry, 160*(8), 1453–1460.

Egeland, B., & Sroufe, L. A. (1981). Attachment and early maltreatment. *Child Development, 52*, 44–52.

Erikson, M. F., Egeland, B., & Pianta. (1997). The effects of maltreatment on the development of young children. In D. Cicchetti & V. Carlson (Eds.), *Maltreatment: Theory and research on the causes and consequences of child abuse and neglect* (pp. 647–684). Cambridge, UK: Cambridge University Press.

Felitti, V. J., Anda, R. F., Nordenberg, D., Williamson, D. F., Spitz, A. M., Edwards, V., … Marks, J. S. (1998). Relationship of childhood abuse and household dysfunction to many of the leading causes of death in adults. The adverse childhood experiences (ACE) study. *American Journal of Preventive Medicine, 14*(4), 245–258.

Fernandez, E. (2008). Unravelling emotional, behavioural and educational outcomes in a longitudinal study of children in foster-care. *British Journal of Social Work, 38*, 1283–1301. doi:10.1093/bjsw/bcm028.

Fernandez, E., & Atwool, N. (2013). Child protection and out-of-home care: Policy, practice, and research connections Australia and New Zealand. *Psychosocial Intervention, 22*(3), 175–184.

Fernandez, E., & Lee, J.-S. (2017). Experiences and outcomes of adults who endured maltreatment as children in care in Australia in the twentieth century. In A. V. Rus, S. R. Parris, & E. Stativa (Eds.), *Child maltreatment in residential care: History, research, and current practice*. New York, NY: Springer.

Fernandez, E., Lee, J.-S., Blunden, H., McNamara, P., Kovacs, S., & Cornefert, P. A. (2016). *No child should grow up like this: Identifying long term outcomes of forgotten Australians, child migrants and the stolen generations*. Kensington, NSW: University of New South Wales.

Find and Connect. (2016). *'Siblings in care'*. Available at https://www.findandconnect.gov.au/guide/vic/E000459. Accessed 8 Oct 2016.

Finkelhor, D., Ormrod, R. K., & Turner, H. A. (2007). Poly-victimization: A neglected component in child victimization. *Child Abuse & Neglect*, *31*(1), 7–26. pii:S0145-2134(06)00334-6.
Fisher, H. L., Jones, P. B., Fearon, P., Craig, T. K., Dazzan, P., Morgan, K., ... Morgan, C. (2010). The varying impact of type, timing and frequency of exposure to childhood adversity on its association with adult psychotic disorder. *Psychological Medicine, 40*(12), 1967–1978.
Ford, T., Goodman, R., & Meltzer, H. (2003). The British child and adolescent mental health survey 1999: The prevalence of DSM-IV disorders. *Journal of the American Academy of Child and Adolescent Psychiatry*, *42*(10), 1203–1211. doi:10.1097/00004583-200310000-00011.
Fries, A., & Pollak, S. (2004). Emotion understanding in postinstitutionalized Eastern European children. *Development and Psychopathology*, *16*, 355–369.
Gilbert, R., Widom, C. S., Browne, K., Fergusson, D., Webb, E., & Janson, S. (2009). Burden and consequences of child maltreatment in high-income countries. *Lancet*, *373*(9657), 68–81. doi:10.1016/S0140-6736(08)61706-7.
Gilligan, R. (2007). Adversity, resilience and the educational progress of young people in public care. *Emotional and Behavioural Difficulties*, *12*(2), 135–145. doi:10.1080/13632750701315631.
Goddard, J. (2000). The education of looked after children. *Child & Family Social Work.*, *5*(1), 79–86.
Greger, H. K., Myhre, A. K., Lydersen, S., & Jozefiak, T. (2015). Previous maltreatment and present mental health in a high-risk adolescent population. *Child Abuse & Neglect*, *45*, 122–134.
Guest, Y. (2012). Reflections on resilience: A psycho-social exploration of the lifelong impact of having been in care during childhood. *Journal of Social Work Practice: Psychotherapeutic Approaches in Health, Welfare and the Community*, *26*(1), 109–124.
Haebich, A. (2000). *Broken circles: Fragmenting Aboriginal families 1800–2000*. Perth, Western Australia: Freemantle Arts Centre Press.
Harvey, A., McNamara, P., & Andrewartha, L. (2016). Towards a national policy framework for care leavers in Australia higher education. In P. Mendes & P. Snow (Eds.), *Young people transitioning from out-of- home care. International research policy and practice* (pp. 93–114). London, UK: Palgrave Macmillan.
Hook, J. L., & Courtney, M. E. (2011). Employment outcomes of former foster youth as young adults: The importance of human, personal, and social capital. *Children and Youth Services Review*, *33*(10), 1855–1865.
Human Rights and Equal Opportunity Commission (HREOC). (1997). *Bringing them home: Report of the National Inquiry into the separation of Aboriginal and Torres Strait Islander children from their families*. Sydney, NSW: Human Rights and Equal Opportunity Commission.
Humphreys, M. (1996). *Empty cradles*. London, UK: Corgi.
IBM Corp. (2015). *IBM SPSS statistics for windows (version 23)*. Armonk, NY: IBM Corp.
Jackson, S. A., & Sachdev, D. (2001). *Better education, better futures: Research, practice and the views of young people in public care*. Ilford: Barnardos.
Kaplan, S. J., Pelcovitz, D., Salzinger, S., Weiner, M., Mandel, F. S., Lesser, M. L., & Labruna, V. E. (1998). Adolescent physical abuse: Risk for adolescent psychiatric disorders. *American Journal of Psychiatry*, *155*(7), 954–959.
Kendall-Tackett, K. (2002). The health effects of childhood abuse: Four pathways by which abuse can influence health. *Child Abuse & Neglect*, *26*(6), 715–729.
Kessler, R. C., Andrews, G., Colpe, L. J., Hiripi, E., Mroczek, D. K., Normand, S. L., & Zaslavsky, A. M. (2002). Short screening scales to monitor population prevalences and trends in non-specific psychological distress. *Psychological Medicine*, *32*(6), 959–976.
Lindsey, D. (1994). *The welfare of children*. New York, NY: Oxford University Press.
Lowell, A., Renk, K., & Adgate, A. H. (2014). The role of attachment in the relationship between child maltreatment and later emotional and behavioural functioning. *Child Abuse & Neglect*, *38*, 1436–1449.
Lueger-Schuster, B., Kantor, V., Weindl, D., Knefel, M., Moy, Y., Butollo, A., ... Gluck, T. (2014). Institutional abuse of children in the Austrian Catholic Church: Types of abuse and impact on adult survivors' current mental health. *Child Abuse & Neglect, 38*, 52–64.

McDowall, J. J. (2009). *CREATE report card 2009: Transitioning from care: tracking progress*. Sydney, NSW: CREATE Foundation.

McFarlane, K. (2008). *From care to crime – Children in state care and the development of criminality*. Second Australia New Zealand critical criminology conference 19–20 June, Sydney, NSW, 2008.

McMillen, J. C., Zima, B. T., Scott, L. D., Auslander, W. F., Munson, M. R., Ollie, M. T., & Spitznagel, E. L. (2005). Prevalence of psychiatric disorders among older youth in the foster care system. *Journal of the American Academy of Child and Adolescent Psychiatry, 44*(1), 88–95.

McNamara, P. (2015). Young people at risk of lifelong poverty: Youth homelessness in Australia. In E. Fernandez, A. Zeira, C. Canali, & T. Vecchiato (Eds.), *Theoretical and empirical insights on child and family poverty – Cross national perspectives*. New York, NY: Springer.

Meltzer, H., Gatward, R., Corbin, T., Goodman, R., & Ford, T. (2003). *The mental health of young people looked after by local authorities in England*. London: Office for National Statistics.

Mendes, P., & Snow, P. (2016). Young people transitioning from out-of-home care. In *International research, policy and practice*. London: Palgrave MacMillan.

Minister for Social Services and Attorney-General. (2016). *Developing a national approach to redress for survivors of institutional child sexual abuse*. Available at https://www.attorneygeneral.gov.au/Mediareleases/Pages/2016/FirstQuarter/29-January-2016-Developing-a-National-Approach-to-Redress-for-Survivors-of-Institutional-Child-Sexual-Abuse.aspx

Moore, S.E., Scott, J.G., Ferrari, A.J., Mills, R., Dunne, M.P., Erskine, H.E., … Norman, R.E. (2015). Burden attributable to child maltreatment in Australia. *Child Abuse & Neglect, 48*, 208–220.

Mullen, P., Martin, J., Anderson, J., & Romans, S. (1996). The long-term impact of the physical, emotional, and sexual abuse of children: A community study. *Child Abuse & Neglect, 20*, 7–21.

Musgrove, N. (2013). *The scars remain: A long history of forgotten Australians and children's institutions*. North Melbourne, Vic: Australian Scholarly Publishing.

Narey, M. (2007). *Beyond care matters: Future of the care population. Working group report*. London: DfES.

Norman, R. E., Byambaa, M., De, R., Butchart, A., Scott, J., & Vos, T. (2012). The long-term health consequences of child physical abuse, emotional abuse, and neglect: A systematic review and meta-analysis. *PLoS Medicine, 9*(11), e1001349. doi:10.1371/journal.pmed.1001349.

Nurius, P. S., Green, S., Logan-Greene, P., & Borja, S. (2007). Life course pathways of adverse childhood experiences toward adult psychological well-being: A stress process analysis. *Child Abuse & Neglect, 45*, 143–153.

O'Connor, T. G., Rutter, M. R., Beckett, C., Keaveney, L., Kreppner, J. M., & ERA Study Team. (2000). The effects of global severe privation on cognitive competence: Extension and longitudinal follow-up. *Child Development, 71*, 376–390.

Okpych, N. J., & Courtney, M. E. (2014). Does education pay for youth formerly in foster care? Comparison of employment outcomes with a national sample. *Children and Youth Services Review, 43*, 18–28.

Pecora, P., Kessler, R., O'Brien, K., Roller, C., Williams, J., & Hiripi, E. (2006). Educational and employment outcomes of adults formerly placed in foster care: Results from the Northwest Foster Care Alumni Study. *Children & Youth Services Review, 28*, 1459–1481.

Pelton, L. H. (1989). *For reasons of poverty: A critical analysis of the public child welfare system in the United States*. New York, NY/England: Praeger Publishers.

Pelton, L. H. (2015). The continuing role of material factors in child maltreatment and placement. *Child Abuse & Neglect, 41*, 30–39.

Penglase, J. (2005). *Orphans of the living: Growing up in "care" in twentieth-century Australia*. Fremantle, WA: Fremantle Arts Centre Press.

Perry, J., Sigal, J., Boucher, S., & Paré, N. (2006). Seven institutionalized children and their adaptation in late adulthood: The children of Duplessis (les Enfants de Duplessis). *Psychiatry, 69*(4), Winter, 283–301.

Radford, L., Corral, S., Bradley, C., & Fisher, H. L. (2013). The prevalence and impact of child maltreatment and other types of victimisation in the UK: Findings from a population survey of caregivers, children and young people and young adults. *Child Abuse & Neglect, 37*, 801–813.

Read, P. (1982). *The stolen generations: The removal of Aboriginal children in NSW from 1883–1969*. Occasional paper no. 1, NSW Ministry for Aboriginal Affairs.

Robson, R. (2008). *Couldn't care less: A policy report from the children in care working group*. London: The Centre for Social Justice.

Rubin, K. H., Dwyer, K. M., Booth-LaForce, C., Kim, A. H., & Burgess, K. B. (2004). Attachment, friendship, and psychosocial functioning in early adolescence. *The Journal of Early Adolescence, 24*(4), 326–356.

Rutter, M., & Quinton, D. (1984). Long-term follow-up of women institutionalized in childhood: Factors promoting good functioning in adult life. *British Journal of Developmental Psychology, 2*, 191–204.

Rutter, M., Quinton, D., & Hill, J. (1990). Adult outcomes of institution-reared children: Males and females compared. In L. N. Robins & M. Rutter (Eds.), *Straight and devious pathways from childhood to adulthood* (pp. 135–157). New York, NY: Cambridge University Press.

Sandelowski, M. (2000). Combining qualitative and quantitative sampling, data collection, and analysis techniques in mixed-method studies. *Research in Nursing and Health, 23*(3), 246–255. doi:10.1002/1098-240x(2000 06)23:3<246::aid-nur9>3.0.co;2-h.

Sansone, R. A., Leung, J. S., & Wiederman, M. W. (2012). Five forms of childhood trauma: Relationships with employment in adulthood. *Child Abuse & Neglect, 36*(9), 676–679.

Savla, J. T., Roberto, K. A., Jaramillo-Sierra, A. L., Gambrel, L. E., Karimi, H., & Butner, L. M. (2013). Childhood abuse affects emotional closeness with family in mid- and later life. *Child Abuse & Neglect, 37*, 388–399.

Schafer, M. H., Ferraro, K. F., & Mustillo, S. A. (2011). Children of misfortune: Early adversity and cumulative inequality in perceived life trajectories. *American Journal of Sociology, 116*, 1053–1091. doi:10.1086/655760.

Sebba, J., Berridge, D., Luke, N., Fletcher, J., Bell, K., Strand, S., … O'Higgins, A. (2015). *The educational progress of looked after children in England*. Oxford/Bristol: Rees Centre/ University of Bristol.

Senate Community Affairs References Committee. (2001). *Lost innocents: Righting the record – Report on child migration*. Canberra, Australia: Commonwealth of Australia.

Senate Community Affairs References Committee. (2004). *Forgotten Australians: A report on Australians who experienced institutional or out-of-home care as children*. Canberra, Australia: Commonwealth of Australia.

Shaw, J., & Tanamas, S. (2012). *Diabetes: The silent pandemic and its impact on Australia*. Canberra: Diabetes Australia.

Silverman, A. B., Reinherz, H. Z., & Giaconia, R. M. (1996). The long-term sequelae of child and adolescent abuse: A longitudinal community study. *Child Abuse & Neglect, 20*(8), 709–723. doi:10.1016/0145 2134(96)00059-2.

Sköld, J. (2013). Historical abuse – A contemporary issue: Compiling inquiries into abuse and neglect of children in out-of-home care worldwide. *Journal of Scandinavian Studies in Criminology and Crime Prevention, 14*(1), 5–23. doi:10.1080/14043858.2013.771907.

Smith, L. J., & McLean, S. (2013). Issues and challenges for service agencies in monitoring educational outcomes for children in out-of-home care. *Children Australia, 38*(3), 100–105.

Springer, K., Sheridan, J., Kuo, D., & Carnes, M. (2007). Long-term physical and mental health consequences of childhood physical abuse: Results from a large population-based sample of men and women. *Child Abuse & Neglect, 31*, 517–530.

Sroufe, L. A. (2005). Attachment and development: A prospective, longitudinal study from birth to adulthood. *Attachment and Human Development, 7*, 349–367.

Sroufe, L. A., & Fleeson, J. (1986). Attachment and construction of relationships. In W. Hartup & Z. Rubin (Eds.), *Relationships and development* (pp. 51–72). Hillsdale, NJ: Erlbaum.

Stahmer, A. C., Leslie, L. K., Hurlburt, M., Barth, R. P., Webb, M. B., Landsverk, J., & Zhang, J. (2005). Developmental and behavioral needs and service use for young children in child welfare. *Pediatrics, 116*(4), 891–900.

Stein, M. (2012). *Young people leaving care: Supporting pathways to adulthood.* London: Jessica Kingsley Publishers.

Stein, M., & Carey, K. (1986). *Leaving care.* Oxford, England: Blackwell.

Styron, T., & Janoff-Bulman, R. (1997). Childhood attachment and abuse: Long-term effects on adult attachment, depression, and conflict resolution. *Child Abuse & Neglect, 21,* 1015–1023. doi:10.1016/S0145-2134(97)00062-8.

Sugaya, L., Hasin, D. S., Olfson, M., Lin, K. H., Grant, B. F., & Blanco, C. (2012). Child physical abuse and adult mental health: A national study. *Journal of Traumatic Stress, 25,* 384–392.

Swain, S., & Hillel, M. (2010). *Child, nation, race and empire. Child rescue discourse, England, Canada and Australia, 1850–1915.* Manchester, UK: Manchester University Press.

Twaite, J., & Rodriguez-Srednicki, O. (2004). Childhood sexual and physical abuse and adult vulnerability to PTSD: The mediating effects of attachment and dissociation. *Journal of Child Sexual Abuse, 13,* 17–38.

Underwood, M. K., & Rosen, L. H. (2011). *Social development: Relationships in infancy, childhood and adolescence.* New York, NY: Guilford Press.

United Nations (UN). (1989). *Convention on the rights of the child.* 20 November 1989, Treaty series, Vol. 1577. Available at http://www.refworld.org/docid/3ae6b38f0.html. Accessed 18 Nov 2016.

van Krieken, R. (1991). *Children and state: Social control and the formation of Australian child welfare.* Sydney, NSW: Allen and Unwin.

Walker, E. C., Holman, T. B., & Busby, D. M. (2009). Childhood sexual abuse, other childhood factors, and pathways to survivors' adult relationship quality. *Journal of Family Violence, 24,* 397–406. doi:10.1007/s10896-009-9242-7.

Wegman, H., & Stelter, C. (2009). A meta-analytic review of the effects of childhood abuse on medical outcomes in adulthood. *Psychosomatic Medicine, 71,* 805–812.

Widom, C. S., Czaja, S. J., Bentley, T., & Johnson, M. S. (2012). A prospective investigation of physical health outcomes in abused and neglected children: New findings from a 30-year follow-up. *American Journal of Public Health, 102,* 1135–1144. doi:10.2105/AJPH.2011.300636.

Widom, C. S., DuMont, K., & Czaja, S. J. (2007). A prospective investigation of major depressive disorder and comorbidity in abused and neglected children grown up. *Archives of General Psychiatry, 64*(1), 49–56. doi:10.1001/archpsyc.64.1.49.

Witt, A., Munzer, A., Ganser, H. G., Fegert, J. M., Goldbeck, L., & Plener, P. L. (2016). Experience by children and adolescents of more than one type of maltreatment: Association of different classes of maltreatment profiles with clinical outcome variables. *Child Abuse & Neglect, 57,* 1–11.

Wolfe, D. A., Jaffe, P. G., Jette, J. L., & Poisson, S. E. (2003). The impact of child abuse in community institutions and organizations: Advancing professional and scientific understanding. *Clinical Psychology-Science and Practice, 10,* 179–191. doi:10.1093/clipsy/bpg021.

Wright, M. (2007). The long-term impact of emotional abuse in childhood: Identifying mediating and moderating processes. *Journal of Emotional Abuse, 7*(2), 1–8. doi:10.1300/J135v07n02 01.

Zielinski, D. S. (2009). Child maltreatment and adult socioeconomic well-being. *Child Abuse & Neglect, 33,* 666–678.

Zimet, G. D., Dahlem, N. W., Zimet, S. G., & Farley, G. K. (1988). The multidimensional scale of perceived social support. *Journal of Personality Assessment, 52*(1), 30–41. doi:10.1207/s15327752jpa5201_2.

Zorc, C. S., O'Reilly, A. L., Matone, M., Long, J., Watts, C. L., & Rubin, D. (2013). The relationship of placement experience to school absenteeism and changing schools in young, school-aged children in foster care. *Children and Youth Services Review, 35*(5), 826–833.

Chapter 21
Congregate Care Settings in the United States

Rebecca D. Webster, Jeremy Wente, Sheri R. Parris, and Adrian V. Rus

There can be no keener revelation of a society's soul than the way in which it treats its children

(Mandela, Asmal, Chidester, & James, 2003, p. 421)

1 Brief History of Congregate Care Settings in the United States

Orphanages began emerging in the United States just prior to the 1800s where relief was needed for displaced children. The first orphan asylum was founded in North America by a group of Ursuline nuns in 1729. This orphanage in Natchez, Mississippi, arose in response to an Indian massacre that left many children without homes and parents to care for them (Gates, 1994). In the cities and towns in the United States, almshouses were built to aid the poor, including children with or without parents. Children were expected to work in these homes to help pay for their stay. The first public orphanage (government supported) was the Charleston Orphan House, founded in 1790 in South Carolina (Murray, 2003), and prior to the 1800s, only five orphanages existed in the United States (Smith, 1995). Quickly the number of orphanages multiplied, and by 1851, there were 77. By 1903, 400 orphanages were in place in the United States. As the general population increased, so did the quantity of institutionalized children (Trotzkey, 1930). The number of children housed in each institution varied from a few children in small settings to large institutions, such as the New York Catholic Protectory that housed 2000 children in 1891. In 1880, the medium-sized institution housed 42 children, and in 1923 the US Census Bureau found that of 960 institutions reporting, 64.7% housed fewer than 80

R.D. Webster (✉) • J. Wente • A.V. Rus
Department of Social and Behavioral Science, Southwestern Christian University, 7210 NW 39th Expressway, Bethany, OK 73008-0340, USA
e-mail: rebecca.webster@swcu.edu; jeremy.wente@swcu.edu; adrian.rus@swcu.edu

S.R. Parris
Texas Christian University, Fort Worth, TX, USA
e-mail: sheri.parris@gmail.com

A.V. Rus et al. (eds.), *Child Maltreatment in Residential Care*,
DOI 10.1007/978-3-319-57990-0_21

children and 27.5% housed fewer than 30. However, approximately 18% (25,350) of all children in care still lived in institutions housing 250 to over 1500 children (US Census Bureau, 1927).

Another answer for the number of children without parents in the United States was the orphan trains. Between the years of 1854 and 1930, more than 200,000 children boarded trains in New York and nearby cities to be transported to states like California, Texas, Oregon, and Washington. Their parents had been immigrants from other countries who died or had abandoned them along the way. In the beginning, the orphans were transported in cars that more resembled those used to transport cattle. Children would often be shipped to homes where farmers needed a hand to raise crops. While this was not always the case, there were reports of abuse and not allowing children to be educated. The orphan trains came to an end with the advent of compulsory education and child labor laws.

In addition to a small number of state and county government institutions, which were found mainly in the Midwest, most US orphanages were opened by religious groups or philanthropists (some of whom wanted to build and endow such institutions as a way to perpetuate their names and achieve a measure of personal immortality and have visible evidence of their generosity; Henry Dwight Chapin, 1929, as cited in Smith, 1995). One reason for religious groups to open such institutions was to preserve the religious heritage of children from specific religious parentage. For instance, as a reaction to the orphan trains that were transporting children west to live and work with Protestant farm families, Jews in New York began opening institutions of their own, and Roman Catholics increased the number of their institutions.

Also, in some instances, civic groups and other organizations took care of orphans as part of the philanthropic mission of their organization and/or as an assistance program to aid the members of their organization. For example, the Masonic Grand Lodge of Texas created a "Widows' and Orphans' Home" for widows and orphans of deceased Masons from across the state of Texas. Members of Fort Worth Lodge no. 148 secured property for the home in Fort Worth, Texas, where it was built. In 1910, a separate facility was opened for widows who were moved to that facility, and in 1913, the orphans' home also became a recognized school district in Texas and was thereafter referred to as the "Masonic Home and School of Texas." Established in 1899, local subordinate lodges contributed to Grand Lodge to supply the funding of this home which continued operating until 2005 (MHS, n.d.; Perkins, 1957).

2 Living Experiences in US Orphanages

In Trotzkey's writing (1930), institutionalized care included "*closed walls, children segregated from the community... commanded by the sound of the cowbell not by word of mouth, every minute of the day from rising to retiring regulated with mathematical precision, the child seldom seen apart from a line but moved in serried ranks, always marching*." Discipline included, "*application of the iron heel and mailed fist which is all the more hideous when applied to defenseless childhood*" (pp. 64–65). Documents provided by those who found themselves at the mercy of the orphanages varied in their reports from positive and loving to impoverished and abusive. Reports of neglect and maltreatment have surfaced over the years, but many stories remain untold. Many reported that the institutions were kept "spotless" at the hands of its occupants. The rooms where the children stayed were often bare, with no furnishings except for a bed to sleep in. Food was limited, and soup, bread, mush, and milk were all common components of the meals. Overeating would never occur for it was forbidden. Many children went without experiencing the feeling of fullness. Additionally, families were often kept apart. Siblings might be separated for great lengths of time since the boys and girls were kept in separate housing (Thurston, 1930).

By the 1920s, some institutions had adopted more child-focused practices and created a more normal living environment, such as exchanging uniform dress for more individualization of clothing, improved food, and sending children to public schools (Hacsi, 1993 as cited in Smith, 1995). Some philanthropists and wealthy institutions provided summer camp and other trips, books and magazines, and birthday presents. Many viewed the finest congregate homes as private schools for the poor, where children could receive more "advantages" than their parents could supply (Reeder, 1929 as cited in Smith, 1995). A number of model programs, praised by professionals at that time, were also developed during the 1920s and 1930s. Such programs included those at institutions such as Edenwald, in Westchester County, New York, and Carson College for Orphan Girls at Flourtown, Pennsylvania (Deardorff, 1924 as cited in Smith, 1995).

Even though the conventional wisdom and recent evidence indicate that children and youth in congregate care have poorer outcomes, quality of care among institutions in the United States varied, and valuable descriptions of orphanage alumni and their recollection of life in some US orphanages have provided more nuanced portraits of life in some of these settings. In 1995, McKenzie surveyed 1589 adults (who were 45 years of age and older at the time of the survey) who graduated from nine private or state-funded orphanages in the South and Midwest in 1967 or before (McKenzie, 1997). In 2002, he conducted another survey of 839 alumni from five private and state-funded orphanages in the same regions who graduated in the late 1960s and before. In both studies, most of the participants were Caucasian and entered the institutions between birth and 17 years of age ($M = 8$ years). Respondents had each lived in their institutions between 1 and 21 years ($M = 9$ years).

Together, the orphanage alumni surveyed by McKenzie reported better outcomes on a large majority of the social and economic indicators than same-age peers in the general Caucasian population (e.g., education, median incomes, unemployment rate, poverty rate, public assistance rate). Overall, 84% of those in the first study (McKenzie, 1997) and 76.3% in the second study (McKenzie, 2003) viewed their orphanage experiences as either somewhat or very favorable. In addition, those in the second study (McKenzie, 2003) reported the top three positive attributes of orphanage care as "personal values and direction" (55.3%); "education, skills development, and guidance" (49.3%); and "basic amenities" (45.5%), and those in the first study (McKenzie, 1997) reported even higher favorability for two of these attributes (for a more complete report, see McKenzie, 2003, pp. 27–28). In the second study, the top negative attributes of orphanage life were reported as "separation from immediate families and siblings" (34.6%), "lack of love and emotional support from institution and staff" (23.1%), and "lack of freedom" (22.9%) (McKenzie, 2003), while the first study found a larger percentage for two of these attributes (McKenzie, 1997) (for a more complete report, see McKenzie, 2003, p. 29) (for additional information about these studies, see also McKenzie, 1996a, 1996b). Myers and Rittner (2001) found similar results in their survey of 94 alumni from the Florida Methodist Children's Home (FMCH). The average age of respondents was 54 years (*SD* = 20.7; range = 17–87), including 52 women and 42 men, and 95% were Caucasian. The average age of entry to the orphanage was 8 years (range = less than 1 year to 15 years old), and the average age upon leaving FMCH was 15 years (SD = 3.20; range 5–20 years). These alumni reported average or above-average results regarding their social and economic achievements (e.g., educational achievement, socioeconomic functioning, personal relationships, personal problems, religious life, satisfaction with foster care received, and life satisfaction).

In recollections of his own congregate care experiences, Dr. Charles Aring wrote about his life from the age of 7 to 15 at a German Protestant orphanage (from approximately 1911 to 1918). He wrote of having his basic needs met, barely including a simple diet and meager portions of food (a piece of fruit was a once-a-year luxury for Christmas) and clothing that was plain and often handed down. Duties of upkeep for the facility were performed by the children, so there was little time for play. However, he does have fond memories of playing with the other children when time allowed, and he did feel a comradery with the other orphans at the institution. Children attended public school and were marched to a local German Evangelical Lutheran Church on Sundays. The orphanage also had a brass band where children learned to play instruments and performed at local events and parades. While life was sparse and regimented at the orphanage, Dr. Aring felt grateful for the opportunity to learn and finish high school in a safe, protected environment, and he went on to become a physician (Aring, 1991). In another account of orphanage life, James Campbell (2000), an alumnus of a North Carolina orphanage who spent 15 years in care during the 1940s and 1950s, also recalls a strict and regimented life and having to perform work at the orphanage by the time he was in sixth grade. This work included rising at 5:00 am to milk, feed, and tend to the cows and steers, as well as cleaning the barn before having breakfast and going to school and then repeating these chores again after school. In high school, his duties consisted of farm work (i.e., working in orchards and produce farms, combining grain and gathering hay). However, the author notes that this work pattern was also consistent with many children's lives outside of congregate care, because in the wider culture in the United States at that time, families believed it wise to instill a strong work ethic in their children. At the same orphanage, girls performed duties such as laundry, prepping food for meals, and assisting caretakers with younger children. In this instance, the orphanage had its own school, and attendance at several church meetings each week was required. Corporal punishment was used for "serious" offenders of rules. Like Aring, Campell remembers his tenure at the orphanage with appreciation for having a warm and stable place to grow up, an opportunity for education and religious training, and an appreciation for the work ethic that was instilled in him; he was thankful that he did not have to live in fear of being moved around from one place to another.

However, by many accounts, younger children seemed to fare less well than older children in orphanage care. For instance, in the early decades of the twentieth century, one-third to three-fifths of children under the age of 12 months died in orphanages, with the primary causes being gastrointestinal and respiratory illnesses that were compounded by malnutrition. Infants and young children in institutional care in the early twentieth century were also reported to suffer from chronic growth stunting and low weight due to malnutrition, as well as other developmental deficits (see Frank, Klass, Earls, & Eisenberg, 1996).

3 Modern Era of US Congregate Care

In 1909, President Theodore Roosevelt convened the first White House Conference on the Care of Dependent Children that served as a protest against institutional care for dependent and neglected children and promoted the concept that all children have the right to a stable, caring family. Also, through this conference, the US Children's Bureau and the Child Welfare League of America (CWLA) were created (James-Brown, 2011; US Children's Bureau, 1967). Although the White House Conference in 1909 marked the beginning of a change in perceptions about institutionalization and a movement toward a focus on family-based alternatives, the number of children in orphanage care did not begin to decline until after World War II, 35 years after the conference. In 1909 the orphanage population was 115,000, and this number continued to grow through the 1920s (Morton, 2000). The growth can be attributed to increases in the US population, and also the Great Depression of the 1930s led to thousands of additional children being sent to orphanages and foster homes. In December of 1933, 102,000 children were cared for in foster homes, and 144,000 (a record number) were in orphanages (Jones, 1993). The depression of the 1930s left many orphanages overwhelmed and financially weakened by the numbers of children in need during that time period. However, on a more positive note, at the time of the third White House Conference of Child Health and Protection in 1930, it was reported that 220,000 needy children had been able to remain in their own homes due to a variety of factors that were emerging to improve children's ability to stay with their own families.

In 1935, the passage of the Social Security Act, including Aid to Families with Dependent Children (AFDC), also provided some support for needy families. After the passage of this act, children were not removed from their homes due to financial difficulties, but only due to increasingly strict standards for inadequate parental care, such as "*abuse, neglect, alcoholism, insanity, prostitution, or uncontrollable behavior on the child's part*" (Jones, 1993, p. 466). Also, with the advent of World War II, the number of children sent to orphanages was reduced as homes became less crowded and the number of available foster homes increased. From the late 1950s to the 1970s, the number of children adopted also continually increased. In addition, by mid-century, the Child Welfare League of America (CWLA) had been established as the central organization for child welfare, and its main purpose was to accredit (or not accredit) organizations that provided out-of-home care for children. Congregate care settings that could not meet their stringent demands were not accredited, and the numbers of "normal" children in institutional care declined, while mainly "disturbed" children remained in institutional settings where professional care could be provided (Jones, 1993). In 1980, the "Adoption Assistance and Child Welfare Act" defined child welfare services as "*(1) Protecting and promoting the welfare of all children; (2) preventing the unnecessary separation of children from their families; and (3) placing children in suitable adoptive homes where restoration to the biological family is not possible or appropriate*". The Act provided support for at-home services aimed at preserving and re-unifying families, for adoptive families, and for "State licensed foster family homes of individuals" or "licensed nonprofit private child-care institutions" (AACWA, 1980; Jones, 1993).

The United Nations Convention on the Rights of the Child (UNCRC), ratified in 1989, names the family as the fundamental group in any society and the natural environment for the growth and well-being of children (UN General Assembly, 1989). According to the UNCRC, families should be provided protection and assistance in order to fully carry out their function in society. Children who are temporarily or permanently separated from their families, or who must be removed from their families for their own best interests, are entitled to special protection and assistance by the State, including assurance of alternative care (UN General Assembly, 1989). The United Nations resolution that provides guidelines for alternative care for young children deprived of parental care, especially those under the age of 3 years, states that such care should be provided in family-based settings. In acknowledging the reality of institutionalization in many places, it states that residential care facilities and family-based care can complement each other in meeting children's needs but also encourages deinstitutionalization and the elimination of large residential care facilities (UN General Assembly, 2010).

In the United States, the child welfare system has adopted a family-service orientation and increased family preventive and differential response services providing early support to families (Gilbert, 2012). The family service orientation conceptualizes child maltreatment in terms of family dysfunction, psychological problems, socioeconomic and marital stress, therapeutic interventions, the use of voluntary out-of-home placements, and a partnership between parents and the state (Courtney, Flynn, & Beaupré, 2013).

In the United States, group care is a commonly used term for residential care. In this chapter, the term "group care" is used to denote any congregate care arrangement: large- and small-scale institutions and group home settings. Congregate care has been defined as "*a placement setting of group home (a licensed or approved home providing 24-hour care in a small group setting of 7 to 12 children) or institu-*

tion (a licensed or approved child care facility operated by a public or private agency and providing 24-hour care and/or treatment typically for 12 or more children who require separation from their own homes or a group living experience). These settings may include child care institutions, residential treatment facilities, or maternity homes" (USDHHS, ACF, & CC, 2015, p. 1). According to the US Department of Health and Human Services, Administration for Children and Families, and Children's Bureau, there were 55,916 children and youth in congregate care in the United States as of September 30, 2013. Of these, 62.7% were males and 37.3% were females, 40.7% were White/Caucasian, 30.1% were Black or African American, and 19.7% were Hispanic; mean age at entry into the current setting was 14 years (*Mdn* = 15 years), and mean time in current setting was 8.1 months. In addition, approximately 24% of children and youth spent more than 1 year in congregate care (USDHHS, ACF, & CC, 2015). Importantly, over the past decade, there has been a 37% decline of children and youth placed in congregate care. Furthermore, this report found that children and youth were placed in congregate care for a variety of reasons. Specifically, 36% of those in congregate care had a DSM (Diagnostic and Statistical Manual of Mental Disorders) or DSM in combination with another (can include child behavioral problems) diagnosis, 25% had a child behavior problem alone (exclude all disabilities), 10.4% had a clinical disability (excludes DSM), and 28.8% had no clinical indicators when they were placed into congregate care (USDHHS, ACF, & CC, 2015).

The Consensus Statement on Group Care for Children and Adolescents: A Statement of Policy of the American Orthopsychiatric Association (Dozier et al., 2014) stated that "*… group care should never be favored over family care. Group care should be used only when it is the least detrimental alternative, when necessary therapeutic mental health services cannot be delivered in a less restrictive setting*" (p. 219). Thus, the authors of this statement consider institutional care to be a non-optimal alternative for children and youth and that smaller group care settings can also be detrimental to their development and well-being. Specifically, to support this strong position on congregate care, Dozier and colleagues (for more information, see Dozier et al., 2014, pp. 220–223) listed ten principles that are explained and supported by research outcomes:

1. Healthy attachments with a parent figure are necessary for children of all ages and help to reduce problem behaviors and interpersonal difficulties.
2. Especially during adolescence, it is critical to balance children's need for parental control and regulation with their developing needs for autonomy.
3. Child-sensitive exercise of adult authority is critical to healthy development.
4. Group care is not an appropriate living arrangement, and it can never substitute for a home environment.
5. Group care itself may be related to an increased likelihood of problem behavior.
6. Group care may cause psychological harm even in typically developing children.

7. Group care for abused and maltreated children also may be physically dangerous.
8. There is no demonstrable therapeutic necessity for group care to be used as a long-term living arrangement.
9. Even children who have never experienced secure attachments can develop them in appropriate family settings.
10. Group care should never be used for young children.

Thus, Dozier et al. (2014) concluded that children in congregate care lack the opportunity to form an attachment to a parent figure or experience child-sensitive caregiving. Because healthy attachment experiences and sensitive caregiving are necessary for optimal development, children reared without such fundamental experiences are at increased risk to develop antisocial and risky behavior. Because foster care, when appropriately supported, can provide a more appropriate caregiving environment, Dozier and colleagues recommend that group care be used only for therapeutic treatment of children and, only when clinically necessary, with a goal of returning children to their families as soon as possible.

4 Brief Review of Literature on Maltreatment of Children and Youth in US Congregate Care Settings

The Child Abuse Prevention and Treatment Act (CAPTA) enacted on January 31, 1974 was the first piece of legislation to provide federal involvement in the protection of children from abuse and neglect. Motivation to create this law developed from the identification of a clinical condition called "battered child syndrome" in 1962 (Overcamp-Martini & Nurron, 2009). Battered child syndrome was described as a condition in which young children receive serious physical abuse, which is a frequent cause of permanent injury or death. Signs of possible battered child syndrome were identified as "*any child exhibiting evidence of fracture of any bone, subdural hematoma, failure to thrive, soft tissue swellings or skin bruising, in any child who dies suddenly, or where the degree or type of injury is at variance with the history given regarding the occurrence of the trauma*" (Kempe, Silverman, Steele, Droegemueller, & Silver, 1962). Thus, after years of growing public interest, in 1974, CAPTA provided federal funding to assist with the investigation and reporting of child abuse and neglect (Myers, 2008). CAPTA also authorized governmental research; created the National Center on Child Abuse and Neglect (NCCAN) within the Department of Health, Education, and Welfare, (Child Welfare Information Gateway, 2012); and mandated reporting of child abuse from professionals (Courtney et al., 2013). The primary focus of CAPTA was initially on abuse within the family and overlooked the issue of maltreatment within congregate care settings. In 1977, the issue of out-of-home care was addressed at the First National Conference on Institutional Abuse and Neglect (Rindfleisch & Rabb, 1984a), though it was until 1989 that the majority of states were compliant with mandated reporting for out-of-home care (Rindfleisch & Nunno, 1992). Throughout the history of CAPTA, there have been multiple amendments and reauthorization bills that have had a broad impact on child protection in the United States. The most recent reauthorization was signed in 2010 titled P.L. 111-320 The CAPTA Reauthorization Act of 2010 ("The Child Abuse Prevention and Treatment Act Including Adoption Opportunities and The Abandoned Infants Assistance Act", n.d.).

Three levels of child abuse were identified by Gil (1975), namely, family, institutional, and societal. The societal level is deemed most severe because what happens at this level also affects children's functioning at the institutional level as well as in their own homes. For the purpose of this chapter, however, our focus is on institutional abuse which according to Gil (1975) includes settings such as daycare centers, schools, courts, childcare agencies, welfare departments, and correctional and other residential childcare settings. He notes that institutional abuse, like abuse in the home, can stem from well-meaning but misguided practices or from hostile attitudes toward children and can occur repeatedly, either occasionally or as part of a regular pattern, or can occur in single instances. Also regarding abuse in these settings, Gil states that "*... acts and policies of commission or omission that inhibit, or insufficiently promote, the development of children, or that deprive children of, or fail to provide them with, material, emotional, and symbolic means needed for their optimal development, constitute abusive acts or conditions. Such acts or policies may originate with an individual employee of an institution, such as a teacher, child care worker, judge, probation officer, or social worker, or they may be implicit in the standard practices and policies of given agencies and institutions*" (pp. 347–348).

The abuse in old orphanages in the early 1900s has been documented (for a review, see Smith, 1995). Also, a valuable description of abuse in orphanages was provided by orphanage alumni who were institutionalized in 1967 or before in South and Midwest US orphanages (other aspects of these alumni surveys were discussed earlier in this chapter) (see McKenzie, 1997, 2003). Of these alumni respondents, 81.5% reported no abuse of any kind during their orphanage stay, while 15.9% reported physical abuse, 9.7% mental or emotional abuse, 1.8% sexual abuse, and 2% other forms of abuse (McKenzie, 2003). In a previous study, McKenzie (1997) found that 87% of the alumni experienced no abuse of any kind, and of those that did, an even lower percentage experienced various types of abuse, namely, physical abuse (10%), mental or emotional (7%), sexual (2%), and other forms of abuse (1%). It should be noted, however, that the various forms of abuse were open to the interpretation of the individual alumni (McKenzie, 2003).

Various researchers found that child and youth maltreatment occurred in congregate care settings in the late 1970s and 1980s (Gil, 1982; Gil & Baxter, 1979; Powers, Mooney, & Nunno, 1990; Rosenthal, Motz, Edmonson, & Groze, 1991) and that this was a significant issue affecting the child welfare system. It was a widespread phenomenon but was often underreported or inconsistently reported (Rindfleisch & Bean, 1988; Rindfleisch & Nunno, 1992; Rindfleisch & Rabb, 1984b). In one study of abuse in out-of-home care in Colorado, Rosenthal and colleagues (Rosenthal et al., 1991) found that a significant number of reports of abuse and neglect were reported in group homes, residential treatment centers, and institutions from 1983 to 1987. Out of 288 reported cases, 55% were for physical abuse, 24% were for sexual abuse, and 21% were for neglect (including emotional and verbal abuse). Most victims of physical abuse and neglect were male, while most victims of sexual abuse were female. The same study found that two-thirds of the perpetrators of all three types of maltreatment were male. Based on limited information available from the late 1980s, Spencer and Knudsen (1992) found that the risk for child abuse and neglect was greater for children in residential or institutional placements than for those in daycare homes and centers and schools settings. Specifically, they found that in Indiana from 1984 to 1990 the rates of substantiated child maltreatment reports were higher for full-time care settings. Blatt (1992) found that younger staff (those under the age of 35) and male staff in these settings were most likely to be reported as perpetrators.

In a study of out-of-home care in Illinois, Garnier and Poertner (2000) examined administrative data to determine the rate of abuse and neglect for children. They found that reports of abuse or neglect during out-of-home care ranged from a high of 2.4% to a low of 1.5% during the 4 years from 1996 to 1999. For those in group homes, abuse rates ranged from 3.5 children per 100 in care during 1997 to 1.1 per 100 children in care during 1998. For those in institutional care, the rate ranged from 4.1 per 100 in care during 1997 to 1.5 per 100 in care during 1999. Additionally, Poertner, Bussey, and Fluke (1999) determined that sexual abuse was the most frequent type of abuse in both institutions and group homes (55.1% in institutions, 60.4% in group homes) from 1993 to 1997, with substantial risk of harm being the second highest category. Physical abuse and neglect consisted of less than 10% of the reports in institutions and just over 10% in group homes. In another study in Illinois, Tittle, Poertner, and Garnier (2008) assessed 302 cases from the total of 691 indicated reports occurring in the year 2000 for children placed in relative care, non-related family foster care, specialized foster care, and institutions (i.e., group homes and hospitals). They found that sexual abuse (74%) was the most prevalent form of maltreatment. This was true for family foster care (74%), relative foster care (76%), specialized foster care (62%), and institutions (89%). The second most prevalent type of maltreatment was lack of supervision (11%). Freundlich, Avery, and Padgett (2007) found a similar trend in an exploratory study that suggested safety is a significant concern in congregate care environments with safety risks taking a variety of forms, including peer-on-peer violence, the stealing of personal belongings, inappropriate conduct on the part of the staff, and poor physical conditions of facilities.

In 2006, the US Government Accountability Office (USGAO, 2008a, 2008b) conducted a survey with respondents from 49 states who reported data to National Child Abuse and Neglect Data System (NCANDS) investigating youth maltreatment in residential facilities, including physical and sexual abuse, neglect, and deaths. The report was developed using multiple methodologies and was limited to residential facilities we defined as those that require youth – ages 12 through 17 – to reside at the facility and that provide program services for youth with behavioral and emotional challenges. Specifically, the review included facilities that provided one or more of the following types of programs: juvenile justice, youth offender, juvenile delinquency, and incorrigibility programs; treatment programs for youth with behavioral, emotional, mental health, and substance abuse issues; homes for pregnant teens; schools for discipline or character education; and therapeutic group homes, such as a home that specializes in supporting and treating youth with severe emotional disorders. Child welfare, health and mental health, and juvenile justice programs that were government operated, privately operated that received government funds, and privately operated with no government funding were surveyed. Results showed that in 2005, there were 1503 incidents of maltreatment by facility staff in 34 states, including physical abuse, neglect or deprivation of necessities, and sexual abuse. Of these incidents, neglect or deprivation of necessities was the most frequent cause of youth maltreatment (44%), followed by physical abuse (24%), sexual abuse (9%), and other incidents of youth maltreatment which included medical neglect and psychological or emotional maltreatment (23%). Examples of physical and sexual abuse included staff hitting youth and slamming them to the ground, staff hog-tying and shackling youth to poles in public places, and girls being forced to eat their own vomit if they threw up while exercising in the hot sun. Staff routinely broke and wired shut the jaws of youth who showed disrespect in another facility. In some facilities, staff engaged in sexual acts with boys. Youth-on-youth violence occurred on an almost-daily basis in some facilities, at times resulting in injuries that required hospitalization. Youth were sexually assaulted and threatened with sexual assault by other youth in some facilities, all without effective intervention from management. Moreover, 28 states responding to the survey reported at least one death in residential facilities in their state in 2006, with accidents and suicides among the most common types of fatalities.

Recently, a study using a small sample of boys from residential programs which provide therapeutic treatment for boys with behavioral and emotional problems showed rates of bullying and victimization were higher for adolescents from residential programs when compared to adolescents from public schools (Wright, 2016). The author of this study concluded that such results underscore the importance of addressing bullying and victimization among adolescents in secure settings as well as the need for developing multicomponent intervention programs aimed at targeting the various risk factors associated with adolescents' involvement in bullying and for considering whether interventions should be sensitive to different populations of adolescents.

5 Causes and Prevention of Maltreatment in Congregate Care Settings

Maltreatment of children and youth in residential settings has been attributed to several factors, including a lack of experienced staff, insufficient staff training, and lack of appropriate supervision – particularly in smaller facilities (USGAO, 2008a). Other institutional factors that have been identified as contributors to abuse are very difficult and stressful working conditions; large caseloads; poor wages, benefits, and undesirable schedules; limited career path and professional development opportunities; inadequate staff to child ratios; seasonal changes in schedules; changes in physical locations; the isolated nature of institutional settings; lack of recreational and leisure activities for children; and the presence of mental retardation, emotional problems, substance abuse, and/or previous familial maltreatment of children (for more information, see Nunno & Rindfleisch, 1991; Powers et al., 1990; Rosenthal et al., 1991). Conversely, the most important factors found to prevent child maltreatment are improvements in staff crisis management training, staff supervision of children, professionalism in childcare, organizational issues, and staff recruitment (Reyome, 1990; Rosenthal et al., 1991).

6 Conclusion

Large numbers of children in the United States receive a child protective services investigation response because they are neglected and/or emotionally, physically, or sexually abused by their caregivers. Consequently, child abuse and neglect are serious concerns of our nation. The well-being of all children, including those who are in congregate or group care, is addressed by the state, tribal, and local agencies which have developed specialized programs to prevent child abuse and neglect. Even though there has been a reported significant decrease in the percentage of children placed in congregate care settings in recent years, still there are tens of thousands of children and adolescents in such facilities across the United States. Knowing that children and adolescents from residential programs experience varying forms of victimization, it is important to further investigate the relationship between the individual (child-level) and contextual (institutional-level) characteristics that facilitate neglect and abuse. Additionally, because children in congregate care (including residential treatment programs) are more likely to have a psychiatric diagnosis or to have experienced trauma prior to placement in these facilities, special attention should be given to address their needs. Evidence-based principles should be employed in organizing residential care facilities in a manner that will decrease the instances of child maltreatment.

Questions for Discussion

1. Study the Dozier et al. (2014) paper (for complete reference, see the reference list at the end of Chapter) titled "Consensus statement on group care for children and adolescents: A statement of policy of the American Orthopsychiatric Association" and identify the ten principles that helped the authors to conclude that institutional care is considered non-optimal for children of all ages. Which principle is most important to you? Why?
2. This chapter presented various causes of institutional maltreatment. If you were an administrator, caregiver, or another specialist working within a congregate care setting, what would you do to protect children and youth from being

neglected and abused (i.e., emotionally, physically, or sexually abused) by staff and/or peers?
3. Determine the number of children and youth in congregate care in your State (or country) and present the most important demographics (e.g., age, gender, race/ethnicity, disability, etc.). What is your State (and country) doing to protect these children and youth? What would you do if you had the authority and resources to protect these children and youth from being maltreated?

References

AACWA. (1980). *Adoption Assistance and Child Welfare Act of 1980 (AACWA)*. Retrieved from https://www.govtrack.us/congress/bills/96/hr3434/summary

Aring, C. D. (1991). Institutions: In defense of orphanages. *The American Scholar*, *60*(4), 575–579.

Blatt, E. R. (1992). Factors associated with child abuse and neglect in residential care settings. *Children and Youth Services Review*, *14*(6), 493–517.

Campbell, J. M. (2000). Looking back to see ahead. *Residential Treatment for Children and Youth*, *17*(3), 95–102.

Child Welfare Information Gateway. (2012). *Major federal legislation concerned with child protection, child welfare, and adoption*. Washington, DC: U.S. Department of Health and Human Services, Children's Bureau.

Courtney, M., Flynn, R. J., & Beaupré, J. (2013). Overview of out of home care in the USA and Canada. *Psychosocial Intervention/Intervencion Psicosocial*, *22*(3), 163–173. doi:10.5093/in2013a20.

Dozier, M., Kaufman, J., Kobak, R., O'Connor, T. G., Sagi-Schwartz, A., Scott, S., … Zeanah, C. H. (2014). Consensus statement on group care for children and adolescents: A statement of policy of the American Orthopsychiatric Association. *The American Journal of Orthopsychiatry*, *84*(3), 219–225. doi:10.1037/ort0000005.

Frank, D. A., Klass, P. E., Earls, F., & Eisenberg, L. (1996). Infants and young children in orphanages: One view from pediatrics and child psychiatry. *Pediatrics*, *97*(4), 569–578.

Freundlich, M., Avery, R. J., & Padgett, D. (2007). Care or scare: The safety of youth in congregate care in New York City. *Child Abuse & Neglect*, *31*(2), 173–186.

Garnier, P. C., & Poertner, J. (2000). Using administrative data to assess child safety in out-of-home care. *Child Welfare*, *79*(5), 597–613.

Gates, D. (1994). History of the orphanage (cover story). *Newsweek*, *124*(24), 33.

Gil, D. G. (1975). Unraveling child abuse. *American Journal of Orthopsychiatry*, *45*(3), 346.

Gil, E. (1982). Institutional abuse of children in out-of-home care. *Child & Youth Services*, *4*(1–2), 7–13.

Gil, E., & Baxter, K. (1979). Abuse of children in institutions. *Child Abuse & Neglect*, *3*(3–4), 693–698.

Gilbert, N. (2012). A comparative study of child welfare systems: Abstract orientations and concrete results. *Children & Youth Services Review*, *34*(3), 532–536. doi:10.1016/j.childyouth.2011.10.014.

James-Brown, C. (2011). Advancing the commitment: Back to the future. *Journal of Public Child Welfare*, *5*, 345–347.

Jones, M. B. (1993). Decline of the American orphanage, 1941–1980. *Social Services Review*, *67*(3), 459–480.

Kempe, C. H., Silverman, F. N., Steele, B. F., Droegemueller, W., & Silver, H. K. (1962). The battered-child syndrome. *Journal of the American Medical Association*, *181*(1), 17–24.

Mandela, N., Asmal, K., Chidester, D., & James, W. G. (2003). Nelson Mandela in his own words. In *From freedom to the future: Tributes and speeches*. London: Little, Brown.
Masonic Home and School of Texas (MHS). (n.d.). *Masonic home and school of Texas – History*. Retrieved from http://www.masonichometx.org/about-mhs/history/
McKenzie, R. B. (1996a). The children of Barium Springs orphanage. *The American Enterprise, 7*(3), 60.
McKenzie, R. B. (1996b). Orphanages: The real story. *The Public Interest, 123*, 100–104.
McKenzie, R. B. (1997). Orphanage alumni: How they have done and how they evaluate their experience. *Child and Youth Care Forum, 26*(2), 87–111.
McKenzie, R. B. (2003). The impact of orphanages on the alumni's lives and assessments of their childhoods. *Children and Youth Services Review, 25*(9), 703–753.
Morton, M. J. (2000). Surviving the great depression: Orphanages and orphans in Cleveland. *Journal of Urban History, 26*(4), 438–455.
Murray, J. E. (2003). Fates of orphans: Poor children in Antebellum Charleston. *Journal of Interdisciplinary History, 33*(4), 519–545.
Myers, J. E. (2008). A short history of child protection in America. *Family Law Quarterly, 42*(3), 449–463.
Myers, L. L., & Rittner, B. (2001). Adult psychosocial functioning of children raised in an orphanage. *Residential Treatment for Children & Youth, 18*(4), 3–21.
Nunno, M., & Rindfleisch, N. (1991). The abuse of children in out of home care. *Children & Society, 5*(4), 295–305.
Overcamp-Martini, M., & Nurron, J. (2009). CAPTA and the residential placement: A survey of state policy and practice. *Child & Youth Care Forum, 38*(2), 55–68. doi:10.1007/s10566-009-9067-9.
Perkins, C. R. (1957). *History of Fort Worth Lodge No. 148, A.F. & A.M.* (Master of Arts, thesis). Texas Christian University, Fort Worth, TX.
Poertner, J., Bussey, M., & Fluke, J. (1999). How safe are out-of-home placements? *Children and Youth Services Review, 21*(7), 549–563.
Powers, J. L., Mooney, A., & Nunno, M. (1990). Institutional abuse: A review of the literature. *Journal of Child and Youth Care, 4*(6), 81–95.
Reyome, N. D. (1990). Executive directors' perceptions of the prevention of child abuse and maltreatment in residential facilities. *Journal of Child and Youth Care, 4*(6), 45–60.
Rindfleisch, N., & Bean, G. J. (1988). Willingness to report abuse and neglect in residential facilities. *Child Abuse & Neglect, 12*(4), 509–520.
Rindfleisch, N., & Nunno, M. (1992). Progress and issues in the implementation of the 1984 out-of-home care protection amendment. *Child Abuse & Neglect, 16*(5), 693–708.
Rindfleisch, N., & Rabb, J. (1984a). Dilemmas in planning for the protection of children and youths in residential facilities. *Child Welfare, 63*(3), 205–215.
Rindfleisch, N., & Rabb, J. (1984b). How much of a problem is resident mistreatment in child welfare institutions? *Child Abuse & Neglect, 8*, 33–40.
Rosenthal, J. A., Motz, J. K., Edmonson, D. A., & Groze, V. (1991). A descriptive study of abuse and neglect in out-of-home-placement. *Child Abuse & Neglect, 15*(3), 249–260.
Smith, E. P. (1995). Bring back the orphanages? What policymakers of today can learn from the past. *Child Welfare, 74*(1), 115–142.
Spencer, J. W., & Knudsen, D. D. (1992). Out-of-home maltreatment: An analysis of risk in various settings for children. *Children and Youth Services Review, 14*(6), 485–492.
The Child Abuse Prevention and Treatment Act Including Adoption Opportunities and The Abandoned Infants Assistance Act. (n.d.). Retrieved from https://www.acf.hhs.gov/sites/default/files/cb/capta2010.pdf
Thurston, J. W. (1930). *The dependent child*. New York, NY: Columbia University Press. Reprinted in Bremner, R. H. (Ed.). *Children and youth in America: A documentary history* (Vol. 11, 1866–1932). Cambridge, MA: Harvard University Press.

Tittle, G., Poertner, J., & Garnier, P. (2008). Child maltreatment in out of home care: What do we know now. Retrieved from https://cfrc.illinois.edu/pubs/rp_20011001_ChildMaltreatmentInOutOfHomeCareWhatDoWeKnowNow.pdf

Trotzkey, E. L. (1930). *Institutional care and placing-out: The place of each in the care of dependent children*. Chicago, IL: The Marks Nathan Jewish Orphan Home.

U.S. Children's Bureau. (1967). *The story of the white house conferences on children and youth*. Washington, DC: U.S. Government Printing Office.

U.S. Department of Commerce, Bureau of Census. (1927). *Children under institutional care, 1923*. Washington, DC: U.S. Government Printing Office.

U.S. Department of Health and Human Services (USDHHS), Administration for Children and Families (ACF), & Children's Bureau (CC). (2015). *A national look at the use of congregate care in child welfare*. Retrieved from https://www.acf.hhs.gov/sites/default/files/cb/cbcongregatecare_brief.pdf

UN General Assembly. (1989). *Convention on the rights of the child*. United Nations, treaty series, Vol. 1577, p. 3. Retrieved from http://www.refworld.org/docid/3ae6b38f0.html

UN General Assembly. (2010). *Guidelines for the alternative care of children: Resolution/adopted by the General Assembly*. A/RES/64/142. Retrieved from http://www.refworld.org/docid/4c3acd162.html

United States Government Accountability Office (USGAO). (2008a). *Residential facilities: State and federal oversight gaps may increase risk to youth well-being*. GAO-08-696T. Retrieved from http://www.gao.gov/products/GAO-08-696T

United States Government Accountability Office (USGAO). (2008b). *Residential facilities: Improved data and enhanced oversight would help safeguard the well-being of youth with behavioral and emotional challenges*. GAO-08-346. Retrieved from http://www.gao.gov/new.items/d08346.pdf

Wright, M. F. (2016). Bullying among adolescents in residential programs and in public school: The role of individual and contextual predictors. *Journal of Aggression, Conflict and Peace Research*, *8*(2), 1–13.

Chapter 22
Best Practices for Residential/Institutional/Group Care of Children: A Harm Reduction Framework

Victor Groza and Kelley McCreery Bunkers

> *The hunger for love is much more difficult to remove than the hunger for bread.*
>
> Mother Theresa

1 Introduction

Residential care, including institutions and group homes, has been one of the main placement options for orphaned, abandoned, or vulnerable children (OAVC) for centuries; in the twenty-first century, most institutionalized children live in low-resource countries (Rosas & McCall, 2009). In high-resource countries, alternative care options are usually family-based (children are in some type of alternative family) and not residential-based (children are in some type of group care); guardianship, subsidized or unsubsidized kinship care, family foster care, and adoption are more readily utilized. In many low-resource countries, family foster care and

The term residential care used in this chapter refers to the short-term or long-term placement of a child into any nonfamily-based care situation. Similar terms referring to institutionalization are residential care, group care, congregate care, or orphanage care. For the remainder of this paper, we will use the term residential care.

V. Groza (✉)
Mandel School of Applied Social Sciences, Case Western Reserve University,
10900 Euclid Avenue, Cleveland, OH 44106-7164, USA
e-mail: victor.groza@case.edu

K.M. Bunkers
Maestral International, Nairobi, Kenya
e-mail: kelleybunkers@gmail.com

A.V. Rus et al. (eds.), *Child Maltreatment in Residential Care*,
DOI 10.1007/978-3-319-57990-0_22

adoption are not the main alternatives due to cultural beliefs against adopting unrelated children, nascent or under-resourced child protection systems that primarily focus on response to problems and not prevention, and lack of political will (Dickens & Groza, 2004; Rosas & McCall, 2009).

Common elements of residential care include care by paid, unrelated personnel working or living with non-related children usually on a rotating basis, children clustered by age groups and gender (i.e., homogenously), periodic transitions to new caregivers and same age peers, a high child-to-caregiver ratio, and lack of or limited stimulating and responsive interactions between children and caregivers (Rosas & McCall, 2009). One of the most common characteristics of residential life is the lack of stable, long-term relationships between a child and a caregiver (Dobrova-Krol et al., 2008; Rosas & McCall, 2009) as well as regimentation and routinization of care that negatively impacts development (Roeber, Tober, Bolt, & Pollak, 2012; Sheridan, Fox, Zeanah, McLaughlin, & Nelson, 2012).

Yet, the reality is that residential care has been and will be one of the main alternative care options for many children in the foreseeable future, particularly in low-resource countries. UNICEF reports that 143 million single orphans (only one parent died) and double orphans (both parents died) were living in 93 countries around the world (Rosas & McCall, 2009), and a United Nations' report (2006) found that 8 million children were in residential care. Many children in low-resource countries with emerging formal child protection systems are living in residential facilities, and there is ample evidence on the proliferation of residential care facilities throughout Africa (Howard, 2008). Drivers that have resulted in the increase of both residential care facilities and the number of children in them include cultural and economic barriers, especially access to education and health care (Rosas & McCall, 2009), donors from high-resource countries funding the establishment of new facilities, as well as the devastation caused by HIV and other diseases, chronic poverty, armed conflict, and a myriad of other political, cultural, and economic factors (Tolfree, 2005).

Based on the considerable research documenting the numerous negative effects of institutionalization, one is led to believe that components of "good institutions" must be an oxymoron. Rosenthal, Bauer, Hyden, and Holley (1999) caution that the danger of improving institutional care may be that it inadvertently strengthens an outdated and less than ideal child protection system. Critics of institutionalization assert that children function better in bad homes than in good institutions. The other side of the spectrum includes those who argue that in certain countries institutions can be a better physical environments than those provided by families (Whetten et al., 2014; Wolff & Fesseha, 1998, 1999). Yet it is imperative to have a pragmatic view that recognizes that institutional care, although not the ideal option for children without parental care, must be acknowledged as a reality and therefore be improved at least in the short term. The long-term goal should absolutely be a system built on family- and community-based services where residential care does not have to exist and the out-of-home care option is used in very rare situations where the child is in need of immediate care and protection for a time bound (i.e., temporary) period of time until another care option is identified. For example, temporary shelters for survivors of sexual abuse require an immediate safe place until their unique caregiving needs can be fulfilled. Until that occurs, concurrent work must focus on the development of strategies to reduce the harmful consequences of residential care using evidence-based guidance. Harm reduction has been used in other public health contexts such as treating substance abuse (Cusick, 2006; Lenton & Single, 1998; Rolon et al., 2013). We use the principles of harm reduction in developing the approach to mitigate the potential adverse consequences of residential care on children's health, development, and social functioning. The primary goal in harm reduction is the development of programs, policies, and interventions to reduce or lessen harm (Lenton & Single, 1998).

Although research exists that would promote the closure of institutions, there is also evidence such as the St. Petersburg-USA Orphanage Research Team study (2008) that demonstrated that residential care can be improved to significantly mediate the detrimental effects to children's physical, intellectual, and psychosocial development. Harm reduction requires redesigning current residential care facilities to incorporate key concepts based on organizational evaluation reports and academic research. Redesigned residential care must be done in conjunction with the development of family-based alternatives such as family preservation and family reunification, kinship care, family foster care, and domestic adoption with a strong focus on quality of care provided in those care settings (Julian & McCall, 2009; Tolfree, 2005) as well as in the context of the United Nations Convention on the Rights of Children (at least in those countries that have ratified the UNCRC). Article 22 of the United Nations Guidelines for the Appropriate Use and Conditions of Alternative Care for Children supports this view by stating that where large child residential care settings remain, alternatives should be actively developed in the context of an overall deinstitutionalization strategy that will allow for their progressive elimination (United Nations, 2010).

This paper, while using a harm reduction framework to discuss improving residential care, leads us down a precarious path. There is a real danger that attempts to modernize child welfare and protection systems to be family-based will be ignored or de-emphasized as efforts and resources are allocated toward improving residential care. From a systemic perspective, the longer a residential care facility runs in a community, the less likely it is to close. It becomes a major employer, it removes from the public eye the plight of OAVC, and it takes on a culture and life of its own. It is perpetuated by foreigners who are willing to donate bricks and mortar but not to sponsor a child or a family to live in the community. We cannot urge enough caution as we make the suggestions that follow.

The chapter is organized into sections by priority of the interventions that should take place in reducing the potential harms of residential care. It starts with the foundation for all types of alternative care – the use of care standards, accreditation of residential care centers regardless of whether they are in the public or private/NGO section, random and planned inspections, as well as a plan for monitoring the quality of care, including developing a system of investigation and sanctions when children die in residential care, are maltreated, or have their rights violated. The United Nations Convention on the Rights of the Child (UNCRC) has had significant impact on child welfare/protection policy development, standards of care, and programming related to institutional care. Many of the standards related to residential care that have been developed in the past two decades have been based on the UNCRC and the articles therein (Browne & Mulheir, 2007; IFCO, SOS Kinderdorf, & FICE, 2007; United Nations, 2010). The Convention was designed to protect children's rights by setting standards in the areas of health, education, protection, and legal services (UNICEF, 2008). This framework has had and will continue to have a significant impact on the way that child protection and child welfare are practiced around the world. It has especially influenced how residential care is implemented and the role it serves within the child welfare continuum.

2 Standards of Care

An essential component of quality residential care is public policy that establishes professional standards for both services and personnel caring for children. Professional standards or guidelines set the type and quality of services to be delivered to the child by the social service agency, in a child-centered/child rights framework. Standards should exist for all alternative care placements within a continuum of care including family preservation and support, kinship care, foster care, domestic adoption, and intercountry adoption (in those countries that permit it) as well as residential care. Personnel standards establish professional employment requirements (criminal background check, education, knowledge, values, and skills) necessary to perform the duties with the highest level of expertise. Standards reflect and promote evidence-based child development strategies and child care practices. Standards provide goals for the continuing improvement of services to children and their families. Standards promote nationwide consistency. They serve as a resource for people in other fields who are concerned with the care and protection of children – legislators, judges, attorneys, educators, health and mental health professionals, law enforcement personnel, opinion shapers in the media, child advocates, faith leaders, and the general public. Standards provide the basis for licensing and accreditation nationwide. From a rights-based perspective, children living outside of parental care have the right to be cared for by qualified personnel who adhere to standards that are based on ensuring quality and conditions of care which are conducive to maximize a child's development (United Nations, 2010).

A best practice model for developing standards is to work through the ministry or central governmental authority level that is responsible for the residential care of children. This is not as simple as it appears. Typically, children of certain ages or children with different disabilities are under the care and management of different authorities, as was the case in Romania in the early 1990s (Gavrilovici & Groza, 2007; Groza, Ileana, & Irwin, 1999) and in Ukraine (Groza, Komarova, Galchinskaya, Gerasimova, & Volynets, 2010). In order to develop standards, it is better for all the children in residential care to be under one governmental authority. When this is not possible, and standards are developed for children under different authorities, it creates inconsistency and derails attempts to improve quality care. Such a situation exists in Ethiopia where accreditation of residential care facilities, supervision, and oversight of those facilities are divided among three different governmental bodies (the Ministry of Justice, the Bureau of Labor and Social Affairs, and the Ministry of Women's Affairs), making it challenging to develop comprehensive standards (Family Health International, Children's Investment Fund Foundation, & UNICEF 2009).

In addition, there is a tendency to develop standards for residential care in isolation from other alternative care options. This stand-alone development of residential care may be problematic as it could keep residential care centers operating and separate from the other care options. If the end goal is a system based on a continuum of care, with residential care being the last option, it is critical that the standards reflect the prioritization of family-based care and that standards for all forms of care are uniform and part of a comprehensive system of care. The foundation of quality care and harm reduction are clear, specific standards of care. It is essential that the standards are concrete, observable, and measurable; vague or broadly defined standards are as problematic as the lack of standards.

3 Accreditation and Licensing

Developing standards is only the first step. Concurrent with developing standards must be a national study/census of residential care facilities. The country must know how many residential care centers they have, where they are located, the sector that they are located (public, private/NGO, faith-based), and how many children are in each residential care center. An example of this type of study is the work of Perez (2008) in Guatemala and the Ministry of Gender and Family Promotion and Hope and Homes for Children (2012) in Rwanda. Up until these studies, there were only estimations of the number of residential care centers and children in residential care. Even in the former communist countries of Romania and Ukraine, getting the specifics about children in residential care was a moving target because not all locations were known and numbers were manipulated based on who was asking and how the information was to be used. For example, if it was to allocate funding, numbers were higher; if it was an investigation, the numbers were lower. When Romania moved to foster family care, court orders were required in some locations to remove children from residential care centers, and only with the authority of the police were the exact number of children discovered.

Once a country has standards, they must move toward accrediting and licensing residential care centers to care for children. Accreditation requires that the residential care center documents, in writing, how they meet or exceed the standard with the evidence to support their claim. Once a written report is received, a review panel of professionals with no ties to residential care staff or political decision-makers should review the report and schedule a visit. The visit is designed to provide further evidence of compliance with stated standards, highlighting strengths and areas for improvement. For example, if the audit of compliance asserts that staff are trained every month, records of the topic of training, who was the trainer, who attended the training, and evaluations of the training must be on file. Children's cases should be randomly pulled by reviewers to ascertain that all the assessment and planning documents are in place, signed, and dated. A predetermined threshold or minimum set of requirements must be met in order to accredit and license a residential care center. If they don't meet the threshold, they are not accredited. A second review can be scheduled in 30 or 60 days to see if the residential care center can change their functioning to meet standards; if it cannot, it must be closed. If it can meet standards, then routine reaccreditation and licensing should be established on a yearly or biannual basis, utilizing established standards with both unannounced and announced inspections and monitoring of the quality of care.

3.1 Inspections and Monitoring Quality of Care

Setting up a system which is able to monitor implementation and adherence to national standards is just as important as developing standards. Ethiopia is an example. The National Guidelines for Alternative Childcare were developed in 2002. The standards were based on the UNCRC, and the development of those standards was viewed as a positive step toward good child welfare practice, especially within child residential care facilities. Unfortunately, the standards have not been formally approved by the government, and an accompanying monitoring system is not established. A 2009 study conducted by Family Health International and UNICEF found that the majority of child residential care centers were not even aware of the existence of the standards. What may be perceived as a positive step forward in developing standards was severely limited by lack of approval, dissemination, and inexistence of necessary monitoring and evaluation systems.

One of the major concerns in the creation of standards and monitoring processes is child abuse within residential care (Hermenau, Hecker, Elbert, & Ruf-Leuschner, 2014; Rus et al., 2013). Children in care are already in a vulnerable state when they enter the residential care center. Children have been abandoned, neglected, spent years in residential care, or in some cases have been living on the streets or in child-headed households. Children in residential care are especially vulnerable to physical punishment from staff, bullying from other residents, and sexual exploitation (Gavrilovici & Groza, 2007). Any mistreatment negatively shapes the environment for all residents whether or not they are a victim of the mistreatment (Groze, 1990). If the mistreatment is a pattern, it undermines the ability of the residential care center to carry out its mission and goals (Sundram, 1984). One problem in determining the incidence and prevalence of mistreatment in residential care settings is the lack of uniform definitions of what constitutes abuse, neglect, or other types of maltreatment such as withholding food or medical care. A second problem is that even if maltreatment occurs, there is no reporting or investigation system in most countries. Fear of reprisal is a major deterrent for staff to report problems, and most governments lack an adequate system for child maltreatment within the family, so a system for documenting, investigating, and remedying maltreatment within residential care is even less likely to exist. If there is no adequate system to respond to the problem, there can never be an accurate assessment of the scope and depth of the problem. There can also never be a solution to the problem. The result is that most OAVC are made even more vulnerable.

It is for this reason that any country using residential care as a major child welfare intervention needs to develop definitions of mistreatment in residential care settings. Sexual abuse means any sexual activity prohibited by law, including sexual exploitation – the use of a child by a person responsible for her or his health or welfare for personal gratification – or procuring or knowingly causing or permitting any person to sexually abuse or exploit the child, *including other children*. Neglect means the willful act of omission that directly results in the child suffering or being exposed to risk of suffering physical or emotional injury. This includes but is not limited to the failure to provide food, clothing, appropriate shelter, bedding, or medical care to the child. Inappropriate treatment means harm or threatened harm to a child's safety, health, or welfare which is caused by violating state, local, or program rules, laws, policies, procedures, or statues. It includes the failure to provide care for the child in a manner consistent with universal professional standards and practices, including anything that violates the right of a child that is not classified as abuse or neglect that injures a child or puts a child at risk for harm (see Groze, 1990).

4 Personnel Standards

All caregivers should have an initial criminal background check that is updated yearly. This includes fingerprinting, when possible, as well as a determination of offenses that exclude caregivers from working with children such as sex offenses, a history of violence, or having their birth children removed from their care.

Caregivers should have a written job description. They should be evaluated, trained, and monitored by appropriate regulating authorities with a special focus on positive caregiving, provision of individualized attention, and cognitive stimulation of children. Article 73 of the UN Guidelines for the Appropriate Use and Conditions of Alternative Care for Children states that special attention should be paid to the quality of alternative care provision, both in residential and family-based care, particularly in regard to the professional skills, selection, training, and supervision of caregivers. Their role and functions should be clearly defined and clarified with respect to those of the child's birth parents, adoptive parents, or legal guardians (UN, 2010).

For optimal developmental outcomes, children need consistent caregivers that are trained and monitored by appropriate regulating authorities. There are challenges to ensuring professional, well-trained staff in low-resource countries. This was the case in Guatemala where Perez (2008) found that 80% of children's residential care facilities operate in accordance with available resources and do not guarantee that ideal, qualified personnel will be present to provide services to the children.

For infants and toddlers, staff training resulting in changed behavior for as little as 5 min a day for 5 days a week from 1 to 6 weeks has a significant positive impact immediately on children's development, cognition, and health (Hakimi-Manesh, Mojdehi, & Tashakkori, 1984; Kim, Shin, & White-Traut, 2003; Sayegh & Dennis, 1965). Staff training and changes in behavior may also have advantages at least up to 6 months after the intervention (Hakimi-Manesh et al., 1984). Rosas and McCall (2009) reported that if these minimal improvements in staff interaction are stopped, the positive effects displayed by children will not continue, emphasizing the need for consistency and continuity of positive caregiver interactions. Even if staff training does not improve child health and developmental outcomes, it might prevent children from getting worse in residential care (Brossard & Décarie, 1971; Casler, 1965).

5 Programming Standards

This next section focuses on the standards necessary for optimal programming, consistent with public policy such as the UNCRC and the best social science evidence to date. It begins with gatekeeping. According to Bilson and Harwin (2003), gatekeeping is a key mechanism used to try to create a better balance between demand for services and supply of services to ensure a more effective and appropriate targeting of services. In this context, it begins with an assessment to identify specific standards to make sure residential care is the only service that can meet the need of the child and the family.

5.1 Assessment at Entry Point

Any child welfare service must begin with a good child assessment; any ongoing service must have continuous, regular child and family assessments in multiple domains of functioning. Regardless of the reason for a child to enter the child protection system, before any long-term decisions can be made, assessments must be completed and recorded in the case file. Of course, this assumes that every child has a file. At a minimum, there should be a medical evaluation (physical exam) by licensed medical staff, developmental assessment by child development specialists, social history by trained and accredited social workers, and, if the child is school age, an educational evaluation by a professionally credentialed educator. Photos should be taken of the child and family. If any relatives are available, a comprehensive family history should be obtained with the names, addresses, and phone number of all relatives recorded. Assessments should be updated monthly for infants, quarterly for toddlers, and every 6 months to a year for older children. The reassessment should include the child's health, development, behavior patterns, social functioning, psychological/psychiatric screening, and educational performance (if appropriate). These assessments and reassessments allow for better monitoring of children, the early identification of problems, and changing services as family and child circumstances change. A report from each assessment, summarizing strengths as well as child's needs, must be written.

Due to the high risk for attachment disorders and disturbances in children from residential care centers (Zeanah, Smyke, Koga, & Carlson, 2005), attachment assessments and early intervention to promote attachment are critical. Attachment may be a pivotal developmental foundation on which many aspects of emotional and behavioral functioning are based (Boris, Fueyo, & Zeanah, 1997). Children raised in residential care have fewer opportunities to develop selective attachments (Smyke, Dumitrescu, & Zeanah, 2002). Of most concern are indications that children in residential care are at greater risk for disorganized attachment, and disorganized attachment is a serious risk factor for later problems throughout the life cycle (Carlson, 1998; Dozier, Stovall, Albus, & Bates, 2001). Programming must allow infants and toddlers to develop and maintain a selective attachment with at least one primary caregiver; this is best done in a family and if not in a birth family, then the extended family or foster family care.

5.2 *Case Management/Planning*

Case management and case planning should begin at the earliest possible time and be comprised of meeting both long-term and short-term needs based on the child assessment as well as congruent with the best interest of the individual child (UNCRC, 2007). Case management has the main objective of getting a child into a family-like, safe, and permanent care in the least amount of time. It follows the value that children should always grow up in the least restrictive setting, and family care is the least restrictive environment. Article 25 of the UNCRC states that children placed outside their own family are entitled to periodic review of all aspects of their placement. This is vital to ensuring that the child's best interest is being pursued. Good case planning is a critical component of keeping residential care temporary; without it, children are much more likely to remain in residential care long term (Perez, 2008). Determining the eligibility and appropriateness of alternative care options for an individual child should be addressed within the case plan that is updated a minimum of every month for infants, quarterly for toddlers, and 6 months for children aged 6 and older.

5.3 *Children's Right to Participate in Decisions*

Incorporating and facilitating appropriate child participation during the time they are in residential care and in the key decisions that must be made (depending on the child's age and competency) are a core component of child rights-based standards.

Children have an opinion that should be heard and recognized (United Nations Convention on the Rights of the Child aka UNCRC, 2007). Children have a right to be consulted and to have their views taken into account in accordance with their evolving capacities. In addition, article 92 of the UNCRC states that "all carers (i.e., *caregivers*) should promote and encourage children … to develop and exercise informed choices, taking account of acceptable risks and the child's age and according to his/her evolving capacities" (UNCRC, 2007, p. 14).

Given the sensitive nature around child participation and the particular role that it plays in different ethnic and cultural environments, it is critical that key personnel such as social workers, psychologists, directors, and caregivers receive training and guidance in how to both promote a child's participation in decisions while at the same time ensuring that the child's safety, permanency, and well-being are a priority. Promoting the participation of children in decision-making processes regarding their care is relatively new, and many countries are still determining how to address this issue within the cultural and legal frameworks of their countries.

5.4 Children's Right to Educational Services

The UNCRC details a child's right to education as a fundamental right. Therefore, it is imperative that residential care centers also respect this right and provide children with educational opportunities appropriate to their age and capabilities. The draft UN Guidelines on Alternative Care makes reference to a child's right to education in Article 83, which states that children should have access to formal, nonformal, and vocational education to the maximum extent possible in educational facilities in the local community (UNCRC, 2007).

Recognizing that early childhood education and development (ECED) is also an important tool for encouraging child development, residential care centers must include ECED programs for young children. Comprehensive ECED promotes cognition, language, social, and emotional development; these skills underpin school readiness and success (Anderson et al., 2003). Over the life span, early development has an impact, and early opportunities to develop as completely as possible establish the foundation for academic success, health, and well-being (VanLandeghem, Curgins, & Abrams, 2002). Early childhood programs can identify problems early, minimize the severity of problems if identified and treated early, and/or stop further deterioration if problems are identified (Blackman, 2002). All education programs in residential care facilities for infants and toddlers should include an early intervention program.

Many children from high-risk situations have learning problems, and children with a history of residential care are more at risk for developing learning difficulties (Dalen, 1995). Specialized testing for learning disabilities and appropriate remedial education must be provided to maximize children's opportunity to learn.

Finally, residential care facilities should promote the inclusion of children in residence into public, community-based educational settings instead of developing their own educational programs. Going to school in the local community fosters community involvement and allows children the opportunity to interact with other children their age in a typical environment. Access to education is not only a right, but it also assists in their later ability to integrate successfully into the community once children leave residential care.

5.5 *Children's Right to Play and Engage in Recreation*

Incorporating a child's right to play and engage in recreation is a best practice in residential care. Article 84 of the draft UN Guidelines states that "Carers should ensure that the right of every child, including children with disabilities or living with or affected by HIV and AIDS, to develop through play and leisure activities" (UNCRC, 2007, p. 15). Promoting opportunities for children to play encourages their physical, psychosocial, and intellectual development. Creating play and recreational opportunities within the community also provides an excellent opportunity for children residing in residential care to interact, in a positive manner, with other children in the community. Residential care facilities should provide and give access to age-appropriate toys for children, which also foster development and creativity. Caregivers and other staff of the residential care facility should also be trained in play techniques. Positive interaction with children during playtime should be included in a caregiver's job description.

5.6 *Children's Right to a Cultural, Ethnic, and Linguistic Identity*

Cultural and religious practices in residential care should be respected and promoted to the extent that a full assessment has shown them to be consistent with children's rights and best interests. The process of identifying and assessing these practices and considering the applicability of other systems should be done in a broadly participatory way, involving relevant cultural and religious leaders as well as professionals and civil society participants working with children without parental care, as well as the children themselves (UNCRC, 2007). The language used in institutions should be the languages of the children. In Guatemala, that could include any and all of the 23 dialects spoken from the indigenous Mayan communities. In Romania where Rroma children are disproportionately in the child welfare system, that means the use of Rroma dialects.

5.7 *Children's Right to Community-Based Care and Community Involvement*

Community integration and inclusion in community activities are the foundation of reforming residential care (see Llorente, Charlebois, Ducci, & Farias, 2003). Children in residential care have a right to be involved with and have access to the community, including local schools, medical services, faith-based organizations, and extracurricular activities. Residential care facilities should be placed within a neighborhood or community as it allows children access to and interaction with local teachers, children, extracurricular activities, and other components of day-to-day life. Allowing children the opportunity to interact with community members may positively affect their ability to integrate into that community once they leave the residential care center. When residential care facilities are placed outside of communities, such as the case of Romanian institutions for children with special needs, the children in care do not benefit from activities, visits, or interactions with community members. They are hidden from view and are frequently prone to neglect and abuse because the potential safeguards provided within a community are absent.

One-on-one interaction between a child in residential care and an adult is frequently limited. To augment this, residential care facilities may utilize community volunteers. These volunteers must be screened and trained before coming in contact with the children to ensure the child's safety and protection. The volunteers provide an opportunity for children to interact with adults outside of the residential care staff. This kind of interaction should enhance the child's development and connections with others, but volunteers should never become primary caregivers. The use of volunteers for key activities where one-on-one contact is important such as bathing, feeding, and play time is a cost-effective way of addressing the needs of children and provides an opportunity for children to interact with members of the community. Although volunteer use may be viewed as beneficial to the facility as it can be seen as a "free" resource, it has potentially negative effects on the children in care. Volunteers, especially short-term volunteers, can and do contribute to instability and prove to be a safety issue as volunteers can be unreliable and often do not have training in child development and other necessary skills (Punaks & Feit, 2014; Rosas & McCall, 2009). Therefore, if a residential care facility is going to incorporate volunteers into their program, they must first have a volunteer training curriculum, a program that a volunteer may complete before working with children, and administrative staff to monitor the volunteer program. A child protection policy must also be understood and agreed to by the volunteer. Ideally, volunteers should be recruited and utilized to support community strengthening activities, not ones that are promotive of residential care and potentially exploitive of the children within those facilities.

5.8 *Children's Right to Life Skills and Transition Services*

Residential centers caring for adolescents must provide youth with the skills, knowledge, and resources necessary to be able to live independently after exiting residential care. Articles 132, 136, and 137 of the draft UN Guidelines for Alternative Care specifically highlight the necessary provision of care, follow-up, and preparation of youth for independent living outside of the residential care facility. Recognizing that residential life often deprives children of the necessary social and educational opportunities that a family setting would provide, residential care facilities should make a concerted effort to provide programs, both educational and vocational, that help young people leaving residential care to become financially independent. Additionally, residential care facilities should have clear policies and procedures related to aftercare and follow-up of children leaving care to ensure support aimed at successful integration of former residents into the community.

6 Conclusion and Recommendations

Fundamental questions to be answered are (1) can residential care facilities be improved to be comparable to family living, and (2) should they be improved? There is growing global consensus on the need to promote family-based alternatives to residential care for children and adolescents. Yet, in the interim, residential care will be a reality for many low-resource countries still working within inadequate or antiquated legal frameworks related to alternative care, cultural attitudes that promulgate only the benefits of residential care and not the negative effects, and a donor community which has been slow to recognize that providing funds for family- and community-based care is more cost-effective and beneficial to the majority of OVAC than residential care. Recognizing these factors does not justify residential care; rather, it is the acknowledgement of current dynamics that must be dealt with in the longer-term goal of promoting family-based care as priority within the continuum of care. Therefore, a pragmatic approach includes the development of a child welfare strategy with both short-term and long-term plans that include a continuum of care approach with the bulk of care options being family-based. Residential care should be considered only in exceptional and emergency circumstances and until a system of family-based alternative care can be established. Residential care should not be the preferred option but rather the last resort. However, when it is provided as an option, there are components to that care that must be included within the organizational and programmatic structure to reduce the harm to children. The components are vital to children's physical, psychosocial, and intellectual development and well-being. Residential care without them can be irreparably harmful. In addition, the components of improving residential care have been outlined in this chapter from a children's rights framework. Harm reduction, children's rights, and modernization of child welfare systems are intricately linked.

Questions for Discussion

There are still untested hypotheses and policy questions that need to be explored in further research. The following are a list of questions to consider:

1. In a continuum of child welfare services, what is the role of residential care, for whom, and how long?
2. What is the place of emergency shelters to provide immediate care and protection to survivors of abuse?
3. How does improving residential care affect the number of children entering residential care? Is the saying, "If you build it, they will come," true in the case of residential care facilities?
4. What is the optimal caregiver-to-child ratio for children of various ages living in residential care?

References

Anderson, L. M., Shinn, C., Fullilove, M. T., Scrimshaw, S. C., Fielding, J. C., Norman, J., … The Task Force on Community Prevention Services (2003). The effectiveness of early childhood development programs: A systemic review. *American Journal of Preventive Medicine, 24*(3S), 32–46.

Bilson, A., & Harwin, J. (2003). *Changing minds, policies and lives: Improving protection of children in Eastern Europe and Central Asia, gatekeeping services for vulnerable children and families*. Florence: UNICEF. Downloaded March 10, 2016 from http://www.unicef-irc.org/publications/pdf/improving.pdf

Blackman, J. A. (2002). Early intervention: A global perspective. *Infants and Young Children, 15*(2), 11–19.

Boris, N. W., Fueyo, M., & Zeanah, C. H. (1997). The clinical assessment of attachment in children less than five. *Journal of the American Academy of Child and Adolescent Psychiatry, 36*, 291–293.

Brossard, M., & Décarie, T. G. (1971). The effects of three kinds of perceptual-social stimulation on the development of institutionalized infants. *Early Childhood Development and Care, 1*(1), 111–130.

Browne, K., & Mulheir, G. (2007). *Deinstitutionalising and transforming children's services: A guide to good practice*. Retrieved 27 July 2016 from http://www.crin.org/en/docs/Deinstitutionaliation_Manual_-_Daphne_Prog_et_al.pdf

Carlson, E. A. (1998). A prospective longitudinal study of attachment disorganization/disorientation. *Child Development, 69*(4), 1107–1128.

Casler, L. (1965). The effects of extra tactile stimulation on a group of institutionalized infants. *Genetic Psychology Monographs, 71*, 137–175.

Cusick, L. (2006). Widening the harm reduction agenda: From drug use to sex work. *International Journal of Drug Policy, 17*(1), 3–11.

Dalen, M. (1995). Learning difficulties among inter-country adopted children. *Nordisk pedagogikk, 15*(4), 195–208.

Dickens, J., & Groza, V. (2004). Empowerment in difficulty: A critical appraisal of international intervention in child welfare in Romania. *International Social Work, 47*(4), 469–487.

Dobrova-Krol, N. A., van IJzendoorn, M. H., Dobrova-Krol, N. A., Bakermans-Kranenburg, M. J., Cyr, C., & Juffer, F. (2008). Physical growth delays and stress dysregulation in stunted and non-stunted Ukrainian institution-reared children. *Infant Behavior & Development, 31*, 539–553.

Dozier, M., Stovall, K. C., Albus, K. E., & Bates, B. (2001). Attachment for infants in foster care: The role of caregiver state of mind. *Child Development, 72*, 1467–1477.

Family Health International, Children's Investment Fund Foundation, & UNICEF. (2009). *Improving care options for children in Ethiopia through understanding institutional childcare and factors that drive institutionalizations*. Received from Family Health International via email on April 10.

Gavrilovici, O., & Groza, V. (2007). Incidence, prevalence and trauma symptoms in institutionalization children. *International Journal of Child and Family Welfare, 10*(3/4), 125–138.

Groza, V., Ileana, D., & Irwin, I. (1999). *A peacock or a crow: Stories, interviews and commentaries on Romanian adoptions*. Cleveland, OH: Lakeshore Communications.

Groza, V., Komarova, N., Galchinskaya, L., Gerasimova, A., & Volynets, L. (2010). Ukrainian adoptive families. *International Social Work, 53*(1), 19–31. doi:10.1177/0020872809348945.

Groze, V. (1990). An exploratory investigation into institutional mistreatment. *Children and Youth Services Review, 12*, 229–241.

Hakimi-Manesh, Y., Mojdehi, H., & Tashakkori, A. (1984). Short communication: Effects on environmental enrichment on the mental and psychomotor development of orphanage children. *Journal of Child Psychology and Psychiatry, 25*(4), 643–650.

Hermenau, K., Hecker, T., Elbert, T., & Ruf-Leuschner, M. (2014). Maltreatment and mental health in institutional care-comparing early and late institutionalized children in Tanzania. *Infant Mental Health Journal, 35*(2), 102–110.

Howard, C. (2008). *Personal correspondence*. Kampala, Uganda: Cure International.

International Foster Care Organization, SOS Kinderdorf, International, FICE. (2007). *Quality4Children standards for out-of-home child care in Europe*. Retrieved August 2, 2016 from http://www.sos-childrensvillages.org/getmedia/1b7397b9-ce47-41e0-8329-3c01a5496c6f/Q4C_colour.pdf

Julian, M., & McCall, R. B. (2009). *The development of children within different alternative residential care environments*. Unpublished manuscript, authors. Pittsburgh, PA: University of Pittsburgh Office of Child Development.

Kim, T. I., Shin, Y. H., & White-Traut, R. C. (2003). Multisensory intervention improves physical growth and illness rates in Korean orphaned newborn infants. *Research in Nursing and Health, 26*(6), 424–433.

Lenton, S., & Single, E. (1998). The definition of harm reduction. *Drug and Alcohol Review, 17*(2), 213–220.

Llorente, M. A. G., Charlebois, L. M., Ducci, V., & Farias, A. M. (2003). *Children in institutions: The beginning of the end? The cases of Italy, Spain, Argentina, Chile and Uruguay*. Florence: UNICEF Innocenti Research Centre.

Ministry of Gender and Family Promotion, Republic of Rwanda (MIGEPROF) and Hope and Homes for Children. (2012). *National survey of institutions for children in Rwanda*. Retrieved August 2, 2016, from http://www.socialserviceworkforce.org/system/files/resource/files/NATIONAL%20SURVEY%20OF%20INSTITUTIONS%20FOR%20CHILDREN%20IN%20RWANDA_FINAL.pdf

Perez, L. M. (2008). *Situation faced by institutionalized children and adolescents in shelters in Guatemala*. Guatemala City, CA: USAID and Holt International Children Services.

Punaks, M., & Feit, K. (2014). Orphanage voluntourism in Nepal and its links to the displacement and unnecessary institutionalisation of children. *Institutionalised Children Explorations and Beyond, 1*(2), 179–192.

Roeber, B. J., Tober, C. L., Bolt, D. M., & Pollak, S. D. (2012). Gross motor development in children adopted from orphanage settings. *Developmental Medicine & Child Neurology, 54*(6), 527–531. doi:10.1111/j.1469-8749.2012.04257.x.

Rolon, M. L., Syvertsen, J. L., Robertson, A. M., Rangel, M. G., Martinez, G., Ulibarri, M. D., et al. (2013). The influence of having children on HIV-related risk behaviors of female sex workers and their intimate male partners in two Mexico–US border cities. *Journal of Tropical Pediatrics, 59*(3), 214–219.

Rosas, J., & McCall, R. B. (2009). *Characteristics of institutions, interventions, and resident children's development*. University of Pittsburgh. Unpublished manuscript, received by email on January 16, 2009.

Rosenthal, E., Bauer, E., Hyden, M. F., & Holley, A. (1999). Implementing the right to community integration for children with disabilities in Russia: A human rights framework for international action. *Health and Human Rights, 4*(1), 82–113.

Rus, A. V., Stativa, E., Pennings, J. S., Cross, D. R., Ekas, N., Purvis, K. B., & Parris, S. R. (2013). Severe punishment of children by staff in Romanian placement centers for school-aged children: Effects of child and institutional characteristics. *Child Abuse & Neglect, 37*(12), 1152–1162.

Sayegh, Y., & Dennis, W. (1965). The effects of supplementary experiences upon the behavioral development of infants in institutions. *Child Development, 36*, 811–890.

Sheridan, M. A., Fox, N. A., Zeanah, C. H., McLaughlin, K. A., & Nelson, C. A. (2012). Variation in neural development as a result of exposure to institutionalization early in childhood. *Proceedings of the National Academy of Sciences, 109*(32), 12927–12932. doi:10.1073/pnas.1200041109.

Smyke, A. T., Dumitrescu, A., & Zeanah, C. H. (2002). Disturbances of attachment in Romanian children. I. The continuum of caretaking casualty. *Journal of the American Academy of Child and Adolescent Psychiatry, 41*, 972–982.

Sundram, C. J. (1984). Obstacles to reducing patient abuse in public institutions. *Hospital and Community Psychiatry, 35*, 238–243.

The St. Petersburg – USA Orphanage Research Team. (2008). The effects of early social-emotional and relationship experience on the development of young orphanage children. *Monographs of the Society for Research in Child Development, 73*(3), vii–295. doi:10.1111/j.1540-5834.2008.00483.x.

Tolfree, D. (2005). Facing the crisis-supporting children through positive care options. *Save the Children UK*. Retrieved January 27, 2009, from http://www.crin.org/docs/3306_FacingtheCrisis[1].pdf

United Nations (UN). (2006). *United Nations secretary general's study on violence against children*. Retrieved July 27, 2016, from http://unviolencestudy.org/

United Nations Children's Fund (UNICEF). (2008). *Draft manual for the measurement of indicators for children in formal care*. Retrieved March, from http://www.crin.org/docs/Formal%20Care%20Guide%20FINAL.pdf

United Nations Convention on the Rights of Children (UNCRC). (2007). Downloaded July 28, 2016, from http://childrensrights.ie/childrens-rights-ireland/un-convention-rights-child

United Nations Guidelines for the Appropriate Use and Conditions of Alternative Care for Children. (2010). Downloaded July 28, 2016 from http://www.unicef.org/protection/alternative_care_Guidelines-English.pdf

VanLandeghem, K., Curgins, D., & Abrams, M. (2002). *Reasons and strategies for strengthening childhood development services in the healthcare system*. Portland, ME: National Academy for State Health Policy. Retrieved August 2, 2016, from http://www.commonwealthfund.org/usr_doc/vanlandeghem_nashp_630.pdf

Whetten, K., Ostermann, J., Pence, B. W., Whetten, R. A., Messer, L. C., Ariely, S., … Eticha, M. (2014). Three-year change in the wellbeing of orphaned and separated children in institutional and family-based care settings in five low- and middle-income countries. *PLoS ONE*. Downloaded May 26, 2016, from http://journals.plos.org/plosone/article?id=10.1371/journal.pone.0104872

Wolff, P. H., & Fesseha, G. (1998). The orphans of Eritrea: Are orphanages part of the problem or part of the solution? *American Journal of Psychiatry, 155*, 1319–1324.

Wolff, P. H., & Fesseha, G. (1999). The orphans of Eritrea: A five-year follow-up study. *Journal of Child Psychology and Psychiatry, 40*, 1231–1237.

Zeanah, C. H., Smyke, A. T., Koga, S., & Carlson, E. (2005). Attachment in institutionalized and community children in Romania. *Child Development, 76*(5), 1015–1028.

Chapter 23
Interventions Designed for Children with Histories of Institutionalization and Placed in Foster or Adoptive Families

Maureen Riley-Behringer and Victor Groza

Primum non nocere

(First, do no harm)

1 Introduction

Worldwide, more than 153,000,000 children are being reared outside of the care of their parents (UNICEF, 2011a). In low-resource countries in particular, reasons for out-of-home care include parental death, child abandonment, child maltreatment (i.e., physical/sexual abuse, neglect, parental addiction, unsafe environment), extreme poverty, famine, parent-child separation due to war or natural disaster, and family-limiting social policies (Roby & Shaw, 2008). Under such circumstances, children may live in one or a combination of the following four environments. First, they may be "taken in" by extended family members or "kin" (those that are "like family" but not related by blood or marriage such as members of the child's tribe). Second, children may survive by living on the streets. Third, they may live within a child-headed household where older children (often siblings) serve as key decision-makers and adults are typically absent from residing in the home. And fourth, children may be placed within state care (Roby & Shaw, 2008); state care is defined as the formal and informal public child welfare system.

M. Riley-Behringer
Department of Social Work, Elizabethtown College, Elizabethtown, PA, USA
e-mail: mriley-behringer@sbcglobal.net

V. Groza (✉)
Jack, Joseph & Morton Mandel School of Applied Social Sciences,
Case Western Reserve University, Cleveland, OH 44106-7164, USA
e-mail: victor.groza@case.edu

A.V. Rus et al. (eds.), *Child Maltreatment in Residential Care*,
DOI 10.1007/978-3-319-57990-0_23

Formal and informal public child welfare services for orphaned and/or abandoned children vastly differ within and between countries based on the availability of financial resources, politics, governmental resources, and infrastructure. Two common forms of public care used in low-resource countries (which often represent "sending countries") are placement in an orphanage/residential care center and/or full-time family foster care (McCall, 2013). Some children only live in institutional-type care while many of those who have been placed in family foster care have also lived a portion of their lives in institutional care.

Globally, there are an estimated two to eight million (USAID, 2009) children growing up in institutional care. The practice of using institutionalization as a method of caring for orphaned and/or abandoned children has been increasing in certain countries such as China (Zhao et al., 2009) and Africa (Foster, 2003) while decreasing in other countries such as Romania. Reasons for these fluxes are country-specific and relate to factors like disease and poverty as well as political, economic, and social reform (Levin, 2010). For example, starting in the year 2004, the Chinese government began opening more institutions to care for the increasing numbers of orphaned children whose parents had both died from AIDS. In Romania, between the years 2007 and 2010, the number of residential institutions declined from 450 sites caring for approximately 160,000 children to 256 sites caring for approximately 10,800 children (Levin, 2010). This was in response to major political pressure, economic development, and social welfare shifts (Levin, 2010) such as laws prohibiting infants from entering residential care, the development of foster family care, and the promotion of domestic adoption (Groza & Bunkers, 2014; Nedelcu & Groza, 2012).

In terms of the number of children living in family foster care worldwide, there is a dearth of research information. Lacking are specific descriptions of the different foster family care environments or the number of children who move from institutional care into family foster care and vice versa. The models of foster care are different globally. The model of children living in short-term foster care prior to permanent family care is followed by North American countries as well as most of Western Europe (Cameron & Freymond, 2006). Many low-resource countries embracing Sharia Law practice *Kafalah* (*see* Williamson & Greenberg, 2010), and countries that do not have a legal framework for adoption such as India where the only legal framework for adoption is for Hindu families (see Groza, Kalyanvala, & BSSK Research Team, 2003), all operate a model of long-term foster care.

Most children living in institutional care are deprived of consistent, sensitive caregiving. Even under the best of circumstances, these environments cannot fully meet individual children's care and developmental needs, particularly among the youngest like infants and toddlers. Institutional care often, but not always, meets perfunctory care needs (food, shelter, clothing), but the quality varies tremendously both within a country and between countries; an exception was the care received by Romanian children residing in orphanages in the 1980s and 1990s which contributed to homogeneity among Romanian intercountry adoption samples (*see* Rutter & the English and Romanian Adoptees [ERA] Study Team, 1998). What is known about institutional care for children is that it is not conducive to their overall health, development, and well-being (Dozier, Zeanah, Wallin, & Shauffer, 2012). For example, being reared in an institution has been linked to delays across several developmental domains. Children often experience immediate and long-term effects over their lifespan, dependent upon a myriad of factors like age at placement, length of time spent in the institution, whether they had a close personal connection to a primary caregiver in the orphanage, and exposure to effective therapeutic treatment/follow-up services post-placement (Albers, Johnson, Hostetter, Iverson, & Miller, 1997; Grönlund, Aring, Hellström, Landgren, & Strömland, 2004).

The various health, developmental, intellectual, and psychosocial effects for children with a history of institutionalization are impacted by an interaction of at least four factors: children's genetic predispositions, exposures to prenatal risk (with consideration to frequency, duration, dosage, and the combination to such risks), the pervasiveness and severity of global and/or social deprivation while in institutional care, and the length of time in institutional care. It is often difficult to decipher which of these factors or combination of factors result in the problematic outcomes reported on children adopted or fostered from institutional care.

Very few studies have examined how prenatal risk, pre-institutional risk, and institutionalization have influenced child developmental outcomes. The dearth of available research in these areas may relate to two key factors: First, there is a lack of reliable documentation about children's birth family history, prenatal history, and pre-institutionalization risk. Second, it is not clear if the risk from these factors is cumulative, exponential, or interactional. These unknown factors likely also contribute to why some results are mixed (Beverly, McGuinness, & Blanton, 2008; Miller et al., 2007).

Although many developmental difficulties have been noted for children exposed to various prenatal and pre-adoptive care risks with the most evidence about the negative impact of institutions (Zeanah et al., 2003), it is difficult to conclude that family foster care always is more positive than institutional care. There are contrary arguments that unregulated foster care or exploitive kinship care can expose children to as many risks as institutional care, even in high-resource countries like the Netherlands (Euser, Alink, Tharner, van IJzendoorn, & Bakermans-Kranenburg, 2014). There may not be enough foster parent training, supervision of foster families, professional expertise in foster care management, or monitoring of the quality of foster care. This is one area of need for further study (van den Dries, Juffer, van IJzendoorn, & Bakermans-Kranenburg, 2010).

In this chapter, we provide guidance on the use of evidence-based and evidence-informed interventions for children with a history of institutionalization before family placement. The interventions are appropriate for adoptive families, foster families, or birth families who regain custody of their children after a period of institutionalization. It is important to remember that adoption, foster family care, and a return to the birth family or to relatives/kinship families are all interventions that can have a positive effect on the health, development, and psychosocial well-being of children (*see* McCall et al., 2016; Van IJzendoorn & Juffer, 2006).

Intervention studies can be placed on a continuum with a progression from efficacy trials to effectiveness trials (Singal, Higgins, & Waljee, 2014). Efficacy can be defined as the performance of an intervention in controlled circumstances whereas effectiveness refers to its performance under "real-world" conditions such as clinical practice (Revicki & Frank, 1999).

To evaluate the interventions suggested in this chapter, we used an evidence-based practice framework. Evidence-based practice (EBP) has been defined as integrating practitioner expertise with the best available research evidence while also considering the values and expectations of the client system (individuals/families/groups/communities) to make decisions about interventions (Johnson & Austin, 2008). A difficulty with such a definition is that any one of the components creates ambiguity as we try to identify EBP: the amount of expertise necessary for a practitioner to make a judgement (Johnson & Austin, 2008), the quality of the research on which that judgement is based (Johnson & Austin, 2008), and the values and culture of the client system (Gambrill, 1999). There are some guides in helping determine EBP such as the Campbell Collaboration (http://www.campbellcollaboration.org/) and the California Evidence-Based Clearinghouse for Child Welfare (http://www.cebc4cw.org/), to name but a few available in the USA, and the Social Care Institute for Excellence (http://www.scie.org.uk/) in the UK. We draw from these sites as well as from published articles in discussion of evidence-based (EBP) interventions for post-institutionalized children.

We also use evidence-informed practice in presenting interventions. Evidence-informed practices (EI) do not have the rigor of EBP but draw from research to guide practice, and the interventions use officially sanctioned or produced guidelines (Johnson & Austin, 2008). Even when research exists about a practice or approach, often there is not sufficient research to understand how to integrate or implement the research into practice (Bellamy, Bledsoe, & Traube, 2006). While a less rigorous standard, EI can be helpful as a parent or professional evaluates the intervention they will use.

A third standard in this continuum is a best practice. Best practices guidelines make standards explicit and often are endorsed by professional organizations or experts in professional organizations. Both evidence-informed and best practices help to meet the demand for practitioners to base decisions on evidence (Bellamy et al., 2006).

This chapter will focus on psychosocial, evidence-based practice intervention models and evidence-informed intervention practice models found to be applicable to working with post-institutionalized children and their adoptive or foster parents. It is organized around the psychosocial and developmental difficulties that commonly bring families to professional intervention. It does not include medical interventions for health problems.

2 Evidence-Based and Evidence-Informed Interventions for Post-Institutionalized Children

Assessment is the foundation of any intervention. For children placed in family care after a period of institutionalization, a multidisciplinary team of professionals with expertise on the effects of institutionalization is critical. Children need a comprehensive health assessment. According to American Academy of Pediatrics (*see* Jones et al., 2012), during the initial physical examination, it is integral to pay particular attention to child welfare systems from which children were placed; some child welfare/child protection systems are underdeveloped and present greater risks for children. The assessment team should include the parent(s), developmental pediatrician, speech and language pathologists, dentists, and a mental health review by a psychologist or social worker. Additional experts may be necessary such as a medical specialist, occupational therapist, etc.

In addition, a family assessment should be conducted related to known histories of birth parents, family adjustment, and an adoptive parents' understanding of medical information and what the information means for their family. Once a comprehensive, multidisciplinary assessment is complete, then interventions can be determined. These multidisciplinary team members may present an array of intervention options to the child's parents in order to address whatever difficulties were documented in the assessment. Conjointly, parents and care team members must coordinate services, work on measureable goals, and develop a strong care plan.

3 Attachment Problems Including Indiscriminate Friendliness

Many foster or adoptive parents worry whether their post-institutionalized children will have the capacity to form trusting, reciprocal attachment relationships. Particularly in the clinical treatment literature, there is tremendous focus on disordered attachment among post-institutionalized children (Stinehart, Scott, & Barfield, 2012; Wimmer, Vonk, & Bordnick, 2009). Much of the research and writing in the area of attachment draws from the seminal works of Bowlby (1958, 1969, 1973, 1980).

The best evidence related to improved attachment outcomes exists for programs that target very young children. Two such programs are *Attachment and Biobehavioral Catch-up (ABC)* (http://abcintervention.com/) and *Video-Based Intervention to Promote Positive Parenting (VPPP)* (http://www.vippleiden.com/en). These interventions are discussed below.

Attachment and Biobehavioral Catch-up (ABC) (http://abcintervention.com/), developed by Dozier and associates (*see* Dozier, Lindhiem, & Ackerman, 2005) at the University of Delaware, is a ten-session intervention aimed at reducing barriers to the development of secure attachment relationships between foster parents and the young children in their care. It is also being used with post-institutionalized children and their parents who formed families via intercountry adoption. Additionally, the ABC program has been adapted and is being evaluated with birth parents whose young children have been maltreated but still reside in their care. That nearly identical versions of this intervention are applied to foster parents, maltreating parents, and adoptive parents speaks to the fundamental attachment needs in young children.

ABC has three components. The first component helps caregivers to reinterpret children's behavioral signals so that they provide nurturance, even when it is not elicited in a typical way. The second intervention component helps caregivers provide a responsive, predictable environment that enhances young children's behavioral and regulatory capabilities. The third intervention component helps caregivers decrease behaviors that could be overwhelming or frightening to a young child.

Developed out of the Netherlands, Video-based Intervention to Promote Positive Parenting (VIPP) is a brief, home-based attachment intervention delivered in four home visits to parents and infants (up to 12 months) whose families are typically considered at-risk for attachment challenges (Juffer, Bakermans-Kranenburg, & van IJzendoorn, 2005). VIPP was drawn explicitly from attachment research and attempts to promote maternal sensitivity through interveners' presentation of written materials and review of in-home, videotaped infant–parent interactions. An expanded version, VIPP-R, provides an additional 3 home visit that focuses on the parent's childhood attachment experiences. Findings are generally supportive of positive program effects on sensitive and nurturing parenting behaviors, attachment disorganization, and externalizing behavior problems during preschool (Juffer et al., 2005; Klein-Velderman, 2005; Klein-Velderman, Bakermans-Kranenburg, Juffer, & van IJzendoorn, 2006). VIPP-SD, a version of VIPP, aims to increase sensitivity and improve discipline strategies of caregivers in order to encourage positive interactions between the caregiver and child as well as to prevent or reduce behavior problems for children ages 1–6. It has demonstrated positive effects on mothers' disciplinary attitudes and behaviors compared to a control group of mothers who did not receive the intervention (van Zeijl et al., 2006).

There are several other interventions where the evidence is either still developing and/or does not reach the level of evidence-based practices. This includes Circle of Security (COS). The Circle of Security (COS) was developed as an intervention to enhance attachment relationships between infants/young children and their caregivers, primarily through work with parents (Marvin, Cooper, Hoffman, & Powell, 2002). Originally created as a time-limited group psychotherapy using video feedback, the intervention has been adapted for individual or family therapy. More recently, parenting DVDs based on the model have been created; these combine education about attachment with an opportunity for caregivers to reflect on their child's needs and the challenges each faces in meeting those needs (Cooper, Hoffman, & Powell, 2009).

For the video-therapy approach, an observational procedure including the standard Strange Situation Protocol (SSP) and the Circle of Security Interview are completed at baseline for treatment planning (Powell, Cooper, Hoffman, & Marvin, 2009). Toward the end of treatment, a second SSP is conducted for additional review. In this treatment, the SSP is used not to classify attachment patterns but rather to illustrate the parent's emotional presence and the child's exploratory and comfort-seeking behavior. The intervention emphasizes the capabilities of young children and draws caregivers' attention to the meaning of subtle behaviors using video review to highlight the positive moments of the parent–child interaction; the goal is to engage the caregiver in increasing the positive moments. This approach builds upon the work of McDonough (McDonough, 2000; Rusconi-Serpa, Rossignol, & McDonough, 2009) and Shaver and colleagues (Mikulincer & Shaver, 2007), both of whom demonstrated that images of positive interactions effectively engage difficult-to-reach parents.

There are preliminary data on the efficacy of the Circle of Security intervention. A pre–post-study of impoverished parents showed significant changes in the proportion of securely attached toddlers. Pregnant women involved in the justice system for non-violent offenses with a history of substance abuse participated in the Circle of Security intervention; outcomes indicated rates of infant attachment security (70%) and disorganization (20%) comparable to those in low-risk samples (Cassidy, Poehlmann, & Shaver, 2010). Although no randomized, controlled trial has been conducted, COS is linked to attachment theory and research and, in its use of video feedback and promotion of caregiver reflection, is an emerging evidence-informed practice.

In addition to the recent development of evidence-based and evidence-informed interventions to improve child–parent attachment, there have been clinical interventions that have been developed with the goal of treating children who have a history of disruptions in early attachment. Proponents of these various treatments designed to promote "reattachment," through coercive holding and rebirthing, for example, have effectively rewritten the criteria for attachment disorders and created a series of loosely related interventions which are coercive and dangerous (*see* Chaffin et al., 2004 for a review and recommendations).

These types of treatment were seen as necessary to "break" these overly willful children. It is important to remember that when stressed, post-institutionalized children continue using the same coping mechanisms that they used in the orphanage, namely, staying in control of the minutest details of their environment (and those in their environment) to feel safe. This is an adaptive skill that likely kept them alive in the institutional environment. Unfortunately, the behavior does not work well in family life, leading desperate and frustrated parents to seek therapies that lacked an evidence base. Treatments which force children to submit to being held against their will, humiliated, or that encourage them to "vent anger" while being restrained are contraindicated (Mercer, Sarner, & Rosa, 2003). In a small number of cases in the late 1990s and early twenty-first century, such treatments had even reportedly led to child injury and death by suffocation (Chaffin et al., 2006; Mercer et al., 2003).

Several professional organizations, in addition to the American Psychological Association, have strong policies against the use of holding therapy and other attachment therapies that lack evidence. A popular website, Quackwatch.com (http://www.quackwatch.org/01QuackeryRelatedTopics/at.html), urges caution when anyone considers attachment therapy. We, too, urge caution when engaging therapists who do not engage in evidence-based or evidence-informed interventions.

4 Sensory Problems and Sensory Integration Therapies

Sensory integration is the process by which individuals organize and interpret information received through their senses in order to successfully meet environmental challenges. Children with a history of institutionalization or any severe neglect before adoption are at-risk for sensory disorders (Cermak, 2009; Cermak & Groza, 1998). Sensory Integration (SI) therapies are forms of occupational therapy in which special exercises are used to strengthen the child's senses of touch (tactile), balance (vestibular), smell, taste, sight, and sense of where the body and its parts are in space (proprioceptive). It can include facilitating adaptive coping and maintaining adaptive routines, teaching parenting skills and behavior management for children with sensory problems, and promoting adaptive developmental progression. In a meta-analysis of SI, Vargas and Camilli (1999) reported that SI therapy was as effective as alternative interventions for treating sensory disorders. In a review of evidence for SI, Davies and Tucker (2010) did not report the effectiveness of treatment but concluded that it was important to conduct comprehensive assessments of sensory-based functions, including multiple measures of sensory integrative functions.

Biofeedback uses electronic instruments to help individuals gain awareness and control over certain psychophysiological processes (Gilbert & Moss, 2003; Schwartz, 2003). Neurofeedback uses a feedback electroencephalogram (EEG) to help an individual control electrochemical processes in the human brain (Evans & Abarbanel, 1999; LaVaque, 2003). Neurofeedback and biofeedback can be efficacious or successful, but the evidence using randomized control clinical trials have yet to demonstrate it is effective. It is probably not harmful, but beware of practitioners who overpromise results or changes in a child or their behavior (*see* http://theconversation.com/brain-training-games-wont-help-children-do-better-at-school-30227).

There is also some controversy about whether sensory disorders exist. A 2012 policy statement from the American Academy of Pediatrics (Zimmer et al., 2012) recommends that pediatricians should not use sensory processing disorder as a diagnosis and communicate with families about the limited data on the use of sensory-based therapies. Because of the policy statement and concerns about efficacy of SI therapies, it was listed as a promising practice with more research needing to be done. The same is true about biofeedback/neurofeedback. Until there is more evidence to support or refute treatment options, it is important that parents use their professional (i.e., pediatrician) and/or foster/adoptive family networking resources (i.e., other foster/adoptive parents' experiences with therapies, support group speakers, reading materials) to make their own decisions about promising practices like sensory integration therapies.

5 Survivor Behaviors: Hoarding and Gorging

Many children placed from institutionalized settings will hoard, gorge food, and be aggressive when first placed in a family. These behaviors helped them survive and even thrive in group care settings even if problematic when living in a family. Over time, the behaviors of hoarding and gorging in particular may decrease, if not stop, without intervention. Other times, it may require some type of intervention, moving from a survival behavior (aka behavior problem) to a clinical problem. There is still not consensus on what constitutes a behavior problem versus a clinical problem (Frost & Hartl, 1996). It has frequently been considered a symptom of obsessive–compulsive disorder, but such a diagnosis may be premature for children with a history of institutionlization. For children who leave institutions or even very neglectful families, the behavior may be linked to anxiety and the change from leaving a relatively depriving environment to a relatively resource rich environment of family life; even if family life is poor, it often has more resources emotionally and psychosocially than what is available in institutional care.

Frost and Hartl (1996) and Steketee and Frost (2003) suggest hoarding is related to information-processing deficits. While their ideas may be appropriate for adults, and may provide some insight into children, the hoarding seen in children who come from depriving situations is different than the hoarding of adults who did not have these early life experiences. It is different than the typical collecting behavior of children because children will hoard seemingly inane objects. Sometimes parents confuse this behavior with stealing, so great care is needed in helping families distinguish between these two different behaviors; sometimes the distinction is not always clear, and it works better for family functioning if parents first assume it is hoarding rather than ascribing the negative connotations of stealing and then punishing children for bad behavior. Hoarding is not bad behavior but a natural reaction for many children who have experiences of neglect.

There is usually a link between hoarding and food problems, such as gorging, although research is still developing. Food-related problems are also prevalent among children in foster care (Casey, Cook-Cottone, & Beck-Joslyn, 2012; Tarren-Sweeney, 2006). It is reasonable to expect that when children leave institutions and join a family, they will have food-related problems. Some of these problems are sensory issues, which were discussed previously. The particular problem we focus on here is gorging.

Regardless of the etiology, depending on the age, *Cognitive Behavior Therapy (CBT)* is the only approach identified as a well-supported, efficacious treatment; it is reported superior to all other approaches in abused, neglected, and traumatized children and has the greatest level of theoretical, clinical, and empirical support. Overall, CBT is one of the most researched interventions (Butler, Chapman, Forman, & Beck, 2006) and should be considered a first-line psychosocial treatment of choice, particularly for anxiety and depression (Tolin, 2010).

There are several variations to the CBT model. There is a CBT model developed by Steketee and Frost (2008) reported to be promising (Pertusa et al., 2010). Another promising CBT model used in the birth, kinship, foster, and adoptive family settings is Alternatives for Families CBT (AF-CBT) (Kolko, 1996). This approach focuses specifically on children ages 5–17 years that have experienced abuse/neglect in their earlier care environment (i.e., institution) who are displaying physically aggressive/oppositional behavior (http://www.afcbt.org/node/104). There is also a trauma-informed CBT model (*see* Mannarino, Cohen, & Deblinger, 2014); a good source for learning about this model is the National Child Trauma Stress Network (http://nctsn.org/) who also lists a number of promising practices that incorporate CBT within a trauma framework (http://nctsn.org/resources/topics/treatments-that-work/promising-practices#q4).

6 Childhood Behavior Problems and Disorders Related to Trauma

By the time children enter an adoptive or foster family, they have encountered one or more traumas. Psychoanalytical and post-psychoanalytical writers suggest the separation from a birth mother may be trauma to the infant (Lifton, 1995; Verrier, 2009). Verrier (2009) specifically relates the newborn's ongoing awareness of his/her birthmother's absence after abandonment as being equally traumatic and indistinguishable as the experience of suffering a parental death. Whether or not relinquished children experience this trauma in the way that Verrier describes, living in an institution is often a traumatic experience. Children may have other negative experiences that can be traumatic while in institutional care such as suffering from neglect, physical abuse, emotional abuse, or sexual abuse.

In addition, even the change from living in an institution to living in a family can be a traumatic experience. Bearing in mind that children organize their world into what is familiar and unfamiliar, they suffer several simultaneous losses when leaving behind all of those people, smells, sounds, tastes/foods, and language that they know; additionally, they lose the safety of their routine. Most people do not recognize these experiences as losses or traumas because the vast majority see moving into an adoptive family as a significant improvement in the life of a child. Still, because of the way children organize experiences, they may be traumatized by such changes which may influence their behaviors once in the adoptive family.

It is often difficult to know the etiology of the behavior problems or disorders. However, there is an evidence-based treatment that we recommend entitled *Parent-Child Interaction Therapy (PCIT)*.

Parent–child interaction therapy (PCIT) has been effective not only with biological dyads (children and parents) but also with foster and adoptive dyads (Allen, Timmer, & Urquiza, 2014; Timmer, Urquiza, & Zebell, 2006). The intervention is rooted in the principles of attachment theory (Bowlby, 1969, 1973, 1980) and Baumrind's developmental theory of parenting (1967). Using an approach of authoritative parenting that brings together the traits of strong consistency, clear communication, and warm/nurturing behavior, parent–child interaction therapy (PCIT) includes two sequential phases, the Child-Directed Interaction and the Parent-Directed Interaction. The goals of the Child-Directed Interaction are to strengthen the parent–child relationship and increase the focus and validation placed on positive child behavior. Parents are taught to use PRIDE skills (Praise, Reflection, Imitation, Description, Enthusiasm) to reinforce positive, appropriate child behaviors and steer away from any type of leading behaviors (i.e., commands, sarcasm, criticism, and negative physical behaviors) to form a solid foundation for productive discipline practices in phase two. The goals of the Parent-Directed Interactions are for parents to learn to communicate effectively while instructing their child and consistently following through with appropriate consequences (i.e., positive reinforcements when compliant; timeouts when non-compliant) (*see* Eyberg, 1988; Funderburk & Eyberg, 2011; Hood & Eyberg, 2003).

PCIT engages both the parent and child to modify the way parents interact with their children in order to diminish child behavior problems, which in turn promotes more positive parenting (Chaffin et al., 2004). The parent wears a "bug-in-the-ear" device which enables them to hear the guidance being provided to them via their PCIT-trained therapist stationed behind the two-way mirror watching the parent–child interaction. At the end of the session, the parent and therapist decide on a homework skill which will be practiced between sessions. Numerous studies have demonstrated the effectiveness of PCIT for reducing specific child behavior problems (Chronis-Tuscano et al., 2016; Eisenstadt, Eyberg, McNeil, Newcomb, & Funderbunk, 1993; Eyberg, 1988; Fernandez, Butler, & Eyberg, 2011).

7 Summary

Foster/adoptive parents who have children with difficulties as a consequence or related to prenatal and pre-adoptive experiences can be desperate to find the "right" intervention, medication, or approach to helping their children. This chapter gives them and those practitioners who work with them some guidance of the evidence-base for the interventions they should pursue. However, parents and practitioners should also be prepared that children's needs continue to evolve. It is not uncommon for families to see marked success with particular interventions and the support of a good therapist. When challenges at home become more managed, families often leave counseling; when new difficulties erupt, some parents feel discouraged about needing to come back for appointments at a later date. This is not failure on the part of the child, parents, or family. On the contrary, it means that each family member is growing and with such growth brings greater sophistication in learning and understanding. The skills learned previously in counseling were designed to meet the learning and understanding level of your child. A return for more advanced intervention and training would be designed to help you and your child with their unique needs as they mature.

If you felt that you made headway with your therapist, reschedule an appointment when you think/feel that life is becoming especially challenging; do not wait until you are feeling increasingly negative towards your child or about your parenting. Consulting other foster/adoptive parents about a therapist they see and who they have had success with is a great way to broaden your provider options. Know that no one therapist will have all of the answers (i.e., a therapist will not manage your child's medications unless they are physician). Also, really competent providers will routinely ask your permission to consult with the other members of your child's/family's care team. Your providers should communicate with one another, bringing together their expertise in order to provide you/your child comprehensive care. To do so, they must always obtain a signed release of information from you; this release may need to be updated every few months.

We are still at a threshold in developing the array of interventions and services that benefit children who experience the various types of early difficulties. We have no doubt that as the field of foster and adoptive care services learns more, the evidence will change and revisions to guides will have to be made.

Questions for Discussion

1. How do families know when to allow time for a problem behavior to disappear and when to seek professional help knowing what we know about development and early intervention?
2. What credentialing process should be put in place for practitioners working with families who have adopted children from institutions?
3. How can we better meet the needs of children and families who do not live in a community with access to adoption-sensitive mental health services?

References

Albers, L., Johnson, D., Hostetter, M., Iverson, S., & Miller, L. (1997). Health of children adopted from the former Soviet Union and Eastern Europe: Comparison with pre-adoptive medical records. *JAMA*, *278*(11), 922–924. doi: 03550110060037.

Allen, B., Timmer, S. G., & Urquiza, A. J. (2014). Parent–child interaction therapy as an attachment-based intervention: Theoretical rationale and pilot data with adopted children. *Children and Youth Services Review*, *47*, 334–341.

Baumrind, D. (1967). Child care practices anteceding three patterns of preschool behavior. *Genetic Psychology Monographs*, *75*(1), 43–88.

Bellamy, J. L., Bledsoe, S. E., & Traube, D. E. (2006). The current state of evidence-based practice in social work: A review of the literature and qualitative analysis of expert interviews. *Journal of Evidence-Based Social Work*, *3*(1), 23–48.

Beverly, B., McGuinness, T., & Blanton, D. (2008). Communication challenges for children adopted from the former soviet union. *Language, Speech, and Hearing Services in Schools*, *39*, 1–11.

Bowlby, J. (1958). The nature of the child's tie to his mother. *International Journal of Psycho-Analysis*, *39*, 350–373.

Bowlby, J. (1969). In J. Bowlby (Ed.), *Attachment and loss, vol. I: Attachment*. New York, NY: Basic Books.

Bowlby, J. (1973). In J. Bowlby (Ed.), *Attachment and loss, vol. II: Separation*. New York, NY: Basic Books.
Bowlby, J. (1980). In J. Bowlby (Ed.), *Attachment and loss, vol. III: Loss*. New York, NY: Basic Books.
Butler, A. C., Chapman, J. E., Forman, E. M., & Beck, A. T. (2006). The empirical status of cognitive-behavioral therapy: A review of meta-analyses. *Clinical Psychology Review, 26*(1), 17–31.
Cameron, G., & Freymond, N. (Eds.). (2006). *Towards positive systems of child and family welfare: International comparisons of child protection, family service, and community caring systems*. Toronto: University of Toronto Press.
Casey, C. M., Cook-Cottone, C., & Beck-Joslyn, M. (2012). An overview of problematic eating and food-related behavior among foster children: Definitions, etiology, and intervention. *Child and Adolescent Social Work Journal, 29*(4), 307–322.
Cassidy, J., Poehlmann, J., & Shaver, P. R. (2010). An attachment perspective on incarcerated parents and their children. *Attachment & Human Development, 12*(4), 285–288.
Cermak, S. (2009). Deprivation and sensory processing in institutionalized and postinstitutionalized children: Part 1. *Sensory Integration and Special Interest Section Quarterly, 32*(2), 1–3.
Cermak, S., & Groza, V. (1998). Sensory processing problems in post-institutionalized children: Implications for social work. *Child and Adolescent Social Work Journal, 15*(1), 5–37.
Chaffin, M., Silovsky, J. F., Funderburk, B., Valle, L. A., Brestan, E. V., Balachova, T., … Bonner, B. L. (2004). Parent-child interaction therapy with physically abusive parents: Efficacy for reducing future abuse reports. *Journal of Consulting and Clinical Psychology, 72*(3), 500–510.
Chaffin, M., Hanson, R., Saunders, B. E., Nichols, T., Barnett, D., Zeanah, C., ... Letourneau, E. (2006). Report of the APSAC task force on attachment therapy, reactive attachment disorder, and attachment problems. *Child maltreatment, 11*(1), 76–89.
Chronis-Tuscano, A., Lewis-Morrarty, E., Woods, K. E., O'Brien, K. A., Mazursky-Horowitz, H., & Thomas, S. R. (2016). Parent–child interaction therapy with emotion coaching for preschoolers with attention-deficit/hyperactivity disorder. *Cognitive and Behavioral Practice, 23*(1), 62–78.
Cooper, G., Hoffman, K. T., & Powell, B. (2009). *Circle of Security: COS-P facilitator DVD manual 5.0*. Unpublished manuscript, Marycliff Institute, Spokane, WA.
Davies, P. L., & Tucker, R. (2010). Evidence review to investigate the support for subtypes of children with difficulty processing and integrating sensory information. *American Journal of Occupational Therapy, 64*(3), 391–402.
Dozier, M., Lindhiem, O., & Ackerman, J. P. (2005). Attachment and bio-behavioral catch-up: An intervention targeting empirically identified needs of foster infants. In L. Berlin, Y. Ziv, L. Amaya-Jackson, & M. T. Greenberg (Eds.), *Enhancing early attachments: Theory, research, intervention, and policy* (pp. 178–194). New York, NY: Guilford Press.
Dozier, M., Zeanah, C. H., Wallin, A. R., & Shauffer, C. (2012). Institutional care for young children: Review of literature and policy implications. *Social Issues and Policy Review, 6*(1), 1–25. doi:10.1111/j.1751-2409.2011.01033.x.
Eisenstadt, T. H., Eyberg, S., McNeil, C. B., Newcomb, K., & Funderbunk, B. (1993). Parent–child interaction therapy with behavior problem children: Relative effectiveness of two stages and overall treatment outcome. *Journal of Clinical Child Psychology, 22*, 42–51.
Euser, S., Alink, L. R., Tharner, A., van IJzendoorn, M. H., & Bakermans-Kranenburg, M. J. (2014). Out of home placement to promote safety? The prevalence of physical abuse in residential and foster care. *Children and Youth Services Review, 37*, 64–70.
Evans, J. R., & Abarbanel, A. (Eds.). (1999). *Introduction to quantitative EEG and neurofeedback*. San Diego, CA: Academic.
Eyberg, S. M. (1988). PCIT: Integration of traditional and behavioral concerns. *Child & Family Behavioral Therapy, 10*, 33–46.
Fernandez, M. A., Butler, A. M., & Eyberg, S. M. (2011). Treatment outcome for low socioeconomic status African American families in parent-child interaction therapy: A pilot study. *Child & Family Behavior Therapy, 33*(1), 32–48.

Foster, G. (2003). *Study of the response by faith-based organizations to orphans and vulnerable children*. Preliminary summary report, World conference of religions for peace and UNICEF, September. Retrieved from http://www.unicef.org/media/files/FBO_OVC_study_summary.pdf

Frost, R. O., & Hartl, T. L. (1996). A cognitive-behavioral model of compulsive hoarding. *Behavior Research and Therapy, 34*(4), 341–350.

Funderburk, B. W., & Eyberg, S. (2011). Parent–child interaction therapy. In J. Norcross, G. R. Vanden Bos, & D. K. Freedheim, Donald K. (Eds.), History of psychotherapy: Continuity and change (2nd) (pp. 415–420). Washington, DC: American Psychological Association. Retrieved from 10.1037/12353-021.

Gambrill, E. (1999). Evidence-based practice: An alternative to authority-based practice. *Families in Society: The Journal of Contemporary Social Services, 80*(4), 341–350.

Gilbert, C., & Moss, D. (2003). Biofeedback and biological monitoring. In D. Moss & A. McGrady (Eds.), *Handbook of mind-body medicine for primary care* (pp. 109–122). Thousand Oaks, CA: Sage.

Grönlund, M. A., Aring, E., Hellström, A., Landgren, M., & Strömland, K. (2004). Visual and ocular findings in children adopted from Eastern Europe. *British Journal of Ophthalmology, 88*(11), 1362–1367.

Groza, V., & Bunkers, K. M. (2014). Adoption policy and evidence-based domestic adoption practice: A comparison of Romania, Ukraine, India, Guatemala and Ethiopia. *Infant Mental Health Journal, 35*(2), 160–171.

Groza, V., Kalyanvala, R., & BSSK Research Team. (2003). Indian families adopting Indian children. *Indian Journal of Social Work, 64*(1), 93–113.

Hood, K. K., & Eyberg, S. M. (2003). Outcomes of parent-child interaction therapy: Mothers' reports of maintenance three to six years after treatment. *Journal of Clinical Child and Adolescent Psychology, 32*(3), 419–429.

Johnson, M., & Austin, M. J. (2008). Evidence-based practice in the social services: Implications for organizational change. *Journal of Evidence-Based Social Work, 5*(1–2), 239–269.

Jones, V. F., High, P. C., Donoghue, E., Fussell, J. J., Gleason, M. M., Jaudes, P. K., … Schulte, E. E. (2012). Comprehensive health evaluation of the newly adopted child. *Pediatrics, 129*(1), e214–e223.

Juffer, F., Bakermans-Kranenburg, M. J., & van IJzendoorn, M. H. (2005). The importance of parenting in the development of disorganized attachment: Evidence from a preventive intervention study in adoptive families. *Journal of Child Psychology and Psychiatry, 46*(3), 263–274.

Klein-Velderman, M. (2005). *The Leiden VIPP and VIPP-R study: Evaluation of a short-term preventive attachment-based intervention in infancy*. Leiden: Leiden University Press.

Klein-Velderman, M., Bakermans-Kranenburg, M. J., Juffer, F., & Van IJzendoorn, M. H. (2006). Effects of attachment-based interventions on maternal sensitivity and infant attachment: Differential susceptibility of highly reactive infants. *Journal of Family Psychology, 20*(2), 266.

Kolko, D. J. (1996). Individual cognitive-behavioral treatment and family therapy for physically abused children and their offending parents: A comparison of clinical outcomes. *Child Maltreatment, 1*(4), 322–342.

LaVaque, T. J. (2003). Neurofeedback, neurotherapy, and quantitative EEG. In D. Moss & A. McGrady (Eds.), *Handbook of mind-body medicine for primary care* (pp. 123–136). Thousand Oaks, CA: Sage.

Levin, A. (2010, November 15). My glimpse of hell and the pitiful children who have been betrayed. *The Telegraph*. Retrieved from http://www.telegraph.co.uk/news/worldnews/europe/romania/8128644/My-glimpse-of-hell-and-the-pitiful-children-who-have-been-betrayed.html

Lifton, B. J. (1995). *Journey of the adopted self: A quest for wholeness*. New York, NY: Basic Books.

Mannarino, A. P., Cohen, J. A., & Deblinger, E. (2014). Trauma–focused cognitive-behavioral therapy. In S. Timmer & A. Urquiza (Eds.), *Evidence–based approaches for the treatment of maltreated children* (pp. 165–185). Dordrecht: Springer.

Marvin, R., Cooper, G., Hoffman, K., & Powell, B. (2002). The circle of security project: Attachment-based intervention with caregiver-pre-school child dyads. *Attachment & Human Development, 4*(1), 107–124.

McCall, R. B. (2013). Review: The consequences of early institutionalization: Can institutions be improved? – Should they? *Child and Adolescent Mental Health, 18*(4), 193–201.

McCall, R. B., Muhamedrahimov, R. J., Groark, C. J., Palmov, O. I., Nikiforova, N. V., Salaway, J., & Julian, M. M. (2016). The development of postinstitutionalized versus parent-reared Russian children as a function of age at placement and family type. *Development and Psychopathology, 28*, 251–264. doi:10.1017/S0954579415000425.

McDonough, S. C. (2000). Interaction guidance: An approach for difficult-to-engage families. In C. H. Zeanah (Ed.), *Handbook of infant mental health* (2nd ed.pp. 485–493). New York, NY: Guilford Press.

Mercer, J., Sarner, L., & Rosa, L. (2003). *Attachment therapy on trial: The torture and death of Candace Newmaker*. Santa Barbara, CA: Greenwood Publishing Group.

Miller, L., Chan, W., Reece, R., Grey, L., Tirella, L., & Pertman, A. (2007). Child abuse fatalities among internationally adopted children. *Child Maltreatment, 12*(11), 378–380.

Mikulincer, M., & Shaver, P. R. (2007). Reflections on security dynamics: Core constructs, psychological mechanisms, relational contexts, and the need for an integrative theory. *Psychological Inquiry, 18*(3), 197–209.

Nedelcu, C., & Groza, V. (2012). Child welfare in Romania. In J. Gibbons & K. Rotabi (Eds.), *Intercountry adoption: Policies, practices, and outcomes* (pp. 91–102). Surrey, UK: Ashgate Press.

Pertusa, A., Frost, R. O., Fullana, M. A., Samuels, J., Steketee, G., Tolin, D., ... Mataix-Cols, D. (2010). Refining the diagnostic boundaries of compulsive hoarding: A critical review. *Clinical Psychology Review, 30*(4), 371–386.

Powell, B., Cooper, G., Hoffman, K., & Marvin, R. S. (2009). The circle of security. In C. H. Zeanah (Ed.), *Handbook of infant mental health* (3rd ed.pp. 450–467). New York, NY: Guilford Press.

Revicki, D. A., & Frank, L. (1999). Pharmacoeconomic evaluation in the real world: Effectiveness versus efficacy studies. *PharmacoEconomics, 15*(5), 423–434.

Roby, J., & Shaw, S. (2008). Evaluation of a community-based orphan care program in Uganda. *Families in Society: The Journal of Contemporary Social Services, 89*(1), 119–128.

Rusconi-Serpa, S., Rossignol, A. S., & McDonough, S. C. (2009). Video feedback in parent-infant treatments. *Child and Adolescent Psychiatric Clinics of North America, 18*(3), 735–751.

Rutter, M., & The English and Romanian Adoptees (E.R.A.) Study Team. (1998). Developmental catch-up, and deficit, following adoption after severe early privation. *Journal of Child Psychology and Psychiatry, 39*, 465–476.

Schwartz, M. S. (2003). Intake decisions and preparation of patients for therapy. In M. S. Schwartz & F. Andrasik (Eds.), *Biofeedback: A practitioner's guide* (3rd ed.pp. 105–127). New York, NY: Guilford.

Singal, A. G., Higgins, P. D. R., & Waljee, A. K. (2014). A primer on efficacy and effectiveness trials. *Clinical and Translational Gastroenterology, 5*, e45. doi:10.1038/ctg.2013.13.

Steketee, G., & Frost, R. (2003). Compulsive hoarding: Current status of the research. *Clinical Psychology Review, 23*(7), 905–927.

Steketee, G., & Frost, R. (2008). *Compulsive hoarding and acquiring: Therapist guide*. New York, NY: Oxford University Press.

Stinehart, M. A., Scott, D. A., & Barfield, H. G. (2012). Reactive attachment disorder in adopted and foster care children: Implications for mental health professionals. *The Family Journal: Counseling and Therapy for Couples and Families, 20*(4), 355–360.

Tarren-Sweeney, M. (2006). Patterns of aberrant eating among pre-adolescent children in foster care. *Journal of Abnormal Child Psychology, 34*(5), 621–632.

Timmer, S. G., Urquiza, A. J., & Zebell, N. (2006). Challenging foster caregiver–maltreated child relationships: The effectiveness of parent–child interaction therapy. *Children and Youth Services Review, 28*(1), 1–19.

Tolin, D. F. (2010). Is cognitive–behavioral therapy more effective than other therapies?: A meta-analytic review. *Clinical Psychology Review*, *30*(6), 710–720.
UNICEF. (2011a). *The state of the world's children 2011: Adolescence an age of opportunity*. Retrieved from http://www.unicef.org/sowc2011
UNICEF. (2011b). *The state of the world's children 2011: Adolescence an age of opportunity*. Retrieved from http://www.unicef.org/sowc2011
USAID. (2009). *U.S. government and partners: Working together on a comprehensive coordinated and effective response to highly vulnerable children*. Washington, DC: USAID.
Van Den Dries, L., Juffer, F., van IJzendoorn, M. H., & Bakermans-Kranenburg, M. J. (2010). Infants' physical and cognitive development after international adoption from foster care or institutions in China. *Journal of Developmental & Behavioral Pediatrics*, *31*(2), 144–150.
Van IJzendoorn, M. H., & Juffer, F. (2006). Adoption as intervention: Meta-analytic evidence for massive catch-up and plasticity in physical, socio-emotional, and cognitive development. *Journal of Child Psychology and Psychiatry*, *47*(12), 1228–1245.
Vargas, S., & Camilli, G. (1999). A meta-analysis of research on sensory integration treatment. *American Journal of Occupational Therapy*, *53*(2), 189–198.
van Zeijl, J., Mesman, J., Stolk, M. N., Alink, L. R. A., van IJzendoorn, M. H., Bakermans-Kranenburg, M. J., … Koot, H. M. (2006). Terrible ones? Assessment of externalizing behaviors in infancy with the child behavior checklist. *Journal of Child Psychology and Psychiatry*, *47*(8), 801–810. doi:10.1111/j.1469-7610.2006.01616.x.
Verrier, N. (2009). *The primal wound: Understanding the adopted child*. Louisville, KY: Gateway Press.
Williamson, J., & Greenberg, A. (2010). *Families, not orphanages*. New York: Better Care Network. Retrieved from http://symposium.jointcouncil.org/wp-content/uploads/2012/04/Williamson-Families-Not-Orphanages-for-JCICS.pdf
Wimmer, J., Vonk, M., & Bordnick, P. (2009). A preliminary investigation of the effectiveness of attachment therapy for adopted children with reactive attachment disorder. *Child & Adolescent Social Work Journal*, *26*(4), 351–360.
Zeanah, C., Nelson, C., Fox, N., Smyke, A., Marshall, P., Parker, S., & Koga, S. (2003). Designing research to study the effects of institutionalization on brain and behavioral development: The Bucharest early intervention project. *Development and Psychopathology*, *15*(04), 885–907. doi:10.1017/S0954579403000452.
Zhao, Q., Li, X., Kalijee, L., Fang, X., Stanton, B., & Zhang, L. (2009). AIDS orphanages in China: Reality and challenges. *AIDS Patient Care and STDs*, *23*, 297–303.
Zimmer, M., Desch, L., Rosen, L. D., Bailey, M. L., Becker, D., Culbert, T. P., … Adams, R. C. (2012). Sensory integration therapies for children with developmental and behavioral disorders. *Pediatrics*, *129*(6), 1186–1189.

Chapter 24
Child Maltreatment in Residential Centers: Summing Up

Adrian V. Rus, Sheri R. Parris, Ecaterina Stativa, and Cosmin O. Popa

1 Introduction

In the following paragraphs, we will provide more detail about these important themes found in the book. We have cited chapters where you can find more information regarding specific types of information; however, other chapters may also contain relevant information on these topics. So, while information may be found in cited chapters, relevant information is certainly not limited to only those chapters cited. In sum, while this chapter provides a small snapshot of the highlights of this book, one must read the whole book to obtain a complete understanding of the topics discussed therein. Finally, there is some overlap of ideas among the different themes discussed in this summary, because many ideas belong in more than one category. Also, while specific statistical results vary among institutions and among countries, there are common themes that permeate among institutions and countries, and many problems that were identified in institutions decades ago still persist based on the results of more recent investigations. Therefore, there is still work to

A.V. Rus (✉)
Department of Social and Behavioral Science, Southwestern Christian University, 7210 NW 39th Expressway, Bethany, OK 73008-0340, USA
e-mail: adrian.rus@swcu.edu; aadrianrus@gmail.com

S.R. Parris
Texas Christian University, Fort Worth, TX, USA
e-mail: sheri.parris@gmail.com

E. Stativa
Social Pediatrics and Obstetrics Research Department, The National Institute for Mother and Child Health "Alessandrescu-Rusescu", Bucharest, Romania
e-mail: ecaterina.stativa@gmail.com

C.O. Popa
University of Medicine and Pharmacy of Tirgu Mures, Tirgu Mures, Mures, Romania
e-mail: cosmin_popa24@yahoo.com

A.V. Rus et al. (eds.), *Child Maltreatment in Residential Care*,
DOI 10.1007/978-3-319-57990-0_24

do to improve living conditions in residential institutions for children, and here we provide a short summary of the findings and conclusions found in this book.

The common themes found in this book include:

- Living conditions in institutions
- Outcomes from institutional rearing
- Standards, accreditation, and licensing
- Recommendations for interventions in institutions
- The role of organizations and communities
- Institutional settings and environment
- Suggestions for future research

2 Living Conditions and Maltreatment in Institutions

Regarding living conditions in institutions, there have been, and continue to be, some modifications to institutional living as traditional prejudices and cultural beliefs give way to new knowledge brought by researchers who are seeking ways to improve children's lives and ensure better outcomes. Historically, and even in some current settings, institutional care environments often provided for children's basic physical needs, but not their psychological, emotional, cognitive, educational, or developmental needs (see Chaps. 2, 10, 14, 19, and 20). Many forms of maltreatment and victimization have been found in institutional care settings, including neglect as well as physical, sexual, and emotional abuse, bullying, severe punishments, exploitation, and witnessing violence. In many cases, children in these settings experience these forms of abuse in more extreme forms than those being reared in typical family contexts and all of which can be perpetrated both by institutional staff or children's peers (see Chaps. 1, 7, 9, 13, and 20). Caregiver-child interactions were often minimal, and children were often neglected, with a social climate and environmental stimulation that were insufficient (see Chaps. 12, 14, 19). Children in institutions often experienced stigma and negative attitudes (often from religious and/or societal perceptions) toward them, which also contributed to the development of emotional and behavioral problems (see Chaps. 9, 12, and 20), and many children were forced into child labor (see Chaps. 20 and 21). In addition, institutions often lacked oversight and regulation, leaving children without advocates to ensure their safety and well-being (see Chaps. 2 and 20).

3 Outcomes from Institutional Rearing

The deprivation experienced in institutions can lead to delays in children's social-emotional, cognitive, and physical development, including severe delays in physical growth (e.g., underweight, stunting, microcephaly) (see Chaps. 5, 14, and 19). These children are also likely to have attachment, sensory, and trauma-related problems and use survival behaviors such as hoarding and gorging (see Chaps. 6 and 23). They are also more likely to experience externalizing (e.g., aggressive and oppositional behaviors, inattention/ADHD) and internalizing (e.g., depression, anxiety) symptoms within the clinical range and at significantly higher rates than non-institutionalized children (see Chaps. 7 and 12). They have also been found to have differences in brain activity (as measured by electroencephalograms–EEGs and event-related potentials–ERPs) associated with internalizing symptoms (see Chap. 6).

Institutionalized children placed in foster care or adopted at younger ages have better outcomes in relation to attachment, cognition, and other domains than those who spend longer periods of time in institutions. In particular, children placed in family settings prior to 24 months of age fare better than those placed after 24 months. This provides evidence that there may be sensitive periods in development for which recovery is optimal and that recovery becomes increasingly difficult after those periods have passed (see Chap. 6). Adults with histories of institutionalization as children have a high prevalence of severe psychological and physical problems (e.g., chronic illness, disability, relationship problems, homelessness, social isolation, anxiety, and depression) and poor educational, career, and financial outcomes throughout their lives (see Chap. 20).

In LMICs (low- to middle-income countries), there is often no difference in well-being (e.g., physical health, emotional well-being, cognitive functioning, and maltreatment [physical/sexual abuse]) among orphans in institution-based vs. family-based care settings, and some children in institutional care fare better than those in family-based care (see Chaps. 16 and 18). Also in LMICs, where harsh punishment and violence against children may be culturally accepted, orphans living in institutions do not report more maltreatment than orphans living in family- or community-based care; therefore, improvements in care are needed not only in institutions but also in other care settings (see Chap. 17). In these countries, it is also imperative to address the needs of street children, who are generally displaced or orphaned children who have not been absorbed by either family-based or institutional care. These children often experience higher levels of abuse and exploitation than their counterparts who are in some type of care setting (see Chap. 16).

4 Standards, Accreditation, and Licensing

Residential settings should be monitored to ensure that quality care standards are maintained, that children's individual needs are being met, and that expectations for accepted behavior among staff and children are clear. There is a need for governmental bodies to develop laws and practices that are funded mandates for appropriate childcare practices (see Chap. 19). These mandates should be based on widely accepted practices, such as the United Nations Convention of the Rights of the Child (see Chap. 2). Standards can then be used to create licensing and accreditation criteria (see Chap. 22) to ensure evaluation and oversight of children's developmental progress, including physical, psychological, and social well-being. Children's risk factors should also be considered in order for preventive steps to be taken. In addition, all partners of the residential facilities should also be monitored, and foster care settings should be supervised and monitored to reduce maltreatment (see Chaps. 7, 12, 13, 15, 16, and 19).

Also, every country should keep current data on all residential care facilities and children within these facilities. Accreditation standards should be developed with inspections and monitoring of compliance by all institutions. Those not meeting the threshold should not be accredited, and those not meeting requirements should be closed (see Chaps. 13 and 22). Risk analyses as well as prevention measures and a complaint management system (including the ability to make anonymous reports to an independent contact person that is not a part of the institution staff) should be implemented in institutions (see Chap. 8). Staff and professionals that work with children and adolescents in institutions should receive ongoing training regarding risks; warning signs; prevention concepts; handling of suspected cases of abuse; intervention strategies, including trauma-focused interventions and therapy; as well as gaining knowledge about the backgrounds and experiences of youth that enter care and ways to effectively engage with these at-risk youth and develop trusting relationships (see Chaps. 8 and 13); and training in child mental health and development, creating a family environment for children in orphanages, and improving the quality of the social environment (see Chap. 10).

5 The Importance of Family and Relationships

Institutionalized children should have the ability to maintain contact with parents and/or other family members, including extended family when possible (see Chap. 12). Also, sibling separation has adverse effects on children, and keeping siblings together when possible should be a priority (see Chap. 18). Caregivers within the institutions should interact with children in a warm, sensitive, nurturing, and responsive manner (see Chaps. 6, 7, 13, 17, and 19). In addition, care should be taken to reduce repeated placements between different institutions (see Chap. 12) and to provide a stable, consistent "family-like" caregiving environment, which includes decreasing the number of children grouped together in institutional settings in order to create more family-like settings (see Chap. 10).

When institutionalization is unavoidable, family-type and foster care settings can provide more favorable and developmentally appropriate settings when operated appropriately and with proper training and oversight of staff/foster parents (see Chaps. 6, 15, and 19), and family reunification should be sought when possible (see Chaps. 15 and 21). For successful reintegration back into a child's biological family, a program to prepare families and children for reintegration, in addition to sufficient follow-up and support after reintegration, is necessary (see Chap. 12). While there is some contradictory evidence in LMICs as mentioned previously, children tend to show better outcomes from being raised in problematic families than in relatively good institutions. The presence of a continuous, sensitive caregiver may ameliorate the detrimental effects of other problems within the family. Thus, providing support for at-risk families, such as community-based early childhood intervention services, and allocation of resources to ensure the safety and support of children and families is recommended (see Chaps. 11 and 15).

6 Recommendations for Interventions in Institutions

Interventions should be theory based and tested using rigorous scientific standards (see Chap. 17), directed at both personal- and institution-level factors and directed at the entire residential community rather than a selected group of perpetrator or victims (see Chap. 13). It is important to have a system for early identification and intervention for attachment, cognition, emotional, and behavior problems and for monitoring of children's psychological and physical well-being. Children should have opportunities to receive social support within the orphanage and to develop competency and achievements across a variety of domains (e.g., developmental, social competence, academic achievement). Also, because most institutionalized children have experienced one or more forms of trauma (sometimes both before and after they enter the institution), interventions should also address trauma (see Chap. 18). Caregivers should receive training to improve the language and cognitive development of infants and young children (see Chap. 12). Interventions should include the addition of therapeutic recreation spaces, appropriate milieu activities, parent-child support groups, and school-child support groups, and support socialization and community integration (see Chap. 12). In addition, children and youth should have increased participation in the institutions where they live, including opportunities to participate in the development of rules and other structures within their institutions (see Chap. 8).

7 The Role of Organizations and Communities

Countries, particularly those with collective and historical trauma, and/or governmentally imposed cultural values that have encouraged institutionalization of children as a preferred method of child rearing, should implement systemic interventions at the national, community, family, and individual levels, to begin to change perceptions, to facilitate a decrease in institutionalization, and to strengthen families (see Chap. 11). Organizations (governmental and nongovernmental) can create public awareness campaigns (see Chap. 8) to reduce stigma and negative attitudes toward institutionalized children, build philosophical foundations for child welfare and child welfare systems that promote the well-being and rights of children, and promote and pilot promising services and interventions. There should be a commitment from the central government to family-based care as the preferred form of care, including the removal of local incentives that work against deinstitutionalization. For instance, on a local level, an institution brings resources and jobs into the community, so there may be local resistance to the closing of institutions (see Chap. 15). In addition, professionals should promote solutions that will work within the framework of their own culture (see Chap. 19).

8 Institutional Settings and Environment

Many long-term residential centers have organizational characteristics and culture that facilitate neglect and abuse by staff and peers, including poor staff training and management; inadequate systems of accountability; lack of resources; ineffective implementation of policies regarding violence, referrals of residents, and capturing children's reports of peer violence; preventing disclosures of abuse; inadequate physical characteristics of living spaces; and a transitional nature of both staff and peers in institutions (see Chap. 1). Approaches should focus on the prevention of violence and abuse in institutional settings. Staff should have specialized training in assessing risk, identifying victims, and addressing developmental victimization (see Chaps. 7 and 17). There should be systematic planning and implementation of programs to reduce all types of victimization found in residential settings, including physical and sexual violence, as well as indirect and verbal violence perpetrated by both staff and peers. Social care systems must scrutinize potential carers, organize training programs, evaluate care systems, maintain high standards of staff conduct, and provide the necessary support and advocates to strengthen children's rights and promote their well-being (see Chap. 12).

9 Suggestions for Future Research

Our authors have identified the following areas where more research is needed to improve the lives of institutionalized children and those in out-of-home care. First, more research is needed to determine caregiver characteristics that lead to best outcomes for children. Such knowledge may help to inform hiring practices, training, and placement decisions (see Chap. 18). Second, while it is recommended that institutionalized children are allowed to maintain connections and relationships with their parents or other family members when possible, empirical testing for models that allow such relationships among institutionalized children are needed to provide a clear evidence base for this practice (see Chap. 18). Third, there should be regular collection and distribution of accurate data regarding institutionalized children (e.g., institutional census data, demographics, and type/quality of care provided). Such data can help track improvements in care settings, both within individual institutions, and across regional or other geographic areas. Data can also help to provide empirical support, or otherwise, for interventions or other modifications to the residential setting and to identify areas in need of further improvement (see Chap. 19). Finally, there is a need to develop consistent and universally accepted definitions for the different types of maltreatment that can become a common language for researchers, policy-makers, and practitioners. While there is currently no universal consensus on specific definitions of the various types of maltreatment, there are some common areas of agreement, and some standardization is occurring with the development of scales that are beginning to be used consistently in research, practice, and policy-making (see Chaps. 1 and 18). Consistency of definitions would bring comparability across studies, improve researchers' ability to combine and build upon each other's knowledge, and better identify and compare types of maltreatment across different institutions; there is a need to improve and find agreement on definitions for the different types of maltreatment (see Chap. 1).

10 Final Thoughts

In sum, our authors have provided an array of thought-provoking information to promote our thinking about institutionalization, maltreatment, and possibilities for improvements in living conditions and outcomes. Both today and in the future, we can foster change and cultivate resources that will enable practitioners, policy-makers, and others to improve the lives and trajectories of all children who are unable to live with their own families. Bringing together empirical knowledge from across the globe will allow us to determine best practices for the children who need us the most.

Index

A.V. Rus et al. (eds.), *Child Maltreatment in Residential Care*,
DOI 10.1007/978-3-319-57990-0

S

T

U

Kolibri 360 GmbH
Ferdinand-Jühlke-Straße 7
99095 Erfurt, Deutschland
produktsicherheit@kolibri360.de